THE MOTOR ENDPLATE

SUMNER I. ZACKS, M. D.
Professor of Patholoy
University of Pennsylvania

ROBERT E. KRIEGER Publishing Company,
Huntington, N.Y.   1973

Original Edition 1964
Revised and Enlarged Edition 1973

Printed and Published by
Robert E. Krieger Publishing Co., Inc.
Box 542, Huntington, N.Y. 11743

© Copyright 1974 by
Robert E. Krieger Publishing Co., Inc.

Library of Congress Catalog Card # 73-84420
ISBN # 0-88275-113-1

All rights reserved, no part of this book may be reproduced in any manner, except for critical review, without written permission of the publisher.

Printed in the United States of America, by
Noble Offset Printers, Inc. New York, N.Y. 10003

DEDICATION

This monograph is dedicated to my father, David Zacks, M.D., for his encouragement past and present.

Table of Contents

Preface to the Second Edition   vii

Acknowledgements

Introduction   xi

Chapter 1:
Anatomy of the Neuromuscular Junction   1

Chapter 2:
Embryogenesis of NMJ   32

Chapter 3:
The Fine Structure of the Neuromuscular Junction   52

Chapter 4:
Ultrastructure of Terminal Axons in the Neuromuscular Junction   71

Chapter 5:
External Lamina in Neuromuscular Junctions   81

Chapter 6:
The Postsynaptic Membrane of the Neuromuscular Junction   97

Chapter 7:
The Soleplate of Neuromuscular Junctions   109

Chapter 8:
  Invertebrate Neuromuscular Junctions   112

Chapter 9:
  Esterases in Neurmuscular Junctions   17

Chapter 10:
  Biochemistry and Physiology of
  Neuromuscular Junctions   149

Chapter 11:
  Denervation and Reinnervation of
  Neuromuscular Junctions   197

Chapter 12
  Nonexcitatory Aspects of Innervation
  Trophic Effects of Axons   248

Chapter 13:
  Effects of Toxins on
  Neuromuscular Junctions   283

Chapter 14:
  The Pathology of Neuromuscular Junctions   318

  Appendix   384

  Bibliography   418

  Index   486

Preface To The Second Edition Of The Motor Endplate

The second edition of The Motor Endplate incorporates many of the advances made in the study of the neuromuscular unit in the nearly 10 years since the first edition. This monograph is a multidisciplinary attempt to collect and interpret information concerning the anatomy and the biochemical physiology of the neuromuscular junction and its alterations that result from laboratory experimentation and the natural experiments of disease. The great volume of new information concerning the neuromuscular unit has necessitated extensive rewriting and reorganization. New or expanded sections have been added on the ultrastructure of the vertebrate and invertebrate neuromuscular junction, the section on embryogenesis of the neuromuscular junction has been expanded to a chapter because of the information obtained from electron microscopy and new chapters have been added concerning denervation and reinnervation of striated muscle and on the "trophic" activity of peripheral nerves.

Experimental data bearing upon current biochemical and physiological controversies have been integrated with the discussion of junctional fine structure in an attempt to make these findings more meaningful. The appendix providing methods for the study of the neuromuscular junction has been brought up to date but routine electron microscopic methods have been deleted. The majority of the original electron micrographs have been replaced because improvements in technique have made them obsolete.

Although the original title, Motor Endplate, has been retained, I have referred to the entire complex of presynaptic terminal and postsynaptic structures throughout the text as the "NMJ" to avoid possible confusion caused by inexact use of "endplate" as a term for both the entire structure and for the "soleplate".

I am grateful to Mrs. Joanne Farno for her help with the manuscript and to the staff of the Robert E. Krieger Publishing Co.

Acknowledgments

I should like to acknowledge my debt to Professor John Welsh, who first interested me in the study of neuromuscular junctions, to Dr. Arnold M. Seligman and Dr. George B. Wislocki, who guided early histochemical investigations, and to Dr. Joe M. Blumberg and the staff of The Armed Forces Institute of Pathology, who collaborated in early electron microscopic studies of the myasthenic NMJ. Also I should like to thank the technical assistants, Mr. Irwin Spiegelman, Mr. Frank Robinson, Mrs. Steven A. Weiss, Miss Marilyn Salscheider and Miss Patricia Rafferty who contributed to these studies and Mrs. Joanne Farno who helped with the preparation of the manuscript. Also, I should like to acknowledge my debt to my students Drs. Alan Kelly and Atsushi Saito who permitted their work to be included. I also wish to acknowledge the help of Mr. Lewis Zacks, who prepared Figures 80, 83 and 105. I should also like to aknowledge permission to use various published illustrations granted by the following journals, institutions, and publishers:

Verlag von C.A. Jenni, Sohn, Bern (Fig. 1)
Annales des Sciences Naturelles (Figs. 2 and 3)
Rockefeller Institute Press, New York (Figs. 4, 31-33, 65-67, 70, 77)
Zeitschrift für Biologie, Urban & Schwarzenburg, Munich (Fig. 6)
Armed Forces Institute of Pathology, Washington (Figs. 7 and 15)
Archiv Für Mikroskopiche Anatomie, Bonn (Figs. 8 and 9)
Journal of Anatomy, Cambridge University Press, London (Figs. 10 and 114)

Revue Canadienne de Biologie, University of Montreal (Figs. 11-13)
Wistar Institute Press, Philadelphia (Figs. 16 and 17)
Trabajos del Instituto Cajal de Investigaciones Biológicas, Madrid (Figs. 19, 20, 83 and 84).
Dr. A.M. Kelly, Dept. of Pathology, University of Pennsylvania, School of Veterinary Medicine, Philadelphia (Figs. 21-30).
The Anatomical Record, The Wistar Institute Press (Figs. 34-37, 406).
American Journal of Anatomy (Fig. 40a).
Journal of Histochemistry and Cytochemistry, Williams and Wilkens Co., Baltimore (Figs. 45-48, 50-54, 63 and 64)
Cambridge University Press, New York Fig. 62)
Dr. S.J. Holt, Middlesex Hospital Medical School, London (Fig. 68).
Drs. R. Davis and G.B. Koelle, Department of Pharmacology, University of Pennsylvania School of Medicine (Fig. 75)
Blackwell Scientific Publications, Oxford (Figs. 77 and 102)
Journal of Physiology, Cambridge University Press, London (Figs. 79 and 80)
Dr. Atsushi Saito (Figs. 86-89, 93-97)
The Journal of Bone and Joint Surgery, Inc. (Figs. 90-92 and 98)
Journal of Experimental and Molecular Pathology, Academic Press, Inc. (Figs. 104-106)
Australian Journal of Experimental Biology and Medical Science, University of Adelaide, Adelaide (Fig. 103)
Journal of Neuropathology and Experimental Neurology, The Association of the Journal of Neuropathology and Experimental Neurology, Inc. (Fig. 107)
Archives of Neurology, American Medical Association (Figs. 108, 121 and 122)
Nature, Macmillan Journals Ltd. (Fig. 109)
Journal of Pharmacology and Experimental Therapeutics, Williams and Wilkins Co., Baltimore (Fig. 110)
Acta Neurologica et Psychiatrica Belgica, Brussels (Fig. 112)
Annals of New York Academy of Science, New York Academy of Science, New York (Figs. 116-118)
Laboratory Investigation, International Academy of Pathology (Figs. 123-127)
Science, American Association for The Advancement of Science (Fig. 82)
Arch. Anat. Microscop. Morph. (Fig. 18)
Developmental Biology (Fig. 81)

This monograph and much of the original work included in it would not have been possible without the support of The John A. Hartford Foundation, Inc., New York, The National Science Foundation and The National Institutes of Health.

Introduction

Although the history of the investigation of the terminal nerve ending on muscle can be traced for 137 years, I believe that the time is ripe for an attempt to bring together available information concerning the various aspects of the neuromuscular junction. Such a review should be useful in indicating possibilities for further research, especially with regard to clinical problems. Pathological investigations of the motor endplate have been few until recently, perhaps because of technical difficulties or the tendency of both general and neuropathologists to ignore this borderline zone between the nervous system and the musculature.

In the early years of NMJ studies, heated controversies were common concerning the detailed anatomy visible with the light microscope after the application of various staining methods, most of which involved the use of heavy metal precipitation. In retrospect, it is not difficult to understand why such arguments arose, considering the complexity and perversity of the staining methods used and the small size of the structure studied. We know now with all the wisdom of hindsight that many of the structures in the NMJ are tantalizingly at or near the limit of resolution of the light microscope. Indeed, the controversies of the past might be taken as a lesson to teach us humility in establishing the verity of our present views. Perhaps in a similar period of time, even the most refined electron microscopic studies of this region obtained by current methods will be regarded as of mere historical interest, because new methods, some still to be invented, will be used further to unravel the chemical ultrastructure of the NMJ.

However, not being equipped with high resolution foresight, but having the advantage of the combined experience of many investigators over the past ten years, we shall attempt to apply information obtained with the electron microscope to reinterpret some of the classical controversies of the past.

Even though many details of the function of the neuromuscular synapse are still uncertain, it is possible now to present a more or less detailed picture of the morphology of the NMJ and some of its histochemical characteristics to serve as a beginning toward studies of NMJs experimentally altered by the laboratory investigator or by the natural experiments of spontaneous disease. This monograph is concerned with the present knowledge of structure of the NMJ and will undertake an exploratory foray into the complex field of experimental evidence relating to the correlation of form and function of this structure. With knowledge of the fine structure of the human neuromuscular junction and some of the changes that occur in disease, it is hoped that these observations will stimulate further investigation of the important group of neuromuscular diseases which now have only begun to be studied.

It is well realized that morphologic study in itself is insufficient to explain the etiology of many of these neuromuscular diseases. However, since at the electron microscopic level of resolution, structure and function are inextricably intertwined, it is hoped that clues to possible chemical abnormalities may be suggested by changes in fine structure. These clues may then suggest appropriate biochemical experimentation. Furthermore, use of labeled substances in conjunction with electron microscopy as well as electron microscopic histochemistry offer additional possibilities for extending our knowledge of these disease entities.

1

Anatomy of the Neuromuscular Junction

THE CLASSICAL PERIOD: 1840-1947

Credit for the first investigations, and incidently the source of a major misconception concerning the Neuromuscular Junction (NMJ), belongs to Valentin (1836) and Emmert (1836), who believed that the termination of the nerve fiber in striated muscle consisted of an arc-like structure with branches dividing and rejoining in a continuing network (Fig. 1). The concept of Emmert, which antedates the Cell Theory of Schleiden and Schwann, seemed particularly quaint to the modern biologist until the discovery of axon transport of macro-molecules. Emmert said:

> "The arc-like ("bogenformige") ending of the motor nerve fiber leads to the conclusion that primitive (nerve) fibers lead from the central part to the periphery and back again from the periphery to the central part (nervous system).
> The appearance of the muscle activity and the arc-like ending of the motor nerve fiber indicates that there is a continuous stream and circulation of the nervous fluid in the motor nerve."

This view was generally well established until 1840, when Doyère first proposed that the nerve fiber came to a complete termination on the surface of the muscle fiber. His studies were carried out in the invertebrate *Milnesium tardigardum,* a species chiefly containing smooth muscle. Figure 1 shows this first illustration of a neuromuscular junction. Three years later, Quartrefages (1843) confirmed Doyère's observations in *Elolidina parodoxa*. Figure 2 remarkably resembles the neuromuscular junction illustrated by Doyère. Careful observations by Wagner of frog muscles (1847) led him to deny the existence of terminal arcs and to recognize the terminal branching of the axon in the junctional region. He also recognized that the terminal nerve fiber lost its myelin sheath before entering the innervation site.

It was not until 1862 that Kühne, one of the outstanding early students of the NMJ, published his first series of observations. He believed that after penetrating the sarcolemma, the nerve fiber branched and formed a complex terminal **arborization**. In the same year (1862), Rouget described a heap of granulated material at the level of the nerve termination in striated muscles of reptiles, birds, and mammals. Although he believed that this was due to the spreading out of the ter-

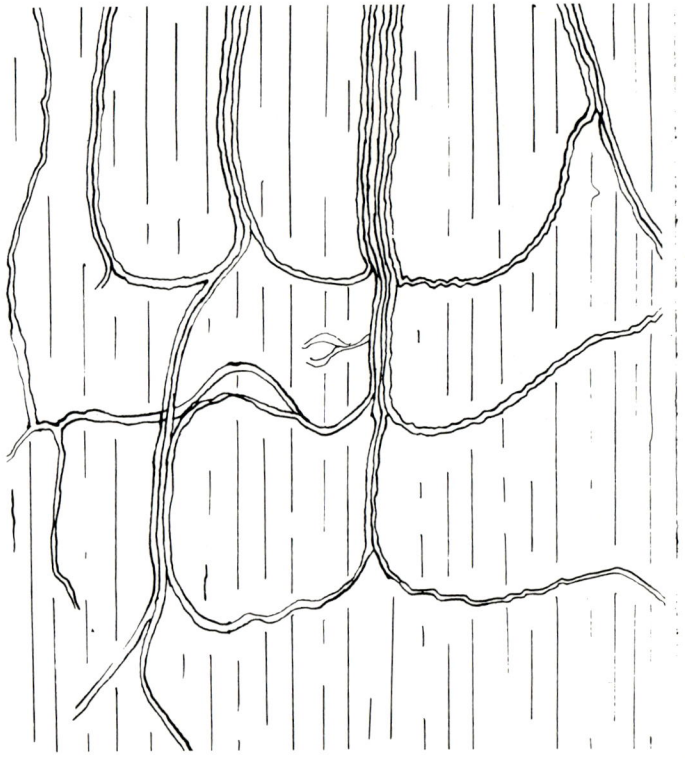

Figure 1. Drawing of the arc-like endings of motor nerve fibers on skeletal muscle according to the concept of Emmert. (After Emmert, 1836.)

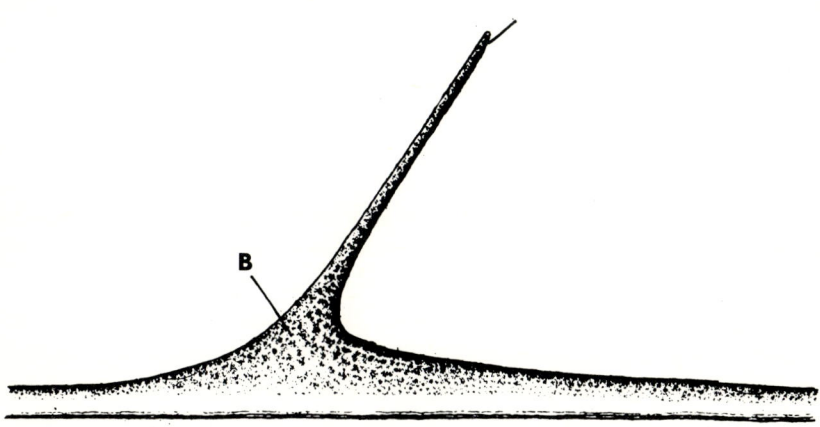

Figure 2. Motor innervation in *Milnesium tardigardum* as described by Doyère. A motor nerve *(a)* is seen to join the muscle fiber at an ill-defined, cone-shaped surface emminence *(b)*. (After Doyère, 1840.)

minal axis cylinders, he did recognize the presence of a specialized region in the neuromuscular junction. This he termed the "plaque terminale." Krause (1863) was the first to use the term "motorische endplatte." He used it to refer to the terminal nerve branching and altered

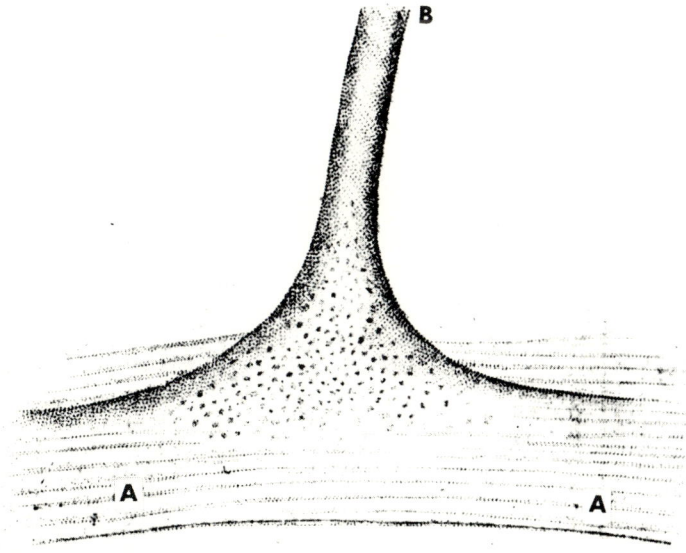

Figure 3. Drawing illustrating the connection between the muscle fiber *(a)* and the nerve fiber *(b)*, according to Quartrefages. Note the similarity to the Doyère illustration. (After Quartrefages, 1843.)

muscle zone observed in the innervated area of cats' eye retractor muscles.

It should be pointed out that the terms "neuromuscular junction" and "motor endplate" are not freely interchangeable. "Neuromuscular junction" is a generalized term referring to all anatomic varieties of specialized junctional regions between nerve terminals and muscle fibers. "Motor endplate" refers to the specialized area on the muscle surface membrane visible in the optical microscope where the terminal axon makes contact with the myofiber. The usage of "terminal plaque" (Rouget, 1862) or motor endplate (Krause, 1863) eventually became a kind of shorthand for the entire neuromuscular apparatus including Schwann cell, terminal axon, and the myofiber surface specialized structures. The staining methods used by Krause and Kűhne tended to emphasize the muscle surface details at the expense of the terminal nerves. To avoid confusion, we will use NMJ for the entire complex and more specialized words for subelements of the neuromuscular complex.

Additional early studies of NMJ morphology in several animals by means of various staining methods were published by Ranvier (1878) and by Kűhne (1864, 1883, 1886a, b, and 1887).

The cause of the intense scientific polemics that occured as additional investigators added their observations on the structure of NMJ can be understood today in terms of the several histologic methods that were used to demonstrate them. Furthermore, we now know that NMJ differ considerably in structural details from one animal to another and indeed in different muscles within a given animal (Cole, 1957).

Before beginning a discussion of the controversial anatomy of the NMJ, a few words must be said about the methods used during the Classical Period of NMJ studies. It was soon apparent that routine staining methods with available dyes showed very few structural details in NMJ. For example, the commonly used hematoxylin and eosin (H & E) stain permits recognition of clustered nuclei in NMJ regions but poorly stains the terminal axons. Consequently, the NMJ are difficult to recognize. Somewhat better for paraffin embedded sections is the PAS-Alcian blue method (Fig. 4) which facilitates recognition of small intra-muscular nerve branches and the aldehyde-fuchsin method that stains the external lamina (see pg. 84). Progress in the study of NMJ began when various metal impregnation methods were used.

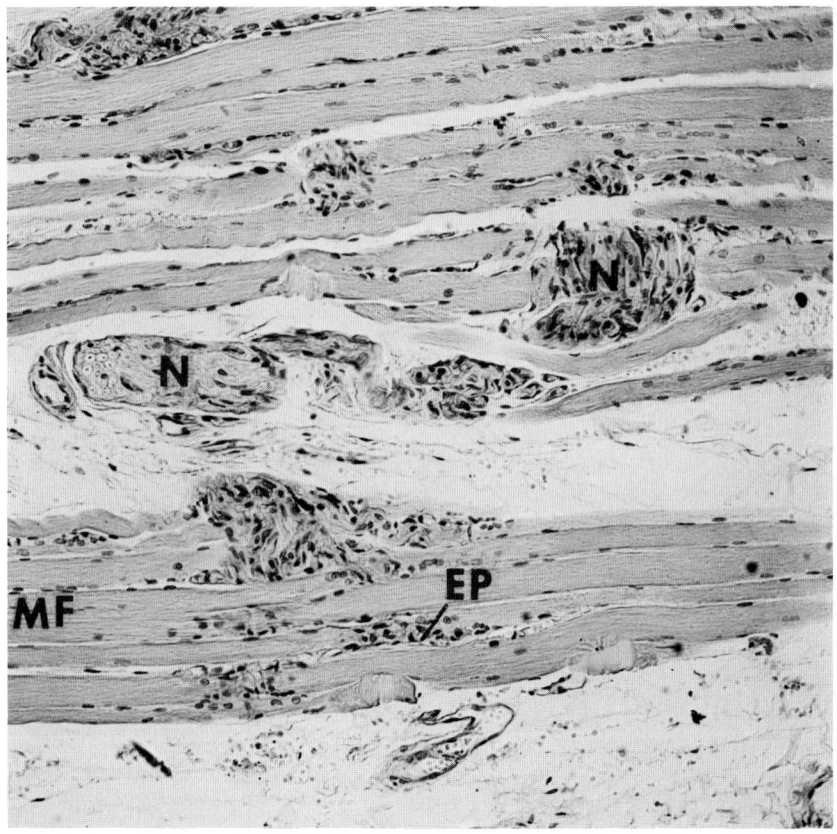

Figure 4. Photomicrograph of human skeletal muscle, illustrating large nerve bundles at N dividing into terminal branches that form areas of innervation on individual myofibers *(MF)*. The area marked *EP* indicates a probable site of a neuromuscular junction. Note that in this PAS-alcian blue stained preparation, little structural detail in the NMJs is visible. (X 100.)

Staining with Gold

One of the favorite techniques was gold impregnation (Ranvier, 1878). Multiple variations were employed by different investigators, although all had the same basic theme. Blocks of muscle tissue bearing nerve fibers were soaked for several hours in solutions of lemon juice. The specimen was then transferred to a solution of gold chloride ($AuCl_3$) for an additional period of time, following which a reducing bath was used. Formulas for several of these procedures are given in the appendix.

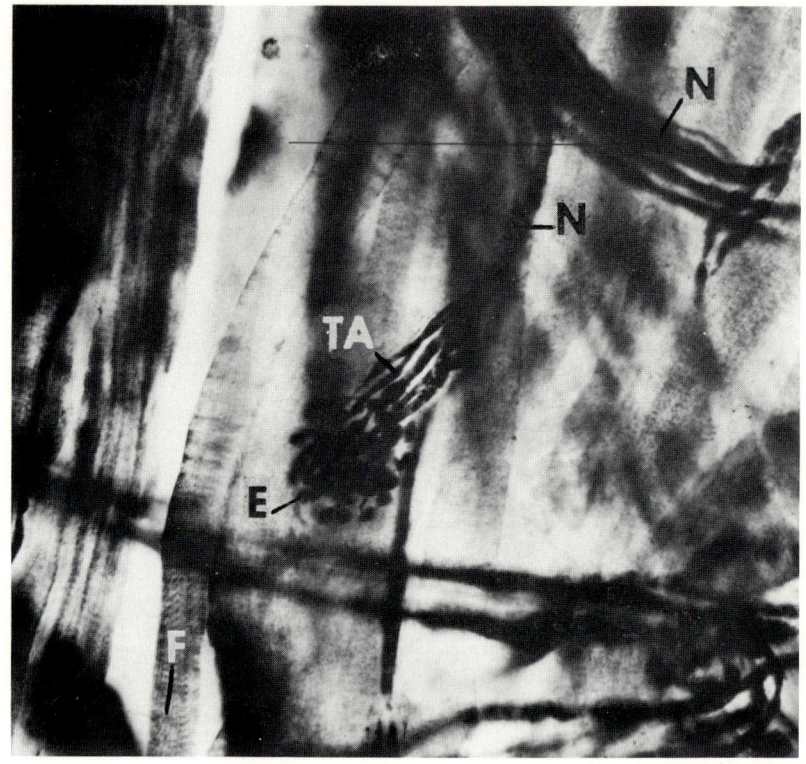

Figure 5. Photomicrograph illustrating the appearance of a gold-stained rat neuromuscular junction. The underlying muscle fibers with striations visible at F are crossed by darkly stained nerve fibers *(N)*. In the center of the photomicrograph, the terminal axons *(TA)* are seen to end in oval end knobs *(E)*. (X 1,000.)

The chemical basis of gold-staining methods is unknown. Because gold-stained NMJs tend to fade, especially if exposed to light for long periods of time, it is unlikely that the color is due to metallic gold. It is more probable that the red color results from a complex with some component of the sole plate subneural apparatus (see pg. 81). Figure 5 illustrates the typical appearance of a gold-stained NMJ.

In a typical gold-staining method such as that used by Kűhne, two major components of the NMJ could be distinguished. The first, representing the terminal nerve branches, stained dark violet and was called the "axialbaum," and the remainder of the junctional region, which appeared red, was called the "stroma." This zone enclosed the axial part. In some preparations, violet-stained material surrounding the axoplasm was recognized. However, the relationship of the "stroma" to the nerve termination always remained more or less uncertain. Several investigators observed that the "stroma" was not entirely homogeneous and that some parts were more granular than others, especially in the periphery. This fringe area in reptilian NMJ was called the "borstensaum" by Kűhne (1883) and was regarded by him as a structure in or on the membrane coating the NMJ. This reference to a specialized structure or fringe in the soleplate was recognized by Couteaux (1960) as an early description of the outcropping of the subneural apparatus in the soleplate. However, Couteaux does not accept the fringe described in frog NMJ by Kűhne as part of the subneural apparatus. Figure 6 illustrates the relationship of the "borstensaum" to other components of the NMJ.

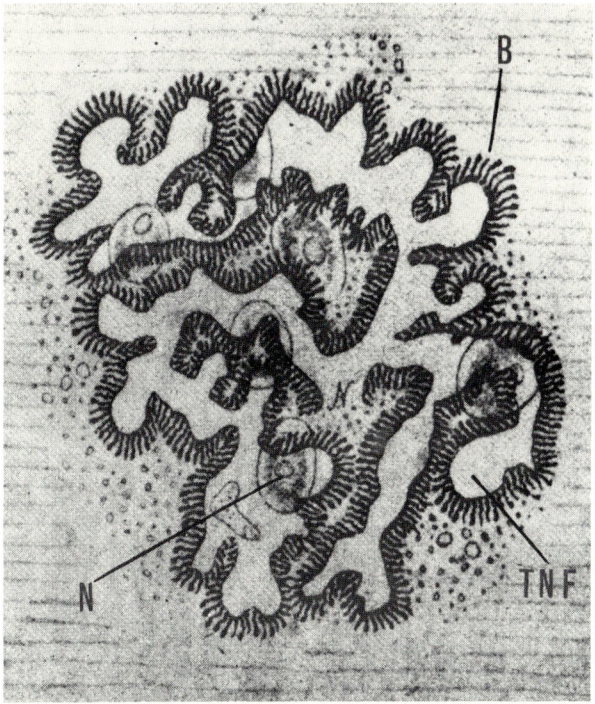

Figure 6. Drawing of a gold stained NMJ from Kűhne illustrating the rod-like "Borstensaum" *(B)* at the periphery of the terminal nerve branches as viewed in the section parallel to the muscle surface. Various nuclei of the soleplate and investing nerve sheaths are also visible at *N*. The terminal nerve fibers would normally occupy the central area indicated at *TNF*. (After Kűhne, 1883.)

Staining with Silver

Those investigators who employed silver-staining methods saw an entirely different picture (Cajal, 1904, 1925; Tello, 1905, 1917, 1944; Boeke, 1909, 1911, 1927; and Lawrentjew, 1928). The silver-stained preparations revealed more delicate structure than those stained by gold chloride methods. For example, the neurofibrils in the axon could be visualized as delicate, tenuous strands, which extended from the axon into the terminal branches. A peculiar button or loop-like structure was often seen at the ultimate termination of each axon branch. Silver staining also demonstrated an unstained zone surrounding the nerve filaments, which was thought by Cajal (1925) to be a peripheral layer of axoplasm devoid of neurofilaments. Also visible with the light microscope in silver-stained preparations were small granules that were more numerous at the level of the nerve ending than in other areas of the motor nerve terminal. Figure 7 illustrates structural details in a silver-stained NMJ.

The Mechanism of Silver Staining. Several investigators have attempted to rationalize the involved technology of staining nerve cells and processes with silver. Gray (1954) in a scholarly review has sum-

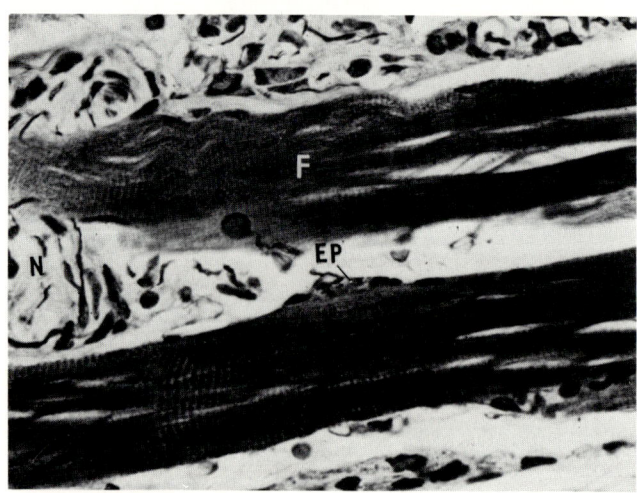

Figure 7. Photomicrograph of human neuromuscular junction *(EP)* in edge view stained by the Gros-Bielschowsky method. The slight Doyere emminence contains silver stained terminal nerve branches. Various nuclei of the soleplate and nerve sheaths are also visible. A moderately large nerve trunk is present at the edge of the illustration *(N)*, and muscle fibers are indicated at F. (X 500.)

marized the bewildering technology of silver staining. Four classes of silver methods can be identified: (1) silver nitrate, (2) silver proteinate, (3) silver diamine, and (4) silver chromate. Perhaps most famous is the "Cajal technique," which consists of many modifications of a basic silver nitrate method.

Although originally compared to the photographic process, silver staining of tissues appears to involve other chemical and physical processes. Gray (1954) suggested that the brown color of the stained tissues was more consistent with silver-protein complexes than reduced matallic silver.

Liesegang (1911), who provided the first theoretical analysis of silver staining, concluded that during impregnation, nuclei of reduced silver are formed in the tissue that serve as centers for further deposit of silver when the sections are developed.

Later studies by Holmes (1943) and Romanes (1950) and Samuel (1953) indicated that two types of reactions occur. The first is binding of unreduced silver to some tissue components, and the second consists of binding of reduced silver in the form of silver muclei. The binding of unreduced silver is probably due to imidazole groups of histidine (Peters, 1955) rather than to carboxyl groups of aldehydes (Romanes, 1950) or lipoproteins (Wolman, 1957). The fraction deposited as reduced silver nuclei is altered by the same factors that determine unreduced silver binding; namely, time, pH, and temperature. Peters (1955) concluded that differentiation of silver staining is dependent on the formation of silver nuclei in a critical pH range of 7.5 to 9.

Gray and Guillery (1961), in an electron microscope study of silver-stained spinal cord synapses, claimed that the neurofilaments form the basis of the argyophilic material that delineates the synaptic rings and clubs observed by light microscopy. Neither cytoplasm, membranes, nor mitochondria and synaptic vesicles were argyrophilic. It is likely that neurofilaments are responsible for silver staining of axon terminals in NMJs, as suggested by Gray and Guillery (1961) for other synapses.

However, whether gold-staining or silver-staining methods were used, it was not easy to be certain whether or not the terminal nerve branches lay on the muscle surface membrane ("sarcolemma" — see discussion on page 16) and were epilemmal or whether the nerve fibers penetrated the muscle surface membrane and were truly hypolemmal. Supporters of the epilemmal theory were Krause, Kolliker, and Retzius, whereas investigators who favored the hypolemmal theory included Kůhne, Gutmann, Young, and Tiegs. Fortunately, this particular point has been settled by the electron microscope, which once and for all has confirmed the Neurone Doctrine of Cajal, there being in effect an epilemmal connection between the nerve and the muscle, which by ordinary methods of light microscopy appears to be hypolemmal. In this way both classical schools of interpretation possessed a partial understanding of the true state of affairs in the NMJ.

Staining with Methylene Blue

The third major method used for demonstrating NMJ was *intra vitam* methylene blue staining. A series of studies by Dogiel (1890), Feist (1890), Kulchitsky (1924), Tiegs (1932), Tello (1944), and Couteaux (1947) employed one of the several variations of this technique. In all the variations the appearance of the NMJ is similar. The terminal axon and its arborization within the soleplate area is stained deep blue. The remainder of the NMJ structures are stained pale blue. Liu and Maneely (1962, 1968) have concluded that the methylene blue method is unreliable for fine details of axon structure since it leads to kinking and beading of the axons.

Although the gold and silver methods have little specificity, because of the more or less indiscriminate formation of heavy metal complexes, it is possible that the methylene blue method yields a bonus

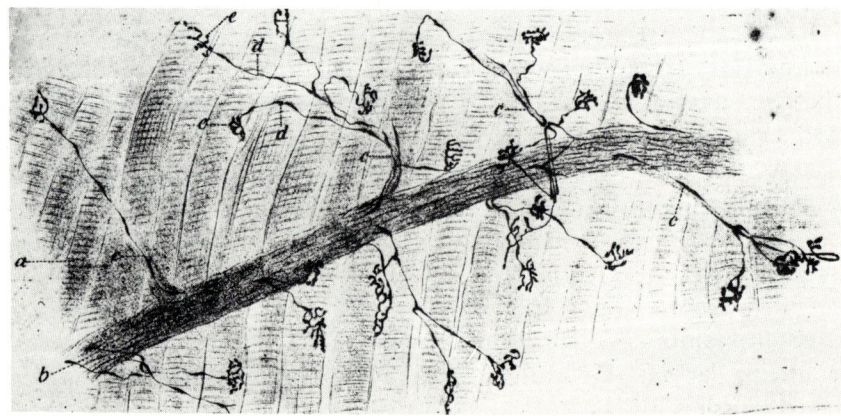

Figure 8. A drawing of motor nerve trunks giving rise to smaller nerve branches, terminal nerve branches, and numerous NMJs stained by methylene blue. (After Dogiel, 1890.)

in the form of information of a truly histochemical nature (Couteaux and Taxi, 1952; Massart and Dufait, 1941). Figures 8 and 9 illustrate the appearance of NMJs stained by methylene blue.

THE STRUCTURE OF THE NEUROMUSCULAR JUNCTION: CLASSICAL VIEW

It will be noted that the early studies of the NMJ were concerned with invertebrate and some amphibian muscles. It was not until 1862 that Rouget reported on the structure of reptile, lizard, and mammalian motor endings in some detail.

As more studies were made, it was soon recognized that there were numerous morphologic forms of NMJs. For example, in snake and lizard muscles, a variety of nerve endings were described by Tiegs (1932), Cole (1955) and Marinskaya (1963).

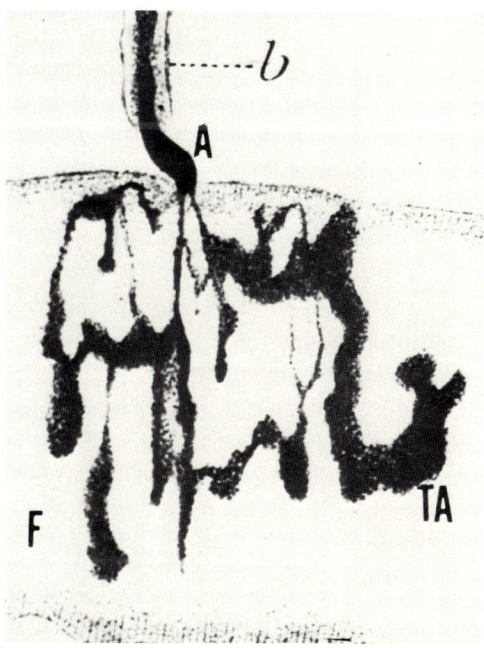

Figure 9. Drawing at high magnification of a NMJ stained with methylene blue, showing the darkly stained axon *(A)* surrounded by the unstained myelin sheath *(b)*. The ramifications of the terminal arborization *(TA)* lie on the surface of the muscle fiber *(F)*. (After Dogiel, 1890.)

Bremer (1882), who used the gold chloride method, found coarse medullated nerve fibers ending in what he believed were hypolemmal branching terminations, that were plate-like ("en plaque") and similar in structure to mammalian NMJ. In addition, there were fine medullated fibers, which ended in simple or complex cluster endings that resembled a bunch of grapes ("Terminaisons en grappe"). Bremer believed that the latter hypolemmal endings might be sensory. Perroncito (1901) and Kűhne (1887), however, believed that they were somatic motor endings.

Without dwelling at length on the numerous forms of motor endings in various animal species and individual muscles that are recognized by more sophisticated methods, we shall describe the structure of an idealized, commonplace mammalian en plaque NMJ visualized by classical staining methods.

In the region of innervation, the surface of the muscle fiber contains a specialized zone of modified sarcoplasm called the soleplate (Kűhne). Because of accumulation of sarcoplasm containing various organelles, the innervated region in some species projects above the myofiber surface forming the eminence of Doyère. The soleplate, which is directly related to the size of the innervated myofiber, may range in size from 20 by 20μ to 50 by 60μ or more. The terminal nerve branch approaches this specialized region of the muscle fiber and loses its myelin sheath. The naked axon branchlet makes contact with the muscle surface and branches extensively to form the terminal arborization. The soleplate underlying the terminal arborization contains numerous granules, chiefly mitochondria.

The NMJ also contains several nuclei of different kinds. These have been the source of an extensive disagreement, which only recently has been resolved. Ranvier (1878) described "arborization nuclei," which were associated with nerve branches, and "fundamental nuclei," which seemed to be a characteristic of the soleplate. These "sole nuclei" named by Kűhne in 1864, were larger, less stainable, and contained larger nucleoli than the arborization nuclei. Still other nuclei, identified as belonging to the endothelial cells of the numerous capillaries typically found in the vicinity of NMJ, were recognized. Ranvier also described "vaginal nuclei," which appeared to be related to a collagenous coating, a prolongation of the Key-Retzius sheath of the nerve fiber, covering the NMJ. Ranvier believed that the arborization nuclei were derived from the endoneural sheath, which was a continuation of the Key-Retzius sheath, and from the soleplate nuclei of Kűhne. Kűhne (1886a, b, 1887) did not accept this interpretation and recognized only the soleplate nuclei and the sarcolemmal nuclei, that is, the membranous coating of the NMJ. Cajal (1909), Tello (1907, 1917), Iwanaga (1925), and Cuajunco (1942) also did not recognize the existence of special nuclei associated with the terminal nerve branches. Del Rio Hortega (1925) believed that the nuclei were of muscular origin. Studies by Couteaux (1938, 1941) established that the arborization nuclei were homologs of Schwann cell nuclei. This conclusion was reached by studies of the embryogenesis of NMJ.

Similar studies on embryonic NMJ were made by Boeke (1949), who used a silver-staining method. Boeke concluded that the arborization nuclei were homologous with the "interstitial nerves" at the level of the terminal plexes. Tello (1944), in a study of NMJ in adult animals, demonstrated that the nuclei were present in a sheath that was a prolongation of the Schwann cell cytoplasm at the level of the NMJ. This sheath accompanied the nerve terminal branches along their entire length. Many workers now agree that the arborization nuclei of Ranvier are in Schwann or perineural epithelial cells (see page 54).

Part of the difficulty in recognizing the nature of the various nuclei in the soleplate was due to misunderstanding of the nature of the periaxonal sheaths of teloglial cells. The term "teloglia" has been used to describe cells which accompany the terminal nerve branches (Couteaux, 1960). The presence of these cells is recognized in classically stained NMJ by their nuclei, since it is difficult to discern cytoplasmic detail in such preparations.

Teloglia

A brief discussion of the teloglia is indicated, since misunderstanding of the relationships of the investing coats of the terminal nerve fibers has contributed much confusion to NMJ studies. For example, lack of appreciation of the nature of the sheaths surrounding the axon (Schwann sheath, and perineural sheath of Key and Retzius or of Henle) has led to the erroneous statement that the neurilemma is structurally continuous with the sarcolemma within NMJ. Kűhne believed that the Schwann sheath was continuous with the sarcolemma, whereas Ranvier disagreed.

Nerve Sheaths and Perisynaptic Cells

Classical neurohistology recognized two sheaths associated with peripheral nerve fibers. The first, immediately adjacent to the axon, is the sheath of Schwann. Theodor Schwann, a pioneer in establishing the Cell Theory, did not originally distinguish between the cell and the membrane that bears his name. However, according to Young (1942) neurilemma, sheath of Schwann, and Schwann membrane are equivalent structures, whereas the Schwann cell is a distinct structure. Schwann's original illustrations show the Schwann cell protoplasm forming the Schwann sheath. Later, when Ranvier (1878) described degeneration and regeneration of peripheral nerves, the separate nature of the Schwann sheath was emphasized. However, Cajal (1928) clearly recognized that the Schwann cell and Schwann membrane were the same structure.

The other sheath of importance that is associated with peripheral nerve fibers lies external to the Schwann cells. It is the perineural sheath of Key and Retzius (1873) or of Henle. This sheath is composed of connective tissue elements. The ultrastructure of these sheaths is discussed on page

The earliest investigators of the NMJ recognized that not all the multiple nuclei in the soleplate region were within the myofiber. Kűhne called these other cells "telolemma" and Renaut (1899) described a nucleated "endothelium" derived from the Henle sheath that formed a bell mouth over the junctional region. Covering sheaths originating around large nerve fasciculi and extending to smaller fasciculi finally reaching the terminal axons had previously been described by Key and Retzius (1876). In 1960, Couteaux, described the NMJ as covered by two kinds of cells; the teloglial cells which he interpreted as terminal Schwann cells and other nuclei that belonged to cells in Henle's sheath outside the NMJ region. This interpretation has subsequently been confirmed in ultrastructure studies. The Sheath of Henle or "perineural epithelium" (Shanthaveerappa and Bourne, 1962, 1964) lies external to the Schwann cells. The terminal cellular processes of the perineural epithelial cells extend to within a short distance of the sarcolemma in junctional regions. However, ultrastructure studies clearly show that it does not fuse with the sarcolemma (Saito and Zacks, 1969). Thus the classical telolemma which partially covers the area of innervation is composed of both Schwann and connective tissue cell processes, both of which may be extremely delicate and neither of which fuse with the sarcolemma (see page 54). These relationships are clearly visible in the electron microscope and during wallerian degeneration when the axoplasm and myelin lamellas are fragmented and only Schwann and connective tissue cells remain, forming the cords of Bungner.

At least three types of nuclei are present in the NMJ: first, the soleplate nuclei representing the modified cells derived from the muscle cell; secondly, the Schwann cell nuclei, which as they lie in close apposition to the innervated zone appear in close relation to soleplate nuclei; and finally, the endothelial nuclei from adjacent capillaries and fibrocytic nuclei (from the sheath of Key and Retzius), which also lie in close approximation to the innervation zone.

Figure 10 summarizes the classical concept of NMJ structure as derived from numerous investigations prior to 1947.

The junctional region consists of terminal nerve branches lying in an area of modified sarcoplasm containing granules and at least three different kinds of nuclei. The intimate relationship of the nuclei to the

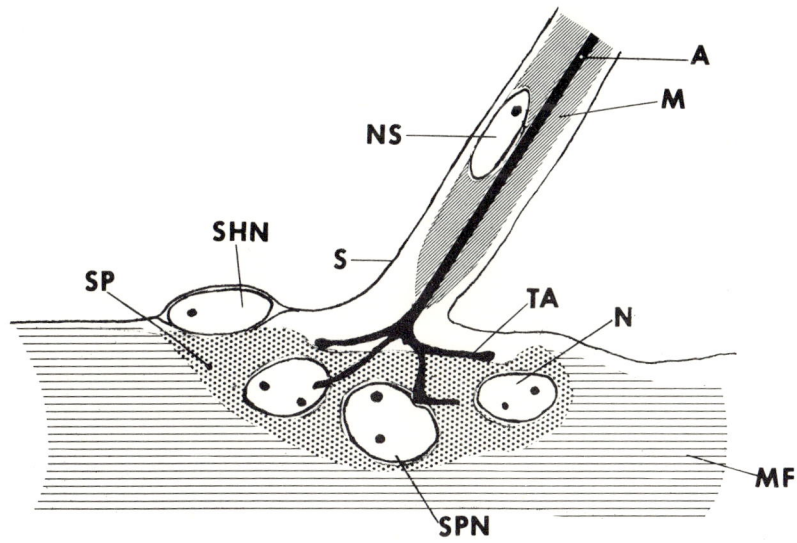

Figure 10. Diagram illustrating the classical concept of anatomic relationships within the neuromuscular junction, redrawn after Gutmann and Young, 1944. A terminal axon *(A)* divides into several terminal branches *(TA)* within the soleplate area, that consists of a depression on the surface of the myofiber. This depression is covered by extensions of the perineural sheath *(S)* which contains a sheath nucleus *(SHN)*. A Schwann cell nucleus is indicated at *NS*. Nuclei of the soleplate are indicated at *SPN*. Myofibers are shown at *MF*. Myelin is indicated at M. (After Gutmann and Young, 1944.)

terminal nerve fibers and the relationship of the nerve fibers to the muscle surface membrane was obscure at this time. However, Gutmann and Young (1944) clearly described the grooves in the sarcolemma in which the terminal nerve branches lay.

In 1947, Couteaux made a major contribution to our understanding of the morphology of the NMJ. By use of supravital staining with Janus green B, he observed new structural details in the subneural region. Radiating from the sides of the terminal nerve branchlets and extend-

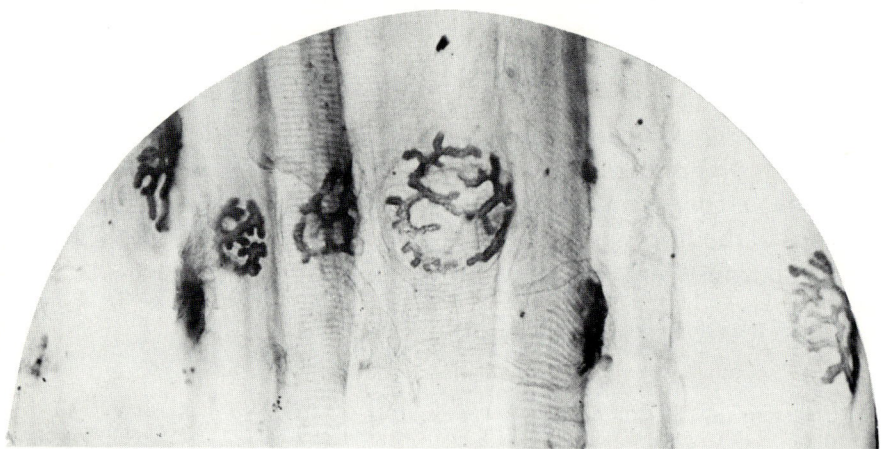

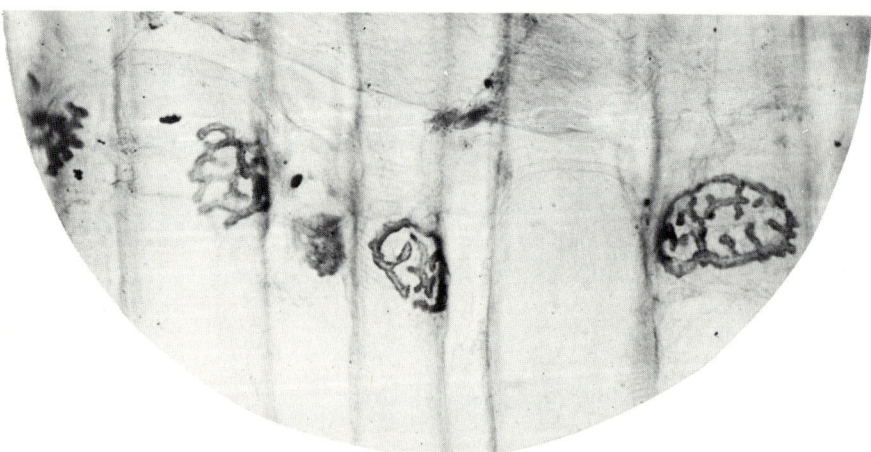

Figure 11. Photomicrograph of neuromuscular junctions stained with Janus green B. Note that the peripheral region surrounding the terminal arborization is more darkly stained than the central portion. The lightly stained myofibers can be seen underlying the NMJs. (X 1,000.) (From Couteaux, 1947.)

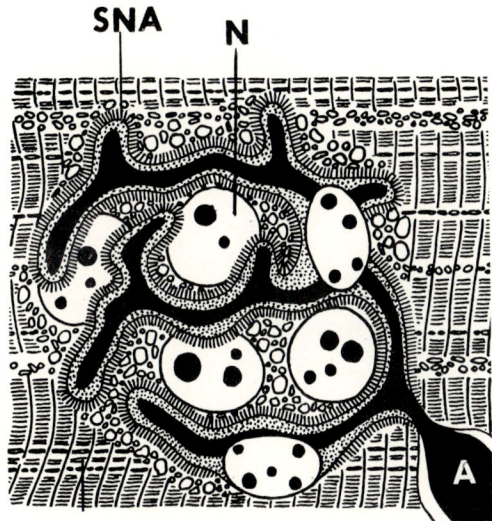

Figure 12. Diagram illustrating a surface view of a NMJ as drawn by Couteaux. The axon *(A)*, after losing its myelin sheath *(M)* enters the NMJ region and divides into the terminal arborization. The axoplasm is shown as solid black. The surface groove is indicated in the stipled portion, and radiating laterally from it is the subneural apparatus *(SNA)*, described by Couteaux. Note the soleplate granules and the several nuclei *(N)*, in the soleplate region. (After Couteaux, 1947.)

ing downwards into the underlying modified sarcoplasm of the soleplate were batonnets or rodlets ("organites"), which stained with Janus green B (Figure 11). This structure was termed the "subneural apparatus" by Couteaux, and the nature of its fine structure was roughly guessed by him despite the resolution limitations of the light microscope. Figures 12 and 13 illustrate Couteaux's concept of NMJ structure.

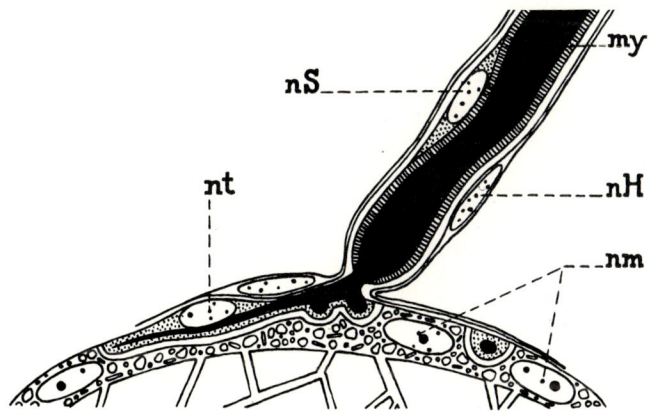

Figure 13. Diagram illustrating a lateral view of relationships within the NMJ. The axoplasm *(A)* breaks up into the terminal branches and lies in a superficial groove on the myofiber surface. The wide black line indicates the region of the subneural apparatus. The Schwann cell nucleus *(NS)*, the myelin sheath *(MY)*, the nuclei of the perineural sheath *(NH)*, and the muscle nuclei *(NM)* are illustrated. Sarcolemma is shown at *SL*. *NT* marks a teloglial nucleus. (After Couteaux, 1947.)

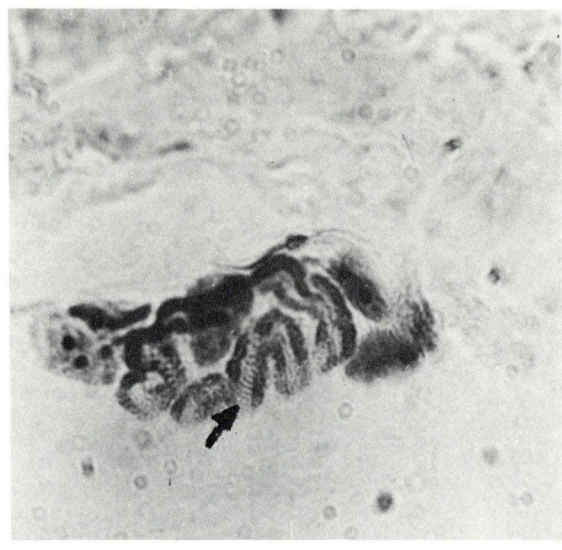

Figure 14. Photomicrograph in phase contrast illustrating a rat intercostal neuromuscular junction stained with lead according to the method of Sávay and Csillik, 1948. Note the dark transverse lines indicating the lead-stained subneural apparatus (arrow). (X 1,000.)

It is probable that the subneural apparatus was observed by Kűhne as early as 1887. He described a peculiar layer of protoplasm in gold-stained preparations that closely followed the outline of the terminal arborization. He believed that it was part of the axon terminal and named it the "stroma." The inner part containing the neurofibrils was called the "axialbaum." Figure 6 illustrates the palisade nature of the "stroma" in methylene blue-stained lizard NMJs. Tiegs stated, "Although it (the 'stroma') is quite distinct from the soleplate protoplasm, it may be merely a condensation of that tissue. But it is also possible that it is homologous with neurolemmal tissue; for in degenerated end organs, from which the axon has completely disappeared, the modified neurolemmal cells (cords of Bungner) can now be seen to be in direct continuity with the perilemma." Thus Couteaux was the first to recognize the existence of the subneural apparatus as a modification of the innervated muscle. This view was later confirmed by electron microscopy. It should be noted that this region may also be seen in whole mounts or thin plastic-embedded sections in the phase microscope with (Figure 14) or without lead impregnation (Figure 15).

Despite the ample documentation offered by Couteaux (1947), Csillik (1960), on the basis of histogenic studies, still claimed a teloglial origin of the subneural apparatus.

Blood Supply of Neuromuscular Junctions

PAS-stained myofibers reveal complex aggregates of capillaries in the region of NMJs, which serves as a useful landmark for finding areas of innervation. Using an injection technique, Marchisio (1964) demonstrated this striking vascularity around NMJs which was thought to be related to the oxygen requirements of the mitochondrial concentrations in this region. A consequence of this vascularity is rapid access of injected drugs to the junctional region.

INNERVATION PATTERNS AND GROSS MORPHOLOGY OF NMJs: THE MOTOR UNIT

As will be recalled, the anterior horn cell representing the lower motor neuron supplies many muscle fibers by branching of the axon.

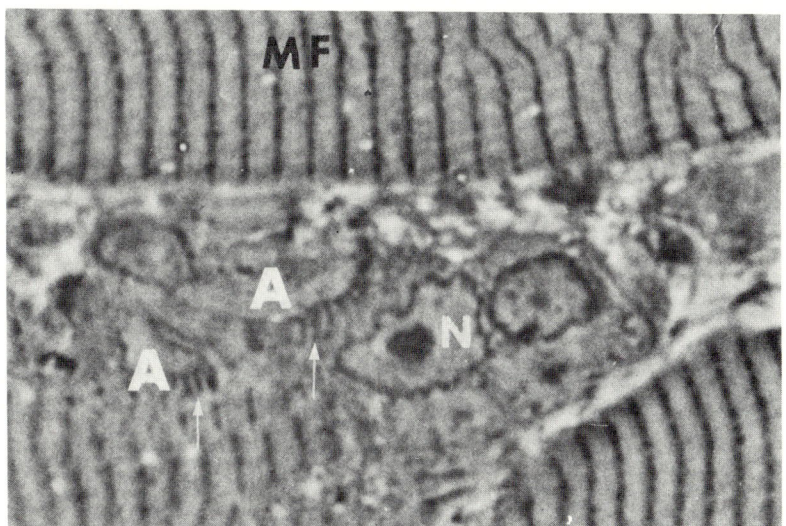

Figure 15. Phase contrast photomicrograph illustrating structural details in a neuromuscular junction. The terminal axons are present at *A* and the rod-like subneural apparatus is indicated at the arrows. Nuclei of the soleplate are also shown at *N*. The myofibers are marked *MF*. (X 4,000.)

The aggregate of muscle fibers supplied by a single neuron is called the motor "unit". Physiologic data obtained by Buchthal et al. (1957) and Krnjevic and Miledi (1958) indicates that individual myofibers are scattered and overlaped in the motor units of a given muscle. This may be a consequence of the pattern of initial innervation when an axon branch forms as the original axon stops growing after it makes initial contact with a myofiber. The branch then innervates subsequent groups of myofibers (Krnjevic and Miledi, 1958). In neurogenic weakness due to peripheral nerve or motor cell disease, there is an increase in the motor unit territory that is attributed to inclusion of surviving motor units that before injury, were located outside the original motor unit. Erminio et al. (1959) suggested that this resulted from reinnervation affected by branching of surviving axons. McComas et al. (1971) has devised an electrophysiological method to estimate the extent of denervation in human muscles by measuring the amplitude of potentials from single motor units and dividing into the action potentials of the whole muscle.

With the discovery of the "checkerboard" pattern that occurs in muscles as a result of differences in the staining properties of individual myofibers, the question of the area of motor unit and its formation has been re-examined. Although differences in individual myofibers are visible in histologic preparations following nearly every enzyme histochemical methods made these differences particularly dramatic. Romanul and Van der Muellen (1967) suggested that during normal development, axons follow a pathway in the nerve and arrive simultaneously at the myotubes of differentiating muscle. The myofibers nearest the tips of the incoming axons are first innervated and as branches form, they are unable to innervate adjacent myofibers and grow further to find non-innervated myofibers in the field of myofibers. This results in wide scatter and overlap. However, ultrastructure studies of differentiating myofibers in conjunction with identification of early neuromuscular contacts (Kelly and Zacks, 1968a, b) indicate that motor unit formation is probably closely linked to the sequence of maturation of myotubes as a system of primary, secondary and tertiary generations (see page 44). As the axons approach the myotubes they are capable of innervating those myofibers that are in an appropriate state of maturation (Lentz, 1969b) and as daughter myotubes differentiate, they receive secondary branches from the original axons or are innervated by terminal axons arising from other neurons. Thus the state of maturation of the myotubes at the time of arrival of the migrating axon sprouts would tend to produce the observed overlapping of motor unit territories. Since all the myotubes are not in the same degree of maturity at the same time, compact motor units rarely are formed.

In the case of nerve regeneration and reinnervation, Romanul and Van der Muellen (1967) have suggested that the regenerating axons traverse new and perhaps tortuous pathways arriving at widely separated points in time. These axons are capable of reinnervating groups of adjacent denervated myofibers thereby producing a compact motor unit. This would explain the groups of myofibers of the same histochemical type found in reinnervated and in cross innervated muscles. Engle (1962), Romanul and Van der Muellen (1967) and Brooke and Kaiser (1970) all considered that the motor units are histochemically homogenous, a concept which presently seems most acceptable. There is no available evidence to support a more complex possibility, namely that an individual motor unit contains myofibers of different histochemical types. In studies of rabbit motor units in rabbit diaphragm, Yasargil (1967) has shown that the typical motor unit consists of 110-120 fibers distributed widely throughout the diaphragm. By employing combined physiological measurements and histochemical staining, Edstrom and Kugelberg (1968) found that motor units of the rat anterior tibial muscle were nearly histochemically uniform (glycogen content, succinic dehydrogenase, phosphorylase and esterase activity) and that the individual myofibers were isolated. A & B motor units contained 80-178 myofibers and accounted for 12-26% of the cross sectional area of the muscle. There was considerable overlapping. Correlation of three histochemical types with three physiologically defined groups was demonstrated by Burke et al. (1971) in the cat gastrocnemius muscle.

Innervation Ratio

The NMJ "innervation ratio" refers to the number of myofibers innervated by a given axon. For many years it has been recognized that nerve branching continues within the intramuscular nerve bundles lying within the perimysium. In infants the "innervation tree" is small and there is increased frequency of branching (Coërs and Woolf, 1959) which nearly always occurs at nodes of Ranvier.

Extensive collateral branching occurs under pathological conditions (see page 238) and appears to be a major compensatory response to injury.

Innervation Bands

A major contribution of these investigations has been the demonstration of localized "innervation bands", even though it has been recognized for many years that NMJ did not occur at random in animal or human muscles (Lapicque, 1931; Pezard and May, 1937; Marnay and Nachmansohn, 1938).

Couteaux (1942, 1947) first demonstrated that NMJ occur in bandlike zones in dog and guinea pig gastrocnemius internus muscles. Later Coërs (1952a) used electrical stimulation and recording to identify areas rich in NMJs.

With the general availability of histochemical methods for the demonstration of AchE (acetylcholinesterase) after 1949, it became an easy matter to locate the zones of innervation in any muscle. Indeed, in work with small animals, thin whole muscles may easily be immersed in the histochemical reagents to delineate the innervation pattern. The thiolacetic acid technique (Barrnett and Palade, 1959) is suitable for this purpose. Such techniques have clearly established that NMJ are located in narrow strips (usually single) in a given muscle. The conformation of the zone depends on the shape and pattern of insertion of the muscle fibers on the intramuscular tendon. For example, in muscles with tendons at each end, the innervation bands run in straight lines perpendicular to the center of the muscle fibers (Fig. 68). In pennate muscles such as the flexor carpi radialis, the line of NMJ follows a curved pattern. It should be stressed that the NMJ always lie in the *mid-portion* of the fiber. This fact can be of considerable importance in obtaining NMJ in human muscle biopsy specimens without recourse to simulation or *intra vitam* staining. Exceptions to this rule occur in the sartorius and gracilis muscles, which have numerous innervation bands scattered randomly throughout the muscles. However, by means of cholinesterase staining to indicate the location of musculotendinous junctions (MTJ) Couteaux (1953) found that numerous MTJ were also present throughout these muscles, which are formed by parallel bundles of short fibers linked together by numerous fibrous bands (Coërs and Durand, 1957). This observation was supported by the microdissection work of Schwarzacher (1957).

When the nerve bundles reach the terminal innervation band, they invest the muscle fibers, crossing them at right angles. Some 5 to 50 nerve fibers emerge as a spray composed of many subterminal fibers. These in turn separate and terminate in small branchlets within the NMJ. Two NMJ may occur on the same muscle fiber as a result of terminal branching, or, infrequently, a NMJ may be supplied by two axons arising from the same cell (Coërs and Woolf, 1959). These investigators never observed evidence of two neurons innervating the same NMJ.

Edds (1950) observed occasional terminal branching of axons in rat muscle. The fact of this branching made it necessary to distinguish between the absolute terminal innervation ratio (ATIR) and a functional terminal innervation ratio (FTIR). The ATIR is defined as the number of *NMJ* associated with a given number of terminal axons divided by the number of terminal axons, whereas FTIR is the number of *muscle fibers* innervated by a given number of terminal axons divided by the number of terminal axons. The work of Coërs (1955a, b) showed the human FTIR to be 1.09: ± 0.059:1, whereas the ATIR was 1.13:1. This means that only 1.5 to 10 per cent of terminal axons supply more than one muscle fiber in limb muscles and that 2.3 per cent of these fibers have two terminal fiber arborizations, that is, double NMJ.

Gross Morphology of Neuromuscular Junctions

Size. According to Coërs (1955b), the mean diameter of human limb muscle NMJ is $32.2\mu \pm 10.5\mu$. Individual NMJ range in diameter from 10 to 80μ with a standard deviation of ± 6.67 to 13.2μ. Coërs and Woolf (1959) were able to demonstrate a close correlation between the diameter of the NMJ and the diameter of the muscle fibers; the larger muscle fibers have larger NMJ. This has been confirmed by Gruber, 1966; Kuno et al., 1971; Morris and Raybould, 1971 and Granbacher, 1971.

Comparative Aspects

It has long been recognized that the gross morphology of NMJ differs in various animals. There are three major varieties of NMJ visible in the optical microscope with traditional staining methods. They are (1) compact NMJ with oval soleplates ("terminaisons en plaque") (2) elongated endings with grape cluster structure ("terminaisons en grappe") and (3) unusual linear junctions that occur in amphibians and reptiles ("terminaisons en ligne").

A comparative study by Cole (1955) illustrates the variations in NMJ structure in several species (Figures 16, 17). He used a single staining method (gold chloride) to permit comparison of the NMJs from various examples of elasmobranch and teleost fishes, amphibians, reptiles, birds, and mammals. Increasing complexity of structure was observed in the phylogenetically more advanced species. The most

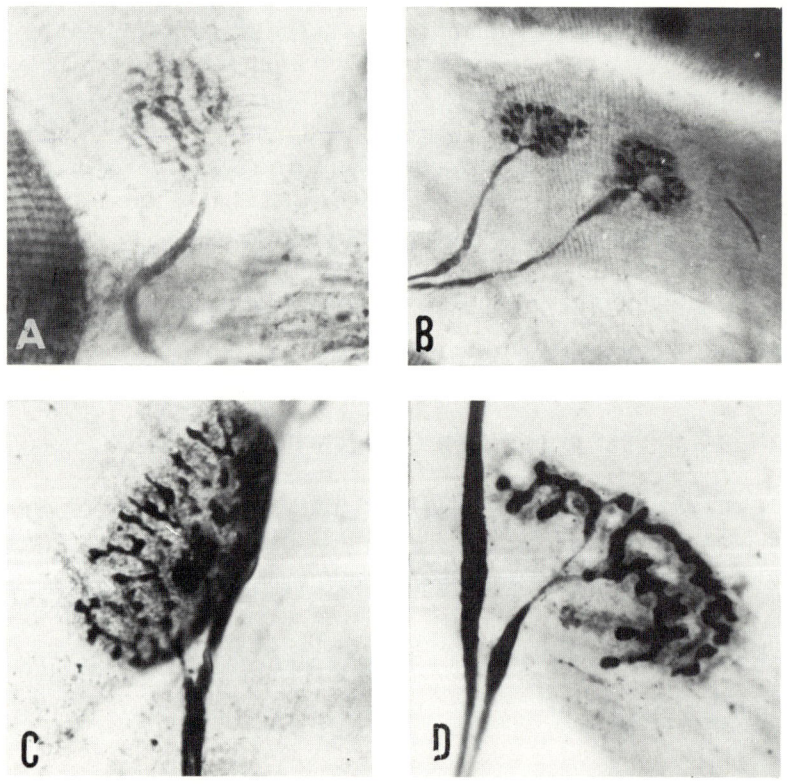

Figure 16. Photomicrographs of neuromuscular junctions from various animal species, stained with gold. *A*, kangaroo rat: Surface view demonstrating oval compact "en plaque" ending. (X 450.) *B*, mouse: The neuromuscular junctions are slightly smaller than those of the rat but are quite similar. (X 450.) *C*, rabbit: NMJ with considerable amounts of granular material in the soleplate. (X 450.) *D*, hamster: Typical hamster NMJ. (X 450.) (From Fig. 6, W.V. Cole, *J. Comp. Neurol.* 102:703.)

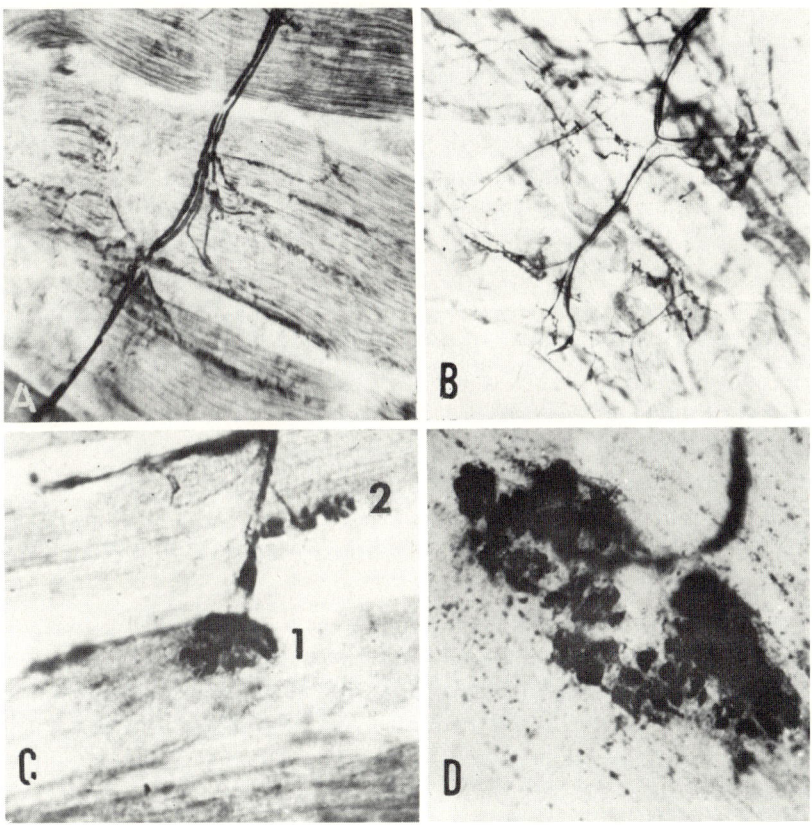

Figure 17. Photomicrographs of neuromuscular junctions from various animal species, stained with gold. *A,* toad: "terminasion en ligne". (X 100.) *B,* turtle: "terminasion en ligne". (X 100.) *C,* snake: *(Coluber constrictor)* illustrating "terminasion en plaque" *(1)* and "terminasion en grappe" *(2)* arising from the same motor nerve. (X 450.) *D,* snake: *(Natrix orthogaster)* "terminasion en plaque". (X 450.) From Fig. 2, W.V. Cole, J. Comp. Neurol. 102:1955.)

primitive endings were terminal rings, whereas in mammals the familiar complex branched structure of the terminal arborization was observed. All the motor endings studied had variable quantities of granular material in the soleplate, which also varied in prominence. The shape of the motor endings conformed to the classical "terminaisons en plaque" and "terminaisons en grappe," with the exception of certain linear endings in amphibians and reptiles for which the term "terminaisons en ligne" was suggested. The snake, lizard, and hamster also had "accessory" endings that differed structurally from the predominant type. However, no explanation for these structures was offered.

Cole concluded that the NMJs appeared to be adapted to the functional requirements of each animal group. The nerve endings of animals requiring well coordinated muscular activity appeared to contain large amounts of granular material and more complicated nerve branching. The "terminaison en ligne" occurred in animals characterized by rapid muscular activity. For example, fish NMJs had rather diffuse terminal nerve branches associated with large amounts of densely staining granular material. On the other hand, the NMJs of *Necturus* had multiple nerve fibers forming an extensive and complex termination. Several snakes demonstrated compact plate-like endings, whereas other snake NMJs were diffuse. Particularly diffuse were the NMJs in the pigeon and chicken. The familiar compact form of NMJ with multiple branched fibers and numerous granules in the soleplate occurs in the rat, mouse, rabbit, hamster, cat, monkey, and man.

Coërs (1957) demonstrated that human NMJ differ from rodent NMJ in that they consist of groups of separate rounded or oval subneural units demonstrated by AchE staining that differ from the compact gutters of rat NMJ subneural apparatus. In man, the cuplet form of subneural apparatus surrounds the terminal axon. Coërs concluded that the whole of the rodent terminal arborization had synaptic membranes were excitatory (Coërs, 1953a). NMJs of the "en plaque" type seemed less complex than those observed in rodents as demonstrated by methylene blue staining.

Although most investigators (Coërs and Woolf, 1959) reported human NMJ were all of the single en plaque variety, exceptions to this rule were found in certain specialized muscles. Wolter (1964) used a combined silver and thiocholine histochemical method to study the innervation of human extraocular muscles. He described three varieties of efferent and six afferent nerves. Of the efferent nerve fibers, only one that was associated with thick medullated nerve fibers had NMJs. The other two kinds of endings were "ring" or "button" formations and delicate spray networks both supplied by nerve fibers with little myelin. Small nerve fibers with ring endings terminated close to NMJs and thus produced double innervation of these myofibers. In some cases, such endings occurred alone. The thin nerve fibers supplying the ring forms also arose in nerve bundles containing thick medullated axons. The thin nerve fibers, which produced fine networks on the myofibers, originated in the walls of small blood vessels. All the NMJs contained

ChE activity whereas the ring type apparently lacked this enzyme when they were in the vicinity of NMJs but not when they occurred alone. No AchE activity was demonstrated in the network type of ending. Wolter suggested that the thin ring ending that was responsible for double innervation of some of the myofibers was parasympathetic or possibly represented a portion of the gamma efferent system since no spindles could be found in these muscles. Other investigators, however, have described spindles in eye muscles (Cooper and Daniel, 1944) and Teräväinen (1969) has demonstrated AchE activity in the multiple endings of rat extraocular muscle.

Unusual innervation patterns have also been observed in human vocal and laryngeal muscles. Rossi and Cortesina (1965) used a histochemical method to study these muscles. NMJs demonstrated by their AchE activity were multiple in the vocalis, cricothyroid and lateral and posterior cricoarytenoid muscles. Multiple innervation was found in 17-80% of the vocalis, 50% of the cricothyroid and lateral cricoarytenoid, and 5% in the posterior cricoarytenoid myofibers. Spiral endings were present in all four muscles whereas muscle spindles were found only in the vocalis muscle. Similarly, Manolov et al. (1965), using silver staining and histochemical techniques, described multiple innervation in 50% of cat vocal muscles.

Functional Significance of NMJ Structure

Although Cole (1955) attempted to correlate functional differences with the presence of en plaque and en grappe NMJs, he was unable to find a consistent pattern. Coërs and Woolf (1959) discussed the possible significance of these differences in terms of the known differences in the response of cat tibialis and soleus muscles to neuromuscular blocking agents (Paton and Zaimis, 1952; Zaimis, 1952). Coërs and Woolf (1959) observed that in rabbit and monkey muscle, the diameter of NMJs differed in "red" and "white" muscles. In red muscles, which are known to be slow reacting and capable of sustained contraction, the NMJ were significantly larger. For example, the soleus, chiefly a red muscle, contains NMJs that have a mean size significantly greater than the NMJs in the gastrocnemius internus and tibialis anterior, which are chiefly white muscles (Coërs, 1955b).

In addition to the correlation between size of NMJs and the different kinds of myofibers, several investigators have attempted to correlate the structure of NMJs with the speed of myofiber contraction initially at the light microscopic, and ultimately at the electron microscopic level of resolution. The latter topic is considered in greater detail on page .

Although it has been known for many years that the responses of red and white muscles differ in many species (Ranvier, 1873; Krűger, 1949, 1950) and that in frogs, tonic muscular responses are associated with small nerves and tetanic responses with large nerves (Tasaki and Mizutani, 1944; Kuffler and Vaughan-Williams, 1953), several investigators claimed that slow and fast myofibers could be distinguished by their morphology (Krűger, 1949; Krűger and Gűnther, 1955, 1958; Hess, 1960, 1961, 1962). According to this hypothesis, the "fibrillenstruktur" muscles with regular separation of myofibrils each surrounded by sarcoplasmic reticulum were regarded as "fast" (tetanic) muscles whereas "felderstruktur" muscles, with irregular spacing and lacking regular distribution of sarcoplasmic reticulum were "slow" (tonic) myofibers. Furthermore, it was claimed that en plaque NMJs were solely associated with "fibrillenstruktur" fibers and cluster like endings ("en grappe") with "felderstruktur" fibers (Krűger, 1949; Gűnther, 1949; Ginsborg, 1960; Hess, 1961, 1962; Hess and Pilar, 1963; Orfanos, 1962; Zenker and Anzenbacher, 1964).

Although there are apparent correlations of the kind of NMJ and muscle structure reported by these investigators, it should be stressed that the muscles studied were in non-mammalian species or extraocular muscles that apparently are highly specialized. Investigations by others (Coërs and Woolf, 1959; Csillik, 1960; Ogata, 1965; Bergman, 1967) have failed to fine similar relationships in other fast and slow skeletal muscles. In a detailed review of NMJs in several species, Barker (1968) concluded that vertebrate striated muscle should be classified as "twitch" and "non-twitch". The former may be "fast" or "slow" and have en plaque NMJs or have en grappe NMJs and also be "fast" or "slow". "Non-twitch" myofibers invariably have en grappe NMJs and are all "slow". More recently, refined histochemical and ultrastructural characterization of different kinds of NMJs have been reported (Padykula and Gauthier, 1970) and more subtle differences have been recognized in the fine structure of NMJs innervating different kinds of muscle (Chapter 3, page 65).

Similar attempts to derive physiologic information from histologic preparations were made by Coërs and Woolf (1959). These investigators observed that in NMJs stained by the methylene blue method, the ramified and plexiform structure of rat and mouse synaptic gutters appeared to receive the entire terminal axon arborization, whereas in man the terminal axoplasm was only partially surrounded by the synaptic gutter. The fine neural filaments that connected the swellings of the terminal arborization appeared to make no contact with the subneural apparatus. These workers concluded that perhaps only terminal and collateral expansions had synaptic function. The objection to this kind of analysis is that physiologic information can not be inferred from silver or methylene blue-stained NMJs.

EVOLUTION OF NEUROMUSCULAR JUNCTIONS: MORPHOLOGIC CONSIDERATIONS

Barets (1952, 1955), Marinskaya (1962) and Coërs (1967) have suggested that phylogenetic progression is indicated by the various kinds of NMJ structure. In the most primitive neuromuscular connections, motor axons are scattered randomly over the muscle surface. A slightly less primitive arrangement is localization of the NMJ at the ends of the myofibers (myoseptal). In the most advanced animals, an en plaque NMJ is located in the mid-portion of the muscle fiber. Figure 18. The disseminated or polar patterns of innervation remain in primitive somatic muscles such as that of the tadpole tail and in the tailless amphibians and reptiles (McKay et al., 1960; McKay and Peters, 1961; Hess, 1963). It is of interest that in adult tailless amphibians, motor

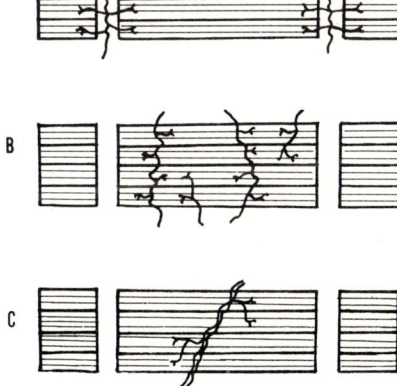

Figure 18. Diagram of kinds of motor innervation patterns in fish muscles. *A.* myoseptal innervation; *B.* scattered innervation; *C.* equatorial innervation. *A & B* are regarded as more primitive stages in motor innervation. After Barets, A. *Arch. Anat. Microscop. Morph. Exptl. 41*:305, 1952.

innervation of two kinds occurs. Some myofibers have a centrally located end bush of Kühne that is similar to an en plaque terminal as well as scattered en grappe endings on the muscles (Gray, 1956). Multiple innervation is observed in several muscles of birds (Ginsborg, 1960; Ginsborg and Mackay, 1961). However, in the higher mammals multiple innervation appears to persist only in the extrinsic ocular muscles and unusual innervation sites such as the inner ear and some of the laryngeal muscles.

In a review, Marinskaya (1962) attempted to trace the evolution of vertebrate neuromuscular junctions. This investigator suggested that the changes in NMJ structure during embryogenesis are a reflection of NMJ phylogenetic history. The compound endings of embryos consisting of several preterminal nerve fibers are replaced in the adult by more compact, single endings. Marinskaya recognized progressive changes in the terminal arborization, size of the soleplate, and structure of the subneural apparatus in the vertebrate phylogenetic series. The terminal arborization tends to become more compact, and the soleplate and the subneural apparatus become more prominent in the higher vertebrates. Furthermore, AchE activity tends to become concentrated at the ends of the axon terminals in the higher vertebrates, unlike the lower forms, in which the enzyme is distributed along the terminal fibers. Although more than one NMJ on a muscle fiber is common in the lower vertebrates, it is quite uncommon in the higher vertebrates.

Although an evolutionary series can be described and functional differences correlated with structure in the case of some tonic and tetanic muscles, the histologic structure of an individual neuromuscular junction appears not to be of reliable significance in defining its functional activity. For example, Gutmann and Young (1944) showed that even immature neuromuscular junctions in the process of reconstitution after denervation were functionally "intact" despite their abnormal and often primitive appearance. It appears that more definitive physiologic correlations with structure will be required to establish the concepts of Cole and Marinskaya, which are based solely upon morphologic observations.

Musculotendinous Junctions

Although not a known component of the excitatory system of skeletal muscle, the musculotendinous junction (MTJ) has caught the attention of several investigators of the NMJ because of its superficial structural resemblance to NMJs and its enzymatic dependence on muscle innervation. Couteaux (1953) called attention to these similarities and demonstrated AchE within the folds of the MTJ. Hess and Pilar (1963) and others have confirmed these findings.

The fine structure of the MTJ consists of invaginations of the muscle surface membrane covered by external lamina of the approximate size or slightly larger than the clefts of the subneural apparatus (Mackay et al., 1969; Mair and Tomé, 1972). Collagen filaments arising from the tendon lie within the invaginations. It is this interlaminated structure of collagen and muscle external lamina with plasma membrane that resembles the subneural apparatus and apparently contributes the strength of the MTJ. Lubinska and Zelená (1967) confirmed the work of Bonichon (1957) and Begliomini and Moriconi (1959) who found the cholinesterase activity developed earlier in the MTJ than in NMJs during embryogenesis. However Couteaux (1953) and Mumenthaler and Engle (1961) observed that enzyme activity appeared coincidently in the NMJ.

Floyd (1970), using a modified Koelle technique for demonstration of cholinesterase activity, observed the enzyme in MTJs and a new palisaded structure similar to the MTJ that were interposed between the ends of two muscle fibers in cat extraocular muscle. These were interpreted as a new kind of cell junction.

Several investigators (Gerebetzoff and Ueten, 1954; Schwartzacher, 1960; Zelená and Szentegothai, 1957; Csillik, 1960) all observed that adult mammalian skeletal muscle under conditions of denervation showed decrease in NMJ AchE activity but no change in the enzyme in the MTJ. However, if the rat muscle was denervated at birth or soon after, no AchE activity could be found in the MTJs (Zelená, 1965). Miledi et al. (1968) have demonstrated that rat soleus muscle (slow) has AchE activity in its MTJs whereas the extensor digitorum longus muscle (fast) lacks this activity. The functional significance of elements of the Ach-AchE system in MTJs is obscure.

2

Embryogenesis of NMJ

Many investigators (Kűhne, 1864; London and Pesker, 1906; Boeke, 1909; Tello, 1917, 1922; Dickson, 1940; Cuajunco, 1942; Couteaux, 1941, 1960; Csillik, 1960; DeAnda et al., 1963) have used classical staining methods to study the formation of NMJs on embryonic muscle as a means of unraveling the complex inter-relationships of nerve and muscle in this region. Primary emphasis was placed on the earliest evidence of NMJ formation and the role of various cells in the formation of the NMJ. Nearly all agreed that neuromuscular contact occurred early in myogenesis during the myotube stage, that complexity of soleplate organization increased with maturation but there was much controversy about the source of the soleplate nuclei. With classical staining methods, the earliest recognizable NMJs were observed at about 11 weeks (Tello, 1917; Cuajunco, 1942; Beckett and Bourne, 1958) a time when the first responses of the muscle to neural stimulation and spontaneous movements begin. NMJ in rat skeletal muscle were reported visible by 16 days in optical microscope studies by East (1931) and Strauss and Weddell (1940).

Definitive answers to these questions were not forthcoming until fine structure studies could be made. The description of NMJ morphogenesis provided by Couteaux (1941, 1960) summarizes the then available information. According to Couteaux, two main phases of NMJ formation occurring during embryogenesis could be identified. In the first, or myotube stage, the muscle nuclei are still in an axial location within the muscle cell and the developing myofilaments still lie in the periphery of the muscle cell. Motor nerve fibers lie close to the surface of the immature myotubes. These have been termed the "exploring fibers." No connections with the muscle are visible at this stage, even though nerve branches lie quite close to the muscle surface membrane.

In the second major phase, when the muscle nuclei have taken up their peripheral location within the muscle cell, adjacent nerve fibers send out terminal sprouts accompanied by Schwann cell nuclei.

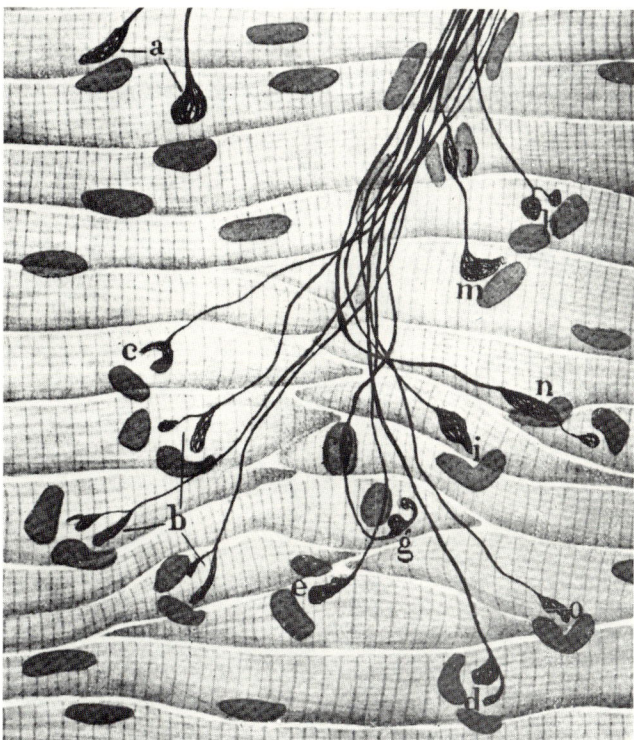

Figure 19. Drawing of developing neuromuscular junctions in a human fetus at term. *a* and *m* illustrate terminal clubs in the vicinity of nuclei. *b*, early development of the terminal arborization is shown. At *N*, a club shaped ending and one like a fish hook is illustrated at *c*. More developed end knobs are shown at *d* and *g*. The tendency of the developing nerve fibrils to enlarge in the vicinity of nuclei is illustrated at *f, l,* and *n*. At *h*, a branched ending is present near nuclei that have divided, and at *i* a nucleus begins to divide in relation to a nerve end knob. (X 1,200.) (From Tello, 1917.)

Each of the small sprouts lies in close relationship to the surface of the muscle fiber at the level of one of its nuclei. Couteaux believed that at this stage, the muscle nuclei divide, probably by amitosis, and accumulate at the site of the future NMJ. Although large nucleoli are prominent features of these nuclei, mitotic figures are never present. There is also increased sarcoplasm in the region of the future NMJ. These components form the "primitive eminence" on the still quite narrow myofiber. In preparations stained with silver by the Gros-Bielschowsky method, the terminal nerve branches seem to be intimately attached to several muscle nuclei surrounded by granular sarcoplasm (Figures 19, 20). These large nuclei, which become the "fundamental

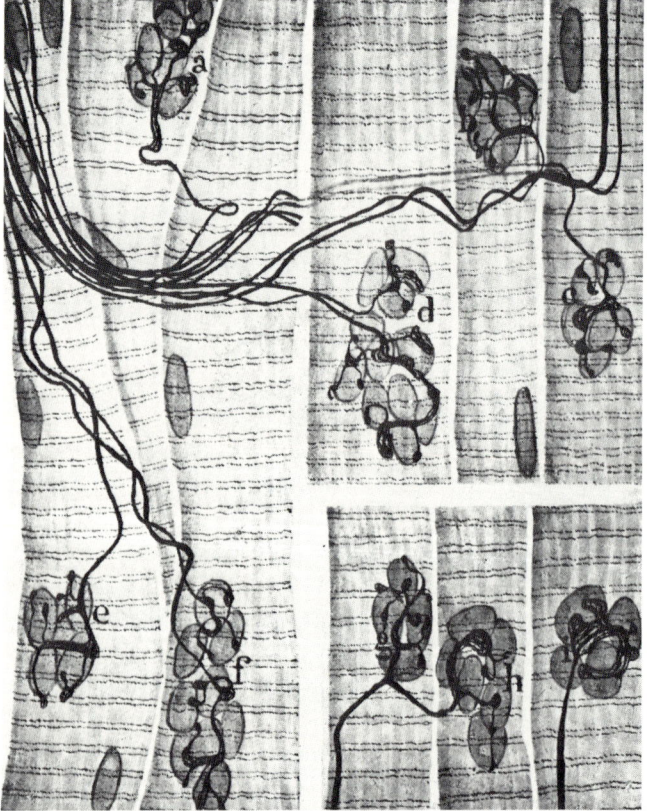

Figure 20. Drawing of NMJs from the tongue of a human fetus at term. NMJs have a, b, c, and e, are single, whereas at d and f NMJs with two separate nerve fibers are shown. NMJs formed by a single fiber are shown at g and h and i illustrates an earlier stage of development. (X 1,200.) (From Tello, 1917.)

nuclei" of the soleplate, are large and more nearly spherical than the oval myofiber nuclei distant from the innervation site. Contact of the nerve fibers with the muscle occurs rather early in development, but full elaboration of the specialized NMJ structure requires additional time. It is likely that the specialized structures of the junctional region are formed by "induction" caused by trophic influences from the nerve because these changes appear to require close approximation or contact with the nerve. There is no evidence to suggest that nerve fibers are attracted to a particular portion of the myofiber cell membrane. Recent studies of NMJ formation in organ culture support this hypothesis. (See below). Thus, formation of the synaptic apparatus is a local phenomenon resulting from some "trophic" influence exerted by the embryonic terminal nerve fiber.

HISTOCHEMICAL AND ULTRASTRUCTURE STUDIES OF NMJ FORMATION

Soon after the demonstration of AchE activity in NMJs by histochemical methods, several investigators used these methods to trace the development of NMJs (Kupfer and Koelle, 1951; Coërs, 1953a; Beckett and Bourne, 1958; Gerebtzoff, 1955, 1959; Zelená and Szentagothái, 1957; Rowinski, 1959; Csillik, 1960, 1965; Lewis and Hughes, 1960; Mumenthaler and Engle, 1961; Drachman, 1963; Wake, 1964; Khera and Laham, 1965; Hirano, 1967a; Filogamo and Gabella, 1967, Juntunen and Terävainen, 1972).

Several of these studies emphasized the time and site of the first appearance of AchE but little new data was obtained concerning the Khera and Laham, 1965; Hirano, 1967a; Filagamo and Gabella, 1967).

Several of these studies emphasized the time and site of the first appearance of AchE but little new data was obtained concrening the process of NMJ formation. In general, these investigations confirmed the earlier studies using impregnation methods that neuromuscular contact occurs early in muscular development (Zelená and Szentagothái, 1957; Mumenthaler and Engle, 1961; Hirano, 1967a; Filogamo and Gabella, 1967). Only Kupfer and Koelle (1951) and Couteaux (1941, 1960) believed that neuromuscular connections are established after the muscle nuclei have completed their migration to the periphery (20-22 days).

In human embryos, the first suggestion of the presence of NMJ as indicated by AchE activity in the subneural apparatus occurred at the 8th week according to Marinskaya (1962 and 8.6 weeks (intercostal muscles and 10 weeks (anterior tibial muscle) (Juntunen and Terävainen (1972)). Using similar methods, Kamieniecka (1968) claimed the first NMJ occurred at the 9th week and Fidziańska (1971) demonstrated the first NMJ at 10 weeks. Additional details of AchE development in NMJ is discussed in greater detail in Chapter 9.

Ultrastructure Studies

Since the first edition of this monograph, several ultrastructure studies of NMJ embryogenesis have clarified this process (Blechschmidt

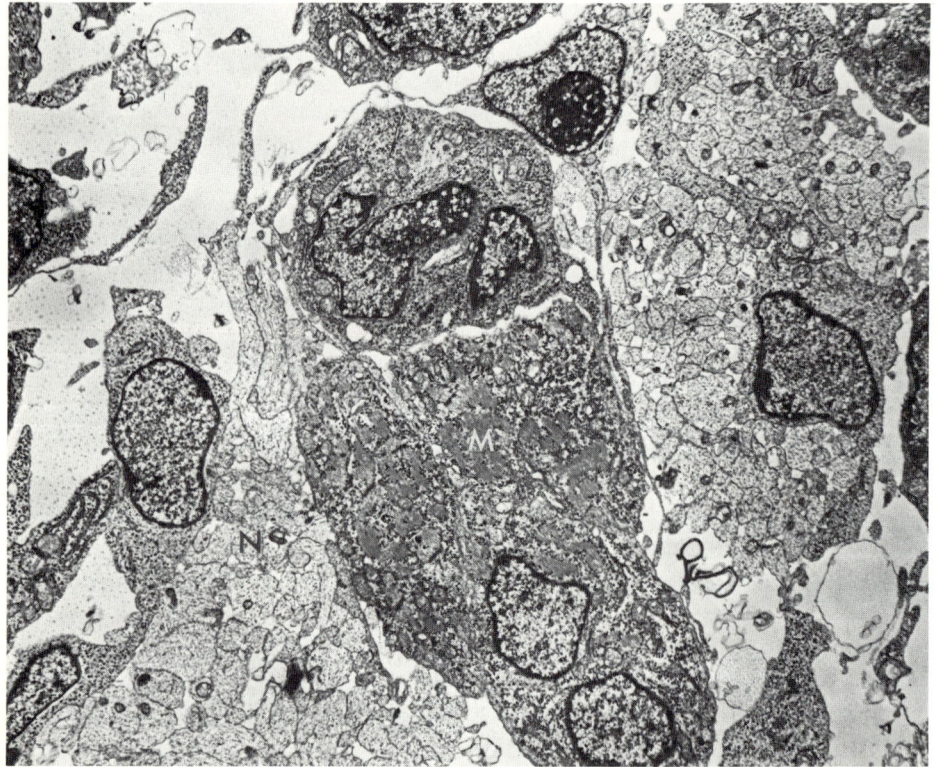

Figure 21. Electron micrograph illustrating a group of small closely related myotubes *(M)* with an intramuscular nerve *(N)* extending diagonally into the illustration. The axons are in contact with each other and loosely wrapped by immature Schwann cells. The nerve appears to make contact with the group of myotubes. (X 7,500.)

and Daikoku, 1966; Kelly, 1966; Teräväinen, 1967a, b; Hirano, 1966, 1967; Kelly and Zacks, 1968; Fidziánska, 1971). The increased resolution of the electron microscope made it possible to trace the earliest events in neuromuscular contact in chicken, rat and human NMJs. The earliest chick neuromuscular contacts observed occurred at 13-20 days *in ovo* (Hirano, 1967), at 16 days in the rat (Kelly and Zacks, 1968) and at 3 to 4 months (Blechschmidt and Daikoku, 1966) or 9-16th week (Fidziańska, 1971) in human fetal muscle. Although not observed by Blechschmidt and Daikoku (1966), Hirano (1967), Teräväinen (1968) or Fidziańska (1971) an initial non-definitive stage of intermediate junctional contact between axon processes and myotubes and between axon processes occurs in the early stages of developing rat muscle. Hirano (1966) observed that the initial neuromuscular contacts occurred in the chick at 13 days (stage 39 Hamilton) when external lamina covered the myotube plasma membrane. First neuromuscular contacts were made by large numbers of axons enclosed by single Schwann cells. These early NMJs had a wide primary cleft (800-1200 A) and occasional secondary synaptic clefts. Also, there was a 300-750 A thickening of the subsynaptic membrane. In a later study, Hirano (1967b) stated that the first indication of NMJ formation in the 13 day chick embryo is the membrane thickening of the postsynaptic membrane. He also suggested that the external lamina formed as the nerve approached. The chick NMJs matured rapidly and by 18-20 days appeared mature. In rat intercostal muscle, Kelly (1966) and Kelly and Zacks (1968) found that the earliest contacts occurred at 16 days. At this stage, the developing intercostal muscles (Fig. 21) consisted of groups of myotubes with little external lamina and between them were minute (0.2-1 μ) loosely clusted axon processes that were interconnected by focal intermediate junctions (Fig. 22, 23). The axons which contained 300 A neurotubules and neurofilaments were loosely and incompletely wrapped by immature Schwann cells. At varying intervals, groups of axons left the nerve trunk accompanied by thin Schwann cell processes and approached groups of myotubes to within 100-150 A (Fig. 21). Occasional intermediate junctions interconnected the cell membranes of both axons and Schwann cells and myotubes and undifferentiated myogenic cells (Figures 22, 23).

These junctions appear to be temporary structures since they were never present once external lamina had formed on the surface of the myofiber plasma membrane. The first definitive evidence of NMJ formation was recognized at 18 days by the presence of the characteris-

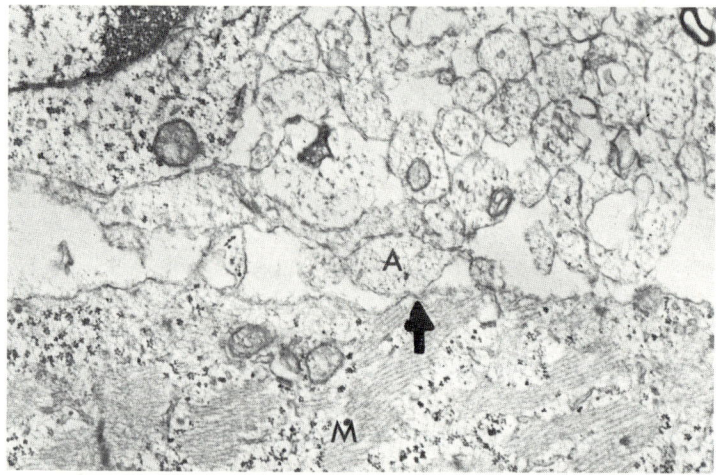

Figure 22. Electron micrograph illustrating close contacts between numerous axon sprouts *(A)* and developing myotube *(M)*. An area of close contact is indicated by an arrow. (X 16,000.)

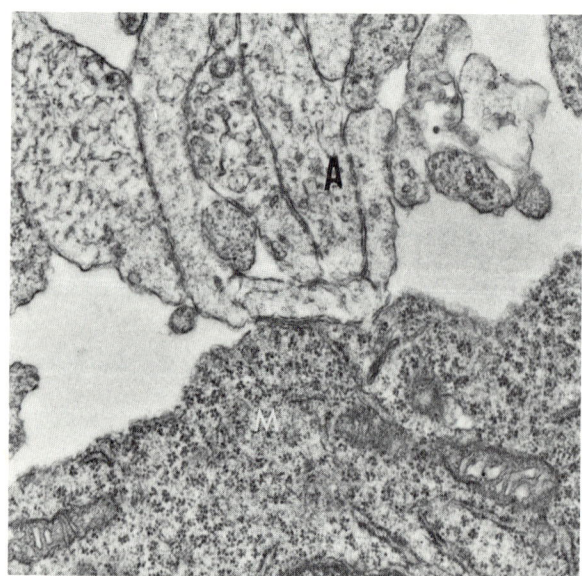

Figure 23. Electron micrograph illustrating detail of an intermediate junction between a developing axon *(A)* and the underlying myotube *(M)*. Note that the axon contains two kinds of vesicles; large vesicles with electron dense cores, and smaller vesicles with faint osmophilic centers. (X 39,000.)

tic thickening in the myofiber plasma membrane underlying the groups of terminal axons (Figure 24, 25). At this time, 3 to 6 terminal axons

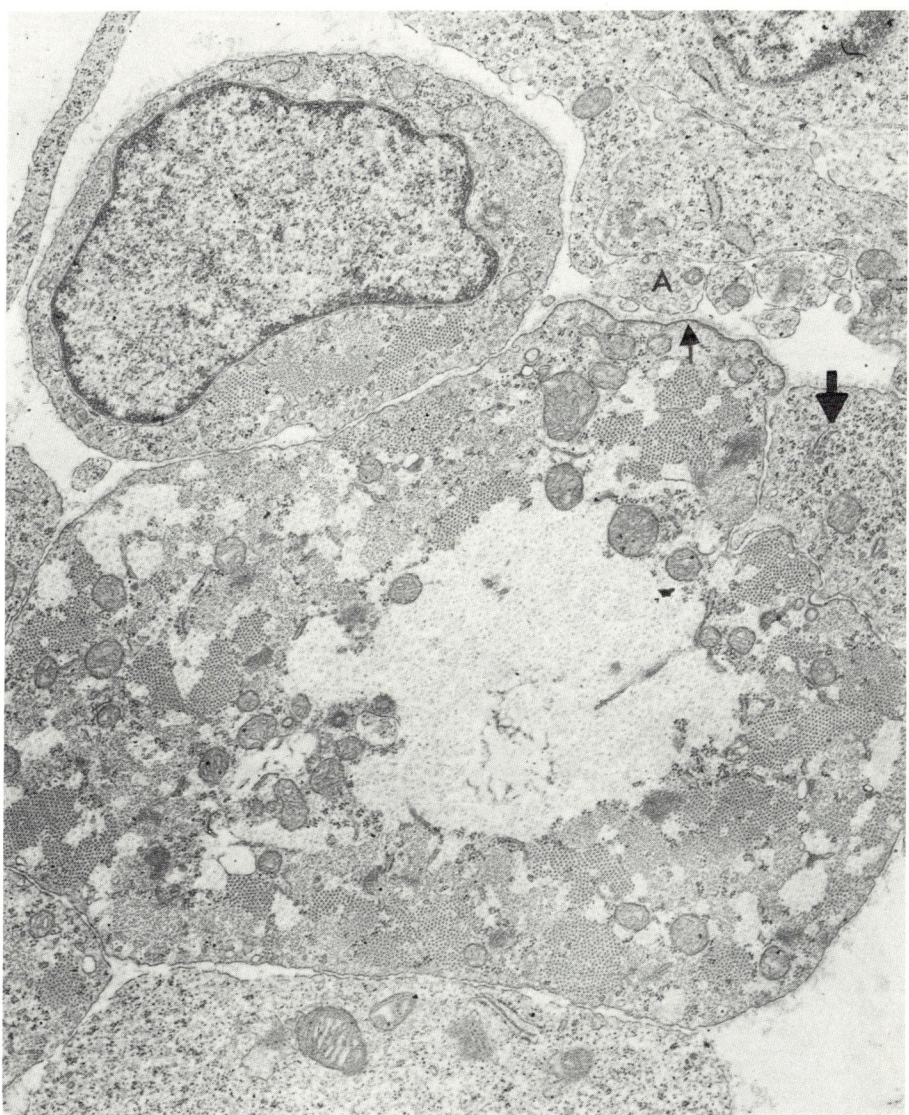

Figure 24. Electron micrograph illustrating a group of myofibers with the most differentiated in the center. Axon sprouts *(A)* approach closely to the myotube plasma membrane which contains focal membrane thickening (arrow). Five accessory cells, some lacking filaments (large arrow) are closely related to the surface of the central myotube. (X 17,000.)

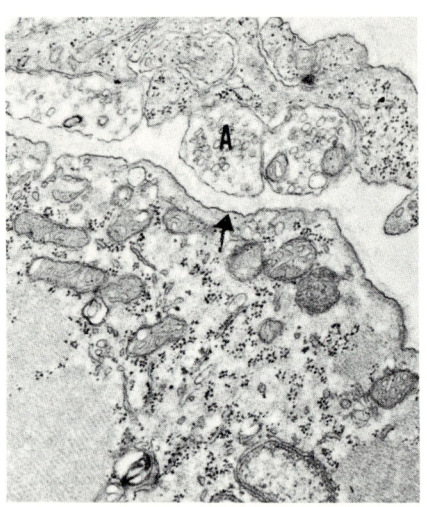

Figure 25. Electron micrograph illustrating detail of approaching axon branches *(A)* to the myotube plasma membrane that displays some membrane thickening (arrow.) (X 24,600.)

innervated individual myotubes within a group of differentiating muscle cells. The axons contained 400-600 Å synaptic vesicles and occasional coated and dense core vesicles. The myotube cell membranes were thickened at sites of innervation and there were small depressions and grooves suggesting rudimentary primary and secondary synaptic clefts (Figures 25, 26). At this stage, the axon was separated from the postsynaptic membrane by 500-900 Å gaps partially filled by external lamina. By 20 days, the subneural clefts were more developed and myotube nuclei were displaced from the cell center to the region of the soleplate. Schwann cell processes isolated individual axons from each other within the intramuscular nerve trunks. NMJs at birth con-

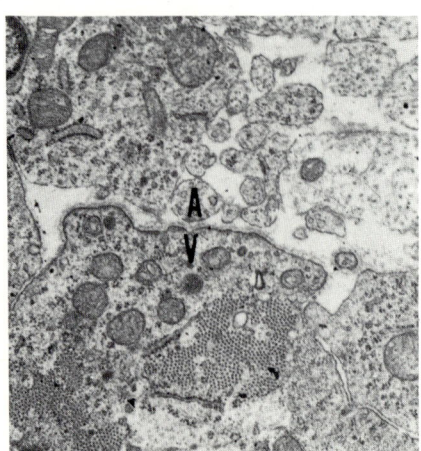

Figure 26. Electron micrograph illustrating detail of developing postsynaptic membrane. The axon branches *(A)* approach closely to the myofiber external lamina that is separated from the thickened postsynaptic membrane (arrow). Note the small invaginated V-shaped pits, the presumptive subneural apparatus at V. (X 17,000.)

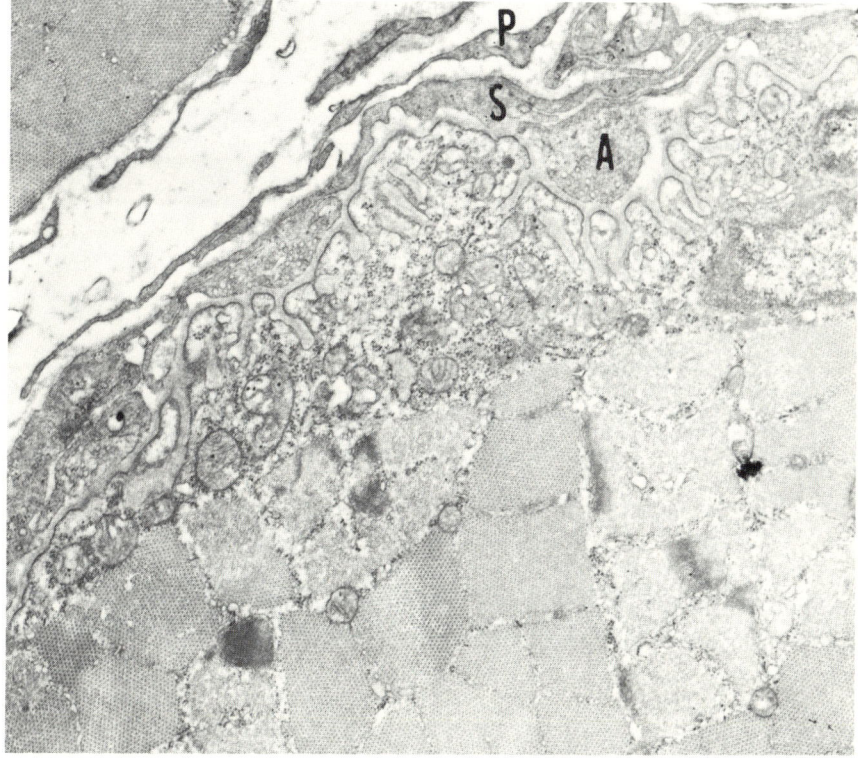

Figure 27. Electron micrograph illustrating nearly adult morphology of a developing NMJ. Note the thickening of the plasma membrane in apposition to the terminal axon *(A)* and the elongation of the clefts of the subneural apparatus. Strands of Schwann cell cytoplasm *(S)* and perineural epithelium *(P)* are also illustrated. (X 17,000.)

tained numerous minute (700-1000 A) axon sprouts containing many synaptic vesicles but few coated and dense core vesicles. The subneural apparatus on large myofibers contained well formed secondary clefts whereas on small myofibers, the NMJs were simpler with poorly developed primary synaptic clefts.

Ten days after birth, the number of terminal axons was much reduced, myelin was well developed and nearly all the axons lay in deep primary clefts similar to the adult pattern (Fig. 27). The diagram (Fig. 28) summarizes this process.

The significance of the initial intermediate junctions between the terminal axons and the future myotube innervation site is unknown. They probably serve as temporary connections to hold the axons in apposition as a seamstress would place a holding stitch. The interme-

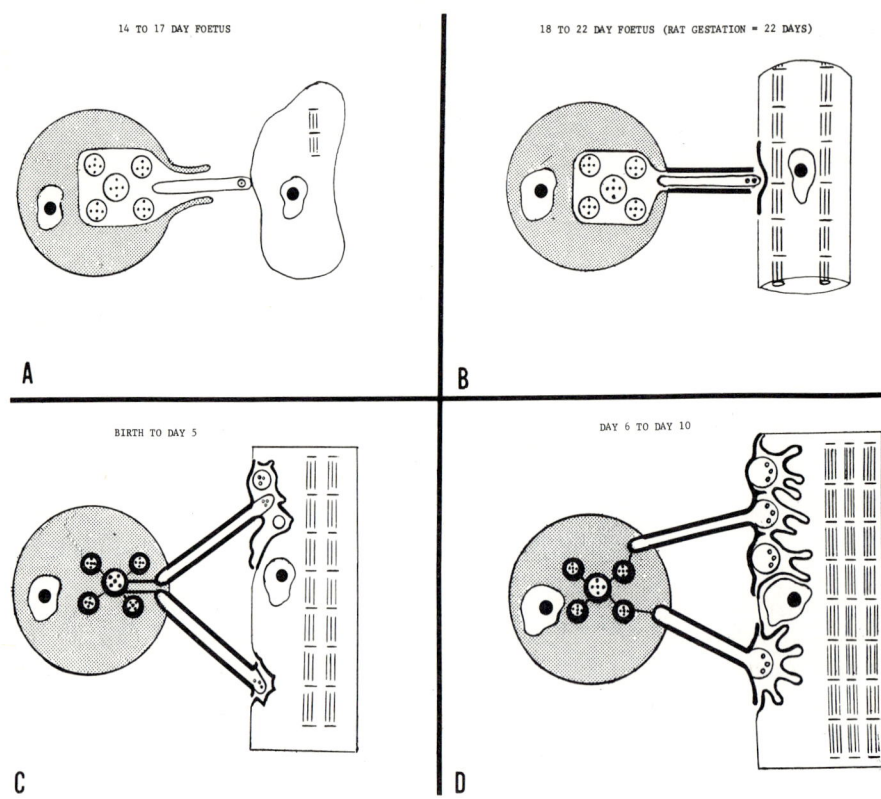

Figure 28. Diagram illustrating the stages of neuromuscular development in the rat fetus from 14-17 days of fetal life to the 10th day after birth. In *(A)*, axon sprouts loosely enveloped by Schwann cell cytoplasm approach the poorly differentiated myotube. At 18-22 days of fetal life *(B)* the axons are more closely surrounded by Schwann cell cytoplasm and surface specialization has occurred on the myotube at the future site of the subneural apparatus. From birth to the 5th day after birth *(C)* the axons are surrounded by Schwann cell cytoplasm and there is axon branching with subsequent formation of additional NMJs. The clefts of the subneural apparatus become deeper and from the 6th to 10th day *(D)* the axon branches within the subneural apparatus are more completely separated by Schwann cell cytoplasm as the subneural clefts acquire their mature appearance. (Kelly, A.M., 1968.)

diate junctions between the axons and myotubes are never observed once external lamina covers the myotube plasma membrane.

Ultrastructure studies indicate clearly that definitive NMJ may be recognized by thickening of the postsynaptic membrane and the development of primitive synaptic clefts (Fig. 24, 25, 26). These criteria, confirmed by NMJ formation in organ culture (page 46), are useful in interpretation of pathologic NMJs. The ultra-structure data indicates that NMJ development occurs earlier than the stage of peripheral nuclear migration (Couteaux, 1941, 1960).

Minute invaginations appear in the thickened myotube plasma membrane that form the presumptive subneural apparatus beneath the aggregates of axon processes. The secondary synaptic clefts begin as small vesicles, similar to pinocytotic vesicles, that appear as v-shaped invaginations of the muscle surface membrane beneath the approaching axons (Fig. 25, 26). Small, smooth walled vesicles occasionally appear to bud from these pits. This data indicates that the secondary clefts may be formed by fusion of vesicles in the fashion suggested for the formation of the myofiber T system by Ezerman and Ishikawa (1967) and Kelly and Zacks (1968). Demonstration of direct connections between the depths of the secondary clefts and the T system (Zacks and Saito, 1970) also supports this hypothesis.

In later stages of development, Schwann cell cytoplasm increases in volume and separates the axon processes from each other as the initial myofiber surface depression deepens. Columns of myoplasm covered by plasma membrane and external lamina elongate to separate the adjacent axons (Fig. 27). Fig. 28 summarized the stages in NMJ differentiation.

Embryogenesis of NMJ and Kinds of Myofibers

The "checkerboard" pattern in skeletal muscles describes the irregular distribution of light and dark staining myofibers in the skeletal muscles of all vertebrates. This pattern is visible after conventional staining, metal impregnation and is most obvious after histochemical procedures to demonstrate various enzymes. It is clear that there are major differences between the several populations of myofibers within a given muscle. Nachmias and Padykula (1958) described three kinds of rat myofibers. Type A were large and contained much glycogen and little mitochondrial enzyme activity. Type C myofibers were small and contained greater mitochondrial enzyme activity, low phosphorylase activity and little glycogen. B myofibers had intermediate characteristics. Similar observations have been made by others (Dubowitz, 1963; Ogata and Mori, 1964; Ogata, 1965) and attempts have been made to correlate enzyme characteristics, myofibrillar structure and physiologic properties. It is now generally recognized that physiologic speed of contraction does not correlate reliably with histochemical or fine structure characteristics of myofibers (Peachey, 1968). Investigators interested in the NMJ have also attempted to correlate the development of NMJ structure with the physiologic responses of fast and slow myofibers.

Nystrom (1968) investigated the postnatal development of motor nerve terminals in slow (red) and fast (white) cat muscles and concluded that NMJs innervating gastrocnemius (fast, white) and soleus (slow, red) were both of the en plaque type and that no en grappe NMJs occurred in these muscles in kittens or cats. In newborn kittens, NMJs were disc-like and matured gradually into typical en plaque endings. There was no evidence that en grappe endings were precursors of en plaque endings as suggested by Krűger (1952).

However, evidence from cross innervation experiments in adult animals (Chapter 12), and data from diseased muscle strongly suggests that the "checkerboard" pattern of skeletal muscle is regulated by the motor innervation despite the grossly similar structure of the NMJs. For example, the "checkerboard" pattern does not develop in aneural chick muscle in tissue culture (Askanas et al, 1972). Ultrastructure evidence for differences in NMJs innervating slow and fast skeletal muscles has been obtained in some species (page 272).

Wirsen and Larsson (1964) demonstrated that the "checkerboard" pattern is present in mouse fetal muscle. Using histochemical staining for phosphorylase activity, they found three kinds of myofibers which they suggested arose as three distinct populations at successive stages of development. Support for this concept was obtained by Kelly and Zacks (1968) who described the formation of successive populations of closely associated myotubes representing different stages of development that were associated with bundles of axon sprouts. In these groups of myotubes, the most mature often had a maturing definitive NMJ whereas less differentiated myotubes in the group had only close contact with the axons (Fig. 22, 24). Since in the early phases of invasion by clusters of axons, they were often tied together by intermediate junctions, it seems likely that a group of axons were responsible for the innervation of a given cluster of myotubes. However, it was impossible to know if the axons arose from a single neuron by branching or represented the contributions of multiple neurons. The latter hypothesis is most consistent with evidence of myofiber type changes following reinnervation. As maturation proceeds, the excess axons are removed by apparent degeneration. The mechanism of contact guidance and "pioneering fibers" suggested by Weiss (1941) could ex-

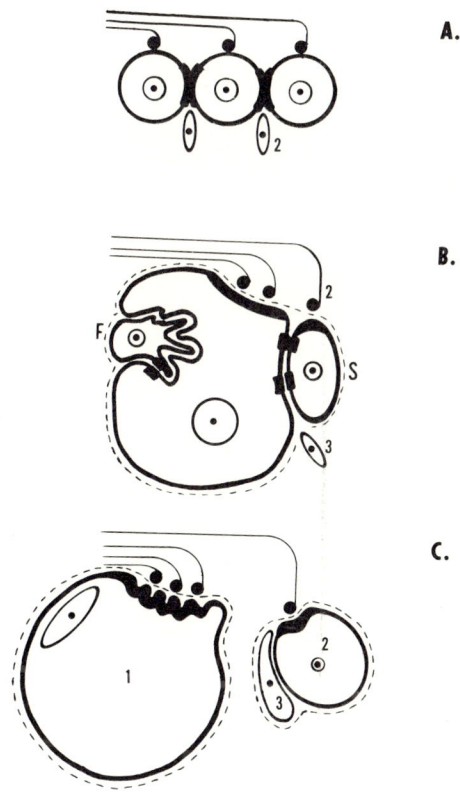

Figure 29. Diagram illustrating neuromuscular relationships during development. In *A*, axon sprouts make temporary specialized contacts with the surface of myotubes. Note the absence of external lamina on the surface of the myotubes at this time and the poorly differentiated generation of accessory or secondary myotubes indicates at *M*. In *B*, myofiber fusion is indicated at *F* and a secondary myotube has begun to separate from the primary myotube at *S*. A tertiary myotube lies beyond the external lamina. An axon, in close association with pre-existing axons that have made initial specialized contacts with a primary myotube, approaches a secondary myotube at 2. In C, this axon has now made independent contact with the secondary myotube and the tertiary myotube is now associated with it within the same external lamina (.....). Continued development of the NMJ on the primary myotube has produced a mature subneural apparatus. (Kelly, 1968).

plain the development of the "checkerboard pattern". If the "pioneering fibers" innervated the initial population of myotubes, successively arriving axons from other neurons guided by the "pioneering fiber" would arrive to innervate the less mature populations of secondary and tertiary myotubes (Figs. 29, 30). Hypothetically, these latter myotube populations could have different biochemical and physiologic properties than the original myotube population and thus explain the "checkerboard" pattern.

NMJ Morphogensis in Organ and Dissociated Cell Cultures

Other opportunities to study the formation of NMJ occur during their differentiation in *in vitro* organ cultures of skeletal muscle and nerve and in regenerating amphibian limbs or during reinnervation of denervated muscle either with specific or foreign nerves.

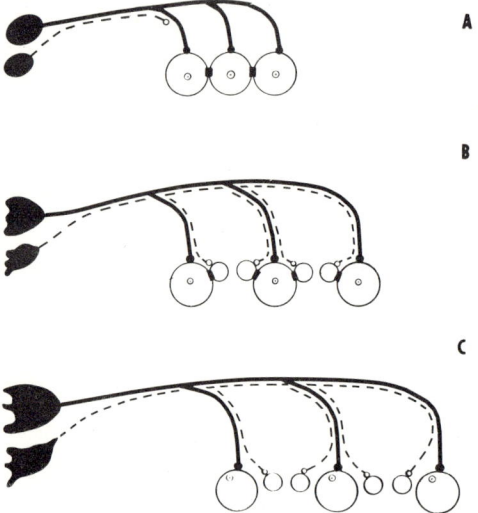

Figure 30. Diagram illustrating the process of innervation of subsequent generations of maturing myotubes guided by the initial relationships between exploring axons and primary myotube generation. This mechanism is proposed as a potential explanation for the "checkerboard pattern" visible in muscels. (See text.) (Kelly, 1968).

Attempts to observe the maturation and differentiation of myofibers and the development of neuromuscular junctions in tissue culture have a history of over 60 years. Early studies were unsuccessful (Harrison, 1910; Weiss, 1934, 1935) because of inadequate technic. However, more recently formation of NMJs in *in vitro* cultures consisting of explanted spinal cord with myotomes, explants of spinal cord and skeletal muscle fragments and monolayer cultures of dissociated myoblasts with spinal cord fragments or dispersed cells has been accomplished (Fig. 31). Also, trans species innervation has been shown to occur in tissue culture (Peterson and Crain, 1970; Shimada and Kano, 1971). Successful cultures were obtained by Nakai et al. (1961) and Nakai (1969) and actual neuromuscular connections were demonstrated by Bornstein et al. (1968), Shimada (1968a), Veneroni (1968, 1969) and by Peterson and Crain (1970), in organ cultures. Formation of NMJ by cultures of separated spinal cord and muscle tissue was demonstrated by James and Tresman (1968, 1969) and Nakai (1969). Veneroni and Murray (1969) and James and Tresman succeeded in obtaining *de novo* formation of NMJs in cultures of spinal cord explants and dissociated myofibers whereas Shimada et al. (1969a, b) found neuromuscular contacts in cultures of dissociated spinal cord and muscle

Figure 31a. Photomicrograph of a silver-stained whole mount preparation of a chick nerve-muscle culture 6 days *in vitro* illustrating multiple bulbous nerve endings in contact with a myotube (X 390).

31b. Photomicrograph of a silver-stained chick nerve ending *(NE)* after 20 days in culture illustrating branched projections on the muscle surface. Probable Schwann cell nuclei *(SN)* and muscle nuclei *(MN)* are illustrated (X 1,200). From Shimada, Y. et al. *J. Cell Biol. 43*:382, 1969 by permission of the Rockefeller University Press.

47

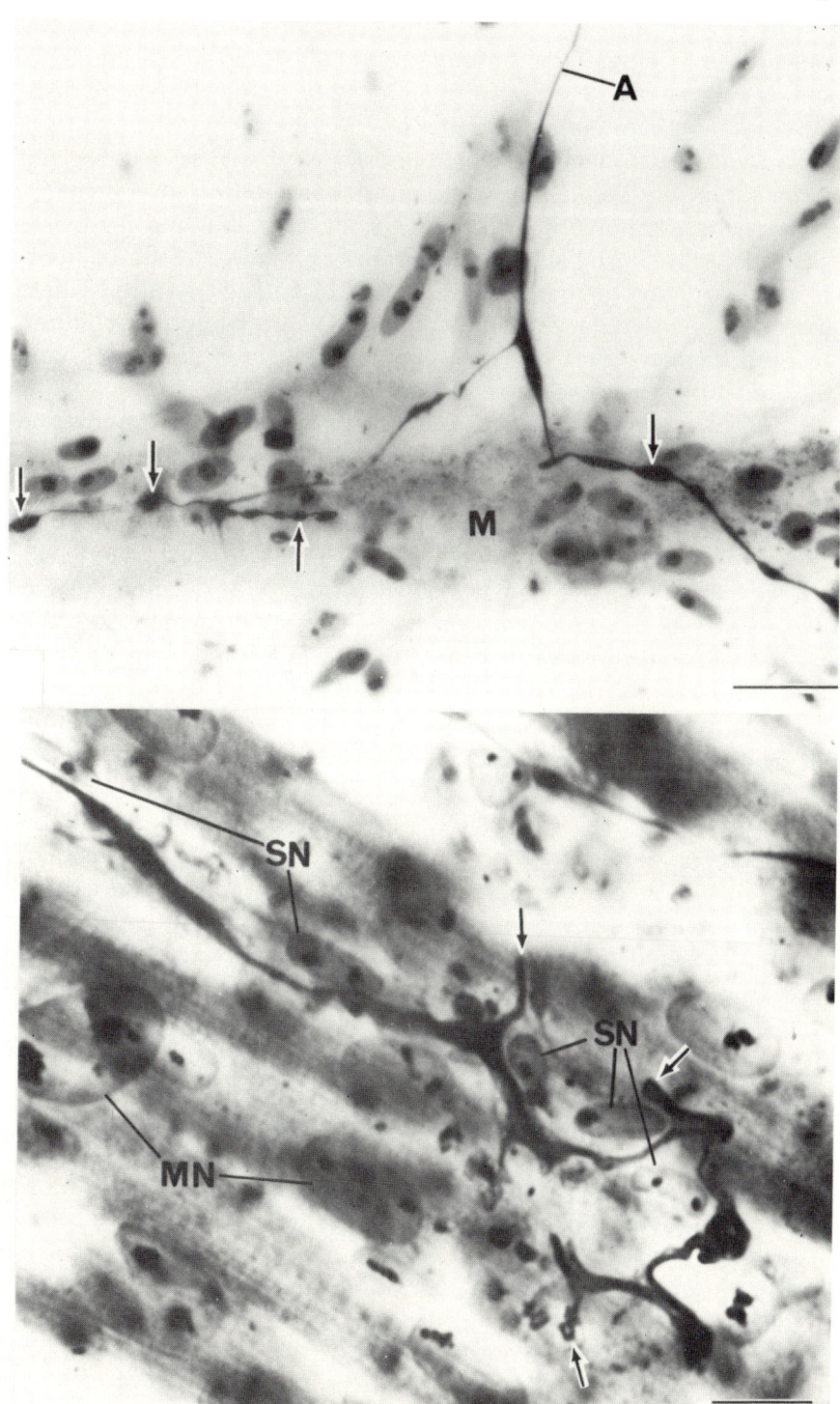

cells. These investigators used monolayer cultures in which the nerve cells are added onto a growing myofiber culture. The NMJs were demonstrated by phase contrast microscopy, AchE activity, silver impregnation and electron microscopy. Shimada et al. (1969a, b) observed formation of en plaque and some en grappe NMJ by silver staining. The argyrophilic nerve fibers grew over the myotubes and tended to align themselves parallel to the myotubes or followed rows of fibroblasts as if guided by them (Weiss, 1941). Thickenings occurred where the nerve fibers contacted the myofibers in these monolayer cultures. By 20 days, complexes of axon terminals contacted the muscle and ultrastructure studies revealed the presence of NMJs.

Junctions resulting in cultures of completely dissociated nerve and muscle cells are simpler than those which developed in the organ cultures. (Shimada and Fischman, 1972.) A possible explanation is that the former lack the Schwann cells which are part of the normal NMJ complex.

Electrical recording from the newly formed NMJ in culture (Crain, 1970; Crain et al., 1970; Peterson and Crain, 1970) demonstrate that functional connections were made. Recently, Kano and Shimada (1971) and Robbins and Yonezawa (1971a,b) demonstrated that functioning multiple innervation is an early stage in the process of innervation. As development procedes this possible vestige of more primitive pattern of innervation is lost (Redfern, 1970).

Dryden (1970) has correlated morphologic maturation with the development of sensitivity to the natural transmitter, acetylcholine (Ach) in cultured chick myoblasts. He found no response to added Ach until the myotubes contained 3 to 10 nuclei and by the time myofilaments appeared at 5 days, the entire surface membrane of the myotubes was responsive to Ach, a response that could be blocked by tubocurarine. The presence of acetylcholine receptors in developing myotubes has been demonstrated by Fambrough and Hartzell (1972) and Hartzell and Fambrough (1973).

However cell culture studies show that neither external lamina nor Schwann cells are required for initial synapse formation. Such systems also permit study of the genetic aspects of neuromuscular transmission (see Seecof, et al, 1972).

Observations on explanted spinal cord and muscle fragments by Bornstein and Breitbart (1964), Bornstein et al. (1968), Crain (1968, 1970), Kano and Shimada (1971) have not solved the problem of specific innervation. Observations from study of developing rodent NMJs indicate that there must be a large degree of randomness in the establishment of the initial neuromuscular contacts.

NMJ in Regenerating Muscle

Another naturally occurring situation where *de novo* formation of NMJs may be observed is in the muscle of regenerating urodele tail or limbs. Liu and Maneely (1968) used an acetylthiocholine histochemical method as well as gold and silver impregnation to study NMJ formation in the regenerating tail of a lizard. Regenerated NMJ were found in the tips of relatively well differentiated myofibers at a time when first movements began. This appearance of NMJ was considerably later than the normally occurring embryonic formation of NMJs in the same animal. Under conditions of original NMJ development, NMJs were formed at the ends of developing myotubes.

Lentz (1969a, b, 1970) studied the fine structure of NMJ differentiation in regenerating newt muscle. The remarkable changes which occur in the stump of this urodele limb following amputation consist of a stage of dedifferentiation followed by redifferentiation. This kind of preparation affords an unusual opportunity to study the *de novo* development of NMJs. In the dedifferentiating muscle, the terminal axons degenerate, as evidenced by loss of axoplasm, clustering of synaptic vesicles with dense cores and vacuoles in the axoplasm. As the number of synaptic vesicles decreases, the axon pulls away from the muscle and the junctional clefts in the subneural apparatus become shorter. To this point, the changes are similar to those produced by denervation in other animals. Ultimately the terminal axon is withdrawn from the muscle surface which becomes covered by Schwann cell cytoplasm. Unlike denervation changes, the dedifferentiated newt NMJ loses all traces of its subneural junctional folds. AchE activity in the subneural apparatus demonstrated by the thiolacetic acid method decreases before marked changes occur in the primary synaptic cleft and decreases sharply as the secondary synaptic clefts disappear and neuromuscular contact is broken. Following withdrawal of the nerve, only a few spots of AchE activity can be recognized. It is of interest that unlike the situation when the nerve is cut, dedifferentiation changes occur before the nerve degenerates. This suggests that withdrawal of some trophic substance may play a role in the loss of NMJ organization.

During reformation of NMJs (Lentz, 1969b, 1970) the earliest evidence of NMJ formation is the arrival of vesicle-filled terminal axons

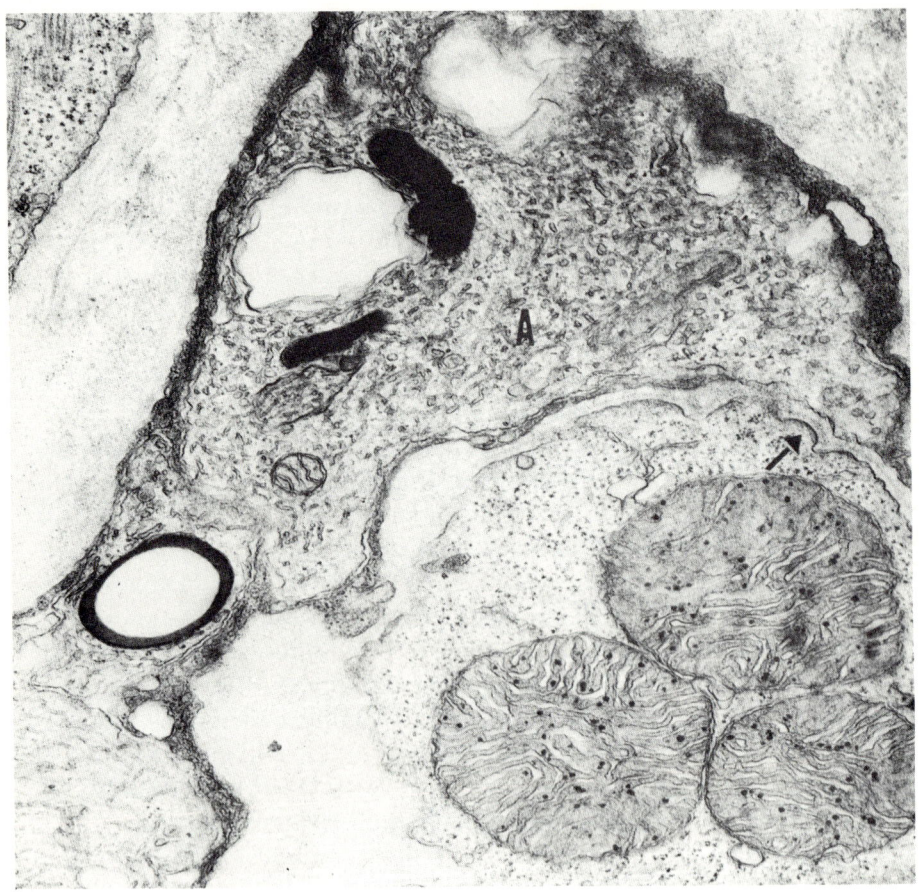

Figure 32. Electron micrograph of nerve fiber and dedifferentiating myofiber two weeks following limb transection. A few junctional folds are present on the myofiber surface at the arrow. The axon *(A)* contains many channels of endoplasmic reticulum but few vesicles. (X 30,000.) (After Lentz, T.L., *J. Cell Biol.* 47:423, 1970.)

that approach the differentiating multinucleated myotubes containing myofibrils. Small ridges appear on the muscle surface and there is an increase in density beneath the plasma membrane (Figs. 32, 33). As the axon approaches closer to the muscle surface, it lies in a shallow depression which will become the future primary synaptic cleft. The surface ridges elongate to form junctional folds. Cholinesterase activity occurs in membranous tubulovesicles in the sarcoplasm near the NMJ and in association with sarcoplasm, especially at the tips of the emerging junctional folds (Fig. 33). Lentz emphasized that both the nerve and the muscle must reach appropriate degrees of differentiation before NMJ formation can occur probably as the result of some kind of "induction." He observed no early intermediate junction apposition of nerve and muscle as occurred in developing rat NMJs (Kelly and Zacks, 1968). In other respects, redifferentiation of NMJ in regenerating newt muscle closely resembled NMJ formation in rodent embryos.

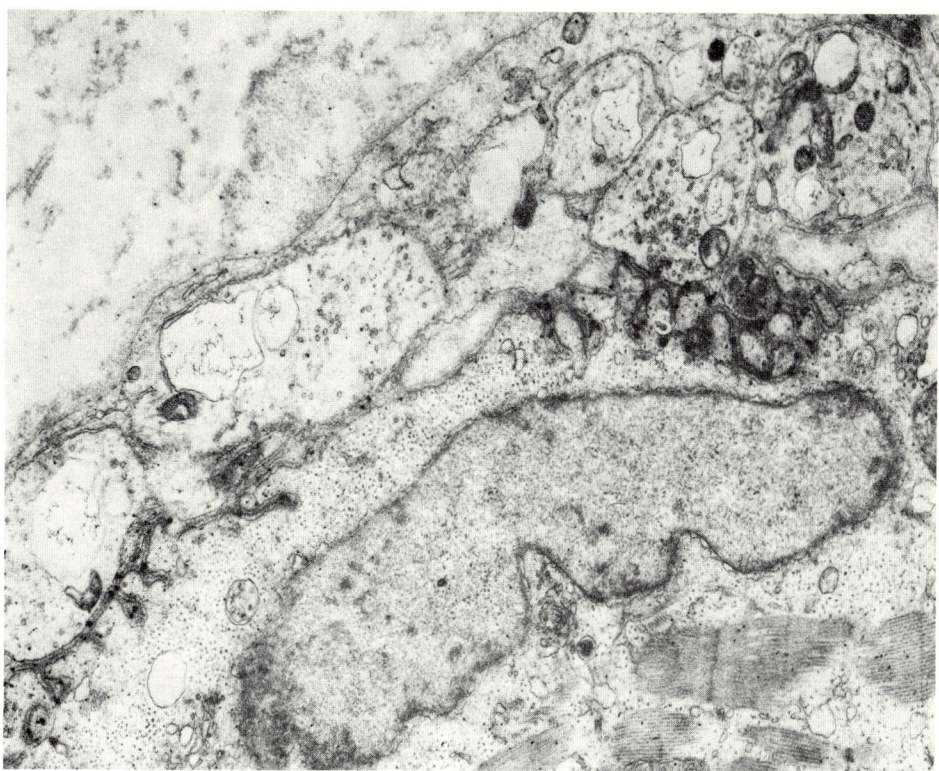

Figure 33. Electron micrograph illustrating cholinesterase activity in a regenerating neuromuscular junction in the limb of the newt, *Triturus*. At two weeks, there are advance signs of dedifferentiation with separation and fragmentation of myofibrils. Cholinesterase activity, indicated by the dense reaction product, is most intense where the subneural clefts *(S)* are elongated, but the intensity of the reaction is reduced compared to normal. (X 13,000.) (After Lentz, T.L., *J. Cell Biol.* 47:423, 1970.)

3

The Fine Structure of the Neuromuscular Junction

In the previous chapters, we have reviewed how the lengthy controversies concerning the anatomic relationships within the NMJ were due to difficulties in fixation and variability of nonspecific staining methods. This body of work established that NMJs are composed of three major components: (1) a terminal nerve branch, (2) the investing Schwann cell and Key-Retzius sheaths, and (3) a zone of modified sarcoplasm beneath the terminal axon. The classical methods of gold, silver, and methylene blue staining, as well as the supravital staining methods with Janus green B and methylene violet (Couteaux, 1947), had established the basic relationships but left many questions unanswered. First, the question whether the junctional region was epilemmal or hypolemmal was still not resolved. A second major question was the relationship of the investing membranes surrounding the terminal nerve branches at the junctional region. Many investigators continued to believe that teloglia lay between the axolemma and the sarcolemma. The nature of the granules in the soleplate was also in question, although most investigators believed that they were mitochondria because they were stained by mitochondrial staining methods. The most pressing question, however, was the nature of the subneural apparatus, the structure that was only partially and tantalizingly revealed by the supravital staining technique of Couteaux. As will be recalled, Couteaux (1947) had shown that the subneural sarcoplasm contained elongated ribbon-like lamellas apparently attached to the cytoplasmic membrane. These lamellas were nearly evenly spaced, yielding a grid-like or fingerprint-like structure. After optimum fixation, iron hematoxylin and Altmann's aniline fuchsin stains also revealed the lamellas (Couteaux, 1947). The shape of the subneural lamellas differed in various animals. In frog NMJ, sections perpendicular to the terminal nerve branches revealed a cross section of the nerve fiber beneath which lay a semicircular area representing the subneural apparatus, whereas the subneural apparatus in mammalian NMJ had a typical radiating pattern on either side of the surface synaptic grooves. Staining of the superficial portion of the lamellas in some NMJ revealed a fringe-like zone similar to that described by Kűhne (1883), which he called the "borstensaum." Couteaux believed that this area corresponded to an outcropping of the edges of the subneural lamellas at the soleplate surface.

The structure of the subneural apparatus revealed by staining methods and optical microscopy can be summarized as follows: The terminal nerve branches lie in surface depressions (gutters) in the junctional sarcoplasm from which radiate peculiar rod-shaped structures which stain with Janus green B (Figs. 12, 13).

The use of the greater resolving power of the electron microscope clarified many of the persistent questions concerning the fine structure of the NMJ. The first attempt to study NMJs with the electron microscope by Beams and Evans (1952) did not greatly advance our knowledge because adequate fixation and sectioning techniques were not available. A few years later, several nearly simultaneous reports contributed greatly to understanding of the structure of the NMJ (Palade, 1954; Reger, 1954, 1955; and Robertson, 1954, 1955a, b, 1956).

Robertson's studies (1954, 1956) of NMJs in the lizard *Anolis carolinensis* answered several of the outstanding questions. First, the endoneural sheath was shown to consist of a thin sheet of cells associated with scattered collagen fibrils, which formed a complete investment of the small nerve fibers. The inside and outside boundaries of this sheath consisted of two dense lines bordering a light central zone. Robertson was not able to decide if cell boundaries were present in the endoneural sheath or whether it represented a syncytium. Nerve fibers surrounded by myelin were observed within small bundles passing between muscle fibers. The investing myelin layers were present within

Schwann cell cytoplasm and were connected to the surface membrane by means of the mesaxon. The Schwann cell plasma membrane consisted of a double membrane complex similar to that observed between endoneural sheath cells. As the terminal axons approached the NMJ, the diameter of the nerve fibers was greatly reduced to less than 1 μ and the myelin layers were lost. In the region of the NMJ, the small unmyelinated axons separated from the investing Schwann cells and lay in depressions or troughs on the surface of the muscle cell. Thin extensions of Schwann cell cytoplasm formed a cover over the trough and appeared to represent the telolemma described by investigators who used optical microscopy. Robertson (1956, 1960) believed the cells surrounding the terminal axon were Schwann cells and Reger (1958) recognized that the neurilemmal or Schwann cells surrounded part of the axon and that other cells in the vicinity were a continuation of the neurilemmal sheath (teloglia). Zacks and Blumberg (1961a) and Brown (1961) as well as Anderson-Cedergren (1959) all interpreted the cells immediately adjacent to the axon as Schwann cells. Shanthaveerappa and Bourne (1962, 1963, 1964, 1965) restudied the layers of cells external to the Schwann cells by a variety of methods. The term, "perineural epithelium" was used by these investigators for the layer of cells previously termed Henle's sheath to call attention to its interesting structural and histochemical properties. They also stated that electron microscopic studies revealed that the perineural epithelial cells envelop the NMJ and are attached directly to the sarcolemma. Review of electron microscopic studies in the 1960's and more recent work has shown that this is incorrect. In the rodent en plaque NMJ, the myelin sheath ends at a final node of Ranvier approximately 1 to 1.5 μ from the muscle surface (Figs. 34, 35). Projections of Schwann cell cytoplasm covered on both sides by BL extend along the axon (Fig. 34) and partially cover the terminal and underlying subneural apparatus (Figs. 34, 35). There is always a gap of approximately 500 A between the Schwann cell plasma membrane and the muscle plasma membrane which is filled with external lamina. The "perineural epithelium" or the terminal elements of Henle's sheath form extremely thin cellular projections external to the Schwann cell processes but these rarely reach the junctional region. Thus there is a gap in which the terminal axon is exposed to the immediate environment. There is no attachment of the Henle sheath to the external lamina or the muscle plasma membrane (Fig. 34-37). In many micrographs, the extremely fine terminal processes of Henle's sheath or "perineural sheath" cells have an inconstant deposition of external lamina. As illustrated in Figure 35, some processes are lined by external lamina on the inner but not on the outer surface (Saito and Zacks, 1969), which may be an artefact.

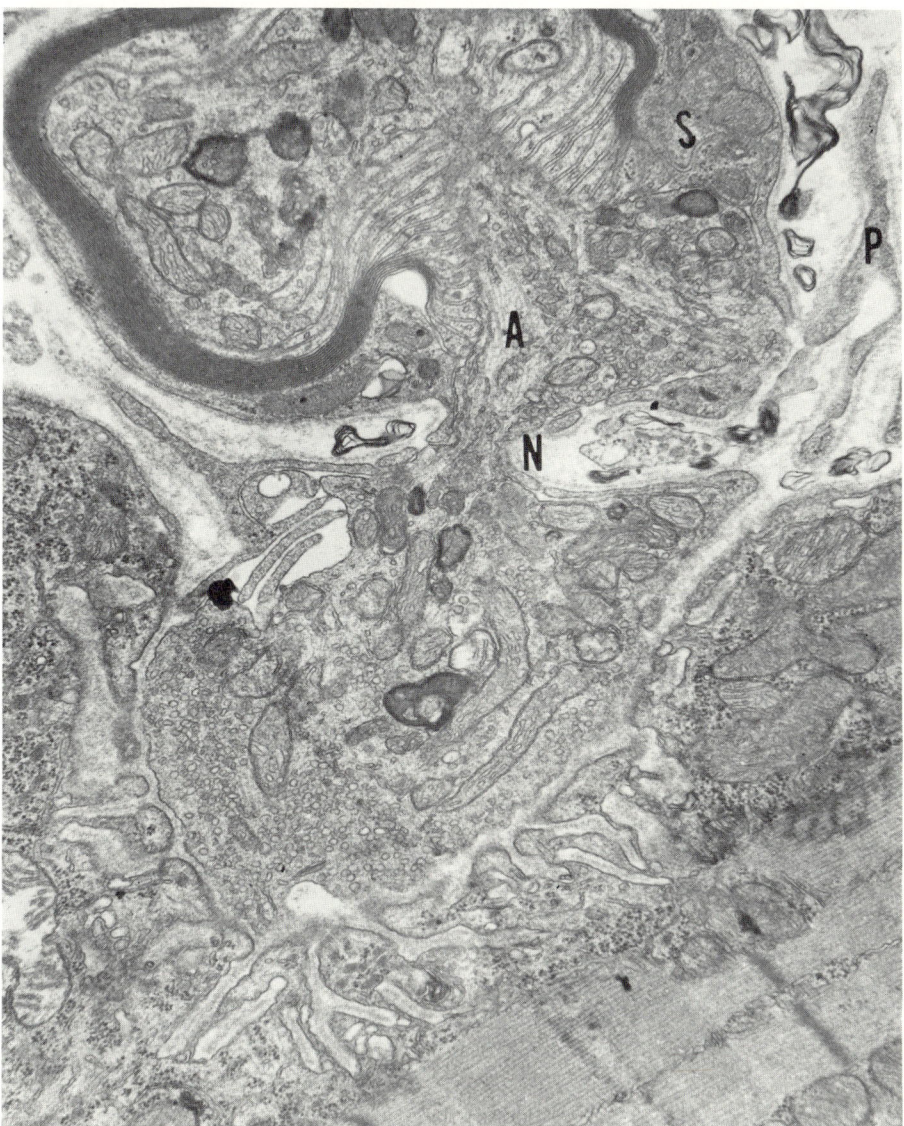

Figure 34. Electron micrograph illustrating the terminal node of Ranvier *(N)* prior to the emergence of the axonal branch to innervate a neuromuscular junction. Note the Schwann cell cytoplasm *(S)* and perineural epithelial cytoplasm *(P)* in relationship to the axon *(A)*. (X 23,300.)

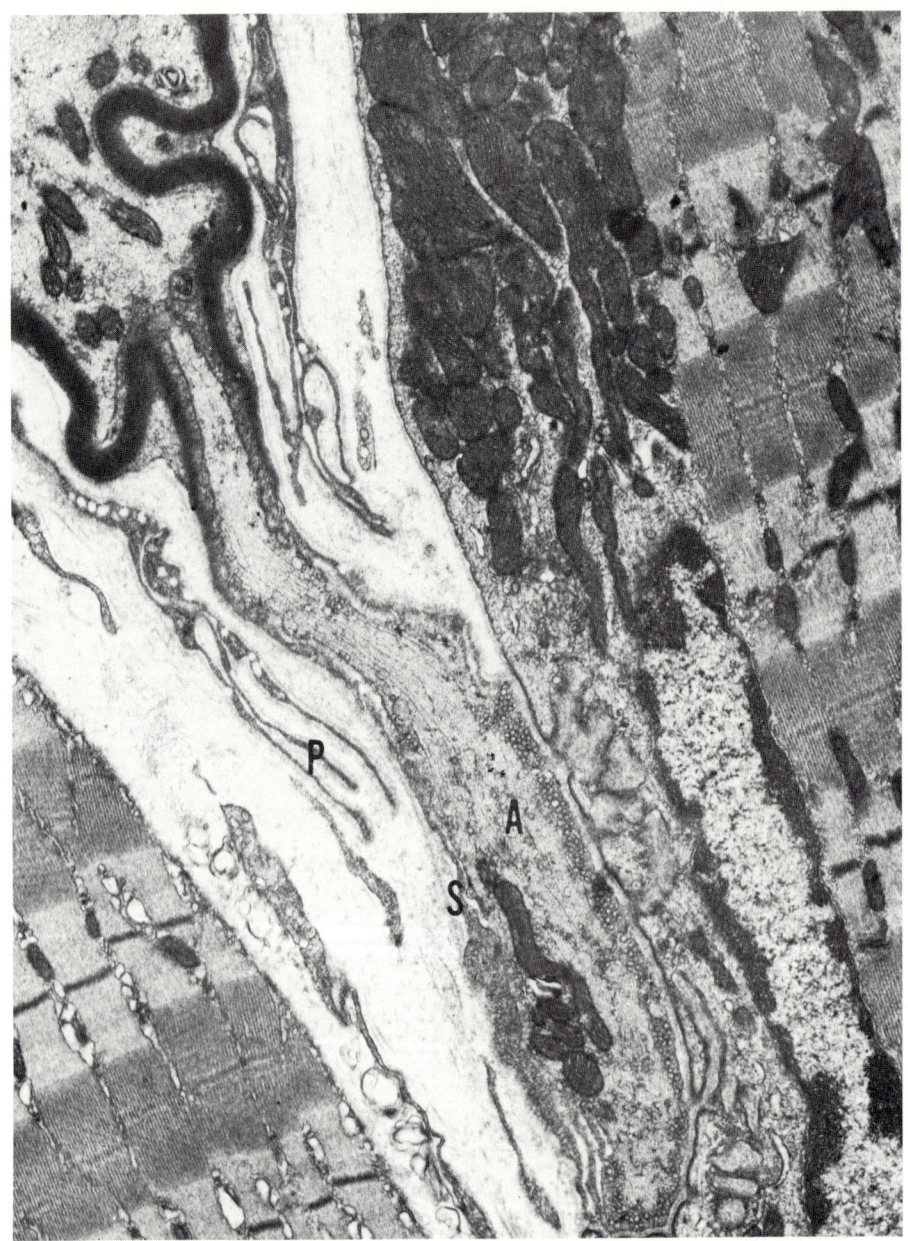

Figure 35. Longitudinal view of an axon *(A)* innervating a neuromuscular junction. Note the final node of Ranvier and the relationships of Schwann cell *(S)* and perineural epithelial cell *(P)* cytoplasm. Clefts of the subneural apparatus and underlying soleplate details are also illustrated. (X 14,200.)

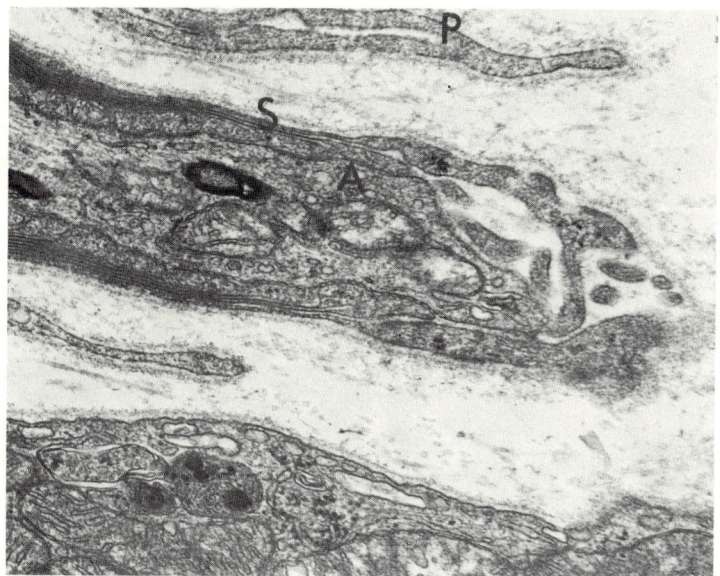

Figure 36. Electron micrograph illustrating details of the investment of a terminal axon *(A)* by Schwann cell *(S)* and perineural cell *(P)* cytoplasm. Note the location of the external lamina external to these cell processes. A myofiber is present at M. (X 26,500.)

Kay et al. (1963 demonstrated that both Schwann cells and connective tissue cells surrounding peripheral nerve fibers are phagocytic by means of uptake of colloidal thorium dioxide and saccharated iron oxide and phagocytosis of axon debris by terminal Schwann cells occurs in degenerating NMJs following denervation.

Subneural Apparatus

Within the synaptic trough, the entire myofiber surface membrane is thrown into folds that are branched and interconnected in a complicated pattern. These "junctional folds" or "secondary synaptic clefts" radiate from the sides and deep surface of the gutter or "primary synaptic cleft." Robertson emphasized that although the clefts were peculiar features of NMJ they were not strictly confined to the synaptic trough but were present in the muscle surface membrane immediately outside the troughs. The junctional folds in *Anolis* NMJs measured 0.5 to 1.0 μ in length and from 500 to 1500 A in width. Characteristically they were narrow toward the axonal surface and were dilated slightly in the deeper portion. The individual folds were separated by

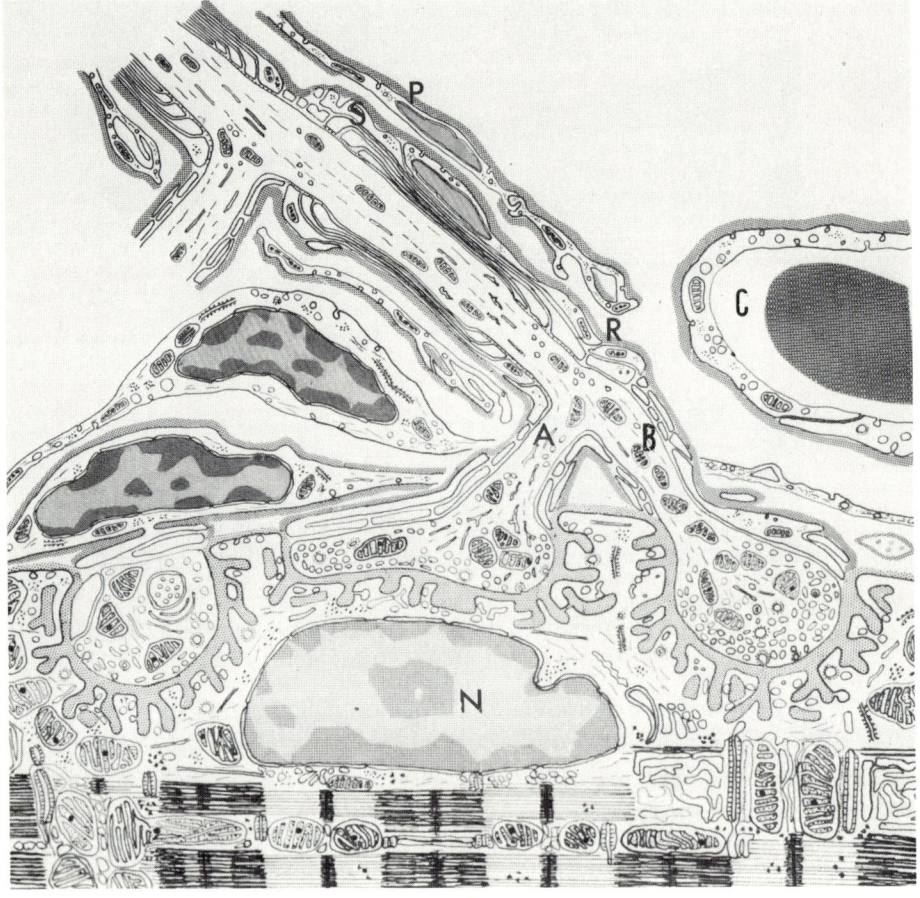

Figure 37. Diagram showing the relationships of the terminal axons to the nerve sheath in the region of a NMJ. The terminal node of Ranvier *(R)* occurs just proximal to the origin of two branches, A and B, which innervate the muscle. Note the relationships of Schwann cell cytoplasm *(S)* and perineural epithelial cytoplasm *(P)* to the axon and the external lamina indicated by hatched lines. A capillary is indicated at C and a myofiber nucleus, at *N*.

distances of 1000 to 3000 A. These clefts, demonstrated by the electron microscope, correspond to the striated border or batonnets of Couteaux's subneural apparatus.

The Membrane Complex

The relationship between the membrane complex of the axolemma and the sarcolemma has been the source of some disagreement. According to Robertson (1956), five distinct layers separate the sarcoplasm from the axoplasm. These layers as identified in order from the axoplasm surface to the sarcoplasm surface are (1) an electron-dense zone less than 100 A adjacent to the axoplasm, (2) a light zone approximately 100 to 200 A in width, (3) a dense zone 200 A wide, (4) another light zone measuring 100 to 200 A, and (5) a dense zone less than 100 A wide adjacent to the sarcoplasm. Altogether, the synaptic membrane complex measures 500 to 700 A in width. Robertson recognized that the middle layer of the "compound synaptic membrane" resulted from the fusion of the outer dense zones of the two closely apposed double surface membrane complexes belonging to the muscle cell and the axon. He observed that in the best preserved preparations, the dense inner edge of the axon membrane complex did not dip into the junctional folds but appeared to cover over the entrance to them. However, in some regions, it appeared that axoplasm did dip into the folds. It could not be decided at the time whether this was an abnormal arrangement. In a later study Robertson (1960) used the term "axon membrane" for the electron-dense membrane surrounding the terminal nerve branch and "muscle surface membrane" for the membrane complex of the underlying muscle fiber. He also pointed out that the terminal Schwann cell was bounded by "hazy granular or delicately fibrillar material" forming an external lamina, which he believed contained mucopolysaccharide or mucoprotein in a hydrated gel largely consisting of water.

Similar observations were made by others. Reger (1959), in a study of degeneration of NMJs in white mice, observed that the synaptolemma (axon membrane) measured 500 to 600 A in width and was composed of five layers of varying electron density. Palay (1958) used the term "synaptic cleft" to describe that space between the axolemma and the postsynaptic surface, and deHarven and Coërs (1959) referred to "primary synaptic cleft" as the space between the axon and muscle surface membranes and "secondary synaptic cleft" for the subneural radiating folds in their study of human NMJs.

In a later investigation of mouse and human intercostal NMJs, Zacks and Blumberg (1961a) observed terminal axon branches lying in depressions (primary synaptic clefts) in the sarcoplasmic surface. Overlying the terminal branches and intimately related to the axon membrane was a mass of Schwann cell cytoplasm that occasionally showed complex infoldings with the axon surface membrane. The Schwann cell cytoplasm, nuclei, and nucleoli had moderate electron

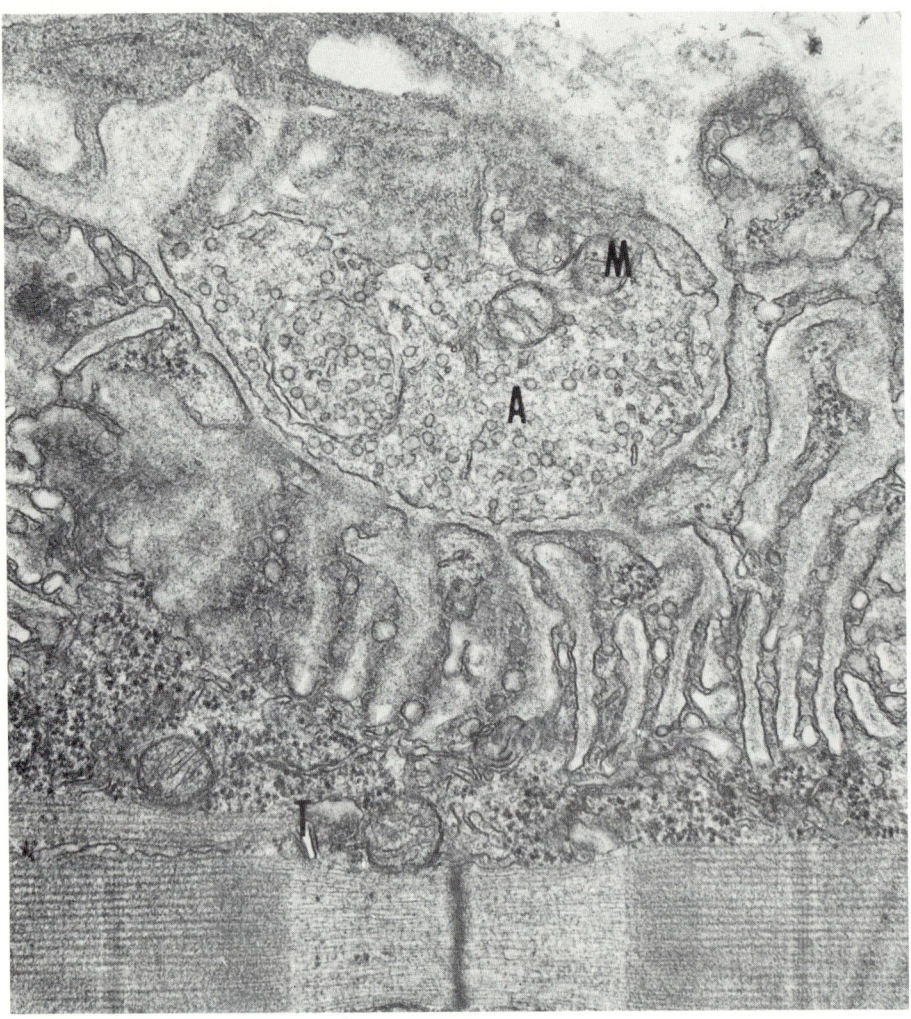

Figure 38. Electron micrograph illustrating the normal anatomy of a mouse NMJ. The axon *(A)* contains a few mitochondria *(M)* and tubules. The axon is separated from the postsynaptic (myofiber) membrane by amorphous external lamina. Thickening of the postsynaptic membrane is indicated at the arrows. The subneural apparatus is composed of elongated clefts that extend deeply into the underlying sarcoplasm. Note the occasional large vesicles in the sarcoplasm between the clefts. Numerous granules, consisting of glycogen and ribosomes, are present in the sarcoplasm. The underlying myofilaments are illustrated in relation to elements of the *T* system *(T)*. (X 31,250.)

density. The primary synaptic clefts (Figs. 38 and 39) in mouse neuromuscular junctions measured 500 to 600 A in width between axon membrane and muscle surface membrane and contained frequently laminated and somewhat granular material of low electron density that has been called "ground substance" (deHarven and Coërs, 1959), "basement membrane" (Robertson, 1960), or "amorphous surface material" (Zacks and Blumberg, 1961a). The term "external lamina" (EL) is now generally preferred. Although sometimes laminated, the EL within secondary synaptic clefts in the best-fixed preparations is amorphous and homogeneous. In human NMJs, this material consists of the fused contributions of two separate layers of EL each approximately 200 A wide. One layer is contributed by the finely granular material that dips down from the surface of the overlying Schwann cell and the second layer of similar material is contributed by the myofiber EL. The two layers join at the edge of the primary synaptic cleft (Figs. 38 & 39). Occasionally two bands of EL separated by a zone of decreased electron density were seen within the primary synaptic cleft

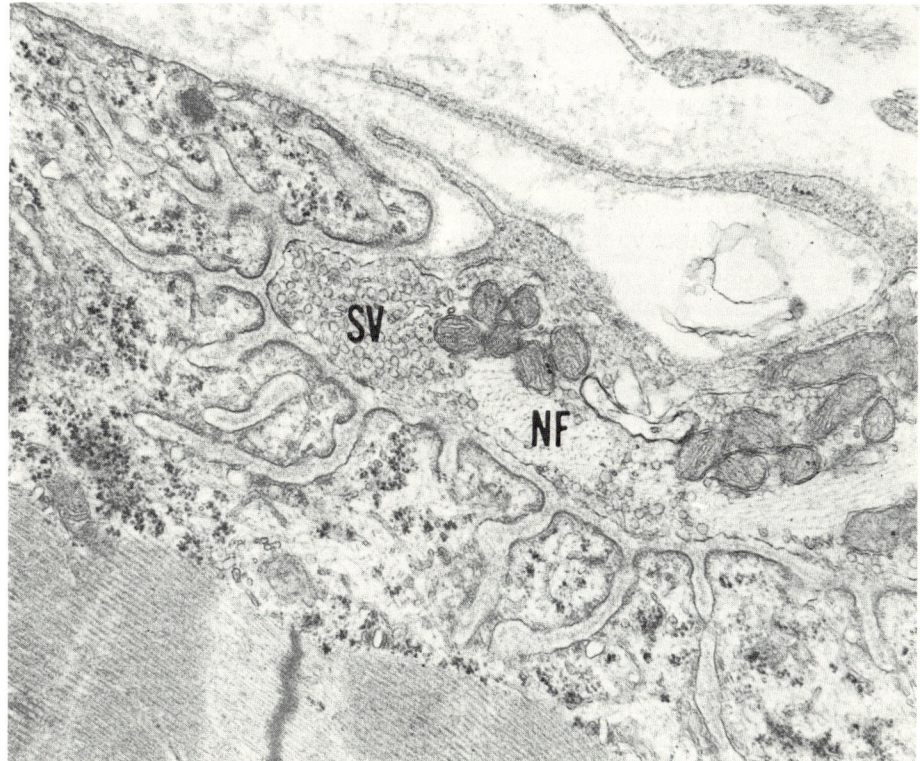

Figure 39. Electron micrograph of a mouse NMJ illustrating details of the synaptic vesicles *(SV)* that are closely opposed to the axoplasmic membrane and the neurofilaments in the terminal axon *(NF).* (X 37,500.)

of human NMJs as described by Bickerstaff et al. (1960). Layering of EL within the secondary synaptic clefts is much less prominent in mouse NMJs than in human NMJs. Subsequent studies indicate that layering is a fixation artefact. The small vesicles and granular material within the EL of rat diaphragm NMJs described by Barrnett (1962) were never observed by the author in normal mouse and human NMJ (Zacks and Blumberg, 1961a).

In human NMJs, the secondary synaptic clefts arise as invaginations from the primary cleft and penetrate from 1 to 0.5μ into the soleplate sarcoplasm. The neck of each secondary cleft is appreciably narrower (500 A) than the more distal portions (700 to 900 A). The muscle cell membrane is wider in the proximal portions of the secondary synaptic clefts than in the more distal portions. The secondary clefts are filled with EL that is continuous with the bands of similar material observed in the primary secondary synaptic clefts. Some electron micrographs reveal bands of EL joined in the proximal portions of the secondary clefts deep within the clefts, forming two distinct layers 150 to 200 A separated by a 100 A zone of decreased electron density. This appearance is similar to that described by Robertson (1956) and Reger (1958). Secondary synaptic clefts frequently lie in close proximity to the myofilaments or are closely related to soleplate nuclei. No connections that might possibly be related to the periterminal network of Boeke have been observed. Furthermore, no teloglial processes are present within the primary synaptic clefts as described by Robertson (1960).

Thus the subneural apparatus consists of narrow columns of infolded sarcoplasm separated by the muscle surface membrane from the EL within the interdigitating secondary synaptic clefts. In some of the older micrographs, interruptions in the axon surface membrane measuring approximately 200 to 300 A were noted, which probably were due to oblique sectioning of kinks in the membrane or fixation artefact. Convincing pores in the axon surface membrane were never seen, although they have been described by Bickerstaff et al. (1959, 1960). However, indentations in the axolemma approximating the size of synaptic vesicles have been reported by some investigators (Couteaux & Pecot-Dechavassine, 1970).

The soleplate sarcoplasm is moderately electron opaque and contains membrane-limited vesicular structures (650 to 700 A) within the sarcoplasmic columns. Although originally thought to connect with the synaptic clefts (Zacks and Blumberg, 1961a) more recent studies utilizing horseradish peroxidase or lanthanum tracers (Saito and Zacks, 1969; Zacks and Saito, 1970) have demonstrated that the majority of these vesicles are intrasarcoplasmic and have no connection with the subneural clefts. Occasional coated vesicles of similar size are also present in the sarcoplasm and these may be identified by their endocytotic activity.

Ultrastructure of En Grappe NMJ

The fine structure of en grappe or multiple NMJ has been described by several investigators in extraocular muscles of the rat (Pilar and Hess, 1966; Terăvăinen, 1969), chicken (Zenker and Krammer, 1967) and monkey (Mayr et al., 1966, 1971). Unlike typical *en plaque* NMJ, the *en grappe* NMJ lacked the characteristic folding of the postsynaptic membrane but membrane thickening was present (Pilar and Hess, 1966; Terăvăinen, 1969). Terăvăinen (1968, 1969) demonstrated that these junctions contain AchE activity and were supplied by unmyelinated nerves. The axon terminals were either grouped or separated. The axons contained 500 A synaptic vesicles and a few, large dense core vesicles. The primary synaptic cleft was 400-1000 A wide and the secondary synaptic clefts were irregular, sparse or in some cases, absent. An unusual feature of some of these NMJs was an axonal protrusion that extended from the terminal axon to lie in an invagination of the postsynaptic membrane. These protrusions contained electron-lucent 500 A vesicles, a few 1000 A dense core vesicles and occasional mitochondria. There was increased density of the underlying postsynaptic membrane but no intervening external lamina. The main terminal was separated from the electron-dense postsynaptic membrane by a 500 A gap whereas the cleft between the axonal protrusion and the plasma membrane was approximately 100 A or less. There was no constant relationship between the axonal protrusion and any myofiber structure. Similar axonal protrusions have been reported by Karlsson and Anderson-Cedergren (1966) in frog intrafusal myofibers. The function of this curious compound type of innervation is obscure. Infrequent subneural clefts were also described by Fernand and Hess (1969) in en grappe NMJ innervating cat inner ear muscles. Figure 40 B illustrates an en grappe NMJ from cat superior oblique muscle.

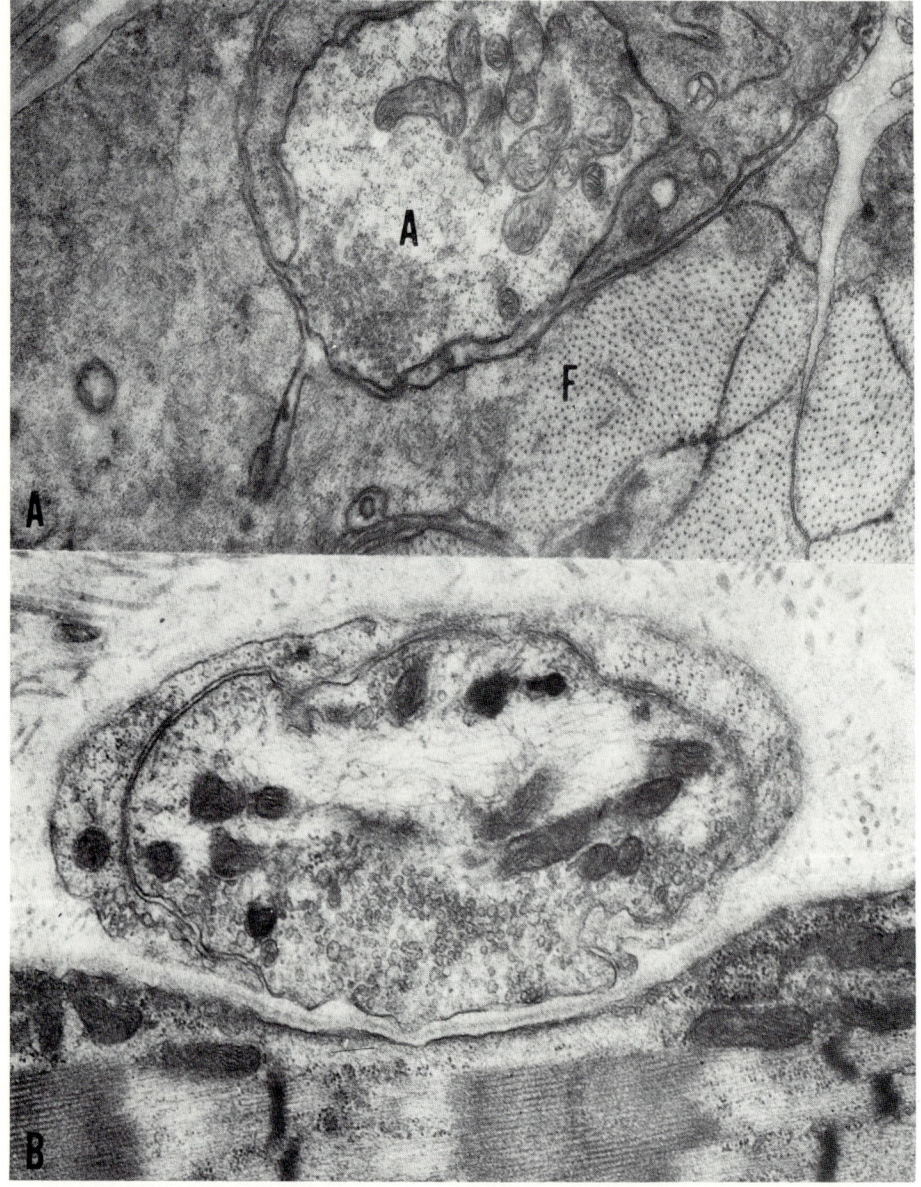

Figure 40a. Electron micrograph illustrating "fast" NMJ in crab muscle. (From Cohen, M.J. and Hess, A. *Am. J. Anat. 121:*285, 1967.)

Figure 40b. Electron micrograph illustrating a "slow" kind of NMJ from cat superior oblique muscle. Note the relationship of the axon *(A)* to the adjacent myofiber *(F)* and Schwann cell components and the absence of typical subneural apparatus. (From Pillar, G. and Hess, A. *Anat. Rec. 154:*253, 1966.)

Ultrastructure of Neuromuscular Junctions and Biochemical and Physiologic Aspects of Myofibers

Attempts to correlate the structure of myofibers and NMJs with physiologic porperties of the neuromuscular unit led to contradictory conclusions when conventional metal impregnation or histochemical staining for cholinesterase activity was used (page 141). Restudy of this problem by electron microscopic methods has yielded somewhat more informative data.

Unlike the frog which has physiologically "fast" and "slow" (tonic) myofibers, mammalian myofibers respond with a twitch to single stimuli but differ in their speed of contraction. Neuromuscular junctions innervating frog slow myofibers lack a subneural apparatus (Page and Slater, 1965) whereas the "fast" myofibers have a regular subneural apparatus that lies across the long axis of the terminal (Birks et al., 1960). However, Zenker and Gruber (1968) reported that some slow myofibers have NMJs with a subneural apparatus. In the snake fish, which has both "fast" and "slow" myofibers similar to the frog (Takeuchi, 1959), Nakajima (1969) found that the NMJ density is more concentrated in the red myofibers than in the white myofibers and that both kinds of myofibers were innervated by multiple en grappe endings. Therefore, although the fine structure of red and white myofibers of the snake fish resembled those of the frog twitch myofiber, the distribution and structure of the NMJs resembled the innervation of frog slow myofibers. In rodents, Duchen (1971a, b) has shown that NMJs innervating "fast" myofibers (gastrocnemius) have more numerous and complex secondary synaptic clefts than "slow" myofibers had large and complicated NMJs compared to the simpler and more compact NMJs on the red myofibers. Intermediate NMJs were also described innervating intermediate myofibers as judged by histochemical staining for succinic dehydrogenase and cholinesterase activity.

Ogata et al. (1965, 1967) claimed that the physiologic properties of rat intercostal red, white and intermediate myofibers could be recognized on the basis of their fine structure and that there were distinct differences in the fine structure of NMJs on the three kinds of myofibers. Red muscle contained many large subsarcolemmal mitochondria, chains of interfibrillar mitochondria and these myofibers had small, poorly developed NMJs with few widely separated subneural clefts. The subneural clefts were shallow and less branched than the clefts in the subneural apparatus of white myofibers. On the other hand, white myofibers usually lacked subsarcolemmal aggregates of mitochondria and chains of mitochondria between the myofibers. The NMJs on these myofibers were large, well developed and had numerous, closely placed subneural clefts unlike the subneural apparatus of red muscle. The subneural clefts were longer, more branched, and appeared generally more complex. Intermediate NMJs innervating intermediate myofibers had moderate numbers of subsarcolemmal mitochondria, fewer intermyofibrillar mitochondria and there was intermediate complexity of the subneural apparatus. These investigators found no differences in the structure or numbers of synaptic vesicles among the various kinds of myofibers they identified. They assumed that the white myofibers identified by their methods corresponded with "fast" myofibers demonstrated by physiological technics.

Using myofiber size and mitochondrial distribution as criteria for myofiber recognition, Ogata and Murata (1969) described red, white and intermediate myofibers in rat "fast", extensor digitorum longus muscle. NMJs on red myofibers were small with few shallow clefts, whereas NMJs on white myofibers were large and had deep and numerous clefts in the subneural apparatus. Murata and Ogata (1969) also studied human intercostal muscle and found some differences from the rat. In human intercostal muscle, the original findings of complex subneural apparatus in white muscle and simple complexes in red myofibers was confirmed. However these investigators also claimed that the terminal axon branchlets in NMJs on red myofibers had oval rather than the usual round profile. Furthermore, human intercostal motor NMJs lacked mitochondrial aggregations near the soleplate and when present, mitochondrial aggregates usually occurred in red myofibers. No correlation between the number of synaptic vesicles in the terminal axons and the kind of muscle innervated by the NMJ was found. The human NMJs also appeared to have more sarcoplasmic vesicles than commonly found in rat NMJs. With the exception of claimed differences in the number of synaptic vesicles in terminal axons, the work of Padykula and Gauthier (1970) is in general agreement with the findings of the Japanese investigators. Padykula and Gauthier (1970) reported differences in the ultrastructure of NMJs in red, white and intermediate myofibers in rat diaphragm (twitch) muscle. The kinds of myofibers were identified on the basis of myofiber diameter, kind and location of mitochondria and width of the Z band. Red myofibers had the least contact between the axon and the muscle, the terminal

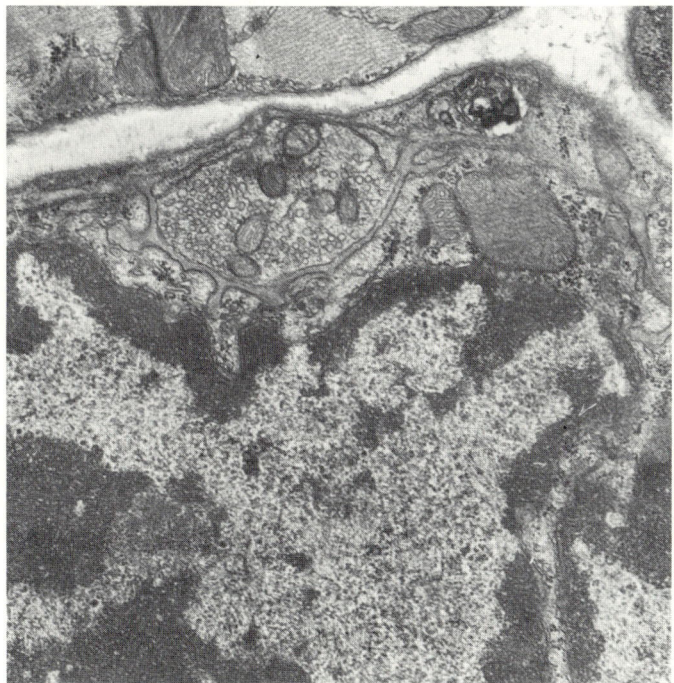

Figure 41. Electron micrograph of a mouse NMJ illustrating typical features of the "slow" kind of junction. Note the relatively few and shallow clefts in the subneural apparatus. (mouse) (X 17,000.)

axons were small and elliptical and contained moderate numbers of synaptic vesicles (Fig. 41). The soleplate contained few sarcoplasmic vesicles. White myofibers had larger areas of contact between the axon terminal and the myofiber, the subneural apparatus had long branching clefts with narrow intervening columns of sarcoplasm and there were numerous vesicles in the axon and the sarcoplasm (Fig. 42). The intermediate muscles had large terminals with the most widely spaced and deepest clefts in the subneural apparatus. Although these investigators called attention to more closely packed synaptic vesicles in axons innervating white myofibers, other investigators have not observed differences in the number or packing of synaptic vesicles, a judgment notoriously difficult to make from random study of thin sections.

Several attempts to correlate NMJ fine structure with the physiologic characteristics of extraocular muscle have greatly clarified earlier studies that were limited by inadequate methodology. The innervation

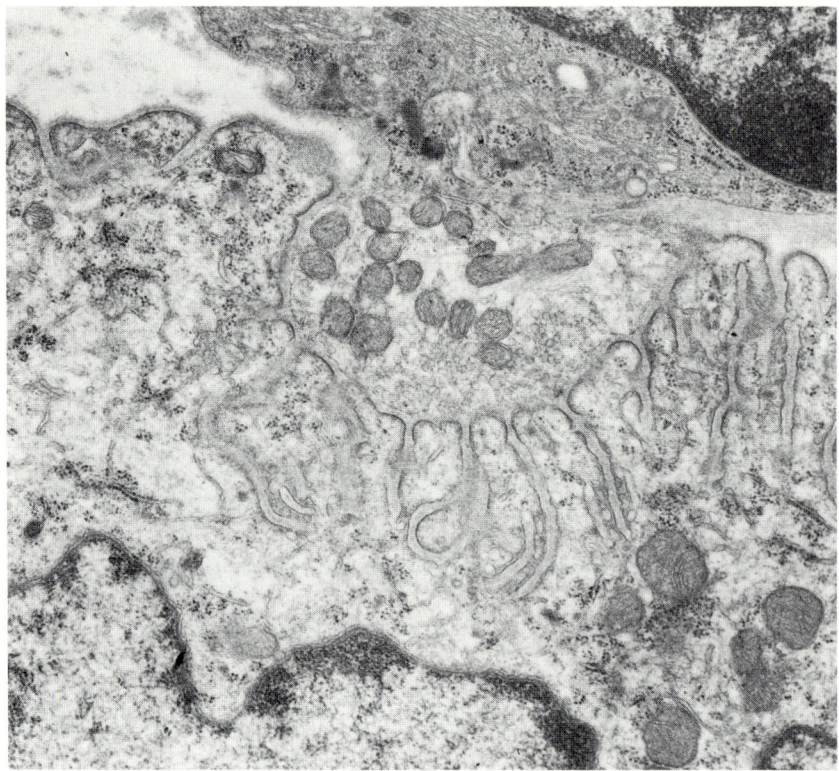

Figure 42. Electron micrograph illustrating the appearance of a "fast" neuromuscular junction with numerous, elongated and branched subneural clefts. (mouse) (x 16,400.)

of extraocular muscle is particularly confusing because of the various kinds of innervation that occur in these muscles. Extraocular muscle is one of the few kinds of muscle in higher vertebrates where both compact and diffuse kinds of NMJs occur and where both singly and multiply innervated myofibers are found. Pilar and Hess (1966) found that twitch myofibers in cat superior oblique muscle could be recognized by the presence of triads at the myofiber A-I junctions and a simple subneural apparatus in the NMJs whereas slow myofibers had reduced sarcoplasmic reticulum and no T system. The subneural apparatus was absent in slow muscle NMJs although postsynaptic membrane thickening was present. From studies of Rhesus monkey eye muscles, Mayr et al. (1966) concluded that singly innervated myofibers with en plaque endings had broad zones of sarcoplasmic reticulum surrounding the myofibrils, numerous mitochondria with irregular arrangement and frequent triads, whereas in multiply innervated myofibers, there was little sarcoplasmic reticulum, relatively few, regularly arranged mitochondria and wider Z discs without M bands or pseudo H zones. Also, the axons were half the diameter of the singly innervated myofibers which resembled frog slow myofibers. Zenker and Krammer (1967) observed that the chicken inner eye muscles (ciliary and iris) were thin and singly innervated. The NMJs supplied by a myelinated nerve from the ciliary ganglion were large, contained typical synaptic vesicles and dense core vesicles but lacked subneural clefts. Mukuno (1966) described few synaptic vesicles in the terminal axons and few subneural clefts in NMJs in human extraocular muscles. In a recent study of rat extraocular muscle, Mayr (1971) has described two muscle layers composed of myofibers of different diameters. Both muscle layers contained singly and multiply innervated myofibers. Multiple innervation was found in larger, "clear" myofibers or on extremely small, "clear" myofibers whereas focal innervation was found on small "dark" fibers, intermediate and large "pale" myofibers. The author identifies as "slow" fibers those which had multiple innervation and lacked a regular T system, and had a poorly developed sarcoplasmic reticulum, irregular fibrils, and Z lines. NMJs on these myofibers lacked a postsynaptic apparatus.

Intrinsic Ear Muscles

Similarly, Fernand and Hess (1969) in studies of cat tensor tympani & stapedius muscles found singly and multiply innervated myofibers. The stapedius, which was singly innervated, has sarcoplasmic reticulum and T system at the A-I junction. The NMJs had extensive soleplates with many subneural clefts. The multiply innervated "slow" myofibers had poorly organized endoplasmic reticulum, jagged Z bands, few T tubules and the NMJs had smaller soleplates with few subneural clefts. When stimulated, the "slow" fibers did not have propagated action potentials and did not yield a twitch response.

Although it is difficult to recognize gross differences in the structure of vertebrate en plaque NMJs that correlate with histochemical types of myofibers, ultrastructural differences are present, particularly with reference to the configuration of the subneural apparatus. Since correlation of the histochemical types of myofibers with physiologic "fast" and "slow" responses is unreliable, so it is also unreliable to attempt to correlate ultrastructure characteristics of NMJs with "fast" or "slow" twitch myofiber responses. Correlation between NMJ structure and myofiber function appears more reliable in the few examples of myofibers innervated by en grappe NMJ such as the extraocular muscles.

As additional information about the various components of en plaque and en grappe NMJ have been accumulated through the work of many investigators, it is more convenient to discuss the terminal axon and its vesicle populations, the external lamina and other components of the junctions in separate sections that include supporting experimental data.

4

Ultrastructure of Terminal Axons in the Neuromuscular Junction

FINE STRUCTURE OF THE AXON

Mitochondria

All observers of the fine structure of NMJs have noted numerous mitochondria, ranging in diameter from 0.25 to 0.5μ and up to 1μ in length. The mitochondria were round, oval, or elongated and folded as viewed in various planes, and all contain a small number of internal double membranes (cristae mitochondrales) typical of vertebrate mitochondria (Figs. 33, 38, 39, 42, 44).

Neurofilaments

One aspect of classical axon cytology that was not confirmed by initial studies of this structure by electron microscopy was the absence of neurofilaments. These filaments, which are so characteristic of terminal axons in classically stained silver preparations, were entirely absent in electron micrographs from tissues prepared by primary osmium fixation. Robertson (1956) suggested that the neurofilaments

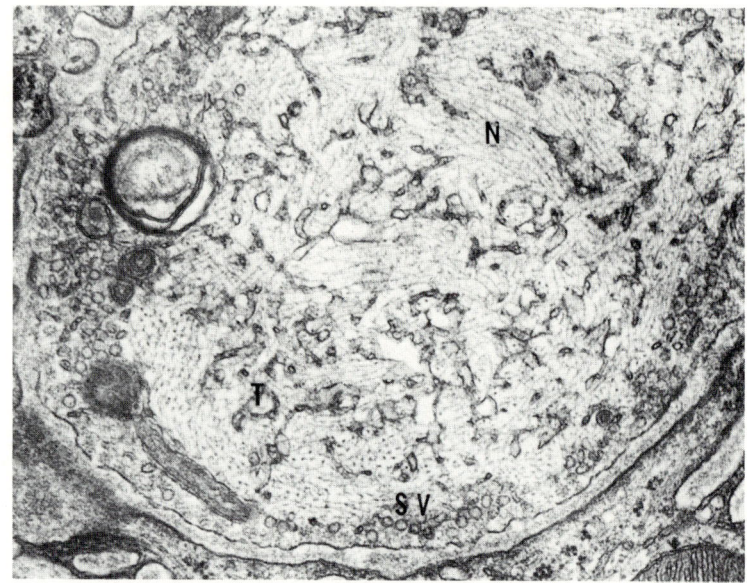

Figure 43. Electron micrograph illustrating synaptic vesicles *(SV)*, branched tubular structures *(T)* and neurofilaments *(N)* within a terminal axon. (X 37,500.)

could not be recognized in the terminal axons because they were converted into tubular bodies that appeared to be vesicular in sections (synaptic vesicles), but the serial reconstructions of Anderson-Cedergren (1959) demonstrated that the synaptic vesicles are not tubules. With improved fixation afforded by perfusion with cold buffered 4-6% glutaraldehyde one can demonstrate various tubules and finer filaments in the terminal axoplasm (Figs. 43, 44). With adequate fixation, the terminal axoplasm contains short 400-600 A as well as smaller 250-400 A tubules and finer filaments of approximately 50 A. As the terminus is approached, the number of tubules are fewer and the fine filaments are relatively more numerous. Some of the smaller tubular structures are present as aggregates of semicircular profiles (Robertson, 1960; Zacks et al., 1962) fill with externally applied horseradish peroxidase tracer and therefore may be directly connected to the subneural clefts or may fill indirectly as the result of endocytosis Figure 45 (Zacks and Saito, 1969; Heuser and Reese, 1973). Also, the axon membrane facing the overlying Schwann cell is frequently invaginated in a series of folds that may appear to be tubules in sectioned NMJs.

Birks (1966) demonstrated that if frog NMJs were fixed with acrolein instead of osmium tetroxide, the occasional short segments of the larger tubules appeared as long winding structures that occasionally

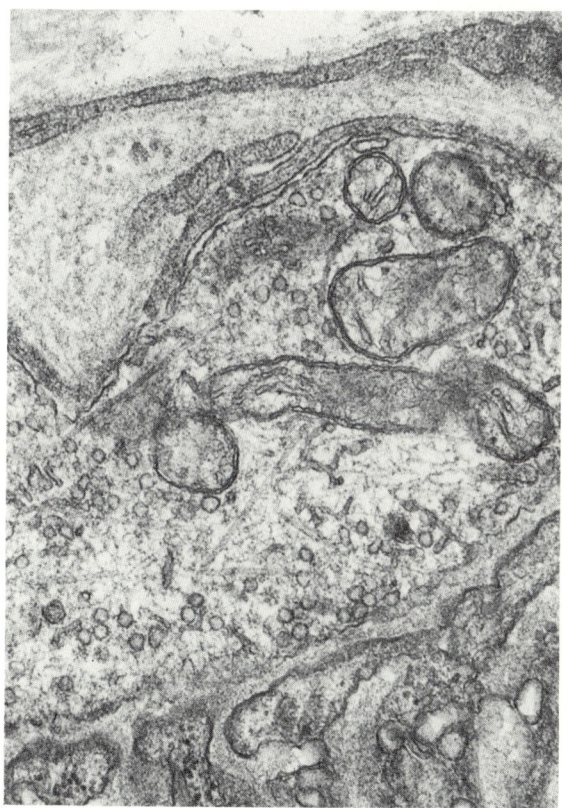

Figure 44. Electron micrograph illustrating details of fine structure of a terminal axon. Note the elongated straight as well as branched tubules of similar width. Synaptic vesicles of various shapes are present on the axoplasmic membrane and neurofilaments of smaller diameter are also present. (X 37,500.)

branched and lay with their long axes at right angles to the long axes of the nerve terminal. Often one end of the tubule was in contact with the axon surface membrane in the region of synaptic contact. When the nerve endings were soaked in a solution of thorium dioxide, thorium particles were found in synaptic vesicles and large diameter tubules as well as in transverse tubules and pinocytotic vesicles in the subsarcolemmal sarcoplasm. Birks concluded that the large diameter tubules open into the synaptic space and the smaller diameter tubules open into the axon-Schwann cell space. Elaborate networks of large tubules of this kind have not been reported by other investigators in the frog or in other NMJs perhaps because of the infrequency of use of acrolein fixation. However, prominent neurotubules were demonstrated in

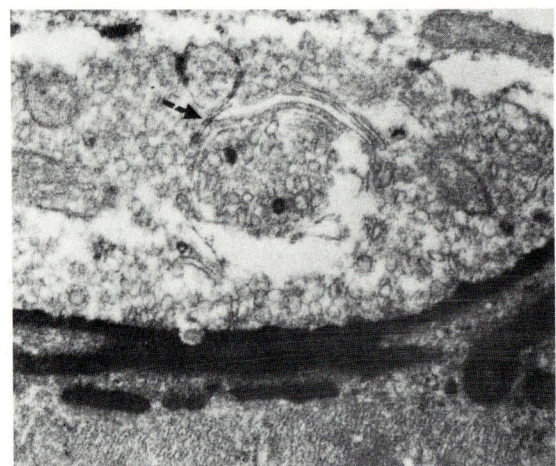

Figure 45. Electron micrograph illustrating horseradish peroxidase *(HRP)* tracer within coiled thin membranes in the axoplasm of a mouse NMJ (arrows). Large amounts of the tracer are present in the primary synaptic cleft and in the *T* system. The *HRP*-containing vesicles within the axoplasm are coated vesicles. (X 32,000.)

stimulated frog NMJs by Heuser (1971; Heuser and Reese, 1973) following glutaraldehyde fixation.

Although neurotubules are closely associated with synaptic vesicles, only a few reports of continuity between the tubules and the vesicles have appeared. Smith (1971) has reported bridge-like connections between axonal microtubules and typical synaptic vesicles in the lamprey spinal cord and Heuser (1971; Heuser and Reese, 1973) has proposed a scheme involving recycling of reabsorbed synaptic vesicle membrane material involving the axonal microtubules. Since the axonal neurotubules visible in electron micrographs are too small to be visible by optical micorscopy, the silver impregnated "neurofilaments" of classical neurocytology are believed to be aggregates of neurotubules.

Vesicles in the Axon Terminals

Improved fixation obtained by vascular perfusion with glutaraldehyde followed by osmium postfixation has revealed a population of several kinds of vesicles in the terminal axons of vertebrate NMJs. In addition to the synaptic vesicles discovered by De Robertis and Bennett (1954, 1955), smaller numbers of "fuzzy" or coated vesicles and dense core vesicles are also present.

Synaptic Vesicles

Early ultrastructure studies revealed that the terminal axon is filled with numerous vesicles, the so-called "synaptic vesicles" (De Robertis and Bennett, 1954, 1955). These measure approximately 300 A in diameter. They are enclosed by a single membrane and contain a central region of low electron density (Figs. 42, 43, 44, 46). After dual fixation with glutaraldehyde and osmium, the synaptic vesicle membrane has been shown to be composed of globular units rather than having typical unit membrane structure (DiCarlo, 1967). The membrane is composed of 40-45 A globules and larger 60-90 A ovals connected by osmiophilic granules. The surface appears to be a mosaic composed of hexagonal polyhedral structures.

Synaptic vesicles arise from endoplasmic reticulum or neurotubules according to Düring (1967) or by dilatation and pinching off of outpouchings from the neurotubules in the advancing axon tips (Blümcke and Niedorf, 1965) or in the Golgi region (De Iraldi and De Robertis, 1968). Heuser and Reese (1973) have emphasized the importance of intraaxonal cisternae. Jårlfors and Smith (1969) were unable to demonstrate direct connections between the 220 A neurotubules and 400-500 A vesicles in lamprey larva but in a later report (Smith, 1971) connections were found in lamprey spinal cord neurons.

Stelzner (1971) used the zinc iodide-osmium tetroxide method to study the origin of synaptic vesicles in the developing lumbosacral enlargement of albino rats. Large numbers of vesicles similar in appearance to synaptic vesicles were found in the vicinity of the Golgi apparatus and intermixed with smooth endoplasmic reticulum. Of these, 10-20% of the vesicles within the Golgi region as well as the majority of the vesicles in other parts of the axoplasm were stained by the zinc iodide osmium method. Of considerable interest was their observation that much of the smooth endoplasmic reticulum was also stained. This data was interpreted to indicate that synaptic vesicles are produced in the Golgi apparatus and smooth endoplasmic reticulum in immature neurons. In adult animals, the number of vesicles are decreased in the Golgi region. However, zinc iodide osmium staining could also be demonstrated in the smooth endoplasmic reticulum of adult axons.

In typical NMJs, the synaptic vesicles are concentrated along the inner surface of the axon plasma membrane facing the synaptic cleft (De Robertis, 1958; deHarven and Coërs, 1959; Birks et al., 1960) and occasionally (scorpion) may aggregate in clusters opposite specialized areas in the postsynaptic membrane (Smith, 1971) (Fig. 33) especially when the nerve is stimulated (Heuser and Reese, 1973). Recently, McMahan et al. (1972) used Nomarski optics to demonstrate varicosities containing synaptic vesicles in frog and mudpuppy terminal axons in living animals.

Although the presence of synaptic vesicles in the synaptic space has been reported (De Robertis and Bennett, 1955; De Robertis and Franchi, 1956; Couteaux and Pecot-Dechavassine, 1970) or in "close association" (Palay, 1956), other investigators have never observed vesicles within the synaptic space (Reger, 1959; Zacks and Blumberg, 1961a), even under conditions of extreme stimulation (Heuser and Reese, 1973; Ceccarelli et al, 1973). Frequently, shallow 300 A indentations in the axolemma can be observed in typical NMJs (Fig. 35, 46), which have been interpreted by some investigators as evidence of opening of a synaptic vesicle into the synaptic cleft. However, there is no requirement for the release of intact vesicles, a most unlikely occurence.

Much attention has recently been given to differences in the shape of synaptic vesicles in central synapses as a means of indicating whether a particular synapse is excitatory or inhibitory (Uchizono, 1965, 1968). With respect to the NMJ, which may have inhibitory innervation in some invertebrates some support for this concept was found in lobster NMJ (Nadol and de Lorenzo, 1968) but Ogata et al. (1967) found no differences in the shape of synaptic vesicles in fast, slow and intermediate types of NMJs innervating corresponding myofibers of rat intercostal muscle.

Synaptic vesicles are found in the central nervous system synapses of mammals, NMJs, the neuropil of arthropods, and the synapses between retinal rod and bipolar cells and are regarded as characteristic features of the presynaptic element of probably all synapses with chemical transmitters (Palade, 1954; Robertson, 1955a, b; De Robertis, 1958). They are now recognized as the storage site of Ach and the release of their contents and subsequent combination with the postsynaptic receptors give rise to the miniature endplate potentials (MEPPs). The importance of these structures was recognized by De Robertis (1958) who stated that the "synaptic vesicles represent the most important (at least quantitatively), constant and specific component of the synaptic terminal". He believed that their location on the proximal side of the synapse was responsible for the polarized functional activity characteristic of synaptic regions. The extensive experimental data concerning the role of the synaptic vesicles in the storage and release of Ach in discussed in chapter

Zinc Iodide Staining of Synaptic Vesicles

De Iraldi and Guedet (1968) found that the classical Champy-Maillet osmium tetroxide, zinc iodide stain (Maillet, 1962) stained synaptic vesicles characteristically. When examined in the electron microscope, the majority of the synaptic vesicles had electron dense cores that did not resemble catecholamine granules, which had pale cores after zinc iodide staining. Nearly simultaneously, Akert and Sandri (1968) described similar staining of synaptic vesicles in cat and rat central synapses and mouse NMJs. Denervated mouse NMJs were also studied after zinc iodide staining (Nickel and Waser, 1969). The nature of the substance in synaptic vesicles that stains by this method is unknown.

Coated Vesicles

Whittaker and Gray (1962) first described coated vesicles in the central nervous system and in a detailed study, Andres (1964) described

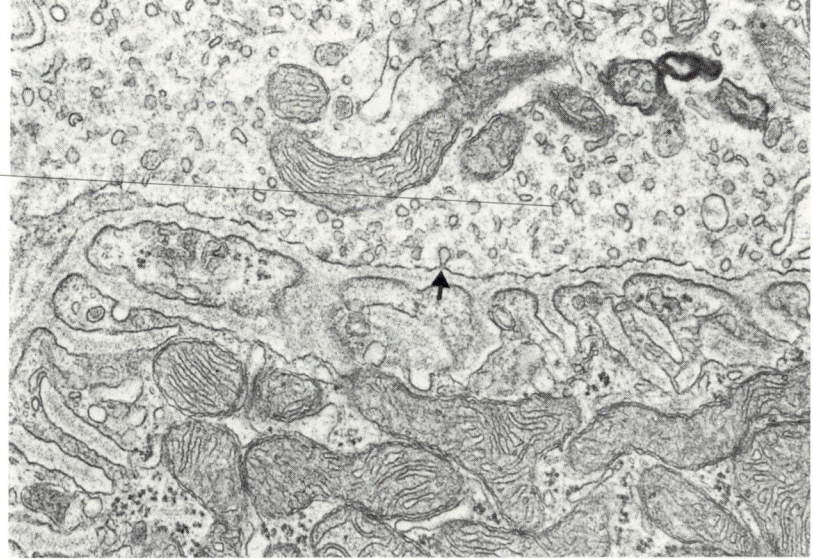

Figure 46. Electron micrograph illustrating the appearance of various kinds of vesicles within the axoplasm. Variously shaped synaptic vesicles are scattered in the axoplasm and a coated vesicle opening to the exterior is indicated by the arrow. (X 37,500.)

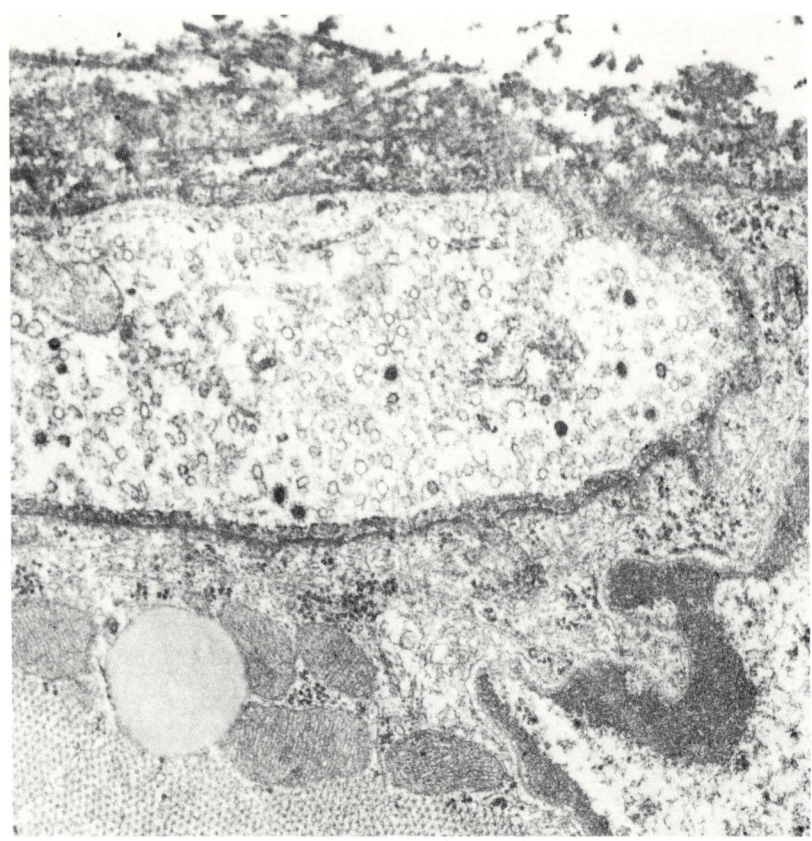

Figure 47. Electron micrograph illustrating HRP tracer within coated vesicles in a mouse terminal axon. The tracer is also present in large amounts in the overlying external lamina and in the secondary synaptic clefts. Note that none of the synaptic vesicles contain the tracer. (X 30,000.)

them as vesicular structures that were enclosed by a unit membrane that had an external "fuzz" or coating that appeared to radiate from the vesicle surface (Fig. 46). These vesicles are similar to structures associated with the uptake of yolk in insect oocytes (Roth and Porter, 1962) and are thought to play a role in the uptake of macromolecules. Both Nickel et al. (1967) and Dűring (1967) described coated vesicles in NMJs. In studies of mouse diaphragm muscle NMJs, these investigators found coated vesicles in the axoplasm facing the Schwann cell as well as opposite the subneural apparatus. The vesicles appeared to connect to secondary synaptic clefts. Coated vesicles were also present in perineural cells, endothelium and sarcoplasm. The coated vesicles appeared to arise as invaginations of the axon surface membrane, possibly in previously coated or specialized areas of the membrane. Earlier ultrastructure studies of NMJs had shown rather large vesicles apparently opening into the subneural clefts from the apposed axolemma. This apparent opening of synaptic vesicles into the synaptic cleft was interpreted as probable anatomic support for the secretion of Ach by rupturing synaptic vesicles. However, Zacks and Saito (1969) demonstrated that horseradish peroxidase injected into mouse muscles appeared only within coated vesicles, which were the only structures that could be demonstrated to open into the synaptic cleft. Scattered coated vesicles containing the tracer were found within the axon 2 minutes after injection (Figs. 47, 48), but none of the typical synaptic vesicles contained the tracer. There was no evidence of horseradish peroxidase in the proximal axoplasm or in neurotubules and, by 24 hours, the tracer had disappeared from the terminal axons. These experiments demonstrate that coated vesicles in the terminal axon can take up a macromolecule of the size of horseradish peroxidase (M.W. 40,000) but we could not determine its fate since enzymatic degradation in the vesicles probably prevents the demonstration of the label after a period of time. There is no certain role of coated vesicles in neuromuscular transmission although recently, they have been considered as part of the mechanism by which the axon membrane is restored after depletion by exocytosis (Bittner and Kennedy, 1970; Holtz-

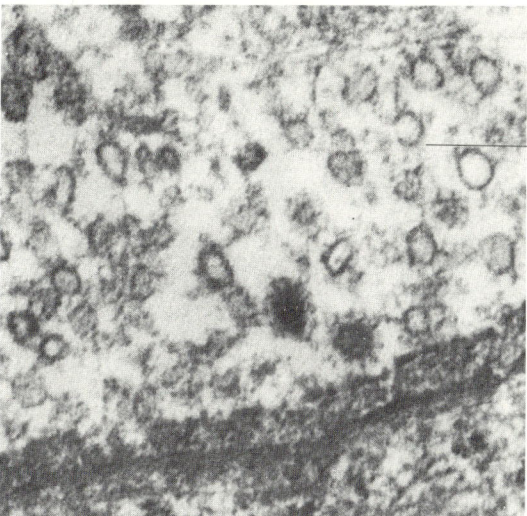

Figure 48. Electron micrograph at high magnification illustrating details of coated vesicles containing HRP tracer in a mouse NMJ. (X 78,000.)

man et al., 1971; Heuser, 1971; Korneliussen, 1972; Korneliussen, et al., 1972; Heuser and Reese, 1973). This is discussed in greater detail in chapter 10.

Dense Core Vesicles in Neuromuscular Junctions

Vesicles with dense cores (700-1100 A) of the kind that initially were thought to contain catecholamines in adrenergic nerve endings (Eranko, 1967) also occur in invertebrate (spider, crayfish, lobster) and vertebrate NMJs. They occur in the terminal axons of NMJs in chicken eye muscles (Zenker and Krammer, 1967), rat esophagus (Gruber, 1968) and rat extraocular muscle (Terävainen, 1969). Dense core vesicles are most common in developing NMJs (Atwood et al., 1971). Kelly (1966), Terävainen (1968) and Kelly and Zacks (1969) observed them in developing (1 day) NMJs of rat intercostal and extraocular muscle (figure 22) and Pappas et al. (1971) observed them in axons in tissue cultures containing rat nerve and muscle. It is of interest in this connection that Csillik (1965b) observed catecholamine fluorescence in immature rat diaphragm NMJs following formalin fixation.

The significance of dense core vesicles in NMJs is unknown. More recent studies utilizing permaganate fixation (Bloom, 1973) reveal small dense core vesicles that are more likely storage sites of biogenic amines. Small dense core vesicles have not been reported in terminal axons of NMJs. If the large dense core vesicles do contain catecholamines, the presence of these vesicles in developing NMJs may indicate the existence of an undifferentiated stage of multipotentiality before cholinergic transmission is established.

5

External Lamina in Neuromuscular Junctions

One aspect of NMJ structure revealed by electron microscopy that has received scant attention until recently, is the nature of the material within the primary and secondary synaptic clefts that separates the presynaptic from the postsynaptic membranes. It seems logical that this "gap substance" might play a significant role in the function of the neuromuscular synapse (Fig. 49).

It has been suggested by Couteaux and Katz (1957) and by Eccles and Jaeger (1958) that the space within the subsynaptic clefts serves as a channel for diffusion of Ach as required by the classical Dale theory. However, we must consider the fact that the synaptic clefts are not merely fluid-filled spaces but contain amorphous hydrated external lamina (EL) material. The EL within the synaptic clefts consists of the fused contributions of a layer of EL covering the overlying Schwann cell and a layer covering the myofiber (Zacks and Blumberg, 1961a). Originally it was thought to be layered (Robertson, 1956), but later work utilizing improved fixation indicates that it is more or less homogeneous. Apparently similar material separates presynaptic and postsynaptic membranes in central nervous system synapses (Luse, 1956; Hess, 1962) and is responsible for the apparently fixed spatial relationship between the opposed synaptic membranes in these synapses and in this regard has been considered to have adhesive properties.

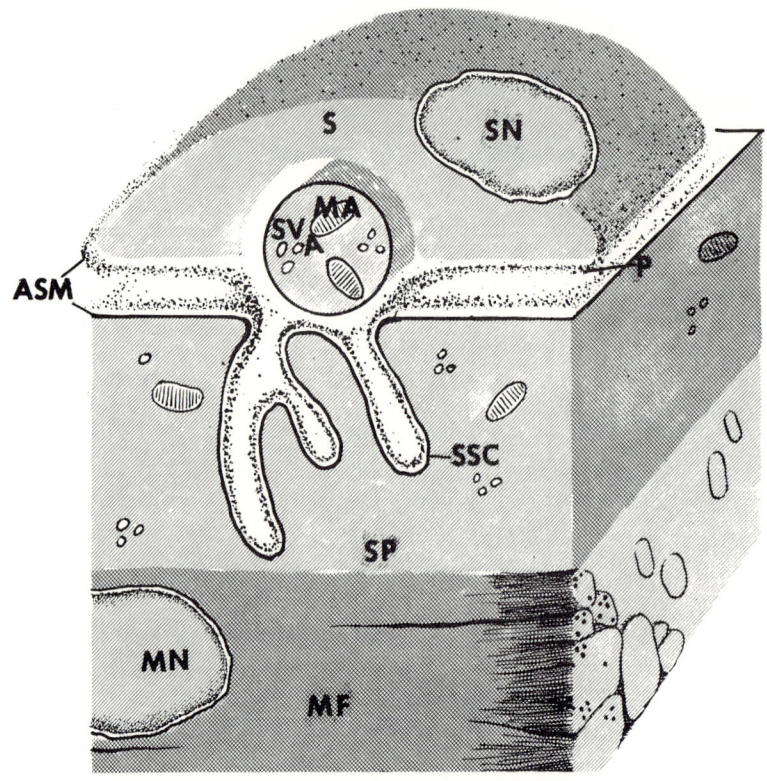

Figure 49. Diagram of a NMJ illustrating the relationship of the layers of external lamina contributed by the Schwann cell *(S)* and by the muscle surface *(ASM)*. Mitochondria *(MA)*, and synaptic vesicles *(SV)* are indicated in the axon. The primary *(P)* and secondary *(SSC)* clefts are also shown. A myofiber nucleus *(MN)* is present within the myofibers *(MF)*.

Histochemical investigations revealed that the muscle EL (Goldstein, 1959) as well as the EL within the NMJ was PAS-positive after amylase digestion (Noël, 1957; Zacks and Blumberg, 1961a; Csillik, 1963; Jonecko, 1970). There is also evidence that more than one kind of PAS-positive material is present. McManus et al. (1950) reported PAS staining of nerve and innervation sites in fresh frozen sections, and Chu (1950) demonstrated that PAS-positive material was present in fresh muscle and brain sections. However, since the PAS-positive material in fresh tissues failed to stain after alcohol extraction, it is unlikely that this material is responsible for the PAS-reactivity in the paraffin or methacrylate-embedded NMJs studied by several investigators. Similarly, McManus et al. (1950) found that paraffin embedding eliminated the selective PAS staining of nerve fibers. Therefore it seems likely that there are extractable substances in fresh or frozen nerve tissue that are capable of recolorizing the Schiff reagent, and that prior oxidation is required to demonstrate staining after formalin fixation and paraffin embedding. These substances are different than the EL material that survives paraffin embedding. As is well known, PAS staining after diastase digestion (to remove glycogen) is not specific for any individual chemical species. Polysaccharides, mucopolysaccharides, mucoproteins, glycoproteins, and glycolipids may all stain with PAS (Pearse, 1960). Although originally stated that localized alcian blue staining occurs in mouse NMJs (Zacks and Blumberg, 1961a) more detailed studies (Zacks et al., 1973) have revealed less staining than originally reported. This stain was used because it is regarded by many investigators as a selective stain for acid mucopolysaccharides at acid pH. Csillik (1963) found that the PAS-staining material in NMJs was lost when the motor nerves were sectioned and concluded that the PAS-staining material is localed in the postsynaptic membrane. Since it is known that EL material persists for long periods of time after denervation (chapter 11), the loss of PAS stainability reported by Csillik indicates that some molecular change in the EL had occurred under conditions of denervation to alter its PAS stainability. However, this work could not be confirmed by Zacks et al. (1973).

Most investigators have concluded that the EL is a hydrated mucopolysaccharide or mucoprotein (Robertson, 1960; Zacks and Blumberg, 1961a; Jonecko, 1970). Luft (1966, 1971) also demonstrated that the EL was stained by ruthenium red, a reagent believed to stain mucopolysaccharides. Additional studies led to revision of this view.

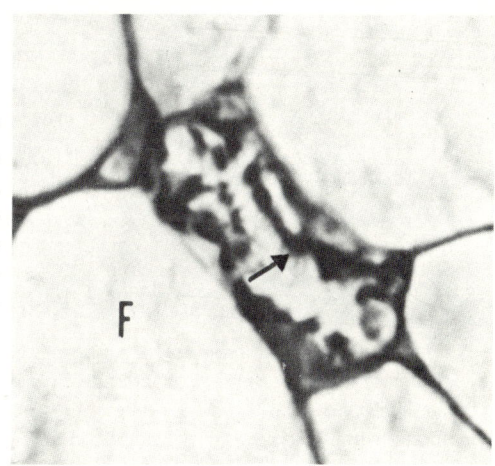

Figure 50. Photomicrograph of a mouse NMJ stained by the aldehyde fuchsin-alcian blue method. Note the dark staining of the myofiber external lamina that extends into the subneural apparatus arrow). The myofibers *(F)* are essentially unstained. (X 1,000.)

Because of its possible role in neuromuscular transmission and the few known differences between EL in innervated and non-innervated areas, Zacks et al. (1973) used a variety of cytochemical methods to investigate the chemical nature of EL within NMJs. For optical microscopy, the technique of staining with aldehyde fuchsin followed or preceded by alcian blue (Spicer and Meyer, 1960) was found particularly useful for demonstrating NMJs in paraffin embedded, formalin-fixed muscle (Fig. 50). This procedure (see appendix) is the most useful means of surveying the structure of the subneural apparatus in routine pathologic tissue such as muscle biopsy specimens that have not been specially fixed for electron microscopy. It was found that stainability of the EL was greatly enhanced by prior sulfation indicating that the EL was poor in intrinsic exposed acidic sulfate groups. Absence of metachromasia after staining with Azure A at pH 1.5-3 (Spicer, 1960) also confirmed this conclusion. Failure to stain with the dimethylphenylene diamine method after periodate oxidation (Spicer and Jarrels, 1961) also indicated that the bulk of the EL was not acid mucopolysaccharide

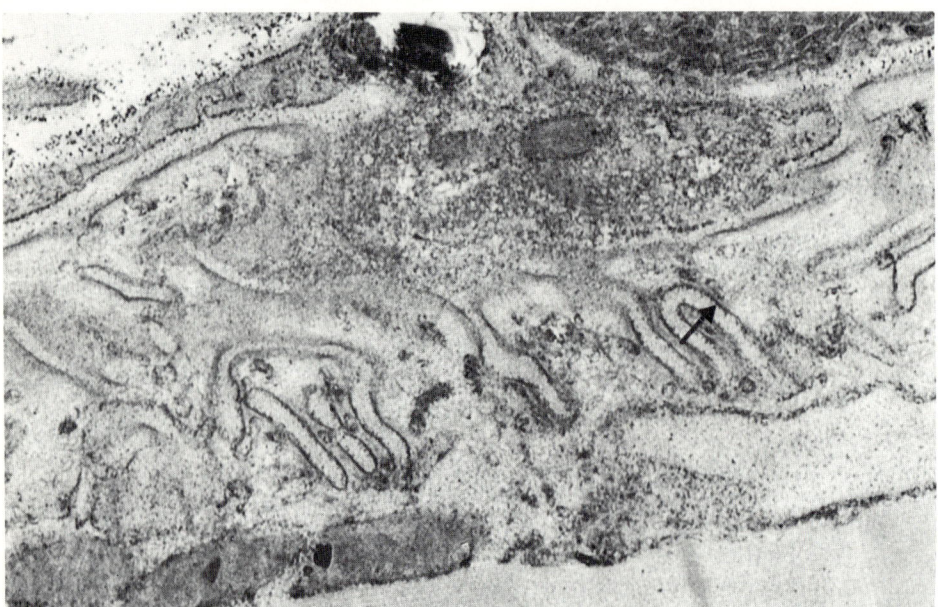

Figure 51. Electron micrograph of a mouse NMJ stained with colloidal iron. Note the deposition of electron dense iron granules in the collagen filaments adjacent to the Schwann cell cytoplasm *(S)* and as fine granules along the external surface of the plasma membrane within the secondary synaptic clefts (arrow). Note that the external lamina within the subneural apparatus is essentially free of iron particles. (X 28,700.)

although some acidic groups were probably present to account for the pale alcian blue staining.

In a series of experiments utilizing stains designed to demonstrate carbohydrates and glycoproteins in fine structure, Zacks et al. (1973) demonstrated that the sarcolemma is a complex composed of the myofiber plasma membrane, a thin "cell coat" (Rambourg and Leblond, 1967; Rambourg et al., 1969) external to the outer leaflet of the plasma membrane that stains with colloidal iron (Fig. 51) and thorium and a thicker external lamina that stains with ruthenium red (Figure 52), methenamine silver (Fig. 53) and phosphotungstic acid in chromic acid (Fig. 54). This cytochemical evidence indicates that the EL covering the myofibers and filling the subneural apparatus of the NMJs is a glycoprotein that is either mixed with, or more likely, contains as an integral part, components with free carboxyl groups. Although the EL stains intensely with ruthenium red, this reaction does not appear

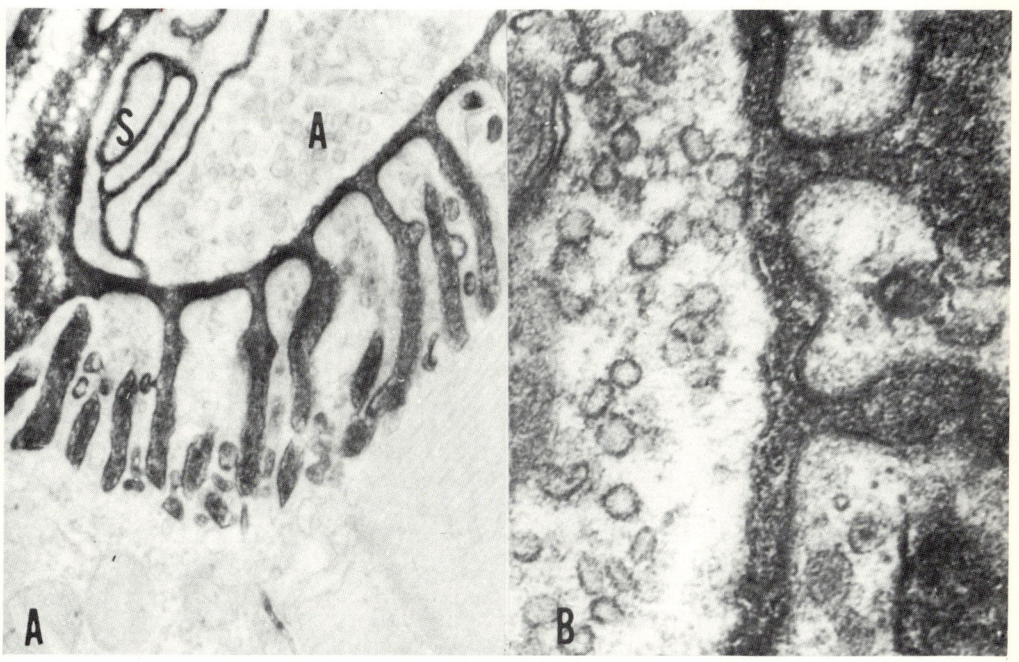

Figure 52. Electron micrograph of a mouse NMJ after staining with ruthenium red. In *A*, ruthenium red is present in the space between the Schwann cell *(S)* and axon *(A)* and within the primary and secondary synaptic clefts of the subneural apparatus. The dye is also present within elements of the *T* system. *B*, electron micrograph at higher magnification illustrating granular precipitate of ruthenium red within primary and secondary synaptic clefts. (*A:* X 24,600; *B:* X 50,000.)

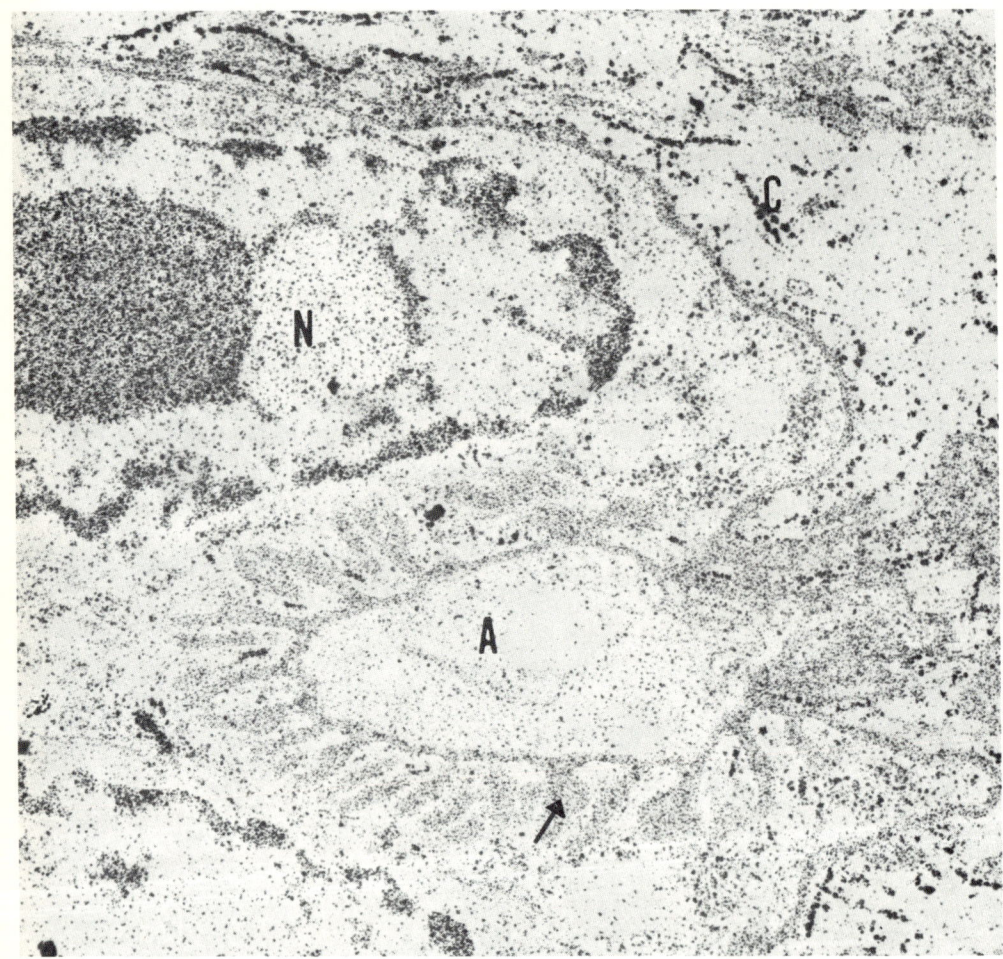

Figure 53. Electron micrograph of a mouse NMJ stained by the PAS-methenamine silver method for glycoproteins. Note the particularly dense stain in collagen filaments in the interstitial spaces *(C)* and the fine granular precipitate of silver particles in the subneural apparatus (arrow). Silver granules are also present in the nucleus *(N)* and sarcoplasm. The terminal axon is indicated at *A*. (X 18,100.)

to be due to acid mucopolysaccharide as suggested by Luft (1966). Recently (1971), Luft has shown that acidic polypeptides also will precipitate ruthenium red.

Early enzyme histochemical studies of acetylcholinesterase (AchE) activity in NMJs suggested that the EL had AchE activity (Zacks and Blumberg, 1961b; Lehrer and Ornstein, 1959; Barrnett, 1962) but more recent histochemical studies (Koelle and Gromadzki, 1966; Zacks et

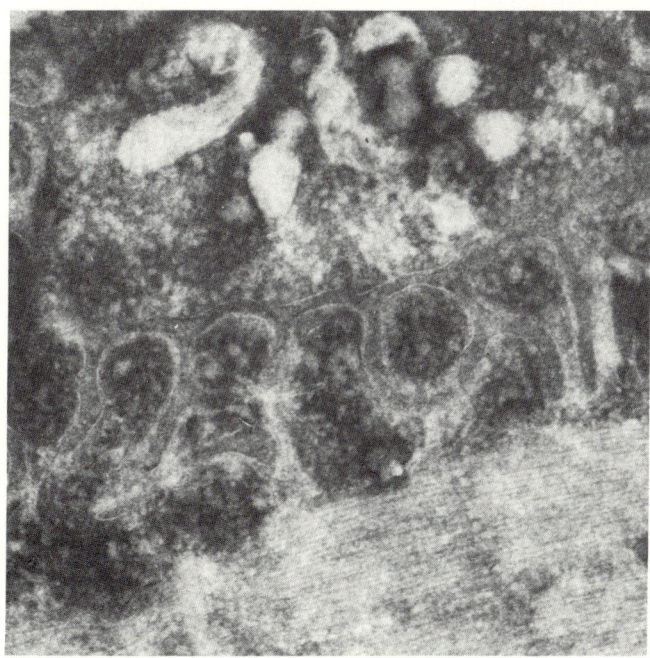

Figure 54. Electron micrograph of a mouse NMJ stained by the chromate-phosphotungstic acid method in tissue embedded in glycol methacrylate. Note the reversed contrast. The synaptic vesicles, axon and muscle membranes, and myofilaments have decreased electron density compared with osmium fixed tissues. There is increased electron density in the external lamina filling the subneural apparatus. (X 24,600.)

al., 1972) (Fig. 61) and investigations employing radioactive cholinesterase inhibitors (Salpeter, 1967, 1969) indicate that the enzyme is localized in close association with the myofiber surface membrane (Fig. 76). Release of AchE from apparently undamaged frog and rat NMJs by collagenase (Hall and Kelly, 1971; Betz and Sakmann, 1971) indicates that the enzyme is incorporated in the cell coats external to the myofiber plasma membrane.

Metal Binding Properties of External Lamina

Until the demonstration of lead reactive substances in NMJs (Sávay and Csillik, 1958) there were no known morphologic or histochemical differences between the EL in NMJs as compared with adjacent non-innervated areas of the myofiber. These investigators demonstrated that when unfixed muscle was treated with 1 per cent lead

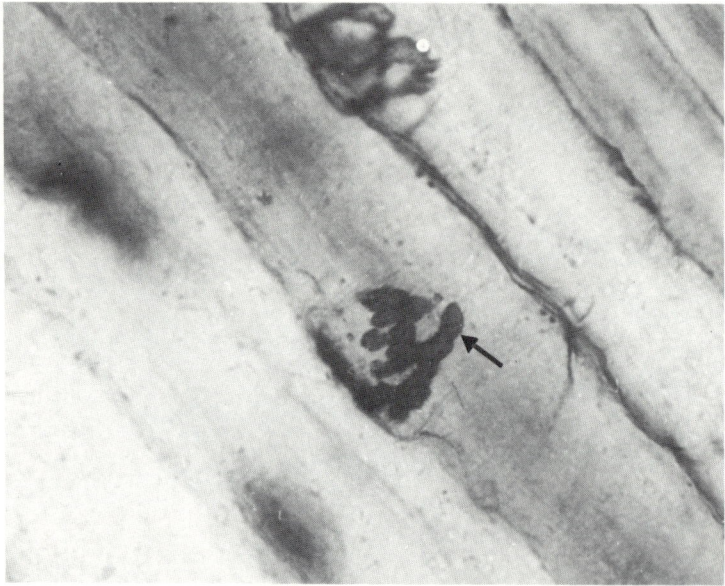

Figure 55. Photomicrograph illustrating the appearance of a NMJ stained with lead nitrate according to the Sávay-Csillik method. Note the deposition of lead sulfide that is most intense at the periphery of the subneural clefts (arrow). (X 400.)

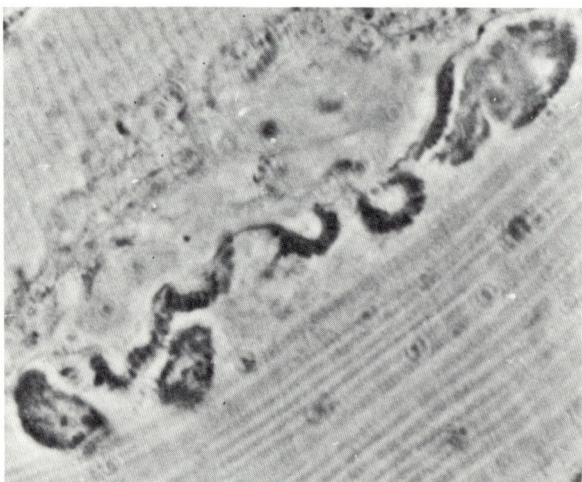

Figure 56. Phase contrast photomicrograph of a semi thin section of a mouse NMJ stained by the lead nitrate technique. Note the density due to lead sulfide precipitate in the subneural apparatus (arrow). The axon is unstained. (X 1,500.)

nitrate in formalin solution followed by ammonium sulfide to trap the lead, the subneural apparatus of the NMJ was as well delineated as when stained with the various methods used to demonstrate cholinesterase activity. The lead staining was prevented by prior freezing or fixation. In a more extensive study, Nakamura et al. (1967) demonstrated that not only lead but many divalent cations are bound selectively by the EL within NMJs. Tin, cadmium, zinc, copper manganese and cobalt were all bound selectively. Although early electron microscope observations on the site of lead binding failed to show localization in the EL within the subneural apparatus (Zacks and Blumberg, 1961b), later studies by Csillik and Davis (1964), Kelly and Zacks (1965) and Zacks et al. (1970) demonstrated that EL in the subneural apparatus selectively binds lead, a reaction many times more intense than in adjacent areas of non-innervated EL (Figs. 55, 56, 57). Using controlled pH, Zacks and Kelly (1968) demonstrated that Pb++ binding was maximal at pH 4.6. These metallic cations are probably bound to the carboxyl groups that are demonstrated by alcian blue and blocked by methylation.

Solubilization of EL with Enzymes

When fresh or fixed mouse muscle was incubated in various concentrations of neuraminidase, hyaluronidase or collagenase under a wide variety of conditions, with or without subsequent staining, there

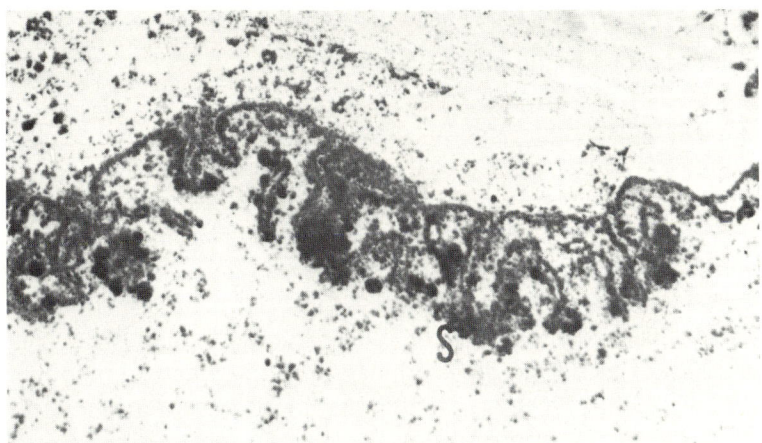

Figure 57. Electron micrograph of lead-stained NMJ illustrating selective precipitation of lead in the subneural apparatus *(S).* (X 17,000.)

was slight reduction of alcian blue staining of the EL only after incubation of fresh muscle with hyaluronidase or collagenase. Electron microscopic studies of these preparations revealed no significant change in the myofiber EL following incubation of thin sections with these enzymes with or without subsequent staining to demonstrate the EL. Similar results were obtained when glycol methacrylate embedding was used to facilitate penetration of the enzyme solutions into the thin sections. Failure to remove myofiber EL with the preparation of collagenase that was demonstrated to hydrolyse gelatin was unexpected since Kono et al. (1964) had reported that an unspecified collagenase preparation removed rat myofiber EL. In our preparations, organized collagen fibrils, recognized by their banding, resisted incubation with high concentrations of collagenase for up to 24 hours at 37°C. but the amorphous coat currounding some of these fibrils was removed.

Gersh and Catchpole (1949) also found that collagenase did not alter purified collagen or collagen fibrils in tissue sections. Our data from mouse and rat muscle apparently do not agree with the results reported for frog muscle by Betz and Sakmann (1971) who were able to solubilize some portion of the EL with enzymes resulting in separation of the terminal axons from the subneural apparatus. Their data indicates that AchE is located in the myofiber cell coat external to the plasma membrane and according to these investigators, EL anchors the terminal axon to the junctional site. This discrepancy may be due to trypsin contamination of the enzyme preparations.

Experiments with Sarcolemmal Tubes

A more satisfactory way of studying the composition of EL involves the isolation of muscle cell "tubes" of sarcolemma that are prepared by extracting the contractile proteins from homogenized myofibers. These tubes consist of the myofiber plasma membrane and its EL.

In our laboratory, a series of experiments (Zacks, et al. 1973) were performed with rat sarcolemmal "tubes" using the basic techniques of Kono et al. (1964) and McCollester (1962). After glutaraldehyde fixation and uranium or lead staining, examination in the electron microscope revealed segments of electron dense muscle cell membrane covered by continuous layers of amorphous EL from which protruded occasional collagen fibrils recognized by their characteristic cross banding. The EL proper is composed of amorphous material arranged in an irregular mesh. Ruthenium red stained the EL intensely as well as the amorphous material coating the collagen fibrils (Fig. 58). However, banded collagen fibrils were never observed within the subneural apparatus. There is no obvious explanation why collagen fibrils are excluded from this region but one may speculate that the presence of the overlying Schwann cell that contributes its EL to the junctional region may be responsible in some way.

In a series of experiments, the isolated sarcolemmal tubes were incubated with various enzymes after which the tubes were sedimented, fixed in glutaraldehyde and examined in the electron microscope. After incubation with collagenase, the EL covering the myofibers remained but the organized collagen fibrils that were embedded in the EL were found in the sediment separate from the membrane fragments. In many preparations, the collagen fibrils appeared partially unravelled with loss of the amorphous matrical material that lies between the strands. Little change was visible after incubation with hyaluronidase or sialidase but pronase removed the EL and papain appeared to hydrolyse the entire preparation.

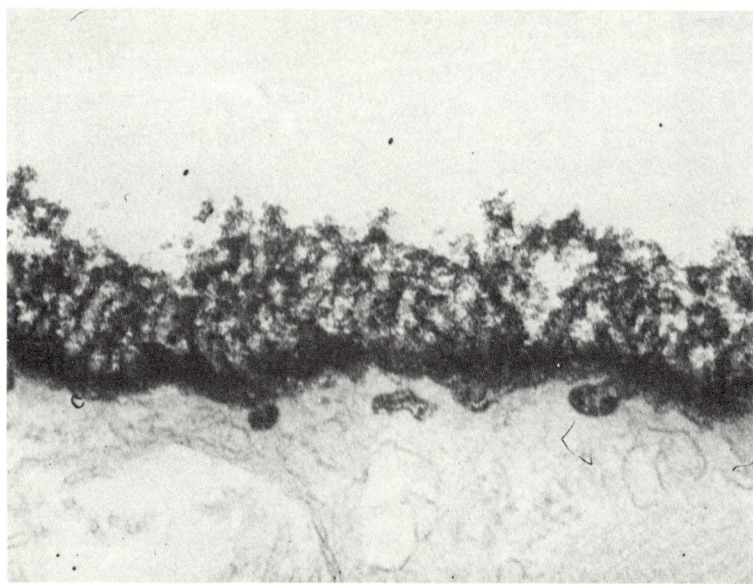

Figure 58. Electron micrograph of mouse sarcolemma stained with ruthenium red illustrating staining of the external lamina and a coating of similar material covering unstained collagen filaments (arrows). Ruthenium red within elements of the myofiber T system is also illustrated. (X 108,000.)

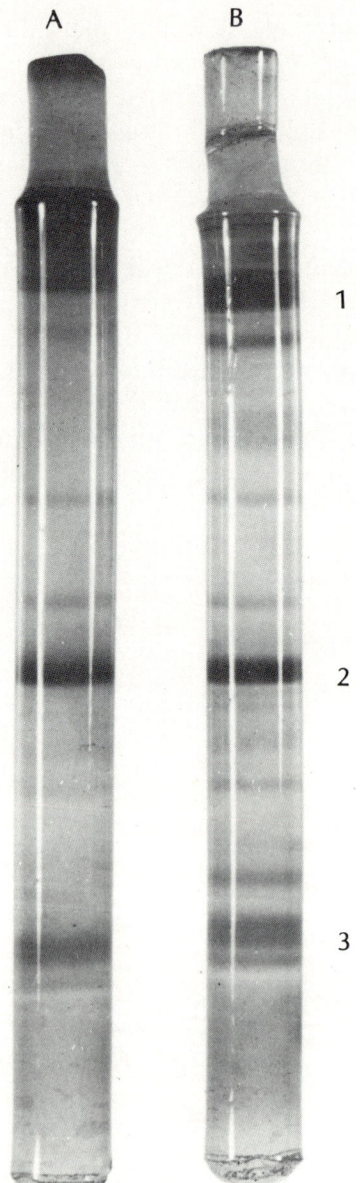

Figure 59. SDS-gel electrophoresis of isolated sarcolemma *(A)* and the LIS extract external lamina substance *(B)*. Gels are stained with Coomassie blue. The molecular weight of the major proteins are *(1)* 170,000; *(2)* 140,000 and *(3)* 44,000.

In studies of rat sarcolemmal tubes, Kono and Collowick (1961) demonstrated the presence of acetylneuraminic acid, glucose, glucosamine, glucuronic acid and xylose. Abood et al. (1966) reported that bullfrog sarcolemma contains 0.9 ±0.2% polysaccharide and 60 ±3%

protein calculated on a dry weight basis. These investigators concluded that amino acid analysis of the sarcolemma excluded the presence of large amounts of collagen. Rat sarcolemmal tubes analysed in our

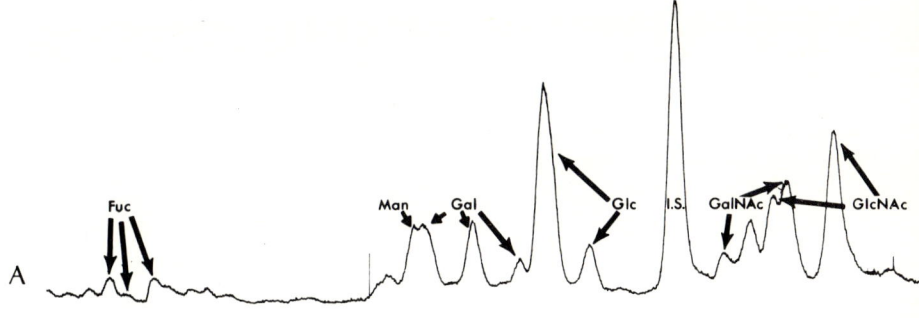

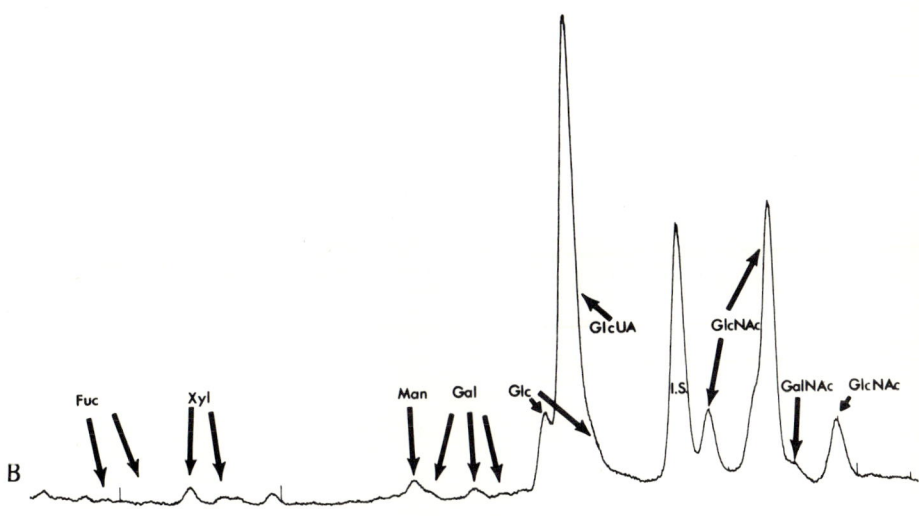

Figure 60a. Gas chromatograph of carbohydrates in isolated sarcolemma. N-acetyl neuraminic acid was detected but elutes after glucosamine and is not shown. Abbreviations: Fuc, Fucose; Man, Mannose; Gal, Galactose; Glc, Glucose; I.S., Internal Standard (mannitol); GalNAc, N-acetyl galactosamine; GlcNAc, N-acetyl glucosamine.

Figure 60b. Gas chromatograph of the LIS extract of external lamina substance. Abbreviations are the same as in Figure 8 with the addition of Xyl, Xylose; GlcUR, Glucuronic Acid.

laboratory (Vandenburgh et al., 1973) contained 78.4% protein, 14.2% lipid and 1.8% carbohydrate. Partial solubilization with SDS-mercaptoethanol and analysis by SDS gel electrophoresis revealed three major and 30-35 minor protein bands (Fig. 59). The three major bands had molecular weights of 170,000, 140,000 and 44,000. Sarcolemmal tube proteins contained large amounts of glutamic and aspartic acid and a glycine, proline and hydroxyproline content intermediate between collagen and non-collagen proteins. The carboxylic amino acids are probably responsible for the polyanionic properties of the sarcolemma such as divalent cation and ruthenium red binding.

Thin layer chromatography to demonstrate sugars indicates the presence of glucuronic acid and some neutral hexose but little amino sugar. There is also a sulfo-sugar present as either keratan or dermatan sulfate. The tightly bound sugar is approximately 5 to 6% of dry weight. Gas chromatography revealed little neutral carbohydrate with the exception of glucose. Large amounts of glucuronic acid and glucosamine were found and a moderate amount of galactosamine. Xylose, the common binding sugar of glycosaminoglycans to protein is present but there was no iduronic acid. (Fig. 60). (Vandenburgh, et al, 1973).

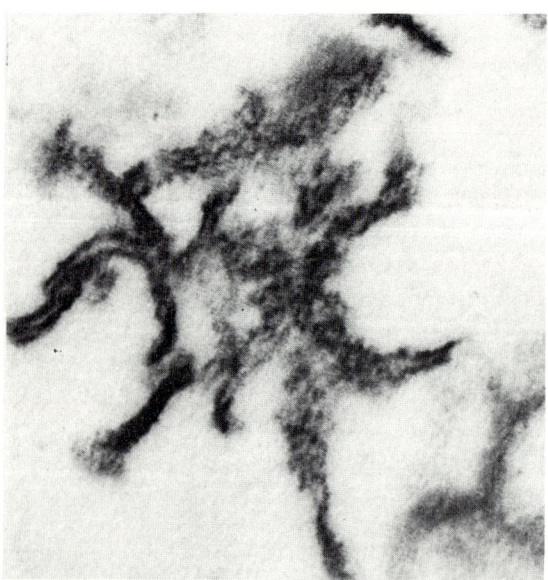

Figure 61. Electron micrograph of isolated myofiber sarcolemmal membranes stained by the thiolacetic acid method. Note the electron dense deposits of lead sulfide on the membrane surfaces forming the subneural apparatus. (X 108,000.)

Acetylcholinesterase Activity in Sarcolemmal Tubes

Isolated rat sarcolemmal tubes stained for AchE activity contained typical subneural apparatuses containing the histochemical reaction product similar to the results obtained by Namba and Grob (1968). In the electron microscope, sarcolemmal tubes stained for AchE activity by the thiolacetic acid method revealed patches of esterase activity in the myofiber plasma membrane, not in the EL (Fig. 61). The most likely site of the enzyme is within the "cell coat" external to the outer leaflet of the myofiber plasma membrane.

Extraction of EL with Lithium Diiodosalicylate (LIS)

Several mechanical and chemical methods were used without success to separate the EL from the myofiber plasma membrane. Only 3.5% lithium diiodosalicylate (LIS) was effective in removing the EL, a reagent successfully used by Marchesi and Andrews (1971) to remove red cell coats and tumor antigens.

After the sarcolemmal tubes were incubated in LIS, the insoluble components were sedimented. Dialysis of the supernatant against water yielded translucent colorless material that spontaneously formed gels containing 100 mg. per cent of EL and a small amount of bound LIS. The gel was somewhat thixotropic; suspensions lowered the pH on stirring. Nuclear magnetic resonance spectroscopy revealed a large chemical shift indicating strong water binding. This appears to explain the findings of England (1970) who demonstrated 200μ white areas of minute ice crystals in zones known to be occupied by NMJs after freezing of the muscle on solid carbon dixide at -1°C. These areas of crystalization were larger than the subneural apparatus demonstrated by staining and were clearly due to ice crystal clusters because they were removed by dehydration. England concluded that the NMJs encouraged the formation of small ice crystals, probably within the glycoprotein EL matrix.

Myofiber EL is insoluble in dilute acids and alcohols and is dehydrated to thin strands without dissolution by chloroform-methanol. Collagenase failed to attack the isolated EL material though it was attacked by pronase and by papain especially after boiling. Hydrolysis with 3N HCl yielded a clear colorless solution. Amino acid analysis of LIS extracted components of EL revealed small amounts of glycine and proline but no hydroxyproline and a considerable quantity of glutamic and aspartic acids. Since isolated, precipitated LIS-extracted EL stains with PAS, alcian blue and ruthenium red, it appears that this material containing carboxylic amino acids is responsible for many of the staining properties of whole sarcolemmal tubes. This material is 94.3% protein and contains less than 0.5% carbohydrate. Thus myofiber EL differs considerably from glomerular basement lamina (Lazarow and Speidel, 1964; Bruchhausen and Merker, 1967; Misra and Berman, 1968). The accumulated data is consistent with the interpretation that myofiber EL contains an acidic protein linked to small amounts of carbohydrate as well as a collagen-like component not extracted by LIS. It is likely that the carboxyl groups of acidic amino acids and/or uronic acids, are responsible for cation binding. We may speculate that these sites may normally be occupied by Ca++ and represent some of the Ca++ released during muscle stimulation (Csillik, 1963). However, cations may also bind to the underlying external leaflet of the myofiber plasma membrane which has been shown to bind colloidal iron. In this connection the physiologic action of uranyl ions (Nastuk, 1967) and lanthanum (Miledi, 1971) on NMJs are of considerable interest. These sites may be more directly involved in the binding of biologically active molecules.

6

The Postsynaptic Membrane of the Neuromuscular Junction

The Subcellular Structure of the Myofiber Cell Membrane

With the exception of the specialized features to be discussed below, the myofiber cell membrane within the subneural apparatus is now recognized to closely resemble unit membranes covering other kinds of cells.

Review of the electron microscopic literature reveals considerable initial disagreement concerning the ultrastructure of the myofiber cell membrane. Bennett and Porter (1955) wrote of the surface layer of the muscle cell (100 A) as the "sarcolemma", apparently excluding the EL material. However, the sarcolemma has long been known to include not only the muscle cell membrane but also a considerable amount of adjacent connective tissue (Peterfi, 1913). Ruska (1954) described two dense lines in the myofiber membrane measuring about 300 A in width which therefore included the EL as a part of the "sarcolemma". On the other hand, Robertson (1955a) referred to the "surface membrane complex" because he was uncertain of the nature of the amorphous material (EL) on the surface of the myofiber and therefore included the entire layer as the cell membrane.

In a most useful early discussion of the ultrastructure of cell membranes and their derivatives, Robertson (1959) pointed out some of the problems of interpretation facing the electron microscopist who

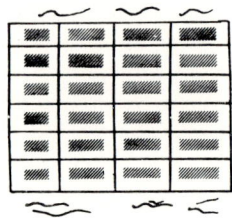
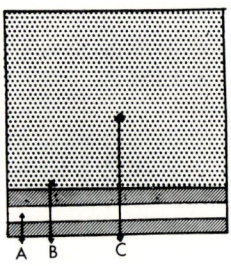

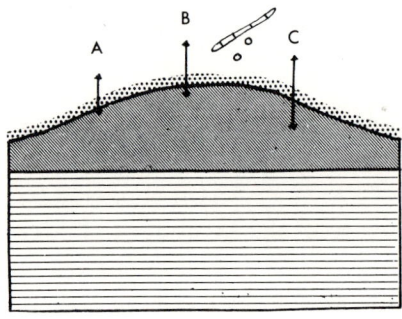

Figure 62. Diagram relating structures visible in the light microscope with membrane structures revealed by the higher resolving power of the electron microscope. In 1, representing the myofiber at approximately 3,600X, collagen fibers and connective tissue are shown as wavey lines at top and bottom and sarcoplasm by the cross hatched squares. The dark line at the top and bottom of the muscle cell represents the cell "membrane". In 2, a low power electron micrograph shows the muscle cell membrane as a complex consisting of a dense inner membrane covered with amorphous external lamina indicated by the stipled area. The membrane may be regarded as the sum of the inner dense membrane, the external lamina and varying amounts of external connective tissue *(A)*; or it may include the surface dense membrane, the external lamina and a larger amount of external connective tissue *(B)*; or as in C it may include a variable amount of the cytoplasmic component beneath the superficial dense line. At greater resolution *(3)*, which represents the surface membrane at 1,000,000X, the dense surface membrane is now resolved into 3 components: 2 dense areas (shaded) and a central low density area represented in white. External lamina is shown in the stipled area. Therefore the membrane might be regarded as the outer single leaflet *A*, the unit *B*, or the unit plus a variable amount of external lamina *(C)*. The "unit membrane" concept refers to the membrane indicated at *B*. (From Robertson, Ultrastructure of Cell Membranes and their Derivatives, *in* The Structure and Function of Subcellular Components, Biochemical Society Symposium (Crook, E.M., ed.) Cambridge University Press, New York, 1959.)

attempts to clarify membrane relations within NMJs. Figure 62, modified after Robertson, illustrates the problems inherent in the interpretation of cellular membranes at various levels of resolution. At 3600 X, the classic characteristics of a myofiber are shown, with A bands and the muscle surface membrane appearing as dense lines in routinely stained preparations. The myofiber cell "membrane" in this preparation appears to be approximately $0.18\,\mu$ or 1800 A wide. When the electron microscope is used, an increase in resolution of approximately two orders of magnitude is obtained. This greatly increased resolution reveals more detail but also raises problems of definition of the "membrane".

At relatively low magnification (50,000 to 100,000 diameters), the cell membrane in conventionally fixed material is composed of two components: an outer, somewhat amorphous granular material of low electron density and an inner, electron-dense line that has been called the "plasma membrane" (deHarven and Coërs, 1959) and the "sarcoplasmatic membrane" (Gutmann and Young, 1944). The "membrane" seen by optical microscopy must include the outer amorphous layer, the dense inner layer, and considerable portions of the external intercellular connective tissue, as well as internal sarcoplasm. Gutmann and Young (1944) recognized that the so-called "sarcolemma" was composed chiefly of endomysium. They described two layers: the "sarcoplasmatic membrane", or muscle plasma membrane, and the thicker connective tissue layer visible in the optical microscope. This fact had been clearly stated as early as 1913 by Peterfi, who recognized that the sarcolemma was composed of supposed "connective tissue" and was therefore not part of the muscle cell. We could decide that the inner, dense line should be called the "plasma membrane" of the "cell membrane", or we might select the double-layered system as the "cell membrane", however indistinct the outer amorphous layer might be. However, higher resolution electron microscopy demonstrates failure of even this simple alternative. At greater resolution, the inner, electron-dense layer is resolved into three layers: an innermost, dense layer of approximately 25 A in width; a middle, less dense layer of approximately the same width; and an external, dense layer of similar width (25 A) that lies adjacent to the outer, amorphous EL material. Here again the question arises which layer is to be regarded as the "membrane". We might regard the innermost dense line at the "membrane", or we might include the middle line and the outermost line in the "membrane". We could also include some or all of the external layer of amorphous material. Robertson (1959) concluded that the "unit membrane" complex, consisting of the dense inner, the less dense middle, and the dense outer "membrane" measuring approximately 75 to 100 A in total width, should be regarded as the "cell membrane".

Sjostrand and Rhodin (1953) and Sjostrand and Hanzon (1954) studied the localization of lipid layers in the double membrane complex and suggested that the low density of 100 to 150 A represented organized lipid layers. However, Robertson (1957) stated that the light areas were more likely to be composed of protein.

It is now known that double membranes are commonly seen in electron micrographs in many sites after osmium fixation. Intercellular boundaries, nuclear membranes, the endoplasmic reticulum, the Golgi complex, the axon-Schwann cell membrane, mesaxons, and synaptic membranes all have this structure. More recent work has also revealed a thin "cell coat" covering the external leaflet of most cell (unit) membranes (Rambourg, 1971).

Specialized Structure of Myofiber Cell Membrane in Neuromuscular Junctions

As discussed in general terms in chapter 6, the myofiber cell membrane underlying the terminal axon in the NMJ has characteristic ultrastructural features that distinguish it from non-innervated areas. Typically, the cell membrane is folded forming clefts 0.5 to 1μ deep and 0.5 to 0.7μ wide that greatly increase and membrane surface area under the terminal axon. The number, width and extent of the clefts differ in different species and in different kinds of muscle. Several attempts have been made to correlate the degree of folding of the myofiber cell membrane in the subneural apparatus with the speed of myofiber contraction. Hess (1961) and Hess and Pilar (1963) have claimed that twitch myofibers have en plaque NMJs with extensive subneural folding and that tonic myofibers with multiple en grappe endings have few subneural folds (Hess, 1961, 1965; Hess and Pilar, 1963; Pilar and Hess, 1966). However there are numerous exceptions (Gray, 1957; Nakajima, 1969; Reger, 1961). For example, Hess in 1966 showed that avian iris muscle has twitch myofibers, yet the NMJs were of the en grappe type and Bergman (1967) showed that the twitch myofibers of the seahorse lack folds in the subneural apparatus as in other twitch fibers. In this species, 0.75 to 1.5μ axons with many electron lucent synaptic vesicles lie in a shallow depression separated by a 750 A gap filled with external lamina. No subneural folds were present in the subneural area. Ogata et al. (1967), Ogata and Murata (1969), Padykula and Gauthier (1970) reported differences in the structure of the subneural apparatus in en plaque NMJs on red, white and intermediate myofibers. In general, white myofibers have more numerous and complex infoldings of the myofiber plasma membrane in the subneural apparatus whereas red muscle NMJs have shallow and infrequent subneural clefts.

Membrane Thickening in the Subneural Apparatus

Analogous to the membrane specializations present in central nervous system synapses, the postsynaptic membrane of typical en plaque NMJs has an area of thickening that appears to be composed of electron dense material attached to the inner membrane leaflet (Figs. 38, 39). In chick sartorius muscle NMJs, the area of postsynaptic thickening is 300 × 750 A (Hirano, 1966) and similar dimensions are found in the NMJs of other species. Membrane thickening also occurs in en grappe NMJs in rat extraocular muscle despite the absence of subneural clefts (Teräväinen, 1968) and in some invertebrate NMJs (page 114).

Postsynaptic membrane thickening is the earliest sign of definitive NMJ formation as the terminal axon approaches the myofiber surface membrane during embryogensis of NMJs (Kelly and Zacks, 1968, 1969) (Fig. 25) and is the first indication of *de novo* formation of NMJs in cross innervated muscle (Zacks and Saito, 1968). Lentz (1969) has also observed that membrane thickening indicates the earliest formation of NMJs in regenerating newt muscle.

Connections between Subneural Clefts and the T System

Although occasional outpouchings of the cell membrane within the clefts have been observed by many investigators and anastomoses occur in some species, use of lanthanum as a tracer is required to demonstrate connections between the synaptic clefts and elements of the T system in the soleplate sarcoplasm (Zacks and Saito, 1970). These are narrow (150 × 1000 A) channels lacking EL that extend from the

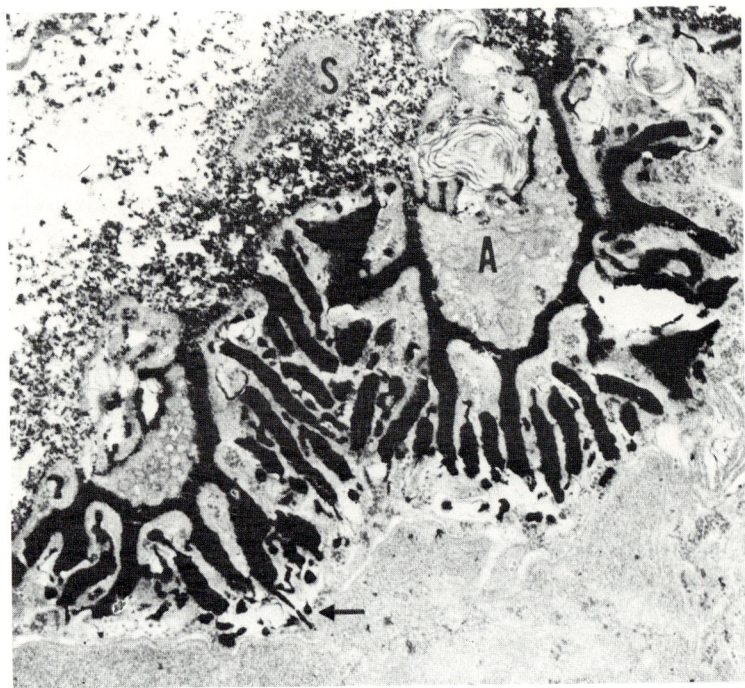

Figure 63. Electron micrograph of mouse neuromuscular junction after impregnation with lanthanum. Note the subneural apparatus filled with electron dense lanthanum particles and elongated tubular structures extending toward T elements in the sarcoplasm (arrow). The axon is indicated at A and Schwann cell cytoplasm is shown at S. (X 24,600.)

depths of the secondary clefts to the T tubules (Figs. 63, 64). Occasionally, these channels appear to be multiple with more than one channel to a single T tubule. These structures were not demonstrated in experiments with ruthenium red and horseradish peroxidase (Zacks and Saito, 1969) used as a tracer probably due to the absence of EL in the tubules that is required for ruthenium red staining and the larger size and surface charge of the peroxidase tracer molecules. It is likely that the intimate relationship between the postsynaptic membrane and the T system plays an important role in the channeling of the wave of depolarization from the subneural apparatus to the contractile elements of the myofiber and the binding of lanthanum to these membranes may indicate sites of Ca^{++} binding because lanthanum ions should be expected to displace bound calcium ions (Leffvin et al., 1964). Furthermore, we suspect that since the subneural apparatus appears to arise during embryogenesis from surface invagination of vesicles with subsequent fusing, it is likely that connections between the secondary

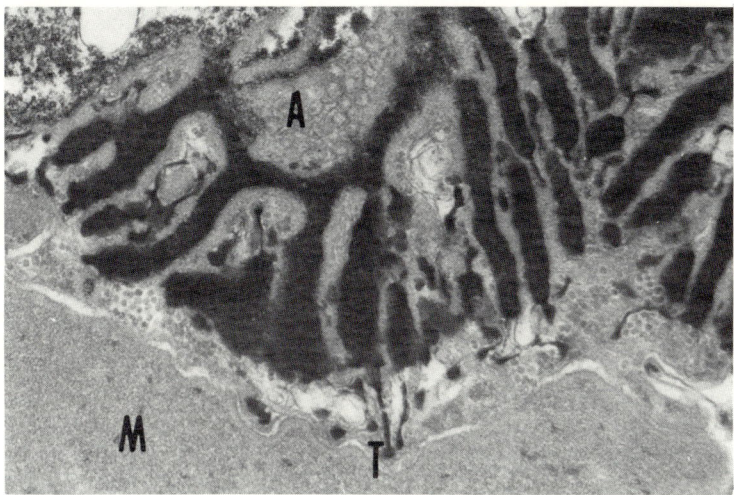

Figure 64. Electron micrograph at higher magnification illustrating lanthanum filled elongated structures extending from the subneural apparatus to elements of the T system. The axon is at A and the myofibers at M. (X 30,000.)

synaptic clefts and the T system are established at the time of NMJ differentiation.

Lead Reactive Substance and Membrane Birefringence

With the exception of areas of membrane thickening, the myofiber cell membrane appears structurally unremarkable in the electron microscope. However, specialized techniques have revealed some properties that may be of functional significance. Csillik (1963) reported that the birefringence conferred on unfixed postsynaptic membranes by lead staining, could be used to investigate the physicochemical properties of the resting and stimulated cell membrane (Fig. 65).

By using mounting media of differing refractive index, Csillik (1963) measured the optic retardation with a polarizing microscope. Plots of the retardation values against refractive index produced "imbibition" curves. In fresh untreated frog muscles, slight transient birefringence was observed in the synaptic area. This was prevented by freezing or formalin fixation. After lead nitrate fixation, strong birefringence was present in the post-synaptic area, but myofibers and myelin were unaltered. The birefringence in frog NMJs appeared within lamellas 3 to 8μ in length arranged in palisade-like rows, that were

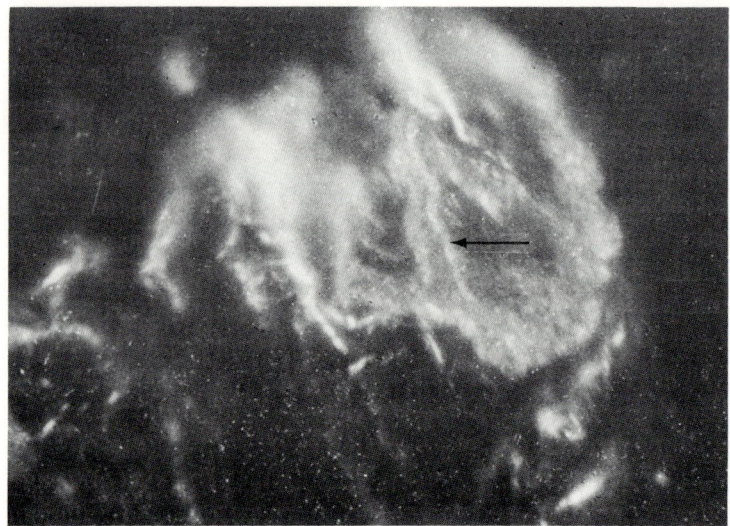

Figure 65. Photomicrograph of a rat NMJ illustrating birefringence of the lead impregnated subneural apparatus. Note that the birefringence is confined to the edges of the clefts. (X 1,000.) (From Csillik, 1963.)

interpreted as part of the subneural apparatus. The birefringence of the folds was positive with respect to their long axis.

When the muscle sections were examined in gum arabic solution (n=1.52), the degree of retardation reached 15 to 18 mμ . Imbibition curves plotted from individual NMJs produced a convex curve never reaching zero at its minimum. Such an imbibition curve is characteristic of structures possessing both form and intrinsic birefringence (Schmidt, 1938). Figure 66 illustrates a typical plot.

Partial extraction of the lipids from the tissue with warm acetone enhanced the optical retardation. The form of the plots was similar but the values were higher. This suggested that the lipids are arranged within the folds in a form similar to other membrane structures and that they lie transverse to the nonlipid part of the complex. On the basis of the form birefringence observed, the micelles in the membrane were thought to lie parallel to the long axis of the synaptic folds.

Csillik found that the birefringence pattern of mammalian NMJs differed from the pattern observed in the frog. In rat diaphragm preparations, where the form of the subneural clefts differs from that of the frog, only the edges of the junctional folds were birefringent and the bottom or central portion of the synaptic gutter was optically inactive. Imbibition curves obtained from rat NMJ were similar to those

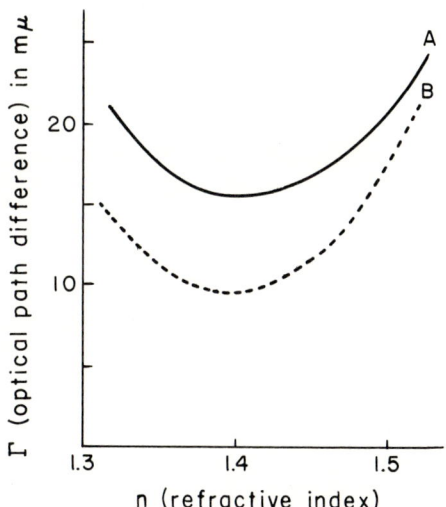

Figure 66. Inbibition curves of junctional clefts in rat diaphragm muscle. Curve A was obtained before treatment with acetone; and curve B after treatment with acetone. (From Csillik, 1963.)

obtained from frog NMJs; both form and intrinsic birefringence was present.

When frog gastrocnemius and rat plantar muscles were subjected to supramaximal electrical stimuli and the NMJs studied in polarized light after lead fixation, no difference between the control and experimental muscles could be identified. Yet when imbibition experiments were performed, a distinct difference was observed. Unlike the controls, lipid extraction of the stimulated NMJs resulted in decreased retardation of polarization instead of the normally expected increase. The imbibition curve declined to zero in frog NMJs and to a minimum of 3 to 4 millimicrons in rat NMJs (Fig. 66). This type of curve indicated that form birefringence predominated and that intrinsic birefringence was minimal. Therefore, electrical stimulation did not appear to alter the micellar organization of the postsynaptic membrane but did alter its intramicellar or molecular organization. Csillik suggested that regular arrangement of polypeptide chains present before stimulation became irregular after stimulation. The organization of lipid molecules also appeared to be altered as a result of supramaximal stimulation.

Experiments employing Ach and eserine also yielded interesting results. When frog muscles were treated with solutions of Ach, the imbibition curves of the experimental and control animals were identical. After lipid extraction, however, increased birefringence, normally observed in control preparations, was also observed in the Ach-treated NMJs. When muscle containing NMJs was exposed to solutions of

Ach (10^{-3}M) containing eserine (10^{-4}M), the imbibition curves resembled those obtained with supramaximal electrical stimuli. Application of eserine alone had no effect. Soaking the muscles in neostigmine also produced alterations in the polarization optical characteristics of the postsynaptic membranes similar to those obtained with electrical stimulation or with treatment with mixtures of Ach and eserine. The only difference was that extraction of lipids with acetone produced a less pronounced decrease in birefringence.

When the sciatic nerve was cut in a series of rats and muscles were fixed with lead nitrate and examined in the polarizing microscope, strong birefringence in the region of the subneural apparatus was present after the tenth postoperative day. The imbibition curves showed marked changes, characterized by higher peaks than normal and decreased birefringence following lipid extraction, that were interpreted as evidence of major molecular alterations in the birefringent material. The less steep curves obtained suggested to Csillik that the micelles were shortened.

Csillik concluded that the post-synaptic membrane contains lipoprotein, on the basis of the acetone extraction experiments and the observation that prior freezing and formalin fixation destroyed the birefringence, precedures known to disorganize lipoproteins. Csillik (1963) also stated that a modified Sudan B-staining method also stained the subneural apparatus indicating the presence of lipids.

In a later investigation, Jod́ et al. (1965) employed a variety of lipid staining methods and a Rivanol precipitation method to study tissue anisotropy as a means of investigating the lipoprotein in the postsynaptic membrane. The subneural apparatus stained with Sudan black, a known phospholipid stain but not with Sudan III, Oil red, Nile blue and Phosphine all of which stain neutral fat. Since acetone extraction failed to remove the Sudan black staining material, the authors concluded that staining was due to lipoproteins. Rivanol-induced birefringence was interpreted as the result of parallel orientation of the dye molecules with lipid particles (Romhanyi and Jobst, 1956). These observations are consistent with the known lipid content of cell membranes.

The major question raised by these studies is the relationship of the birefringent structures observed in the polarizing microscope to the fine structure of the subneural apparatus. Polarized light photographs of lead-fixed NMJs in the original study (Csillik, 1963) do not show sufficient detail to permit a conclusion as to what elements of the

NMJ are birefringent. Certainly the general region of the subneural apparatus is birefringent, but we cannot be certain whether the muscle surface membrane of the synaptic clefts or the EL within them is responsible for the birefringence. Csillik concluded that the EL material within the clefts was not the site of binding of the lead-reactive material. He based this conclusion on his observation that PAS stainability disappeared five to eight days after denervation, and that therefore this material could not be the part of the subneural apparatus that was stained. These observations are subject to other interpretations. Electron microscopic studies (Reger, 1959; Bauer et al., 1962; Saito and Zacks, 1969a, b) have shown that both the EL and the myofiber cell membrane persist for a long time after denervation and Csillik and Davis (1964), Kelly and Zacks (1965) and Zacks et al. (1972) have shown that the major site of lead binding by unfixed NMJs is the EL. We have also found that PAS and ruthenium red staining persists in denervated mouse NMJs. The possibility remains that noncrystalline lead binding also occur in the myofiber cell membrane as suggested by Csillik (1963) and Zacks and Blumberg (1961a) under the conditions of staining with lead recommended by Csillik and that this relatively small quantity confers the birefringence observed despite the large quantities of lead that may be bound by the overlying EL.

Csillik (1963) hypothesized that intrinsic changes in birefringence following supramaximal electrical stimulation are due to alterations in the protein micelles in the membrane during activity and might be the basis for changes in ionic fluxes through the synaptic membrane, which are thought to occur during neuromuscular transmission. A similar result obtained with Ach combined with eserine might be caused by temporary coupling of Ach to the protein of the receptor substance in the postsynaptic membrane, leading to molecular deformation, a mechanism of coupling producing alteration of protein structure suggested by Nachmansohn (1955). Csillik suggested that the lead-reactive material may be the Ach receptor described by Langley (1909). To support this argument, he cited his observation that neostigmine produces changes in the birefringence of the postsynaptic membrane, whereas there were no changes in the polarization optical properties of the membrane after application of eserine or tubocurarine. Thus substances that depolarize the membrane (Ach plus eserine) alter the orientation of the membrane micelles, whereas nondepolarizing agents (tubocurarine) do not alter the micellar orientation and therefore do not alter the membrane birefringence. Csillik suggested that the changes observed after denervation indicate a subtle alteration in the postsynaptic membrane that makes the intrinsic lipids less resistant to solvent extraction. Although subject to several serious questions, especially concerning the precise localization of the lead-reactive material, these ingenious experiments have provided the first experimental approach to possible molecular derangements of the postsynaptic membrane. If changes in polarization optical characteristics of the membrane can be better localized and more easily repeated, this method should be of great value in studying NMJs in neuromuscular disease. These interesting techniques have proven difficult to use in our laboratory, and this is the probable reason why this work has not been used by other workers.

Csillik concluded that the subneural clefts contain both lead-reactive material and AchE. He did not believe that the AchE was responsible for lead binding because AchE survived freezing and formalin fixation, whereas lead binding by the subneural apparatus was reduced or abolished by these procedures. Current data indicates that the enzyme is probably located in the postsynaptic membrane or the narrow cell coat covering the external leaflet of the cell membrane rather than in the outer thicker layer of the myofiber external lamina.

7

The Soleplate of Neuromuscular Junctions

The soleplate is the area of modified sarcoplasm beneath the junctional membrane. The unique characteristics which distinguish it from sarcoplasm in non-innervated sites was recognized in the earliest studies of NMJs.

Mitochondria in the Soleplate

The junctional sarcoplasm was known to contain numerous granules from the early studies of Rouget (1862, 1864) and Kŭhne (1887). Later studies (Boeke and Noël, 1925; Noël, 1950), in which mitochondrial stains were used, led to the conclusion that the granules were mitochondria and this was later confirmed by electron microscopy. These mitochondria contain few transverse cristae and a small number of intramitochondrial dense granules. They resemble mitochondria present in non-innervated regions of the myofiber.

Soleplate Granules

In addition to mitochondria, the soleplate sarcoplasm contains scattered electron-dense granules measuring approximately 150 A which are visible only in the electron microscope. These granules occasionally occur in clusters but show no particular relationship to any of the other components of the soleplate. Soleplate granules were observed in NMJs of the frog (Birks et al., 1960), the mouse (Reger, 1954, 1958, 1959; Zacks and Blumberg, 1961a; Andersson-Cedergren, 1959), the lizard (Robertson, 1956), and in man (de Harven and Coërs, 1959). Granules with similar dimensions described by Edwards (1959) in insect neuromuscular junctions were called "aposynaptic granules." Reger (1958) suggested that the granules were glycogen, in accordance with the observations of Fawcett (1958). However, many of the particles are ribonucleoprotein (ribosomes), as suggested by Andersson-Cedergren (1959) and confirmed subsequently by many investigators. Staining with lead citrate perferentially increases the contrast of the glycogen particles whereas uranyl acetate stains the ribosomes more intensely.

Periterminal Network

None of the students of NMJ fine structure have found evidence of fibrils in the junctional sarcoplasm forming attachments to the myofiber Z bands, despite the suggestion of Reger (1955) that the penetration of the "Z membranes" extended for an indefinite distance into the soleplate sarcoplasm. Electron microscopic investigations have also failed to show evidence of Boeke's (1911, 1932) "periterminal network," a system of neurofibrils that were once thought to connect the terminal nerve fiber to the underlying myofibrils. Although neurotubules and thin filaments are present in terminal axons, there are no filaments traversing the synaptic gap in NMJs.

Golgi Apparatus

Although the Golgi apparatus is a component of striated muscle, and Andersson-Cedergren (1959) illustrated this structure within the soleplate sarcoplasm, it is not a prominent feature. Occasional straight or coiled pairs of electron dense membranes 70-80 A in width are also found randomly scattered in the soleplate. These are segments of smooth endoplasmic reticulum. They are probably part of the interfibrillar sarcotubular system.

Vesicles in the Soleplate

Various vesicular structures occur in the soleplate. Outpouchings and anastomoses of the secondary synaptic clefts often appear as empty thin walled vesicular profiles. Also, occasional coated vesicles are present in the soleplate sarcoplasm. These are easily recognized in NMJs dually fixed by glutaraldehyde and osmium (Fig. 37) and are easily found in tracer studies utilizing horseradish peroxidase.

Thin channels connecting the depths of the secondary synaptic clefts to superficial elements of the T system are also demonstrated when lanthanum is used as a tracer (Fig. 63, 64) but are not seen otherwise.

8

Invertebrate Neuromuscular Junctions

Since the first edition of this monograph, sufficient information about the structure and physiology of invertebrate NMJ has accumulated to warrant a discussion of this subject. Although neuromuscular transmission in invertebrates differs significantly from transmission in vertebrates, a description of various kinds of invertebrate NMJs may yield useful comparative data.

Davis et al. (1968) described simple apposition junctions between ganglionic cells and epithelio-muscular cells of Hydra. No specialized synaptic features were found with the exception of possible increased membrane density. The presynaptic terminal lacked synaptic vesicles.

Apparently the first occurrence of NMJ analagous to those which occur in vertebrates is in worms. For example, the motor innervation of the segmental muscle of *Nereis* is polyneuronal and multiterminal similar to that seen in arthropods. The structure of the nerve endings is similar to the en grappe fibers that occur in some vertebrate muscles. These muscles are capable of fast twitch-like contractions to effect escape and slower graded contractions that are associated with ambulation (Dorsett, 1964). In a study of *Ascaris,* Reger (1965) observed peculiar long processes extending from the body wall cells. These processes arose from the basal myofibrils and ended on dorsal and ventral nerves. The myofibers appeared to be extending to the nervous system instead of the usual circumstance where the nervous tissue extends to the muscle. Several of these muscle processes were in apposition on a single axon with an intervening synaptic cleft of 350-500 A. Layered membranes were present in both the axon and the sarcoplasm forming a triple 75-80 A complex. Electron dense patches were present at intervals along the opposed membranes due to increased thickness of the intermembrane leaflets similar to the junctional membrane specialization that occurs in vertebrates. At NMJ, there was close apposition of the membranes forming a 5 layered 170-200 A complex. Presynaptic endings contained mitochondria, microtubules and two kinds of vesicles. The first, measuring 200-600 A, had a single 3 layered membrane and a central area of low density whereas the larger vesicles measuring 600-1200 A contained a dense 500-800 A central granule. The postsynaptic area had occasional, elongated and branched myofiber membrane invaginations. The "close junctions" in this synapse suggested the possibility of electronic transmission at these sites (Jarman, 1959) although the presence of two kinds of synaptic vesicles would indicate that neurohumoral transmission probably also occurs. Similar structure is seen in the larval ascidian tail (Tannenbaum and Rosenbluth, 1972).

Histochemical studies failed to show ChE activity in lamellibranch (mollusc) nervous systems (Nagy and Salanki, 1965) yet the enzyme does occur in the sarcolemma and endomysium of *Anodonta* (Kerkut and Cottrell, 1963). This enzyme is more common in gastropods.

Barrantes (1970) described the fine structure of NMJs in the tentacle of the slug *Vaginula soleiformis*. One kind of nerve ending consisted of a presynaptic element separated from the sarcolemma by a primary synaptic cleft. Projections of the sarcolemma containing sarcoplasm extended into deep invaginations of the presynaptic terminal. Profiles resembling synaptic vesicles as well as larger bodies measuring 855 A containing dense granules were also present. The other kind of ending consisted of a presynaptic element closely opposed to the sarcolemma with a simple intervening synaptic cleft. The presynaptic terminal contained clear vesicles as well as larger (1190 A) vesicles enclosing large, dense granules. There were numerous subsarcolemmal cisterns on the postsynaptic surface that were interpreted as possibly analagous to the T system of skeletal myofibers. The most primitive type of nerve-muscle ending in lamellibranches was described by Graziadei and de Rubeis (1963) who observed simple expanded neural processes lying on the surface of unipolar cells in the mantle of *Ostrea*. No NMJs could be demonstrated and no attempt was made to show esterase activity. Lacking fine structure data, there is no information concerning membrane specializations.

A fine structure study of the innervation of tentacles in *Helix* and *Limax* smooth muscle, (Rogers, 1968) demonstrated close junctions with single, usually naked axons and cytoplasmic intrusions of the muscle. The presynaptic axons contained both 500 A and 800-1000 A vesicles. Some of the axons appeared to form multiple, simultaneous close junctions in addition to the membranes separated by a synaptic gap of 200 A. External lamina filled the gap between the presynaptic and postsynaptic membranes in these simple synapses. However, no cell membrane specializations were demonstrated in either pre- or postsynaptic membranes. A very primitive arrangement of innervation was demonstrated in an ultrastructure study of the sucker of octopus by Graziadei (1965, 1966). In this location, optical microscopy and ultrastructure studies demonstrated fine nerve fibers innervating the helical smooth muscles. These neurites, measuring 0.1 to 1μ in diameter, were enclosed in a common Schwann-like cell. The thin nerve fibers ran in free contact with the myofiber surface or within a groove in the surface of the myofibers. In some cases, up to 5 nerve fibers ran through tunnels in the myofiber enclosed by a mesaxon-like structure that was formed by enfolding of the myofiber surface membrane. These nerve branches contained synaptic vesicles, mitochondria and had increased membrane density in the area where the nerve and muscle membranes were opposed. The synaptic vesicles in the axons also tended to clump near the apposed 200 A membrane complex. The width of the synaptic gap was of the order of 100 A. Peculiar perpendicular structures crossed some of the gaps between the apposed membranes. In all junctions, the postsynaptic membrane was in close relationship to sarcoplasmic reticulum. Loe and Florey (1966) found both Ach and ChE activity in the nervous system and other structures of octopus but were not able to demonstrate cholinergic transmission with certainty.

Myofiber innervation is relatively simple in crustacea. Cohen and Hess (1967) described NMJs in "fast" and "slow" crab muscles. The number of Schwann cell processes were diminished as the terminal axon approached the muscle surface and some of the processes spread out over the surface of the myofibers. The terminal axon, containing mitochondria and synaptic vesicles, and still covered by Schwann cell processes lay in a deep invagination of the muscle surface. There were occasional dense thickenings of the apposed axon and myofiber plasma membranes and synaptic vesicles appeared to be aggregated in such areas. In the subneural area were occasional invaginations of the myofiber cell membrane but no regular system of clefts as those which occur in vertebrate NMJs. All the myofibers, both "fast" and "slow", had multiple nerve terminations although they were most numerous on "fast" myofibers (Fig. 39A). In a study of the eye raising muscle, Hoyle and McNeill (1968) demonstrated axons lying losely within Schwann-like cells that came to lie in simple grooves or invaginations of the underlying myofibers. In some instances, the axons lay deeper within the myofibers in a space formed by extension of the myofiber cell membrane. Both pre- and postsynaptic membranes were thickened in regions of apparent synapses. However, no secondary synaptic clefts were present. A similar situation where nerve endings are buried in simple clefts or embedded beneath the surface was demonstrated in an ultrastructure study by Atwood and Johnston (1968). In their investigation of the fast motor innervation of the crab *Pachygrapsus crassipes,* they found low density synaptic vesicles, thickening of pre- and postsynaptic membranes but no secondary synaptic clefts in the NMJs.

There has been considerable interest in the morphology of lobster NMJs because of the physiologic evidence indicating the existence of both excitatory and inhibitory endings (Fields and Kennedy, 1965; Alexandrowicz, 1967). Peterson and Pepe (1961) concluded that there were no morphologic differences between excitatory and inhibitory axodendritic synapses but Uchizono (1967) found that crayfish excitatory motor endings had round synaptic vesicle profiles whereas inhibitory endings in the central nervous system had oval or elongated synaptic vesicle profiles. Nadol and DeLorenzo (1968) also found anatomic evidence for two kinds of lobster NMJs. One contained spherical synaptic vesicles (500-900 A) and the other had elongated vesicles (200 × 400-600 A) similar to the axodendritic presynaptic endings present in the central nervous system. Nadol and DeLorenzo suggested that the endings containing elongated vesicles were inhibitory and that the endings containing spherical synaptic vesicles were excitatory. One kind of lobster NMJ had both pre- and postsynaptic membrane thickenings but neither kind had secondary synaptic clefts.

Sherman and Fourtner (1972) described multi-terminal innervation of the walking leg of the horseshoe crab *Limulus polyphemus.* These junctions consisted of an evagination of myofiber sarcoplasm, multiple axon branches and accompanying glial cells. As in other arthropod NMJs, the fine structure of the synapse was characterized by closely apposed pre- and postsynaptic membranes, presynaptic clustering of a granular synaptic vesicle and an extensive postsynaptic complex in the myofiber. Lang (1972) has described the fine structure of several kinds of NMJs in *Limulus* heart.

There is some evidence of cholinergic transmission in the insect central nervous system but the NMJs are not cholinergic (Treherne and Smith, 1965; Hill and Usherwood, 1961; Usherwood and Grundfest, 1965).

In the locust NMJ, a terminal axon containing electron lucent synaptic vesicles is separated by a gap less than 200 A wide containing dense material. The postsynaptic membrane lacks specialized structure. In general, NMJs in orthoptera have a simple synapse without a subneural apparatus. However, small mitochondria and moderate numbers of synaptic vesicles are present in the presynaptic axon (Faeder et al., 1970).

In amphioxus, Flood (1966) has described complex NMJs consisting of projections from muscle fibers to the surface of the spinal cord. The ventral root fibers of muscle origin are interconnected by many "tight" junctions and terminate as conical expansions on the surface of the spinal cord. There is an intervening cleft filled with EL that separates the myofiber cell processes from numerous boutons arising from the cord axons.

Rosenbluth (1972) has described the fine structure of two kinds of NMJ in the earth worm body wall muscle. Type I junctions resemble cholinergic junctions in vertebrates whereas type II junctions resemble adrenergic junctions present in vertebrate smooth muscle.

9

Esterases in Neuromuscular Junctions

The existence of an enzyme responsible for the destruction of the humoral transmitter in the vicinity of NMJs was suspected by Loewi (1921, 1922) early in his studies of the "vagusstoff" and was later demonstrated by Loewi and Navratil (1926a) and Marnay and Nachmansohn (1937) found that there was enough AchE in the NMJ region of the frog to destroy the calculated amount of secreted Ach during the few milliseconds of the refractory period. Similar studies by Feng and Ting (1938) led to the same conclusions for the toad. Couteaux and Nachmansohn (1940) demonstrated that portions of skeletal muscle that had a high concentration of NMJs also contained the most AchE and although there was some AchE activity in the terminal nerve branches, most of the enzyme activity was localized in the subneural region. Microchemical investigations by Boell and Nachmansohn (1940) confirmed earlier data that AchE was intimately associated with NMJs.

HISTOCHEMICAL DEMONSTRATION OF ESTERASES IN NEUROMUSCULAR JUNCTIONS

An ideal histochemical method for demonstration of esterase activity should use a physiologic rapidly hydrolyzed substrate that can be converted into an insoluble fine grained colored or electron dense product. The method should be suitable for frozen sections to avoid possible inhibition by fixatives and conditions of temperature and ionic concentration, pH, and other factors optimal for enzyme activity should not be too different from conditions suitable for the reaction designed to produce the final pigment. Of course, if a coupling agent is used, it should not inhibit the enzyme. Although numerous basic procedures, each with several modifications have been proposed and used for staining of esterases in NMJs, the localization and kinds of esterases in this location remains complex and controversial. It proved difficult to prepare synthetic substrates with ideal properties largely due to the quaternary "head" that characterizes substrates resembling the normal activator, Ach. The quaternary group of these molecules limits penetration of the substrate before hydrolysis by the enzymes and encourages diffusion before and after hydrolysis. Thus, negatively charged structures, such as the nucleus, bind such charged complexes because of their phosphate groups. Substrate molecules that lack the quaternary "head" are not physiologic and may also fail to meet ideal requirements for other reasons.

ESTERASE ACTIVITY IN NEUROMUSCULAR JUNCTIONS

An early attempt by Gomori (1945) to demonstrate lipase activity utilized esterified fatty acids and hexitol anhydrides derived from sorbitol (Tweens) as substrates. The fatty acids liberated by enzymatic hydrolysis were precipitated as calcium soaps. These in turn were converted to lead soaps, which were made visible in tissue sections by conversion to lead sulfide. Tween 60 (stearic ester of polymannitol) and Tween 80 (oleic acid ester of polymannitol) were used, the latter particularly for "true" lipase. For NMJ cholinesterases, Gomori (1948) recommended myristoyl choline as a substrate. Thin tissue slices were embedded in celloidin and paraffin after fixation in cold acetone. Sections from these blocks were then incubated for periods up to 16 hours at 37°C. in a buffer solution (pH 7.5) containing myristoyl choline, cobalt, calcium, magnesium and manganous ions. The hydrolysis product, fatty acid combined with cobalt, was made visible by treating the sections with yellow ammonium sulfide.

Several practical and theoretical limitations of this procedure soon became evident. Gomori showed that rat brain extracts, containing considerable AchE activity (Mendel and Rudney, 1943) failed to hydrolyze the higher choline esters. Furthermore, purified red cell and electric organ AchE did not hydrolyze myristoyl choline. Adams and Whittaker (1949) concluded that myristoyl choline (a C_{14} acid) was hydrolyzed by ChE but not AchE, whereas Koelle and Friedenwald (1949) believed that the myristoyl choline method demonstrated only "nonspecific esterases." Later experience indicated that acetone destroyed cholinesterase activity and at least part of the difficulty in demonstrating cholinesterase by this method was due to varying degrees of inhibition of the enzyme prior to hydrolysis of the substrate. Thus staining of NMJs by the myristoyl choline method yields uncertain results.

This early attempt at AchE localization required long incubation periods and produced rather diffuse staining of NMJs as judged by later standards.

Azo Dye Methods

Because of the problems encountered in utilizing a chromogenic substrates resembling the natural substrate Ach, other methods were designed, which utilized the acetyl esterase function of AchE. Mendel and Rudney (1943) had demonstrated that tributyrin and methyl butyrate are hydrolyzed by AchE at low rates, and Bodansky (1946) added triacetin to the list of substrates attacked by AchE. Other substances hydrolyzed by AchE include ethylchloroacetate (Myers and Mendel, 1949), β-naphthyl acetate (Ravin et al., 1953), and indoxyl acetate (Barrnett and Seligman, 1951). All these investigators showed that AchE would hydrolyze substrates other than Ach. These esterases were inhibited by physostigmine and diisofluorophsphate (DFP) in appropriate concentrations, justifying their classification as cholinesterases.

To take advantage of the acetyl esterase function of AchE, an entirely different method was introduced by Nachlas and Seligman (1949). These investigators used the less specific substrate β-naphthyl acetate in the presence of a coupling agent, diazotized β-naphthylamine. Early attempts to stain NMJs by this method were unsatisfactory owing to lipid solubility of the final colored reaction product and

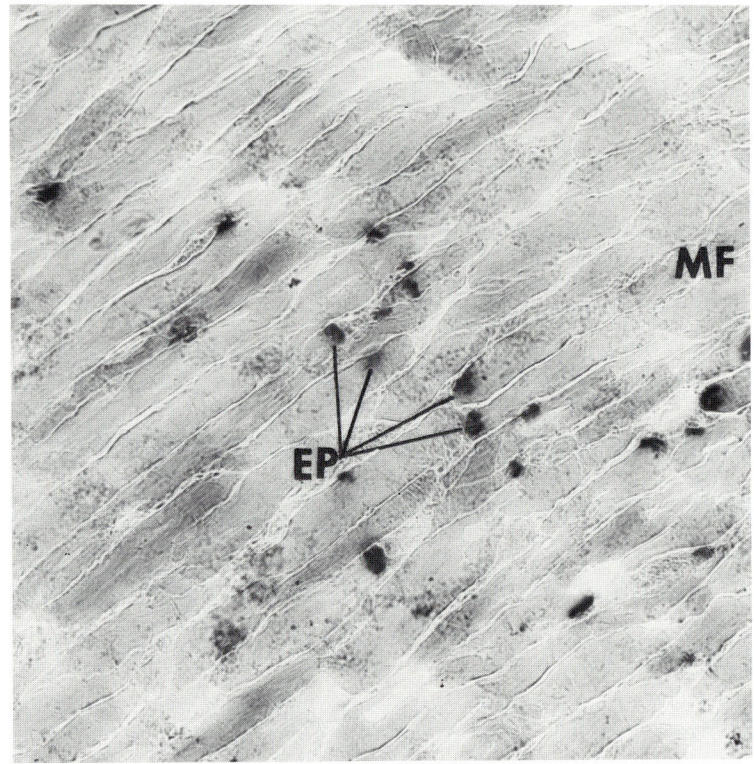

Figure 67. Low power photomicrograph of rat intercostal muscle showing several NMJs *(EP)* stained by the β-naphthyl acetate method for cholinesterase. The NMJs are stained blue-purple. There is slight background staining of the myofibers *(MF)*, probably the result of diffusion of the dye product. Note that the details of the subneural apparatus are not visible. (X 150.) (After Ravin et al., 1953.)

some tendency of the final dye product to diffuse (Chessick, 1953). Selection of less soluble coupling agents yielded better localization of AchE in NMJ (Ravin et al., 1953). Various inhibitors were used to distinguish cholinesterases from aliesterases and lipases.

Gomori (1952a, b) modified this basic method by recommending the use of β-naphthyl acetate, which he claimed reduced diffusion artefacts. Later As-acetate was successfully used (Gomori, 1952a, b) to stain NMJs. All the naphthyl ester methods demonstrated marked cholinesterase activity in the region of the subneural apparatus, although rarely were individual batonnets of Couteaux (1947) visible. Figure 67 illustrates the appearance of NMJs stained by the β-naphthyl acetate — Fast blue RR method.

Hexazonium Pararosanilin Method

A method developed for both optical and electron microscopic visualization of AchE (Lehrer and Ornstein, 1959) utilized β-naphthyl acetate as substrate and "hexazonium pararosanilin" as coupler. When applied to cold formalin-fixed tissues, the result is red staining of the subneural apparatus. After postfixation in buffered osmium tetroxide, electron micrographs from NMJs stained in this way demonstrate moderately increased electron density at the sites occupied by the coupled dye. The product of the "hexazonium pararosanilin" method was localized in the subneural apparatus within the primary and secondary synaptic clefts.

Personal experience has indicated that all the histochemical methods for demonstrating AchE activity lose a great deal of their sensitivity when they are applied after various fixatives. This is sometimes done to obtain a prettier picture (Barrnett, 1962) although in many cases areas of low enzymatic activity may be missed. The β-naphthyl acetate method applied to fresh frozen sections is highly sensitive, as is the thiolacetic acid method to be described. Formalin fixation inhibits cholinesterase activity to varying degrees under various conditions (Taxi, 1952) and therefore the sensitivity of methods employing prior formalin fixation is reduced. Many fixation routines allow survival of sufficient enzyme activity to yield histochemical localization of cholinesterases (Chessick, 1954; Coupland and Holmes, 1957; Lehrer and Ornstein, 1959). Glutaraldehyde has been used successfully as a fixative prior to application of histochemical demonstration of various enzymes including AchE (Sabatini et al., 1963).

Indoxyl Acetate Methods

Another histochemical procedure for the demonstration of esterases was introduced by Barrnett and Seligman (1951), which was based on the hydrolysis of indoxyl acetate by esterases. The resulting indoxyl auto-oxidized to form a blue insoluble precipitate of indigo blue. Early results with this method were unsatisfactory because of a tendency to form large crystals which seriously interfered with cytologic localization. Later modifications (Holt, 1052, 1954; Holt and Withers, 1952) in which substituted indoxyl esters (5-bromo indoxyl

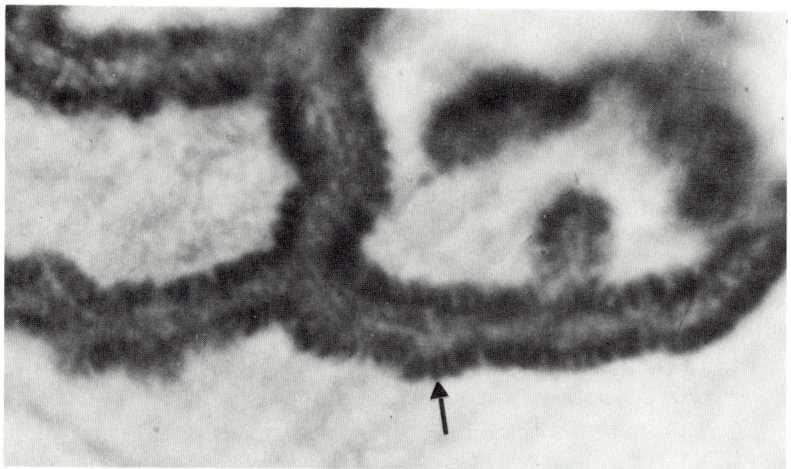

Figure 68. Photomicrograph of a rat intercostal NMJ stained by the method of Holt and Withers. The dye forming substrate was di-indoxyl diacetate, which was allowed to react with tissue sections in the presence of a ferri- ferrocyanide redox buffer. The subneural apparatus (arrow) is well illustrated. (X 3,050.) (Photograph courtesy of Dr. Stanley J. Holt, Courtauld Institute of Biochemistry, The Middlesex Hospital Medical School, London.)

acetate) were used with the addition of oxidizing agents (ferricyanide, ferrocyanide) reduced the size of the dye crystals and greatly improved localization. These latter modifications demonstrated esterase activity within individual batonnets of Couteaux in the subneural apparatus. Figure 68 illustrates cholinesterase activity in NMJ stained by the method of Holt and Withers (1952).

It should be stressed that both the β-naphthyl acetate and the indoxyl acetate methods lack specificity for cholinesterases. A series of inhibition controls are required to identify the type of esterase responsible for histochemical staining.

Acetylthiocholine Methods

A major technical advance was made in 1950 when Koelle employed acetylthiocholine as a chromogenic substrate. After hydrolysis of this substrate (which closely resembles the normal substrate, Ach) the thiocholine moiety was precipitated with copper. The resulting precipitate, situated, it was hoped, at the sites of enzyme activity, was made visible by placing the sections in ammonium sulfide to con-

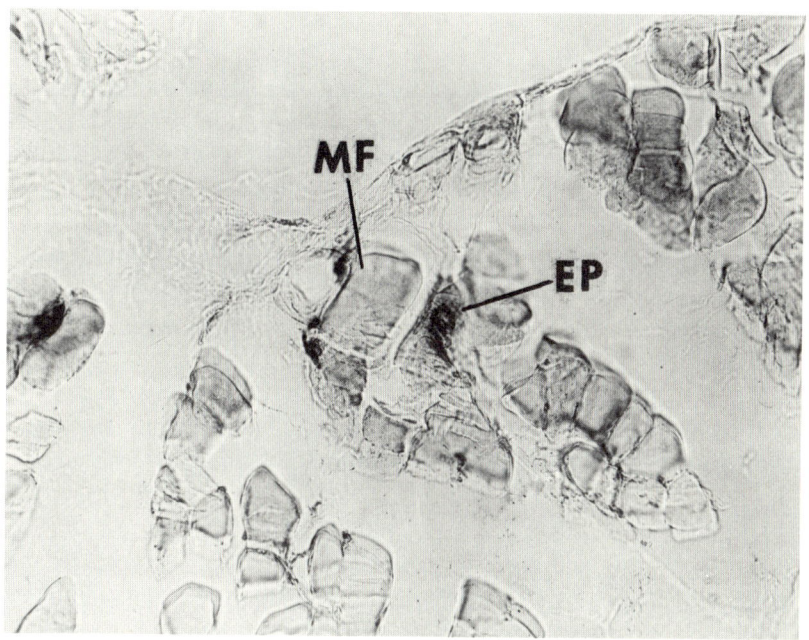

Figure 69. Photomicrograph of mouse neuromuscular junctions *(EP)* stained by the Koelle copper thiocholine method. The myofibers *(MF)* are unstained and the NMJs *(EP)* are darkly stained owing to deposits of copper sulfide in the region of the subneural apparatus. (X 265.)

vert the resulting copper thiocholine sulfate (Malmgren and Sylvén, 1955) to copper sulfide (Figure 69). Specificity of the staining reaction for AchE was claimed when acetylthiocholine was used as substrate. Butyrylthiocholine was the substrate employed to demonstrate ChE.

Staining of NMJs with the original method demonstrated AchE activity not only within the NMJs but in adjacent soleplate nuclei as well. This suggested that the final reaction product, copper thiocholine, was diffusible, although Koelle (1951) believed that nuclear staining was due to *enzyme* diffusion. Migration of the thiocholine probably was due to the positive charge ($-N^{+4}$) present in the reaction product. This cationic group tended to bind to cell structures that did not contain enzyme activity but that had free negative groups (PO_4^{-3}). In 1951 Koelle modified his original method to include sodium sulfate, which eliminated the nuclear staining. The improvement in localization was apparently due to partial inhibition of enzymatic activity. A large number of modifications of the acetylthiocholine method have appeared in 20 years. To a greater or lesser degree, however, all share the limitations of the original, somewhat cumbersome, method. These methods are to a large extent all characterized by a tendency of the final dye product to diffuse, due to the charged molecule and a rather coarse granular precipitate with distinct limitations for high resolution localization of enzymatic activity in some of the original modifications of the method. More recent procedures designed for ultrastructure studies yield finer precipitates. Naik (1963) reviewed several aspects of the thiocholine method and more recently, Eränkö and Terävainen (1967) and Eränkö et al. (1967) have considered the various modifications.

Of the numerous modifications of the basic Koelle and Freidenwald technique (1950), a few major points of histochemical interest are worthy of consideration. The first modification of the original method was the addition of sodium sulfate to reduce diffusion of the substrate and reaction products (Koelle, 1951) and the use of selective inhibitors with the selective substrates (Koelle, 1955). Prefixation with formalin and the use of low pH was introduced by Couteaux (1951) and omission of the conversion to copper sulfate was suggested by Holmstedt (1957) and also used by Brzin et al. (1966). Modifications were developed to improve localization of the histochemical reaction product for use in ultrastructure studies. For example, Birks and Brown (1960) attempted to use the Koelle method as an electron microscopic histochemical procedure. Silver sulfate replaced the usual copper sulfate, and glycine was omitted in their modification of the Koelle method. Localization of the thiocholine complex was demonstrated in Schwann cells and axonic mitochondria, in the subsynaptic clefts, and on nuclei. The greater resolving power of the electron microscope unfortunately accentuated the limitations of the thiocholine method. Lead was substituted for copper as the trapping ion by Joó et al. (1965) and gold was substituted for copper by Koelle and Gromadzki (1966), yielding greatly improved resolution.

Douglas (1966) attempted to reduce diffusion artefacts by pretreating the sections with copper glycinate before incubation with the histochemical reagents. He also suggested heating the tissue to inactivate esterases on the surface of the tissue pieces thus permitting deeper penetration of the histochemical reagents.

A new principle based on this method was introduced by Karnovsky and Roots (1964) in which a complex of copper with citrate and ferricyanide was used to form a precipitate of copper ferrocyanide (Hatchett's brown) in the tissues. The ferricyanide is reduced to ferrocyanide and copper as the acetylthiocholine substrate is hydrolyzed by cholinesterase to form thiocholine. Eränkö et al. (1967) in turn modified the Karnovsky-Roots procedure. Eränkö et al. (1967) used a lead complex with tris-acetate buffer to trap the ferrocyanide ion formed by selective reduction of ferricyanide by thiocholine formed as a result of enzymatic hydrolysis of acetylthiocholine. This reaction produces a colloidal white precipitate of $Pb_2Fe(CN)_6$ that can be observed directly in the light microscope or after conversion to lead sulfide. This yields finer localization suitable for optical as well as electron microscopy.

In a study of the effect of several variables (fixation, reaction time), Teräväinen (1969) demonstrated a disturbingly variable deposit of the enzyme reaction product with the modified thiocholine method. After 30 minutes fixation in 2.5% buffered glutaraldehyde, the histochemical reaction product was found in the subneural apparatus, on the myofiber plasma membrane, in the axon and Schwann cell as well as in association with collagen fibers. Diffuse distribution of the reaction product was greater if the incubation temperature was elevated to 20° from 4°C. Much better preservation of ultrastructure occurred after 120 minutes fixation and there was greatly reduced reaction product outside of the NMJ. Under these conditions, the reaction product was found in the subneural apparatus and there was less precipitate between the axon and the Schwann cell. The final localization of the reaction product largely depended upon the direction of penetration of the histochemical reagents into the fixed tissue blocks. After 2 hours fixation and 30 minute incubation, the reaction product occurred exclusively on the sarcoplasmic surface of the myofiber cell membrane within the NMJs. This was interpreted by the author as evidence that sites of greatest AchE activity were located in this location, a conclusion that seem unwarranted by the demonstrated diffusibility of the reaction product. DFP had been used to inhibit ChE so that it was unlikely that hydrolysis of the substrate by soluble ChE was responsible for the diffuse reaction.

Koelle and Gromadzki (1966) substituted gold for copper or lead in the basic thiocholine method as the capturing agent (Figure 70). This improved the discreteness of the precipitate and its electron density. The precipitates formed in these procedures were gold thiocholinephosphate and gold sulfide respectively.

A remote derivative of the thiocholine method is the technique of Nyberg-Hansen et al. (1969). This is basically similar to the Koelle and

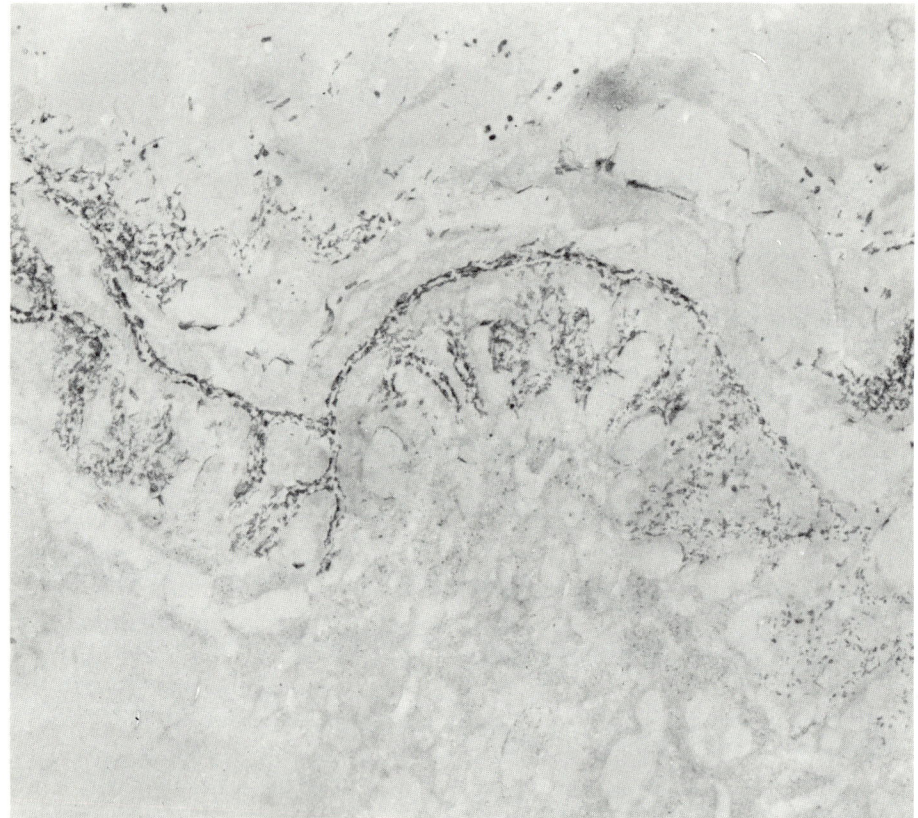

Figure 70. Electron micrograph of mouse intercostal NMJ stained by the gold thiocholine method of Davis and Koelle for AchE activity. Note the deposition of electron dense reaction product in the membranes of the overlying axon and the subneural apparatus. Note the absence of reaction product within the external lamina. (X 31,000.) (From Davis, R. and koelle, G.B., *J. Cell Biol.* 1967.)

Freidenwald (1949) procedure with the substitution of a quaternary carbon analog of acetylthiocholine, 3,3 dimethyl butyl thiolacetate (DMBTA). This substrate is electrically neutral and therefore should penetrate biological membranes more easily than substrates with quaternary nitrogen groups. Aarseth et al. (1968) and Nyberg-Hansen (1969) have used this method to demonstrate ChE activity in pre- and postsynaptic membranes of NMJs.

Bergman et al. (1967) introduced two new histochemical substrates in histochemical techniques employing the use of osmiophilic reagents and reaction products (Hanker et al., 1964). In this basic procedure, thiolesters are employed as substrates and fast blue BBN is the coupling agent. Following hydrolysis by the esterase, the thiol is captured to form an osmiophilic diazothioether that is converted to osmium black by exposure to osmium vapor (Hanker et al., 1966). The histochemical reaction product, osmium black is electron dense and allows localization of the sites of activity. However, these substrates though selective are not highly specific. Preferentially hydrolyzed by AchE are 2-naphthylthiolacetate (NTA) and 2-thiolacetoxybenzanilide TAB). On the other hand, ChE selectively hydrolyzes the third substrate 2-thiolpropionoxybenzanilide (TPB). This procedure does not greatly increase resolution over that available with other methods. Most of the AchE activity was localized in the postsynaptic membrane of the NMJ and none in the presynaptic membrane. The external lamina and synaptic vesicles were free of enzyme activity. A new finding was the demonstration of nonspecific esterase activity beneath the subneural apparatus with the TPB substrate.

Mednick et al. (1971) have introduced a new principle for the histochemical demonstration of cholinesterase. In this procedure, an enzyme susceptible thiolester group is incorporated into a molecule that also contains a diazonium group. Thus after hydrolysis of the thiolester by the enzyme, an osmiophilic polymer results due to formation of diazothioether linkages. Thiolacetate substrates with diazonium groups are specific substrates for cholinesterase because of a strong positive charge on the diazonium group. After exposure to osmium tetroxide, sites of AchE activity in NMJs are visible as black deposits by optical microscopy and as electron dense granules in the electron microscope. The ingenious aspect of this technique is the use of a single agent as both substrate and trapping reagent to form a polymer. The resulting molecule is insoluble in water and lipid before osmication. Specificity is conferred by production of a positively charged nitrogen group via diazotization immediately before use. However, such charged molecules are limited by the objections of diffusion and spurious binding. A polymerizing substrate 3-acetoxy-5-indolediazonium has also been suggested by this group (Davis et al., 1972).

The illustrations provided by Mednick et al. (1971) show extremely large discontinuous masses of histochemical reaction product overlying the subneural membranes in NMJs. These masses are so large as to seriously raise the question whether they can be interpreted as being on the inner membrane surface, as claimed. This is particularly true of the ATBD reaction whereas with ATTD, the discontinuous

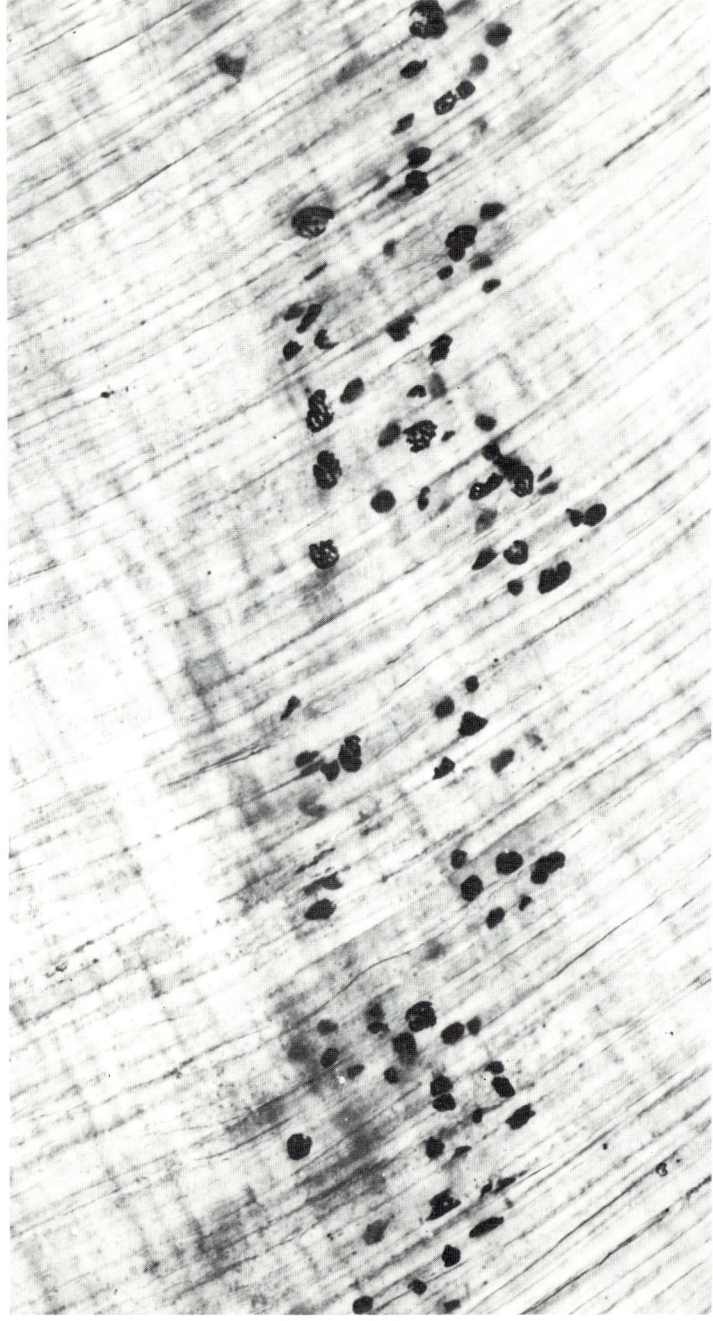

Figure 71. Photomicrograph of mouse intercostal muscle showing an innervation band composed of numerous NMJs stained by the lead thiolacetic acid method. (X 100.)

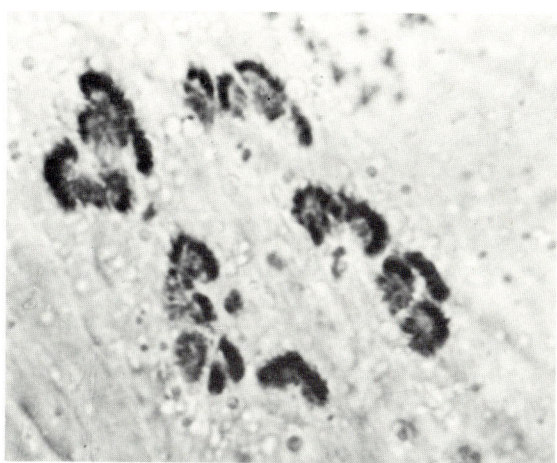

Figure 72. Photomicrograph at higher magnification illustrating NMJs stained by the lead thiolacetic acid method. Note the deposition of dense lead sulfide particles in the region of the subneural apparatus (arrows). (X 400.)

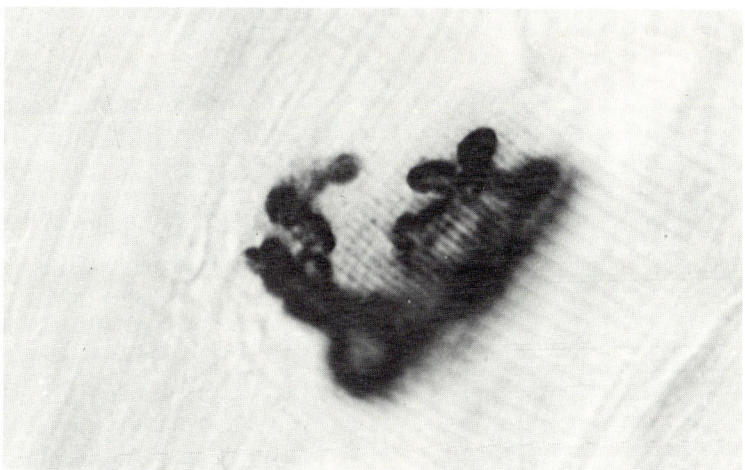

Figure 73. Photomicrograph of mouse NMJ stained by the lead thiolacetic acid method showing deposition of lead particles in the subneural apparatus. (X 1,000.)

masses of reaction product extend on both sides of the membrane and well into the EL within the clefts.

Instructions for staining with this method using p-acetylthiolbenzenediazonium ion (ATBD) and α-acetylthiol-m-toluenediazonium ion (ATTD) are included in the appendix.

Thiolacetic Acid Methods

An additional nonspecific substrate for the localization of cholinesterases in NMJs was reported by Crevier and Belanger (1955). In this method tissue sections are incubated with the substrate, thiolacetic acid (CH_3COSH) in the presence of lead, magnesium, manganese, and calcium ions. The lead is used to precipitate lead sulfide at the sites of AchE activity as hydrogen sulfide is released by the hydrolysis of Ach. Magnesium, manganese and calcium ions are employed as enzyme activators.

With some modifications, this method has been adapted for the study of the localization of AchE in the fine structure of muscle (Barrnett and Palade, 1959) and NMJs (Zacks and Blumberg, 1961b). The electron opaque lead sulfide precipitate is a good indicator of sites of esterase activity (Fig. 71). This method yields a high degree of resolution, producing unusually sharp images of NMJs with individual clefts visible in the light microscope (Figs. 72, 73). In the electron microscope, at least 500 A resolution can be obtained.

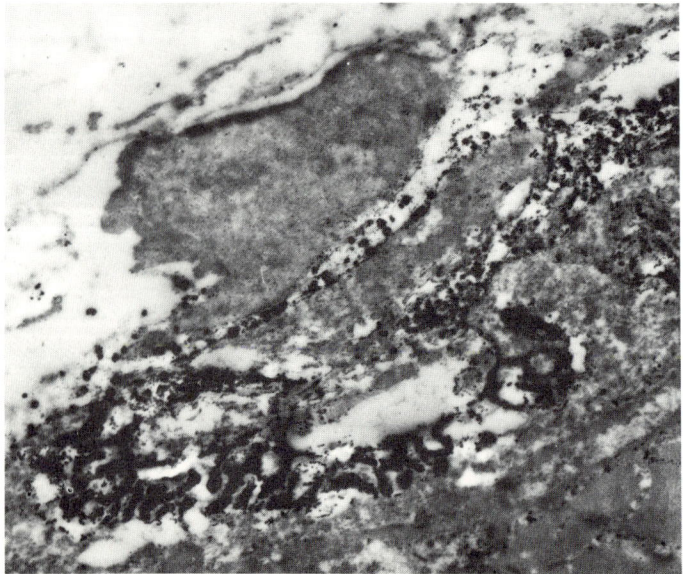

Figure 74. Electron micrograph of mouse NMJ stained by the lead thiolacetic acid method. Note the electron dense reaction product in the subneural apparatus. (X 11,000.) (From Zacks and Blumberg, 1961b.)

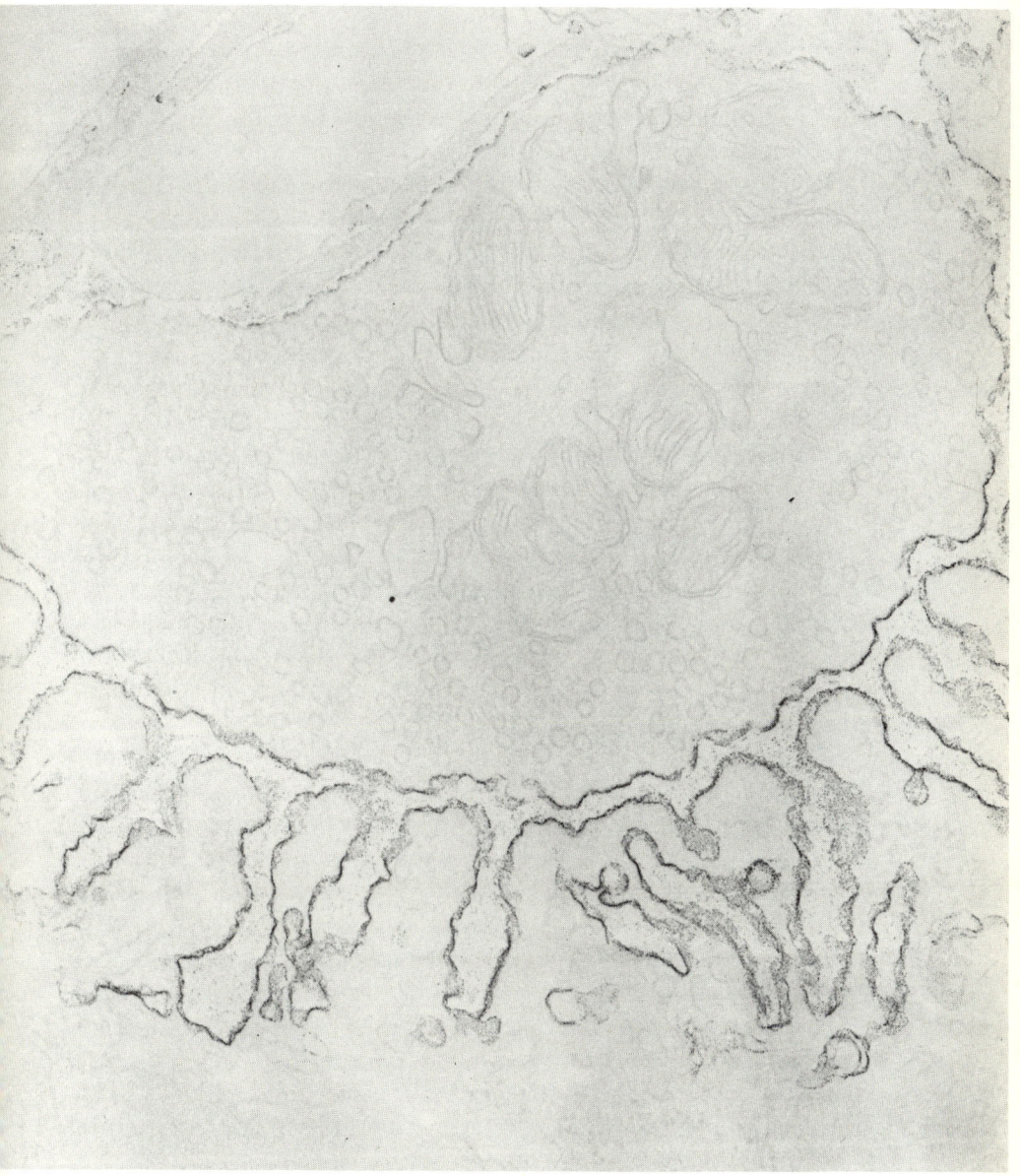

Figure 75. Electron micrograph of mouse intercostal NMJ stained by the gold thiolacetic acid method. Note the deposition of extremely fine granules of the histochemical reaction product in the membranes of the overlying axon and the subneural apparatus. The external lamina filling the clefts of the subneural apparatus is generally free of reaction product. Note also that the axon surface that faces away from the junctional region also displays enzymatic activity. (X 50,500.) (From Davis, R. and Koelle, G.B., unpublished.)

When fresh muscle containing NMJs is stained by the thiolacetic acid method, lead sulfide particles indicating sites of cholinesterase activity are found in the primary and secondary synaptic clefts of the subneural apparatus (Zacks and Blumberg, 1961b). In early work with this method, the histochemical reaction was applied to unfixed tissue with resultant loss of fine structural detail (Fig. 74).

When prior fixation is used (0.25 per cent osmium tetroxide containing 0.4 M sucrose), there is some loss of enzyme activity and the histochemical reaction product is found in the plasma membrane of the muscle covering the junctional folds, the synaptic clefts, parts of the plasma membrane covering the terminal axon, and vesicular structures in the terminal axoplasm (Barrnett, 1962). Similar results, with considerably better resolution were obtained when lead ions used by Barrnett (1962) were replaced by gold (Davis and Koelle, 1965, 1967; Koelle and Gromadzki, 1967). (Fig. 75). This modification failed to demonstrate esterase activity in synaptic vesicles as claimed by Barrnett (1962). Many investigators agree with Koelle and Gromadzki (1967) that the reaction product obtained with the gold thiolacetic acid method is finer and yields more discrete localization at the cost of enzyme specificity when compared to results obtained with thiocholine methods.

Although it was believed initially that dissociated complexes between lead and gold and thiolacetic acid were formed in this staining reaction, more recent studies (Koelle and Horn, 1968; Koelle et al., 1968) indicate that thiolacetic acid may not be the actual substrate. These investigators observed that a highly purified preparation of thiolacetic acid was less active as a histochemical substrate for AchE in NMJs of mouse intercostal muscles than impure thiolacetic acid or the residue from distillation. The crude substance contained 92-94% thiolacetic acid by iodimetric titration and only 70-72% after storage. Column and thin layer chromatography revealed that the active material was an acidic, polar substance with disulfide groups. Koelle and Horn (1968) found that addition of acetyl disulfide to the three times distilled thiolacetic acid greatly increased the staining activity to approach the reaction of 0.03 M unpurified thiolacetic acid. Reduction with sodium ascorbate or sodium borohydride decreased the activity of both the mixture and the impure thiolacetic acid but not the triple distilled material. Thus it appeared that the active material in the thiolacetic acid method is acetyl disulfide rather than thiolacetic acid. Differences in the histochemical reaction using gold (Au+) or

$Au(S_2O_3)_2^{-3}$ as capturing agent were attributed to combination of acetyl disulfide with AchE at both anionic and esteratic sites in the absence of the free heavy metal ion. Whereas when Pb++ or Au+ are present, acetyl disulfide attaches only at the esteratic site.

Consideration of these histochemical procedures for the demonstration of esterases indicates a clear dilemma; substrates that are reasonably specific in that they have a quaternary nitrogen "head" that will fit the AchE anionic site tend to diffuse in aqueous media and bind to other anionic sites therefore preventing discrete localization whereas other synthetic substrate molecules provide discrete localization but poor specificity. Several investigators have stressed the other major drawback of quaternary ammonium substrates, namely their poor penetration of membranes. The seriousness of this objection depends upon whether one believes that the esterase active sites are on the postsynaptic membrane, embedded in the postsynaptic membrane with the active sites exposed or actually within the membrane complex with no exposure of the active sites to the synaptic space. According to classical Dale theory, Ach released in the synaptic cleft is hydrolized presumably in the postsynaptic membrane by enzyme molecules that must be exposed on the surface. On the other hand, Nachmansohn (1955) has suggested that the entire Ach mechanism is within the membrane suggesting that the esterase sites are not exposed. Under these circumstances, a nonpenetrating substrate would be a distinct drawback in demonstrating the enzyme sites. Recent studies by Hall and Kelly (1971) and other data indicate that the enzyme is exposed on the membrane surface. The question of penetrability of the substance must also be considered in terms of how the histochemical procedure is carried out. Penetration of the substrate is of most importance in procedures where fresh muscle is exposed en toto to the histochemical reagents prior to fixation. This technique has been used by relatively few investigators (Koelle, 1951; Zacks and Blumberg, 1962a). In the majority of histochemical methods, histochemical staining is performed on sections after fixation (Couteaux, 1951; Karnovsky and Roots, 1964; Koelle and Gromadzki, 1966; Davis and Koelle, 1967; Holt and Withers, 1952; Bergman et al., 1967). Under these circumstances, the histochemical reagents might be expected to have easy access to surviving enzyme proteins within the tissue sections without interference by membrane barriers. Also, prior fixation with formalin would be expected to alter many of the membrane proteins bringing about changes in their binding properties as well as their permeability.

Kinds of Esterases

Although a long and complex story in itself, the nature of the various esterases and the substrates they act upon will be reviewed briefly.

Alles and Hawes (1942) discovered cholinesterase in erythrocytes, and Stedman et al. (1932) demonstrated cholinesterase activity in blood sera. The work of Richter and Croft (1942) and Mendel et al. (1943) led to the recognition that there were two kinds of cholinesterase: namely, specific or acetylcholinesterase (AchE — EC 3.1.1.7) of the nervous system and erythrocytes, and nonspecifie or serum cholinesterase (ChE — EC 3.1.1.8), found in the tissues and sera of many animals. In addition, even less specific aliesterases (aliphatic esterases) or nonspecific esterases (NsE) and lipases were also found in sera and many tissues. The comparative distribution of cholinesterases was reviewed extensively by Augustinsson (1948).

In addition to studies of esterases in isolated cell systems, much contradictory data has accumulated as the result of histochemical studies. To a large degree, the particular esterases demonstrated and their sites of localization were dependent on the methods used. It was soon evident that the original Tween method of Gomori had limited specificity for cholinesterase and numerous variants and substitutes were proposed. Although α-naphthyl acetate methods (Nachlas and Seligman, 1949; Gomori, 1952a, b) and variants of these methods permitted demonstration of esterases in NMJs, the resolution was less than satisfactory due to diffusion and the specificity was questionable. Development of indoxyl methods by Holt (1951, 1952) and by Barrnett and Seligman (1951) offered better resolution of fine structure in the subneural apparatus, but generally gave way to the numerous more specific variants of the Koelle and Freidenwald technique that employed acetylthiocholine and butyrylthiocholine.

During the early period of the development of esterase histochemical methods (1951-1961), occasional attempts were made to improve the specificity of the histochemical reactions. For example, Denz (1953, 1954) and Holmstedt (1957) used various substrates and inhibitors to demonstrate two kinds of cholinesterase in NMJs. Present in greatest activity was a "true" cholinesterase (AchE), and in addition there was lesser activity due to nonspecific cholinesterase (ChE). However, it is notable that in most of these reports, few attempts were made to distinguish AchE from ChE and NsE since inhibitors were generally not used (Snell and McIntyre, 1956; Waser and Hadorn, 1961; Manolov, 1963; Lewis and Shute, 1964 and Miledi, 1964).

In the ten years that have now elapsed since this subject was considered in the first edition of this monograph, a complex literature has developed describing several new substrates for the histochemical localization of various esterases and the use of several inhibitors to distinguish one enzyme from another.

Histochemical studies using thiocholine substrates with physostigmine as inhibitor to distinguish kinds of cholinesterases from noncholine esterases were published by Hines (1960), Birks and Brown (1960) and Brzin and Majcentkačev (1963). Methods utilizing naphthyl acetate without inhibitors failed to distinguish nonspecific esterase from cholinesterases in the junctional region (Lehrer and Ornstein, 1959; Zacks and Blumberg, 1961b; Bauer et al., 1962; Barrnett, 1962; Guth and Zalewski, 1963). In the later 1960's, diisopropyl fluorophosphate (DFP) was used histochemically to discriminate AchE from ChE (Gerebtzoff et al., 1954; Silver, 1963; Filogamo and Gabella, 1966). However DFP alone is inadequate to distinguish the various enzymes (Eränkö, 1959; Holmstedt and Sjoqvist, 1961). More selective inhibitors including tetra isopropyl pyrophosphoramide (iso-OMPA) were introduced to increase specificity. Iso-OMPA inhibits ChE selectively and thus offers the possibility of distinguishing AchE from ChE activity in tissue sections. A second inhibitor 1,5-bis-(4-allyl dimethylammonium phenyl) pentan-3-one diiodide (2484C51) was introduced as a specific inhibitor of AchE (Tuncbay, 1964; Koelle and Gromadzki, 1966; Lewis and Shute, 1966). It also became possible to distinguish between an organophosphorus-resistant and sensitive ChEs that were capable of hydrolyzing α-naphthyl acetate by use of another inhibitor, diethyl-p-nitrophenylphosphate (E600).

Another attempt to improve the specificity of the thiocholine method was that of Kokko et al. (1969) in which acetyl-β-methylthiocholine was used to increase the specificity of the method for AchE. The basic Karnovsky-Roots (1964) principle was used in this method with the addition of acetylselenocholine to reduce ferricyanide to ferrocyanide. The histochemical reaction product was found in the endoplasmic reticulum of neuronal perikarya and in nuclear envelopes as well as in dendrites and fibers in the neuropil but no details of NMJ staining were reported.

Nonspecific Esterase in NMJ

In addition to AchE and ChE, focal concentrations of NsE in rat NMJs has been reported by Barron et al. (1968), Eränkö and Terävãinen (1967) and Terävãinen (1967, 1968), and in NMJs in human vastus medialis and peroneus brevis muscles (Chokroverty et al., 1971). Barron et al. (1968) has suggested that the enzyme in this location may be related to membrane metabolism.

The study of NMJs on isolated myofiber sarcolemmal membranes permits the measurement of several enzyme parameters undisturbed by other sources of muscle esterases. Namba and Grob (1968) found that isolated muscle membranes chiefly contained AchE activity although ChE was also detected as a minor component. The membrane AchE had a pH optimum of 8, a Michaelis-Menten constant (K_m) of 3.1 MM and a maximal activity velocity (V_{max}) of 23.1 Mm Ach/30 minutes/mg. N. These investigators found that the cholinesterase activity of the muscle membrane was localized entirely within the NMJs.

Solubility of Cholinesterases in the NMJ

Koelle et al. (1970) studied the AchE activity in frozen sections of stellate and ciliary ganglia and in intercostal muscle NMJs, after exposure to a detergent, Triton X. After extraction with 0.3% Triton X, AchE activity in the ganglia was eliminated whereas the AchE activity in intercostal muscle NMJs was apparently increased. Koelle concluded that there were different AchE isozymes in the two kinds of tissue although differences in binding or the nature of the insertion of the active enzyme protein in the cell membrane must also be considered in interpreting these results.

Localization of Esterases in Neuromuscular Junctions

Of importance in evaluating theories concerning the mechanism of transmission was the precise localization of the AchE activity within the NMJ. Early attempts to settle this question by biochemical means led to confusing results for various reasons. Marnay and Nachmansohn (1938) described an increase in cholinesterase activity in denervated guinea pig muscles, an erroneous conclusion resulting from ignoring the coincident muscle atrophy. Later Couteaux and Nachmansohn (1940) showed that there was an actual decrease in AchE activity three to four weeks after nerve section. Similar results had been reported by Martini and Torda (1937) and Feng and Ting (1938). Another factor that was not considered is that the NMJ is not the only source of AchE in muscles. The musculotendinous junctions contain AchE (Couteaux, 1953) and the muscle (myosin) itself contains a cholinesterase (Varga et al., 1954).

Histochemical methods applied to the question of AchE localization in NMJ yielded more precise information although some of the initial data were contradictory.

Many investigators believed that the AchE activity would be found solely within the terminal nerve branches, but several histochemical studies demonstrated that AchE activity survives for considerable periods of time after nerve section which produces complete degeneration of the terminal nerve branches. Sawyer et al. (1950) found decreased but persistent AchE activity in NMJs after denervation, whereas Snell and McIntyre (1956) observed complete disappearance of the enzyme approximately 45 days after nerve section. Similar results were obtained by Coërs (1953, 1955a), Gerebtzoff and Vandermissen (1956), Kupfer and Koelle (1951) and Savày and Csillik (1956). Histochemically demonstrable AchE activity persisted in denervated muscle for 45 days in the guinea pig to 3 months (Coërs, 1953c) or 4 months (Savày and Csillik, 1956) in the rat. This indicated that the enzyme was at least partially synthesized in the postsynaptic area. However, the possibility remained that localization of AchE activity within the subneural apparatus might be due to artefactual diffusion of the enzyme or the products of the histochemical reaction. Couteaux (1958) showed that this was not the case by demonstrating that mechanical isolation of the subneural apparatus before incubation with the histochemical reagents resulted in staining of the subneural apparatus.

As Couteaux (1960) pointed out, the possibility still persisted at this point that the AchE activity of the postsynaptic region could possibly be due to teloglia. Histochemical evidence of esterase activity within teloglial cells was also reported by Zacks and Blumberg (1961b); Davis and Koelle (1965) and Lewis and Shute (1966). Barrnett (1962) and Miledi (1964) also found cholinesterase in synaptic vesicles unlike many other investigators.

As a result of these experiments, it was clear that much of the myofiber esterase activity was located in the region of NMJs (Couteaux,

1947; Couteaux and Taxi, 1952; Holt and Withers, 1952; Coërs, 1953a, b; Gerebtzoff, 1953; Denz, 1953; Holt, 1954; Gerebtzoff et al., 1954; Woolf and Till, 1955; Crevier and Belanger, 1955).

In general, ultrastructure studies of esterase localization in NMJs confirmed optical microscopic evidence that most of the enzyme activity was in the subneural apparatus (Lehrer and Ornstein, 1959; Birks and Brown, 1960; Zacks and Blumberg, 1961b; Lewis and Shute, 1964; Iwayama, 1966).

These earlier studies revealed histochemical reaction product on pre- and postsynaptic membranes as well as in the intervening EL. Also, several investigators commented on the presence of extrajunctional esterase activity and, as we have discussed, differentiation of AchE, ChE and NsE was uncertain. Use of more refined methods combined with various inhibitors increased both resolution and specificity.

Iwayama (1966), who used the thiocholine lead nitrate method with DFP to inhibit ChE, demonstrated AchE activity in the subneural apparatus but not the terminal axon or soleplate. Eränkö and Teräväinen (1967) found both AchE and ChE in NMJs. AchE was principally located within the subneural apparatus whereas ChE was found in the axon and was nearly equal to AchE in the subneural clefts and in the region adjacent to the subneural apparatus. ChE however, was the only cholinesterase present in the Schwann cells.

Davis and Koelle (1967) demonstrated AchE activity in the presynaptic and the postsynaptic membranes of mouse intercostal muscle NMJs. ChE was present in low activity in both sites and greater enzyme activity was found in the Schwann cells adjacent to the nerve terminal. No reaction product was found in the EL. (Fig. 75). The new self polymerizing histochemical substrates used by Mednick and Seligman (1971) show enzyme localization solely in the postsynaptic membrane of NMJs in rat diaphragm and intercostal muscles.

Esterase activity demonstrated by the lead thiolacetic acid method was found in the external cell coat of isolated sarcolemmal membranes from areas of intercostal muscle rich in NMJs (Zacks and Sheff, 1968) (Fig. 61).

Radioautographic Localization of Sites of Cholinesterase Activity

Ostrowski et al. (1963) employed tritium-labeled DFP to localize the sites of cholinesterase activity in NMJs. The resolution however of this early attempt was less than that obtained with the better histochemical methods. Rogers et al. (1966) used radioactive DFP to study the distribution of the enzyme in mouse sternomastoid and diaphragm muscles. They found that there are $7\text{-}10 \times 10^7$ and $2.5\text{-}3.5 \times 10^7$ sites that bind radioactive DFP. Approximately 35% of these were active AchE sites and an estimated 10% or less were ChE sites. Of the AchE sites, approximately 85% were located in the junctional folds and 10% in the overlying connective tissue. Approximately 5% of the activity was found in the terminal axon. The remaining sites probably represented noncholine esterases.

More recently, improved radioautographic methods have been used to attempt accurate quantitization of the number of AchE active sites in NMJs by using the technique of radioactive specific inhibitors. Salpeter (1967, 1969, Salpeter et al, 1972) used tritiated DFP to demonstrate AchE molecules in mouse diaphragm and sternomastoid muscle. She found that 85% of the AchE activity was localized in the junctional folds of the subneural apparatus with a concentration of somewhat greater than 20,000 active sites per μ^3. However, the resolution was insufficient to determine with certainty if the terminal axon contained any of the label. However, if present, it constituted less than 10%. The specificity of the method is based upon the selective reactivation of DFP inhibited or phosphorylated AchE by 2-PAM (pyridine-2-aldoxime). Using an average NMJ size of $50 \times 30\mu$ and assuming a spheroid with an estimated volume of 1,000-2,000 μ^3, Salpeter calculated the total number of AchE molecules in an NMJ as $1\text{-}2 \times 10^7$ which compares well with the estimate of Rogers et al. (1966) who obtained a value of $2\text{-}3 \times 10^7$ using P^{32} or tritiated DFP. These studies revealed a 14 times greater labelling of membranes in NMJ than in nonjunctional membranes. Figure 76 illustrates sites of esterase activity demonstrated by radioactive DFP (Salpeter, 1969). In her later study (Salpeter et al, 1972), the number of DFP binding sites in NMJs of diaphragm (red muscle) were nearly identical with the number of binding sites in the previously studied sternomastoid (white) muscle.

Cholinesterases in En Grappe Neuromuscular Junctions

NMJ cholinesterase histochemistry with or without electron microscopy has been used to investigate en grappe and en plaque NMJs innervating mammalian extraocular muscles. Haggqvist (1962) using

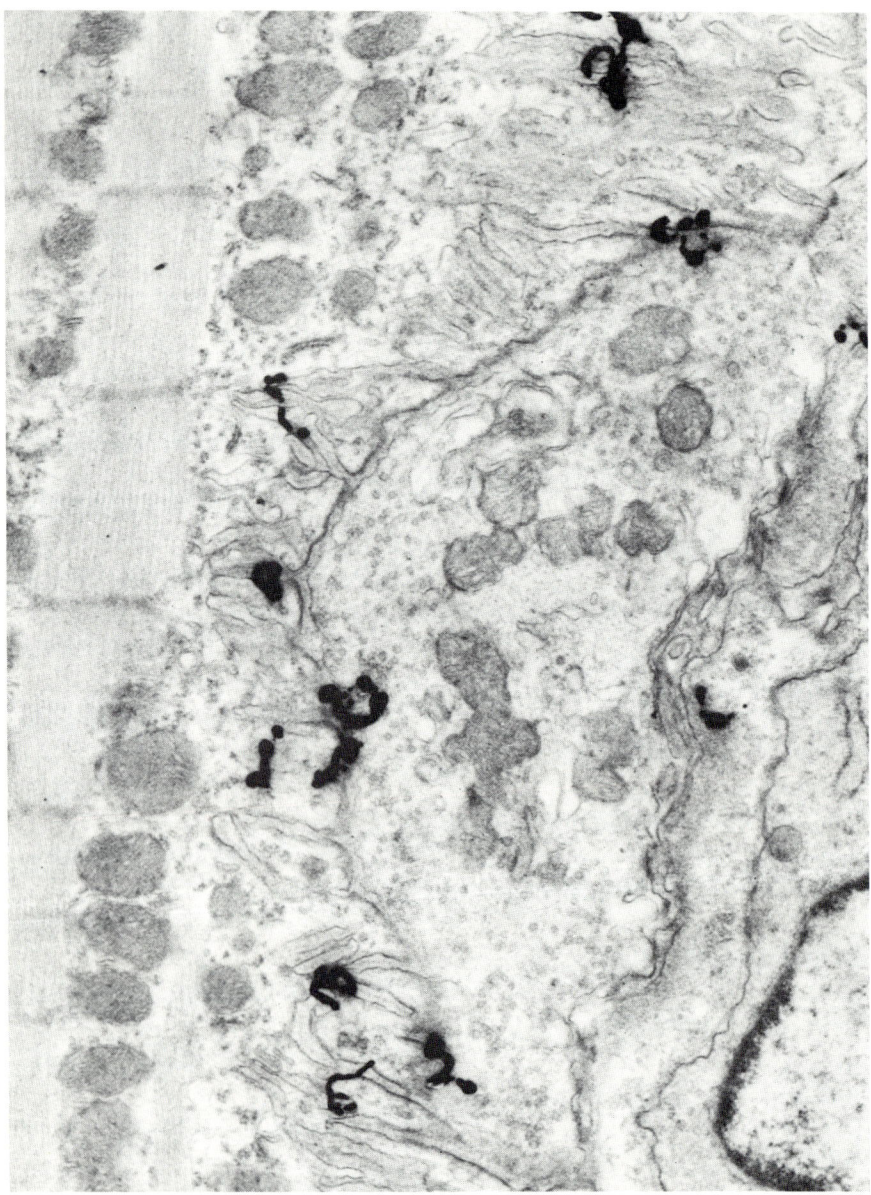

Figure 76. Radioautograph of DFP-3^H at a NMJ after the incubation sequence DFP-^{H}-2 PAM. Developed silver grains are present over junctional folds *(JF)* and teloglial cap (SCH+CT), but not over the nerve terminal *(N)*. (X 20,000.) (Fig. 21. From Salpeter, M.M., Electron Microscopic Radioautography as a Quantitative Tool in Enzyme Cytochemistry. II. The distribution of DFP reactive sites at motor endplates of a vertebrate twitch muscle. *J. Cell Biol. 42*:122, 1969, by permission Rockefeller University Press.)

the Holmstedt method reported that AchE was present in en plaque NMJs supplied by coarse nerve fibers whereas ChE was present in en grappe NMJs supplied by fine nerve fibers. Teräväinen (1968b) studied esterases in rat extraocular muscles and found singly innervated twitch myofibers with en plaque NMJs conatining AchE, ChE and NsE activity. In addition, large and small multiply innervated myofibers were described. The larger measured about a third the size of typical en plaque NMJs and were composed of 2 to 5 axon terminals associated with a few subsynaptic folds which contained slight AchE and ChE activity. The smaller multiple endings contained both AchE and ChE. These consisted of multiple synaptic contacts arising from unmyelinated axons along the myofiber at variable distances. The subneural apparatus had few synaptic folds but a postsynaptic membrane density was present.

Namba et al. (1968) described AchE activity in both en plaque and en grappe NMJs in superior rectus muscle and Buckley and Heaton (1968, 1970) found both enzymes in zones of focal and multiple innervation in rat and guinea pig extraocular muscles. Quantitative measurement of cholinesterase activity was accomplished by acetyl ^{14}C, acetyl thiocholine in which the ^{14}C acetate was extracted and counted by liquid scintillation. These investigators found that the focal endings contained considerably greater AchE activity than the fine motor endings and suggested that differential enzymatic activity might be related to the speed of contraction. Barnard and Rogers (1967) had shown that in mouse extraocular muscle, the number of cholinesterase sites in twitch myofibers was five times the number in tonic myofibers. They attributed this to the less extensive synaptic folding of the tonic fiber NMJs. No difference in the kinds of enzymatic activity was found; both kinds of NMJs hydrolysed acetylcholine and butyrylcholine.

Cholinesterase and Skeletal Muscle Physiology

NMJ cholinesterase activity in fast and slow, and red and white muscles has been studied in attempts to correlate the enzyme activity with the physiologic responses of the muscle. Nyström (1968) used histochemical methods to study kitten and cat gastrocnemius muscle ("fast", white) and the soleus muscle ("slow", red) and found differences in enzyme content and structure that appeared gradually with increasing development. Both AchE and ChE activity was found in the NMJs. Nyström concluded that the structure of the subneural apparatus and differences in NMJ esterase activity did not explain differences in post tetanic potentiation in soleus and gastrocnemius muscles. Buckley and Heaton (1971) demonstrated that the posterior latissimus dorsi muscle of the chick, a twitch muscle, contained nearly 4 times the cholinesterase activity of the anterior latissimus dorsi muscle which consists of "tonic" myofibers and frog tonic muscle NMJs have less ChE activity than twitch myofibers (Heaton, et al, 1972).

Species Differences in Cholinesterase Activity in Neuromuscular Junctions

Namba (1971) has measured cholinesterase activity in man and several laboratory animals. The greatest activity was found in rat NMJs followed in declining order by human, guinea pig, chicken, mouse and dog NMJs.

Morphogenesis of Cholinesterase Activity in Neuromuscular Junctions

Of considerable interest are studies demonstrating the development of AchE activity in embryonic neuromuscular junctions (Kupfer and Koelle, 1951; Couteaux, 1960; Mumenthaler and Engel, 1961). Couteaux (1960) has shown that in the 80 millimeter embryo, the guinea pig NMJ contains demonstrable AchE activity in the zone of the subneural membrane, a degree of activity greater than that present in other parts of the muscle fiber. This increased histochemically detectable cholinesterase activity occurs in parallel with the formation of immature subneural clefts. These clefts, though shorter than in the fully matured guinea pig NMJ, are present in the muscles of newborn animals. The subneural region, as revealed by AchE staining, is cup-shaped when the initial contact between the nerve fiber and the muscle is first established. Later the subneural apparatus branches out and becomes more complex, finally forming the familiar adult subneural apparatus.

In chick embryo skeletal muscle (Mumenthaler and Engel, 1961), ChE activity first appeared in muscle fibers on the sixth day and could be demonstrated as a diffuse deposit of pigment granules after histochemical staining. NMJs were recognizable on the fourteenth day and were easily demonstrated in sixteenth and seventeenth day embryos.

In the development of human NMJs, a similar sequence is observed. In the newborn infant, histochemical staining for AchE activity reveals the subneural apparatus as a simple circle with radiating batonnets (Coërs and Woolf, 1959), and later more complex NMJs were found. (Fig. 77).

Gerebtzoff (1953, 1954), Beckett and Bourne (1958), and Mumenthaler and Engel (1961) noted that the shape of immature NMJs differs considerably from the shape of adult NMJs in various species. As they mature, more NMJs containing larger, lobulated areas of subneural apparatus appear. The mature NMJs consist of numerous gutters with the subneural apparatus outlined by cholinesterase activity. Figure 74 diagramatically illustrates these stages.

Application of histochemical methods that permitted enzyme localization in the fine structure of NMJs has greatly increased our knowledge of this subject.

Wake (1964) observed the first NMJs in chick embryos at 12-13 days *in ovo* by means of silver and thiolacetic acid staining. The cholinesterase activity was present in the junctional surface and at 15 days, in relationship to the subneural sarcoplasm and fundamental soleplate nuclei. Using the copper ferrocyanide method of Karnovsky

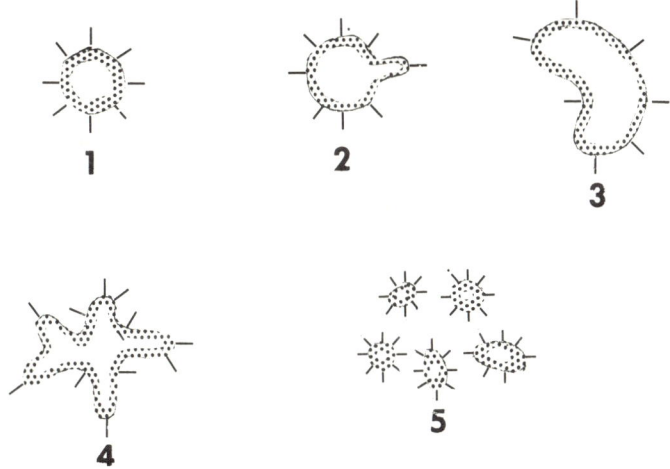

Figure 77. Diagram illustrating progressive stages (1-5) in the increasing complexity of subneural apparatus resulting from the fragmentation of an original single unit during maturation. (After Coërs and Woolf, 1959.)

and Roots (1964), Hirano (1967) examined chick embryo lower limb and pectoralis muscles 5-21 days *in ovo* and 1-2 days *ex ovo*. The earliest junctional AchE activity was observed at seven days (Hamilton stage 30) as a single curved line of the histochemical reaction product. Later, NMJs appeared to differentiate in 3 stages: a. initial formation 7-13 days, subsequent formation 13-18 days, and early maturation, 20 days. Using eserine (10^{-4}M) inhibition and the selective substrates, acetylthiocholine and butyrylthiocholine, Hirano demonstrated that the esterase in the subneural apparatus was AchE. Atsumi (1971) appears to have found the earliest cholinesterase activity at 6 days and NMJ formation by 8 days. Rowinski (1959) found activity at 9 days and Gerebtzoff (1959) at 10 days *in ovo*. Mumenthaler and Engel (1961) were able to demonstrate activity only at 14 days and Visintini and Levi-Montalcini (1939) found enzyme activity at 13 days. Wake (1964) found earliest activity at 17 days and Khera and Laham (1965) demonstrated ChE in 19 day duck embryos.

In the rat, Terävainen (1968) observed the first occurrence of AchE at 18 days in the plasma membranes of the mid portion of myofibers and ChE appeared at 21 days. ChE first appeared one day after birth. The first AchE activity was found in the depression formed on the surface of the myofiber, the presumptive primary synaptic cleft. It was not until 5 days later (7-9 days after birth) that the enzyme could be demonstrated in the clefts and ramifications of the subneural apparatus. However, Terävainen emphasized that the earliest demonstrable AchE activity appears in the terminal axon. Thus according to this investigator, the development of AchE activity begins after the morphologic characteristics of the NMJ are established. This was confirmed in rat intercostal NMJs by Kelly (1966) who found esterases in soleplates at 18 days. Lead staining by the Savay and Csillik method (1958) had shown indications of earlier selective lead binding in presumptive innervation bands when the first specialized membrane structures occurred (Kelly and Zacks, 1968).

By means of radiometric assay of AchE, Buckley and Heaton (1970) have demonstrated increased enzyme activity with age that is proportional to myofiber size and NMJ area.

In an investigation of embryogenesis and regeneration of lizard NMJs, Liu and Maneely (1968) found the first appearance of cholinesterase activity in the intersegmental connective tissue at stage 7 followed by disappearance of the enzyme by stage 10. It is not clear if

AchE or ChE were demonstrated because specific substrates and inhibitors were not used. Neuromuscular junction-like structures containing cholinesterase activity were found at the ends of myotubes near intersegmental zones in stage 8 and in the mid portion of the myofibers by stage 10. These morphologic findings correlated with slight movements of the tail at stage 8 and vigorous spontaneous movements at stage 10. At stage 8, myotubes were most numerous in the developing muscles whereas early myofibers with myofilaments were present at stages 9 & 10. During regeneration, the pattern was similar with cholinesterase-positive structures present in the 14 mm. regenerate, increasing in the 16 mm. and disappearing in the 22 mm. The NMJs were not demonstrated at the myotube stage of myogenesis (6 mm. regenerate) nor early myofiber stage (14 mm. regenerate). The first NMJs were found at the tips of myofibers in the 19 mm. regenerate coincident with early tail movement. In these myofibers, the NMJs occurred at the mid portion of the myofibers (27 mm.).

Bornstein et al. (1968) and others have observed the development of cholinesterase in NMJs formed in organ culture of explanted mouse embryo somites and spinal cord. Development of discrete sites of AchE activity in differentiating NMJs studied in embryos and tissue culture appears to correlate with the approach of the axons as if the enzyme was neurally induced (Couteaux, 1960; Wake, 1964).

Origin of Cholinesterases in Neuromuscular Junctions

The origin of cholinesterase activity has been considered by several investigators. Some have suggested that the enzyme is synthesized in the cell body (Tennyson and Brzin, 1970) from which it migrates to the junctional region by means of centrifugal axonal flow (Zelená and Lubinská, 1962; Barondes, 1964; Kristensson, 1970) whereas others have concluded that the enzyme is synthesized in the axons (Zelená and Szentagothai, 1956; Shen, 1958; Koenig, 1965). Others have suggested that the enzyme is synthesized in the innervated muscle (Koelle, 1961; Wake, 1964; Lentz, 1969). This hypothesis is strengthened by the long persistence of cholinesterase activity in NMJs after sectioned axons have degenerated and the apparent induction of enzyme activity in developing myofibers as axons approach future sites of innervation (Wake, 1964). There is little support for

Csillik's (1960, 1965a) idea that cholinesterase is formed in "teloblasts" (Schwann cells) that participate in the formation of new NMJs (Mumenthaler and Engel, 1961). It is likely that both the neuron cell body and the innervated muscle can synthesize cholinesterases. Koelle (1961) suggested that there are two types of neuronal AchE: namely, "internal" or "cytoplasmic" AchE and "external" AchE at the neuronal cell membrane. The former is thought to be synthesized in the granular endoplasmic reticulum within the cell body and subsequently transported by means of the agranular reticulum to all portions of the neuronal cell membrane. Within the membrane the active sites are thought to be oriented outwardly. The "external" AchE is the normally active enzyme, whereas the "internal" enzyme represents a reserve form. The role of AchE in the presynaptic membrane might be destruction of Ach liberated during activity or possibly destruction of Ach that "leaks" from the presynaptic terminal during inactivity. However, Koelle (1961) was not able to explain the origin or the intense postsynaptic AchE activity in terms of neuronal secretion. He suggested that cholinesterase in that location is produced by muscle cells, possibly under the influence of the presynaptic nerve terminals. In either or both cases, it is not clear how the active sites of the enzyme molecules become exposed on the surface of the synaptic membrane.

Experimental studies employing inhibition of cholinesterase have also been performed. For example, Koenig (1965) concluded that AchE could be synthesized in axons because enzyme activity reappeared in distal axons and in the stump of cut nerves after inhibition by DFP. Similarly, Sonesson and Thesleff (1968) attempted to determine the source and rate of formation of cholinesterases in NMJs by means of irreversible inhibition by DFP and observation of the recovery of enzyme activity after denervation. The sciatic nerve was cut and tied and after one week, DFP was injected into the anterior tibial muscle of the denervated leg. The opposite leg served as control. The rats were sacrificed at periods of 1-27 days. The anterior tibial muscle was weighed, fixed and NMJ cholinesterase activity was demonstrated by the Koelle-Freidenwald method. The index of activity was the length of time required to demonstrate enzyme staining. After a week, the cholinesterase activity in the muscles was increased since the incubation time required to demonstrate histochemical staining was decreased: Two weeks after DFP inhibition, the normally innervated muscles had normal cholinesterase activity. Resynthesis in the soleplate sarcoplasm was the probable means of the rapid restoration of cholinesterase activity. Furthermore, reduced rates of restoration of cholinesterase reconstitution were observed after denervation or poisoning with botulinum toxin. The authors suggested that the appearance of enzyme activity in the NMJ may be dependent on some trophic substance carried by the nerve. This also could explain the apparent induction of the enzyme in the postsynaptic region during embryogenesis.

COMBINED STAINING METHODS

Axon Impregnation with Silver and AchE Staining

In order to facilitate studies of collateral branching and pathologic changes in NMJs, it is necessary to demonstrate not only the sub-

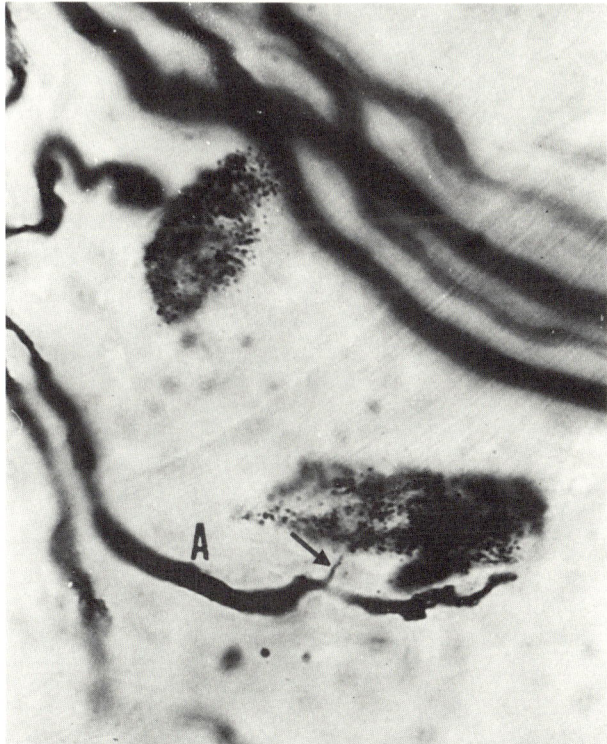

Figure 78. Photomicrograph illustrating mouse NMJs stained by a combined silver and cholinesterase method. The axon *(A)* including fine branches (arrow) are made opaque by silver impregnation and esterase activity in the subneural apparatus is made visible by lead sulfide granules (thiolacetic acid method). (X 1,000.)

neural apparatus by means of cholinesterase staining but also the axons innervating the endplates. A variety of techniques have been employed by several investigators (Gwyn and Heardman, 1965; Namba et al., 1967; Ip, 1967; Nakata and Nishijima, 1971). The majority of these methods utilize thiocholine or thiolacetic acid to stain esterases in the subneural apparatus prior to impregnation of the axons with silver (Fig. 78). Details of some of these methods are given in the appendix.

Catecholamine and Cholinesterase Staining

In applications where it is desirable to demonstrate both cholinesterase and epinephrine, Badawi and Schenk (1967) have developed a combined method utilizing the acetylthiocholine ferrocyanide reaction (Karnovsky and Roots, 1964) with a paraformaldehyde technique to demonstrate catecholamines in U.V. light. Both consecutive and simultaneous staining procedures were used successfully by these investigators.

10

Biochemistry and Physiology of Neuromuscular Junctions

The study of synaptic function has contributed several new and fundamental concepts to modern biology. The peripheral synapse, as exemplified by the NMJ, has been the focus of extensive biophysical and biochemical investigations directed toward understanding the mechanism by which information is transmitted from the central nervous system to a peripheral effector organ, the skeletal musculature. In this respect the peripheral synapse serves as a useful, albeit imperfect, model for the anatomic and physiologic characteristics of the less accessible central synapses. Understanding of the latter constitutes a major step in placing the normal and abnormal function of the central nervous system on a rational basis. The present discussion of NMJ biochemistry and physiology is concerned with several major topics but does not attempt to be complete. The reader is referred to the monographs of Katz (1966), Hubbard and Llinas (1969) and McLennan (1970) for a more detailed consideration of this subject.

Early Investigations

Sherrington was the first to explore systematically the significance of the anatomic independence and interdependence of each neural unit (neuron doctrine) in the functioning of the nervous system.

He clearly set forth the aspects of neural transmission that required explanation: (1) the delay in the reflex pathway, (2) less close correlation between the instant of cessation of stimulation and the cessation of the results of stimulation (after discharge), (3) increased ease of transmission with a chain of impulses (temporal summation), (4) one-way transmission, and (5) fatigability and sensitivity to chemical agents, anoxia and anesthesia. Many of these characteristics of central synapses were most easily studied in peripheral synapses.

The early investigators were preoccupied with whether transmission at peripheral synapses was electrical or chemical in nature. The electrical argument was summarized by Lapicque (1926), and others continued this controversy well into the 1940's (Eccles, 1945; Kuffler, 1948; and Rosenblueth et al. (1939). Rosenblueth (1950) summarized the evidence for the two contending theories and concluded that the bulk of it favored his choice of the chemical transmission hypothesis.

The history of the concept of chemoreceptor function at NMJs began in 1904. Elliott (1904, 1905), who was aware of the work of Lewandowsky (1899) and Langley (1901) on the physiologic action of adrenal extracts, noted the similarity between their results and the results of sympathetic nerve stimulation. He therefore suggested that epinephrine probably was released by nerve endings. Dixon (1906, 1907) suggested that a similar material must be present in parasympathetic nerve endings. Dixon (1907) succeeded in inhibiting isolated frog heart preparations with extracts from dog hearts excised during vagal stimulation. The effect of these extracts on the frog heart was blocked by atropine, a result similar to that obtained when atropine was given to the intact animal during vagal stimulation. In retrospect the identity of the material in Dixon's extracts is unclear because it is unlikely that significant amounts of Ach would survive the high concentration of cholinesterases present in blood. To repeat such an experiment and demonstrate Ach reliably one must add an AchE inhibitor such as eserine to the extracts.

About the same time, another experimental approach was destined to provide the essential link in interpreting the action of the parasympathetic nervous system. In a search for inhibitors in adrenal gland extracts, Hunt (1901) concluded that an ester of choline might be involved. "Evidence was obtained that aqueous extracts of the suprarenal contain at least one other blood pressure lowering body in addition to choline, the presence of which in the extracts of the suprarenals causes a fall in blood pressure. This second body differs from choline in its physiological effects chiefly in that it caused a fall of blood pressure after the administration of atropine. By repeated precipitation with platinum or mercuric chloride, or by treating the filtrates from these precipitates with hydrogen sulphide this second body disappeared; at the same time the amount of choline seemed to be increased ...Hence it was considered probable that some body was present which yielded choline on decomposition. It was suggested that this precursor of choline might be some ester-like body containing choline in its molecule."

Five years later Hunt and Taveau (1906) found an acetate ester that had 1000 times the depressor activity of choline. Dale (1914), displaying great insight, suggested that something was present that must also destroy the active principle and thus prevent its detection in simple experiments. An enzyme in the blood was to be sought. Dale stressed the similarity between the action of Ach and normally occurring parasympathetic effects. He also distinguished "nicotinic" and "muscarinic" types of receptor response to Ach, the former being blocked by atropine whereas the latter was not.

Still another chapter in the early study of chemical receptor action at the NMJ was provided by the work of Loewi (1921), who in his famous heart experiment demonstrated that the fluid from a stimulated heart contained something that inhibited a second heart. This effect was blocked by atropine. Loewi concluded that stimulation of the vagus nerve leads to release of some material ("vagusstoff") in the perfusing solution that was either formed or liberated from the cells. In a later paper (1922) Loewi compared the "vagusstoff" with the properties of Ach and showed that there was choline in the perfusion fluid. He also demonstrated that choline was relatively inactive and therefore not the "vagusstoff." Loewi and Navratil (1926a) compared the rate of destruction of Ach with that of the "vagusstoff" and later showed inhibition of the destructive mechanism by eserine (1926b).

Four years passed before Englehart and Loewi (1930) and Matthes (1930) established that the action of eserine was to inhibit the enzyme that destroys Ach. It was found that eserine was effective in inhibiting the Ach-destroying enzyme even when greatly diluted (10^{-5} to 10^{-6}M).

Dale and Dudley (1929) finally put the completing link in the chain of evidence when they isolated Ach from the spleen and thereby established it as a normally occurring substance. Thus there was great probability that Ach and the "vagusstoff" were the same substance.

Dale and Dudley therefore concluded that Ach was the parasympathetic mediator. However, the critical reader might say that this assertion is still based upon indirect evidence and that many subtle phenomena could be hidden from view in such a crude structure of circumstantial evidence. Subsequent studies by numerous investigators have added many confirmatory data. The assertion that Ach is the chemical transmitter at parasympathetic synapses and at the NMJ is based on the following evidence:

1. Ach occurs in man and other animals.
2. Ach is released during neural stimulation.
3. An enzyme, AchE, is present and the products of its hydrolysis are relatively inactive.
4. Chemicals that potentiate (eserine) or block (curare) the effects of neural stimulation are also active in isolated preparations when Ach is added exogenously.

To return to the five characteristics of synaptic transmission described by Sherrington, we might ask how these are accounted for by the hypothesis of Ach chemoreception at the NMJ. Certainly delay in the reflex pathway (synaptic delay) is understandable in terms of the time required for Ach to be mobilized and diffuse from the presynaptic terminal to the postsynaptic membrane. One-way transmission, fatigability, and sensitivity to chemical agents are all explicable in terms of the theory.

Various investigations by the end of the 1920's had established fairly well what the transmitter was (Ach) and what happened to it (hydrolysis by cholinesterase), but not where it came from, how it was stored or released, or how it reacted with the hypothetical "receptive substance" (Langley, 1905, 1909).

The more modern history of this complex subject is conveniently considered under a series of headings corresponding approximately to the sequence of events beginning with the synthesis of Ach in the axon terminal, its storage in and release from the synaptic vesicles by the presynaptic stimulatory potential (PSP) as facilitated by the presence of cations followed by its diffusion across the synaptic gap to the specific receptors (AchR) of the postsynaptic membrane (PSM). The resulting alteration of these receptors generate the miniature endplate potentials (MEPPS) which when summated, generate the endplate potential (EPP) that in turn causes depolarization of the PSM. The properties of these potentials and their molecular substratum as well as the nature and reactions of the specific receptor sites will be considered.

Synthesis of Acetylcholine

Determination of the site of Ach synthesis in the terminal axons of NMJs is a particularly difficult problem considering the small size of the NMJs and the large amounts of muscle that they must be separated from in order to perform biochemical studies. The presence of AchE may be used as a general indicator of cholinergic synapses (Koelle, 1968) but it is not involved in Ach symthesis. The enzyme that is responsible for the synthesis of Ach from choline and acetyl CoA is choline acetylase (choline acetyl transferase). Histochemistry has been of little help in localizing either Ach or choline acetyltransferase. There is no method available for demonstrating Ach and only recently have new procedures been developed to demonstrate choline acetyltransferase (Burt, 1970). However, using biochemical analyses, Tuček (1972) demonstrated that most of the enzyme activity in muscle is in intramuscular nervous tissue.

Ach Localization in Nervous Tissue

Because of the difficulty of isolating subcellular components from NMJs, the early investigations were devoted to the study of central nervous system synapses using variations of the differential sedimentation techniques described by Claude (1938) and Schneider and Hogeboom (1950). Still later, these techniques were turned to the investigation of Ach synthesis in the electric organ of the electric eel *Electrophorus* or fish *Torpedo,* a structure which in its derivation and physiology is a model of the vertebrate NMJ. Formation of Ach by brain homogenates had been demonstrated by Quastel et al. (1936), and in 1943 Nachmansohn and Machado discovered the enzyme responsible for the synthesis of Ach, choline acetyltransferase.

Early studies of sedimented particles from brain yielded 3 particulate fractions: a nuclear fraction, isolated at low centrifugal forces; a mitochondrial fraction, requiring somewhat higher g forces for sedimentation; and lastly, the "microsomes", which required considerable centrifugal force to sediment. Hebb and Smallman (1956) reported that Ach was synthesized in axonal mitochondria and Hebb and Waites (1956) suggested that AchE and possibly Ach were synthesized in the cell body and carried to the axon terminals by means of axoplasmic flow. Hebb and Whittaker (1958) used gradient sedimentation (0.32-1.6M sucrose) to study particles sedimented from rabbit brain homogenates. They concluded that both choline acetyltransferase and Ach were present in the same fraction as the mitochondria but within different particles. They could not determine which particles were involved since no electron microscopic control was provided in this study. In a subsequent investigation, Whittaker (1959) employed density gradient sedimentation and electron microscopic control of the sediments. This procedure is essential to permit correlations between biochemical activity and morphology. Such control of particulate sediments is now routine in current research. Whittaker (1959) isolated three fractions by sucrose density gradient centrifugation. The fractions consisted of (1) a fraction less dense than 0.8M sucrose, containing particles measuring 2. to 5μ ; (2) a fraction more dense than 0.8M sucrose and less dense than 1.2M sucrose, with particle diameters ranging from 0.02-0.3μ and (3) a fraction denser than 1.2M sucrose containing particles measuring 0.02-1.0μ (median; 0.25μ). This latter fraction (3) contained mitochondria when examined in the electron microscope. Most of the particle-bound Ach was found in the 2 layers containing 60% of the particles in the 0.02-0.08 μ size range. In the electron microscope, these structures resembled synaptic vesicles observed in tissue sections. Whittaker also demonstrated that freezing and thawing or changing the osmolarity of the suspension media resulted in two forms of bound Ach: a labile fraction and one more stable.

Bellamy (1959) reported that the mitochondrial fraction from rat brain contained 70% of the total bound Ach and a roughly similar percentage (54%) was found in pigeon brain mitochondria. Choline acetyltransferase activity was present in all the fractions except the supernatant. The activity of this enzyme was greater in the mitochondrial and microsomal fractions than in the whole homogenate. Although brain mitochondrial preparations incubated with choline failed to synthesize Ach, there was an unexpected release of bound Ach into the medium: 64% of the bound Ach from pigeon and 46% of the bound ester from rat mitochondrial preparations.

In a study of sucrose homogenates from guinea pig forebrain, Gray and Whittaker (1960) found most of the Ach in 500 A particles obtained after sedimentation in a 0.8-1.0M sucrose density gradient system. Their electron micrographs show structures which they interpreted as "pinched off nerve endings" or synaptosomes which contain mitochondria, synaptic vesicles and still adhering portions of the postsynaptic membrane. They concluded that there was a probable relationship between the transmitter and the synaptic vesicles.

In a later study, De Robertis et al. (1962) also employed sucrose gradient sedimentation and electron microscopic control of the sediments to study Ach and AchE activity in subcellular components of rat brain. As in previous studies, nuclear, mitochondrial, and microsomal fractions were separated. By application of a discontinuous sucrose gradient of 1.4, 1.2, 1.0 and 0.8 M sucrose, these investigators separated the mitochondrial fraction into four subfractions. The first, which was found in the supper limit of the 0.8M sucrose level, contained 29 per cent of the total protein and was shown by electron microscopy to consist chiefly of myelin. The second fraction, grayish in color and less compact, was found at the approximately 1.0M sucrose level. It contained 10 per cent of the total protein and was heterogeneous, containing myelin, microsomal particles, vesicles, curved membranes, small dense bodies, and fragmented nerve endings. The third fraction was more compact than the second. It separated at the 1.0 to 1.2M sucrose level and contained 12 per cent of the total protein. It appeared more homogeneous than the second fraction and contained whole and fragmented nerve endings, synaptic vesicles, and a few mitochondria. Subsynaptic membranes were attached to many of the nerve endings. The fourth layer, at the 1.4M sucrose level, contained 24 per cent of the total protein and was composed of a mass of compact nerve endings. The bottom sediment, which was grayish with a dark orange portion, contained 25 per cent of the total protein and was composed of free swollen mitochondria and a few nerve endings. The third mitochondrial subfraction studied by De Robertis and associates (which contained nerve endings and other structures) contained the greatest concentration of Ach and AchE activity. However, relatively large concentrations of both Ach and AchE were also found in the second mitochondrial subfraction, which was composed of microsomal particles, vesicles, and curved membranes, as well as fragmented nerve endings. Thus, even with more refined techniques, it was not possible to be certain which particles contained the Ach, choline acetyltransferase or AchE activity.

To release synaptic vesicles from the "synaptosomes" (nerve endings), De Robertis et al. (1963) added distilled water to "mitochondrial preparations" obtained from rat brain. When sedimented, the synaptic vesicle fraction contained 6.3 per cent of the protein and had the greatest concentration of Ach and choline acetyltransferase activity. Takeno et al. (1969) described two fractions of bound Ach in rabbit brain homogenates. One fraction was stable and the other, roughly equal in quantity, was labile. Approximately 28% of the initial total Ach was recovered in the fraction of bound Ach after disruption of the nerve endings. These investigators concluded that the stable fraction of bound Ach is the portion within the synaptic vesicles whereas the labile fraction is cytoplasmic.

Ach Synthesis in the Electroplax

Since the electroplax of the electric eel resembles NMJs in many ways, (Feldberg and Fessard, 1942; Grundfest, 1957; Luft, 1958) Ach synthesis in various fractions obtained from this structure have been studied extensively. Sheridan et al. (1966) obtained fractions composed of small vesicles and granules that contained large amounts of bound Ach. In later studies, Israël and Gautron (1969) concluded that Ach is bound to the synaptic vesicles isolated from the electric organ of *Torpedo* and that choline acetyltransferase (and AchE) are not associated with the vesicles. Israël (1970) isolated synaptic vesicles from *Torpedo* that contained 50-300 times more Ach than the equivalent fraction obtained from the brains of rats or guinea pigs. Most of the choline acetyltransferase activity was found in the supernatant fraction but because it was not possible to completely inhibit the esterase activity of the homogenates, the level of Ach in the soluble component could not be determined accurately. Ach synthesis appears to occur in the cytoplasm of the axon terminals, not within the vesicles.

A criticism applicable to all of these studies is the difficulty in controlling possible nonspecific absorption of the Ach and enzymes from the disrupted nerve terminals onto the exceedingly large surface area provided by the particulate material freed by homogenation and centrifugation. Thus it is difficult to be certain whether enzyme activity associated with a given fraction represents material that was there prior to disruption of the cells. This is of particular importance when the objective is to distinguish between the enzyme activities of several particles that vary moderately in size. Another theoretically possible source of false localization is change in the particle membrane resulting from the technical procedures used to separate the particles.

It should be emphasized that these data all concern particulates isolated from brain or electric tissue and do not refer to NMJs. It is obvious that isolation of synaptic vesicles from NMJs poses technical difficulties of greater magnitude than the isolation of subcellular particles from brain or electric tissue.

Ach Synthesis in NMJs

That most (78-90%) of the choline acetyltransferase activity of skeletal muscle is located in the intramuscular nerve fibers has been demonstrated by loss of the enzyme activity after denervation (Hebb et al., 1964; Emmelin et al., 1966; Israël, 1970). There is a very rapid decline of enzyme activity in the first 80 hours after nerve section after which there is a slower loss of activity (Tuček, 1968).

In a different approach to the problem of where in the terminal Ach is synthesized, Csillik et al. (1970) used ^{14}C labeled hemicholinium, a substance known to prevent choline uptake by the terminal. Radio-autography and optical microscopy used to localize sites of hemicholinum binding demonstrated silver grains in areas of the central nervous system known to contain considerable quantities of Ach. Neither neuron cell bodies or larger dendrites were reactive but silver grains were observed in the vicinity of some of the larger neurons. In skeletal muscle, silver grains were localized in the NMJs, apparently in the terminal axons. However, the resolution limitations of optical microscopy and the absence of correction for scatter resulted in little new information from this approach that assumes an intracellular site of action of hemicholinium.

Burt (1970) devised a histochemical technique to localize choline acetyltransferase activity by means of forming a mercaptide of acetyl CoA, a product of the enzyme reaction, by means of lead precipitation. The specificity of this reaction for choline acetylase is based upon the observation that most of the acetyl CoA hydrolysis in NMJs is coupled to Ach synthesis and nonspecific hydrolysis of acetyl CoA can be localized by inhibition of choline acetyl transferase with Cu^{++} or by selectively releasing the choline acetyl transferase from the tissue sections by 0.1M KNO_3 in the incubation medium. The "HEPES" reagent (N-2-hydroxy ethyl piperazine-N-2) ethane sulfonic acid was used to form the mercaptide. The reaction product was found on the perikaryon of rat spinal neurons, particularly anterior horn cells. This report did not include a description of NMJs.

There is no conclusive evidence contrary to the view that choline acetyltransferase is synthesized in the neuron cell body and is transported down the axon to the nerve terminal (Hebb and Waites, 1956; Hebb and Silver, 1961).

Site of Ach Synthesis and Packaging of Ach

Mann (1938) and Birks and MacIntosh (1961) suggested that Ach must be segregated in the terminal axons, probably within the synaptic vesicles, to protect it from hydrolysis. Although many studies of brain particulates had shown that Ach and choline acetyltransferase were associated with synaptic vesicles (DeRobertis et al., 1962, 1963), there also was evidence that choline acetyltransferase was present only in the cytoplasm (Israël and Gautron, 1969; Israël, 1970) of the electroplax nerve endings. Whether choline acetyltransferase is bound to synaptic vesicles or is free in the synaptoplasm largely depends upon the means of isolation used and the particular animal species. Localization of choline acetyltransferase either within synaptic vesicles or in the synaptoplasm is important in deciding where Ach is synthesized. For example, Burton (1964) reported that the synaptic vesicles took up radioactive Ach after presumed synthesis in the synaptoplasm and Marchbanks (1968) demonstrated free exchange of synaptoplasmic Ach with external radioactive Ach but not with Ach in synaptic vesicles. Marchbanks believed that the Ach was synthesized in the synaptoplasm but not in the vesicles that appeared not to take up the neurohumor. Data was also obtained by Kuriyama et al. (1968) and Chakrin and Whittaker (1969) that there also is rapid exchange of Ach between the synaptoplasm and synaptic vesicles from brain. Kuriyama et al. (1968) demonstrated that radioactive Ach was bound to purified synaptic reaction that could be prevented by several inorganic ions and organic molecules. In this work, binding was defined in terms of the association of radioactive Ach with synaptic vesicles after separation either by centrifugation or gel chromatography. Guth (1969) reexamined the problem and defined bound Ach as that fraction which exists within the synaptic vesicles and which therefore should be protected from hydrolysis by AchE in the homogenate. Guth therefore briefly exposed the synaptic vesicle preparations to AchE to hydrolyze the free extravesicular Ach and preserve the intravesicular Ach. Enzyme hydrolysis was stopped by adjusting the pH to 4.0. Using this technique on guinea pig cortex synaptic vesicle preparations, Guth demonstrated that there is an extremely rapid uptake of Ach by vesicles from the medium in a period of 15-30 seconds that occurs against the concentration gradient. In this time, the Ach concentration in the vesicles became 3 times that of the supernatant. He also found that some Ach synthesis occurred in the synaptic vesicle suspension but this apparently was not a requisite for incorporation of the neurohumor within the vesicles. Similarly, Ritchie and Goldberg (1970) studied the uptake of radioactive Ach and choline by synaptosome preparations from rat brain in which the synaptic vesicles had been released by hypoosmotic shock in the presence of physostigmine to prevent AchE hydrolysis. These investigators reported that the amount of radioactive Ach in the synaptoplasm and synaptic vesicles was a linear function of the radioactive Ach in the incubation mixture. The greatest quantity of Ach was found in the synaptoplasm and only 1.5% within the synaptic vesicles. Even after incubation for 30 minutes at 38°C., there was only 1.2 times more Ach formed than in the samples incubated at 0°C. It appeared that Ach entered the vesicles by passive diffusion rather than active uptake. When synthesis of radioactive Ach was studied, it was found to be linear when the synaptosomes were incubated with radioactive choline at 38°C. for 60 minutes. Subsequent analysis showed that the amount of radioactive Ach in the synaptic vesicles constituted approximately 15% of the amount synthesized in the synaptoplasm compared to the approximately 1.5% present as a result of binding of the radioactive Ach or by contamination. Therefore, it was clear that there was more newly synthesized radioactive Ach in the synaptic vesicles than could be attributed to contamination from the Ach in the synaptoplasm. These investigators concluded that Ach was synthesized in both synaptic vesicles and synaptoplasm although the greater part of the synthesis occurred in the latter.

It has been demonstrated that there is a rapidly available Ach fraction in axons constituting 15-20% of the total and a much larger, less readily available fraction that can be released on prolonged neural stimulation. A morphologic correlate of this may be that the synaptic vesicles near the axon cell membrane facing the postsynaptic membrane are the first released and that the less readily available Ach is contained in the synaptic vesicles distant from the membrane surface (Hubbard, 1970; Birks and MacIntosh, 1961). In the electric organ (Whittaker, 1971) two fractions containing radioactive choline are also found. These appear to consist of a rapidly available population of vesicles in the vicinity of the presynaptic membrane and a second less labeled and less available fraction of vesicles more distant from the membrane.

In the current view (Kása et al., 1970a, b) choline acetyltransferase is localized with ribosomes in the neuron cell body, associated with neurofilaments in the axons and between the synaptic vesicles in nerve terminals but not in mitochondria. It is conveyed to the axon terminal synaptoplasm (Fonnum, 1968, 1970) where it is responsible for the transfer of the acetyl group from acetyl CoA to choline. However, acetyl CoA, a mitochondrial enzyme (DeDuve et al., 1962) cannot penetrate the mitochondrial membrane (Lowenstein, 1964). Thus to get the various components of the synthetic system together in the synaptoplasm, it is suggested that acetyl groups from the mitochondria are transported to the cytoplasm in the form of citrate mediated by citrate synthetase and when reaching the terminal axoplasm in the presence of ATP and citrate lyase, forms acetyl CoA (Potter, 1970). With choline and choline acetyltransferase present, Ach is synthesized and taken up by synaptic vesicles.

It is also clear that the store of choline in the nerve terminal is small (Potter, 1970) and that the choline utilized in Ach synthesis must be provided continuously from outside the terminal. It probably enters the terminal by means of a carrier (Potter, 1970) that apparently is the mechanism that is blocked by hemicholinium (MacIntosh, 1961). Choline resulting from hydrolysis of secreted Ach probably is reabsorbed by the terminal and utilized for re-synthesis of Ach, a process that is accelerated by nerve stimulation (Potter, 1970). We may also speculate that some choline from membranes of synaptic vesicles may be reutilized in this way. In the presence of anticholinesterase drugs, there is also evidence that Ach itself may be reabsorbed by the terminals, a process that iy considered to be abnormal (Potter, 1970). Koike, et al (1972) have shown Ach synthesis in the cell bodies of *Aplysia* neurons and transport of labelled Ach down the axons.

Experimental evidence for the role of synaptic vesicles in synaptic transmission

To obtain evidence that synaptic vesicles were essential for neuromuscular transmission, De Robertis (1956) studied changes in the synaptic vesicles in the ventral acoustic nerve ganglia of guinea pigs after destruction of the cochlea.

After 22 hours the nerve endings were swollen, there was decreased electron density of the "matrix", and most of the synaptic vesicles had clumped together or disappeared. After 44 hours there was more marked agglutination of synaptic vesicles, and after 48 hours the mitochondria were fragmented, the vesicles were gone, and the membrane was focally disrupted. This particular investigation does not seem to answer the central question: namely, whether the known decrease in Ach following degeneration is associated with the decreased numbers of vesicles. Furthermore, since changes occurred in several subcellular components, including the mitochondria, synaptic vesicles, and membranes, it was impossible to determine which disordered component was associated with the known biochemical defect.

Another attempt to alter synaptic vesicles was reported by De Robertis and Franchi (1956). In this study rabbits were kept in darkness for 24 hours to nine days and the synaptic vesicles in the retinal rod and cone synapses were examined in the electron microscope. In normal retinas, spherical synaptic vesicles were present in the presynaptic cytoplasm, which were concentrated near the synaptic membrane. The vesicles ranged in size from 200 to 650 A with a mean diameter of 386 A. The synaptic vesicles in retinas of animals kept in darkness for 24 hours had accumulated near the synaptic membrane. There was a slight increase in their mean diameter, but changes in the number and size of the synaptic vesicles were not conspicuous. After 48 hours in darkness, there was slight decrease in synaptic vesicle size, the mean diameter being 281 A. After nine days of darkness, the size of the synaptic vesicles was greatly reduced. The range was 50 to 400 A with a mean diameter of 195 A. This is compared with the 396 A mean diameter observed in the control (light-exposed) animals. The number of vesicles in the controls was approximately similar to the number of synaptic vesicles in the dark-adapted retinal synapses.

Synaptic vesicles within cone synapses ranged in diameter from 150 to 550 A with a mean of 338 A when exposed to the light. After being kept in the dark for nine days, the range of vesicle size was 50 to 400 A with a mean diameter of 236 A. De Robertis and Franchi interpreted these results as supporting the concept that identified the synaptic vesicles with the hypothetical Ach-containing packets. In subsequent investigations, De Robertis (1958, 1959) claimed that there was a decrease in size and number of synaptic vesicles after electrical stimulation, but this was not confirmed by deHarven and Coërs (1959) and Birks et al. (1960). Mountford (1963) concluded that the appearance of change in vesicle populations visible in electron micrographs could be deceptive. He found no statistically significant change in the size of synaptic vesicles in guinea pig receptor biopolar synapses under light or dark conditions. There were large variations in vesicle size between individual animals and individual synapses.

However, were it possible to demonstrate changes in synaptic vesicle diameter after dark adaptation, such data would still fail to clarify the functional role of the synaptic vesicles. Certainly many other biochemical processes related to reception of visual impulses and their synaptic transmission must be at a low level of activity during dark adaptation.

In an attempt to correlate changes in the synaptic vesicle population with changes in the ionic environment known to alter MEPPs (page 170), Hubbard and Kwanbunbumpen (1968) soaked rat phrenic nerve-diaphragm preparations in the solutions of saline, KCl and $MgCl_2$. The preparations were then fixed, prepared for electron microscopy and the relative numbers of synaptic vesicles adjacent to the synaptic clefts were studied. Soaking in salt solution increased the proportion of subneural clefts that were related to presynaptic membrane densities with associated synaptic vesicles. After exposure to 20 Mm KCl, both the specific synaptic vesicle population and the whole population of terminal vesicles within the terminal axon were depleted. This effect was prevented by increasing the concentration of $MgCl_2$. Solutions with increased osmotic pressure reduced the number of specific vesicles, (with relationship to the axoplasmic membrane), but not the general vesicle population. The authors suggested that this data supports the vesicle hypothesis and that the specific vesicle population is part of a feed-back mechanism that adjusts transmitter synthesis and mobilization to the rate of transmitter release. However they failed to explain why there was no change in the number of synaptic vesicles per unit area.

In a later study, Landau and Kwanbunbumpen (1969) observed changes in synaptic vesicles produced by electric current. Bass and Moore (1966) had previously suggested that the electric charge on synaptic vesicles played a role in excitation-release coupling. Using the rat phrenic nerve-diaphragm preparation, stimulation via the nerve produced an accumulation of synaptic vesicles and mitochondria in the presynaptic terminal and a decrease in the width of the synaptic gap. With hyperpolarizing currents, there was a decrease in number of synaptic vesicles and a wider gap. These changes were thought due to the flow of current. Similar changes did not occur when the effect of K^+ was studied. The authors concluded that both mitochondria and synaptic vesicles probably carry positive charges. Several investigators have suggested that the charge on the synaptic vesicles is important in bringing about their migration to the synaptic membrane. The time required for this migration could partially explain the delay that occurs between the onset of depolarization of the axon terminal and the arrival of the Ach quanta at the postsynaptic membrane (Samojloff, 1967; Katz and Miledi, 1965). The several milliseconds that elapse are primarily utilized by a series of presynaptic events because Ach diffusion across the synapse is very rapid. Some controversy has been generated over whether the synaptic vesicles bear negative or positive charges. Vos et al. (1968) stated that synaptic vesicles from brain are negatively charged, a finding which would fit with the original hypothesis whereas Landau and Kwanbunbumpen (1969) concluded there were positive charges on synaptic vesicles in *in vitro* experiments utilizing stimulation by polarizing currents.

Despite these repeated attempts to prove the correspondence of synaptic vesicle fusion and MEPPs, definitive evidence has been elusive. More recent work by Jones and Kwanbunbumpen (1970a, b) demonstrated an increase in terminal axon vesicles on tetanic stimulation. If hemicholinium were included in the bathing medium during tetanic stimulation, MEPP amplitude decreased and depletion of synaptic vesicles occurred. This procedure is more informative since it relates known parameters of the normal function of the NMJ. Certainly in vertebrate NMJ, there can be great numbers of recorded MEPPs without visible depletion of the synaptic vesicle population. Heuser and Miledi (1971) found that La++ increased MEPP frequency without alteration of the terminals after 1 hour and Heuser (1971; Heuser and Reese, 1973) has reported anatomic evidence for depletion and rapid reformation of synaptic vesicles in stimulated frog NMJs. Furthermore, it appears that recently synthesized Ach is released preferentially (Collier, 1969; Potter, 1970). This problem has also been considered by Korneliussen (1972; Korneliussen et al, 1972).

Perhaps most convincing of the role of synaptic vesicles in the generation of MEPPs is the work of Jones and Kwanbunbumpen (1970a, b) and the experiments with black widow spider venom (Longenecker et al., 1970; Clark et al., 1971; Ceccarelli et al., 1972; 1973) and β-bungarotoxin (Chen and Lee, 1970) that show destruction of synaptic vesicles and coincident loss of MEPPs. The former work excludes the possibility of nonspecific action of non-neurotoxic components in the experiments with impure spider venom.

Changes in synaptic vesicles under conditions of degeneration due to denervation are considered in chapter

Exocytotic Release of Acetylcholine from Synaptic Vesicles

In the first description of synaptic vesicles, De Robertis and Bennett (1955) noted that they were oriented with respect to the synaptic surface of the terminal axon. Occasional vesicles appeared to be attached to the inner leaflet of the terminal axon plasma membrane and there were occasional indentations of the external leaflet, suggesting that Ach is transferred from its storage form in the synaptic vesicles to the synaptic cleft by means of exocytosis. In this hypothesis, the vesicles would fuse with the axon plasma membrane after which they would open into the synaptic cleft allowing discharge of the enclosed Ach. It is difficult to prove directly that this occurs. Although indentations in the axon plasma membrane have been demonstrated by several investigators, these could as also be interpreted as evidence of endocytosis. Convincing evidence of fusion of synaptic vesicles to the axon plasma membrane has now been obtained in NMJs poisoned by spider venom (Clark et al., 1971) and in similar data reported by Couteaux and Pecot-Dechavassine (1970) for NMJs at rest. A particularly convincing demonstration of fusion of synaptic vesicles to the axon membranes and opening onto the synaptic cleft has recently been obtained in freeze-etched electric organ of *Torpedo* (Nickel and Potter, 1970). Because there is no direct means of labeling the vesicles, we must depend on indirect evidence to support this hypothesis. If exocytosis does occur at a rate sufficient to release the quantities of Ach known to be secreted by terminal axons, the fate of the large amount of vesicular membrane involved must be considered. For example, Bittner and Kennedy (1970) concluded that 24mm^2 of membrane per hour per crayfish neuron is produced, a quantity that necessarily precludes loss of the membrane or permanent incorporation into the terminal axon membrane. If the surplus membrane from the synaptic vesicles is not added to the axon plasma membrane, it could be reincorporated into the axon by means of reverse exocytosis or endocytosis, a mechanism that appears to operate in some gland cells. Endocytosis is known to occur in both central and peripheral synapses but there is little indication that it correlates well with increased Ach secretion produced by neural stimulation. Birks (1966) found little correspondence between thorotrast uptake and stimulation of frog NMJs and Zacks and Saito (1969) found that only coated vesicles and narrow tubular structures in unstimulated mouse terminal axons took up horseradish peroxidase (HRP) used as a tracer (Fig. 47). Holtzman et al. (1971) found rare or no up-take of HRP in terminal axons of lobster NMJs but after continuous or periodic electrical stimulation of the motor nerves, many synaptic vesicles contained HRP but few coated vesicles with HRP were found.

Recently, Heuser (1971; Heuser and Reese, 1973) stimulated frog sartorius NMJs at 10 CPS and observed reduction in the number of synaptic vesicles, increase in axolemmal membrane area and membrane-bound cisternae associated with increased numbers of coated vesicles in the axoplasm. HRP was taken up by coated vesicles and cisternae during the initial minute of stimulation. Only during recovery from stimulation, when the cisternae returned to normal, did he find synaptic vesicles containing HRP. These findings suggested that newly formed synaptic vesicles arose from the cisternae. Heuser suggested a cycle in which membrane is added to the axon plasma membrane by fusion of synaptic vesicles and is recovered by invaginations of coated vesicles which then transfer the material to the cisternae where new synaptic vesicles are formed. This hypothesis suggests a constant renewal of axon surface membrane that is consistent with the quantitative data of Bittner and Kennedy (1970). In this view, membrane is added and subtracted from the axon surface membrane as Ach quanta are released. Data that may be interpreted as contrary to this hypothesis is the structural (diCarlo, 1967) and enzymatic (Israël and Gautron, 1969) differences between synaptic vesicle membrane and the axon surface membrane. The synaptic vesicle membranes lack unit membrane structure and may be less stable than the axon plasma membrane. If the synaptic vesicles were coacervates of Ach enclosed by phospholipid, their fusion with the axonal membrane would not pose a problem of addition of membrane protein. Disruption of the vesicle phospholipid could release choline that might be recycled by the terminal along with the choline released by the hydrolysis of Ach. Furthermore, data indicating prolonged interference of Ach secretion by botulinum toxin may be cited as evidence contrary to rapid turnover of axon membrane. Available data indicates that the toxin binding is presynaptic in gangliosides (Simpson and Rapport, 1971) and is not easily reversible. Only when new axon terminals form following crush injury and reinnervation (Duchen, 1970) or as the result of sprouting (Duchen, 1971a, b) is the botulinum toxin induced block reversed.

Present information indicates that synaptic vesicles do discharge their Ach content by exocytosis, that there is only transient addition of their membrane to the axon plasma membrane, but that the mechanism proposed for recycling of membrane and resynthesis of the vesicles is still hypothetical.

ELECTRICAL ASPECTS OF ACH RELEASE AND BINDING BY POSTSYNAPTIC RECEPTORS

Miniature Endplate Potentials

A new aspect of the chemoelectrical phenomena that occur at NMJs was discovered by Fatt and Katz (1950, 1951). These investigators found that when microelectrodes were placed in NMJs, "unexpected signs of continuous spontaneous unrest" were present. These potentials differed from the endplate potentials (EPPs) discovered in curarized frog muscle by Gopfert and Schaefer (1938). Whereas the EPP was the immediate electrical result reflecting the depolarization of the NMJ due to chemical stimulation of the muscle receptors, the miniature endplate potentials (MEPPs) represented what appeared to be spontaneous subthreshold activity that rarely developed sufficient amplitude to depolarize the NMJ. These 1 mv. miniature potentials resemble normal EPPs in many respects except amplitude. The MEPPs were propagated electrotonically for short distances (1-2 mm.) from the NMJs and they were monophasic and had a consistent time course, rising in 1-2 milliseconds and declining by 50% in 3-4 milliseconds. Their constant shape and slightly varying size indicated an "all or none" response. This evidence of a highly localized phenomenon occurring in only certain points of the NMJ was thought to indicate that Ach was being released in subthreshold quantities or quanta. In a summary of their experience with MEPPs, Fatt and Katz (1952) concluded that intact nerve endings were required for their production because the MEPPs were abolished by nerve section.

Since previous calculations indicated that 1 million Ach molecules were necessary to trigger an impulse at the NMJ (Acheson, 1948), the MEPPs, which were 1/100 as large as EPPs, might require the release of several thousand Ach molecules. This led to the concept that the MEPPs were due to discharges of Ach packets. That the MEPPs were not an artefact was indicated by their electrotonic spread. When the recording electrodes were at some distance from the NMJs, they could not have damaged the nerve endings, yet the MEPPs could still be recorded. The size of the MEPPs proved to be very resistant to various pharmacologic and physical agents. Similar observations were made by Liley (1956a) and Del Castillo and Katz (1954a).

The amplitude of the MEPPs was found to be independent of the condition of the nerve endings and was altered chiefly by postsynaptic factors. Substances that did affect the nerve endings altered the *frequency* of the MEPPs. Thus it appeared that once the quantal package was released, it could not be altered by environmental conditions, but alterations in the environment could influence the release of the quanta or the postsynaptic receptors. Katz (1958) concluded that the size of an Ach quantum depended on some fixed property of the nerve terminal.

When the synaptic vesicles were first described, neurophysiologists including Del Castillo and Katz (1954a, b), Boyd and Martin (1956a), and Liley (1956a) agreed with the microscopists that the synaptic vesicles might be the Ach packets predicted by the physiologic investigations. Katz (1958) suggested that the synaptic vesicles may represent the storage form of Ach and their release in quantal increments may be the anatomic basis of the MEPPs. Thus the MEPP hypothesis was widely accepted; that MEPPs result from the random discharge of "quanta" or packets of Ach from the presynaptic terminal (Boyd and Martin, 1956a; Liley, 1956a; Katz and Miledi, 1965a; Gage and Hubbard, 1965). Local excitation of the terminal axon branches as a source of MEPPs was excluded because unrelated MEPPs occurred a short distance apart in a single nerve terminal and were observed even after depolarization by K^+. The MEPPs were generated by a transient local increase in conductance of the postsynaptic membrane of the order of 10^{-7} mho (Del Castillo and Katz, 1956b; Takeuchi and Takeuchi, 1960) as a consequence of the release of one quantum from the presynaptic terminal. The similarity of the MEPP and the EPP generated by normal nerve stimulation was stressed by Fatt and Katz. In their hypothesis, MEPPs are local depolarizations of the postsynaptic membrane which are insufficient to depolarize the entire postsynaptic membrane. Only when they summate in sufficient number, as occurs during nerve stimulation, is there sufficient depolarization of the postsynaptic membrane to produce a propagated muscle action potential. The EPP is generated as a result of simultaneous arrival of a sufficient number of Ach quanta at the postsynaptic receptors following their release from the axon terminal caused by nerve depolarization. The function of axonal depolarization is to increase the probability of discharge of any single quantum. For example, Liley (1956b) demonstrated that incremental electrotonic depolarization of the axon terminal increased the average frequency of MEPPs. Approximately 15 mv. of depolarization produced a 10 fold increase in MEPP frequency. With a potential change of 90 mv., the frequency increased 10^6, which was sufficient to generate an EPP. Gage and Hubbard (1965) also demonstrated that the size of a MEPP, that is the number of Ach molecules per quantum, can be reduced without altering the probability of its release.

According to Thies (1965), the quantum content of EPPs is reduced for a while after stimulation but concurrently there is mobilization of Ach in the terminal that is also stimulated by the previous neural activity. This may be due to movement of synaptic vesicles from reserve areas distant from the axon membrane to the vicinity of the membrane. Mobilization of the reserve quanta is apparently independent of previous release of transmitter that may be observed in Mg++ poisoned terminals where an initial stimulus yields no transmitter release and no response but a second stimulus following soon upon the first generates an EPP. It appears that each stimulus of the presynaptic terminal produces Ach release as well as mobilization of Ach. However, Mallart and Martin (1967) have suggested that facilitation in frog NMJs may also include a postsynaptic component.

The facilitation and depression of EPPs that occurs during repetitive stimulation may be due to changes in the number of released Ach quanta rather than to their size (Del Castillo and Katz, 1954c). With prolonged hyperpolarization of the axon terminal, there is an increase in EPP amplitude due to an increase in the number of quanta released per stimulus. Apparently, hyperpolarization produces electrophoretic movement of Ach quanta according to the hypothesis of Hubbard and Willis (1968).

Response of the MEPPs to various pharmacologic agents also supports the hypothesis that they arise as the result of release of Ach from the presynaptic terminal and subsequent binding to postsynaptic receptors. For example, the MEPP amplitude is reduced by curare (Ach block) and increased by neostigmine and other anticholinesterase drugs. That the MEPPs were not due to single Ach molecules was indicated by experiments that showed smooth graded reduction of the membrane potential, rather than in quantal increments, when Ach was added to the external solution. Furthermore, Ach applied in this way failed to affect the rate of discharge of the MEPPs.

Various other experimental agents applied to the external medium revealed additional characteristics of the MEPPs. If sucrose or NaCl was added to the muscle bath to increase the tonicity of the external solution, there was marked increase in the frequency of discharge of MEPPs and correspondingly, reduction of the tonicity reduced the rate of discharge (Fatt and Katz, 1952). However, increased rate of discharge produced by increased tonicity was not accompanied by an increase in the size of the Ach quanta. Del Castillo (1960) suggested that not all random contacts of the Ach-containing quanta with the presynaptic membrane were successful and he postulated that there were "weak spots" or pores that could serve as "special channels" for the released quanta.

Del Castillo and Katz (1954d) altered the state of polarization of frog presynaptic membrane by externally applied electronic currents. When cathodic currents were used, there was a graded increase in the rate of MEPP discharge, which increased in parallel with the current strength. Anodic polarization with weak currents failed to reduce the rate of spontaneous MEPP discharge, whereas strong anodic currents produced bursts of discharges. Similar studies on mammalian NMJs by Liley (1956b) demonstrated graded effects on the rate of MEPP discharge by both cathodic and anodic currents.

Kuno et al. (1971) have demonstrated that the area of the frog NMJ correlates with the diameter of muscle fiber it innervates as well as with the mean quantum content. The amount of Ach released on nerve stimulation is related to NMJ size. Furthermore, Miledi and Stefani (1970) have found different MEPP patterns in fast and slow frog myofibers.

Recently, Negrete et al. (1972) have obtained evidence in frog sartorius muscle that tangental diffusion of Ach causes recruitment of AchRs within the subneural apparatus. They concluded that a single Ach packet activates the AchR population in the postsynaptic membrane in an area comparable to the width of the synaptic cleft, a process that requires more time than radial diffusion across the cleft. Therefore varying Ach packet size is reflected in the amplitude and rise time of the changes in conductance and potential.

The Role of Calcium and Magnesium in the Release of Ach

Del Castillo and Stark (1952) demonstrated that increased concentration of Ca++ in the external bathing solution increased MEPP amplitude without alteration of the sensitivity of the postsynaptic membrane and Del Castillo and Engbaek (1954) found that Mg++ has an opposite effect.

Several hypotheses have been offered to explain the mechanism of Ca++ facilitation of Ach release from the terminal axon. Del Castillo and Katz (1954b) suggested that Ach release from frog NMJs is regulated by two precesses: one that is dependent on Ca++ and is initiated by the nerve impulse and another process that regulates spontaneous release of Ach that is not Ca++ or Mg++ dependent. In the first process, Ca++ and Mg++ may compete for some specific molecular locus in the presynaptic membrane. The resulting complex with Ca++, but not with Mg++, would be dissociated by depolarization of the axon. The activated molecule released Ach and allowed its passage through the membrane. Del Castillo and Katz (1956b) suggested that the contents of the vesicles were released at sites where binding was facilitated by Ca++ and Boyd and Martin (1956a) hypothesized that Ca++ enters the terminal axon, combines with fixed negative charges on the inner surface of the membrane and allows the negatively charged synaptic vesicles to approach the membrane releasing sites where they would be bound by Van der Waal's forces. This concept of neutralization of charges is also supported by work showing effective substitution of a limited number of other species of cations in this process. Data obtained by Jenkinson (1957) indicate that the concentrations of Ca++ and Mg++ required to maintain the EPP at a given level agree with this hypothesis. Hodgkin and Keynes (1957) suggested that the depolarization of the nerve terminals caused by the nerve action potential was produced by influx of Ca++ following which the synaptic vesicles were broken down releasing Ach. Hubbard (1961) found that the spontaneous release of Ach was affected by altering the [Ca++] or [Mg++] in the bathing medium and that these ions affected only a portion of the spontaneous release of Ach. Studies of spontaneous MEPP production by rat diaphragm NMJs exposed to Ca++-free bathing solutions revealed decreased rate of spontaneous potentials, an effect enhanced by adding a Ca++ chelating agent, EDTA to the medium. Under these conditions, MEPPs were eliminated in most fibers after 6 hours exposure to EDTA. Spontaneous MEPP production was restored by Adding Ca++ or Ba++ to the bathing solution or by local iontophoretic application of Ca++ the area containing NMJs (Feldman, 1965; Elmqvist and Feldman, 1965). Exposure to caffein or g-strophanthin, substances believed to release Ca++ from intracellular stores, increased the rate of MEPPs in Ca++ free solutions with marked reduction of this response in the presence of EDTA. It was concluded that Ca++ is required for spontaneous release of Ach and that bound intracellular Ca++ can also be made available for this function under appropriate conditions.

Cohen et al. (1970) suggested that structural changes occur in the nerve membrane during the action potential an hypothesis that is supported by data indicating that the entry of Ca++ into the nerve terminal is increased by depolarization (Keynes and Lewis, 1956). According to Heuser and Miledi (1971), during depolarization of the axon membrane, receptors for calcium on the external axon surface membrane become altered so as to be accessible to Ca++ into the bathing medium. These combine with calcium and after a series of processes involving calcium migration inward to the inner surface of the membrane, transmitter quanta are released. Blockade of Ach release by La+++ appears to be due to prevention of the inward movement of Ca++. The increased release of Ach quanta caused by La+++ may therefore be due to replacement of Ca++ by La+++ or displacement of Ca++ inward as a result of La+++ binding. Since MEPP production is temperature dependent and the delay caused by lowered temperature is presynaptic (Katz and Miledi, 1965), Hubbard et al. (1971) has suggested that the temperature dependent reaction is the rate of Ca++ removal from intraaxonal sites where it plays a role in the release of the Ach quanta. They found no evidence that a metabolic reaction was involved. Blioch et al. (1968) concluded that at constant temperature, MEPP frequency (frog cutaneous pectoris muscle) depends only on the concentration of the various cations inside the axon terminal that possibly regulate adhesion of the synaptic vesicles to the inner presynaptic membrane. It is clear that under physiologic conditions, Ach is not released by the nerve action potential without Ca++ present in the external medium before the depolarization begins and the entry of Ca++ from the bathing solution into the terminal axon is an essential step that occurs between the depolarization of the axon terminal and the release of the

Ach quanta. Furthermore, the amount of Ach released is a function of the external Ca++ concentration either as a result of stimulation or spontaneous secretion (Dodge and Rahimoff, 1967; Hubbard et al., 1968a, b) and intracellular stores of Ca++ are capable of maintaining spontaneous release of Ach quanta (Elmqvist and Feldman, 1965) which explains the persistence of MEPPs at NMJs in the absence of external Ca++. Quantitative studies by Kita and Van der Kloot (1973) have shown that in Mg++ blocked terminals, the effect of [Ca++] changes on EPP amplitude is non-linear.

Although Mg++ opposes the action of Ca++ when both are present in the external medium, Mg++ can replace Ca++ if external Ca++ is absent (Hubbard et al., 1968a, b). Hurlbut et al. (1971) has shown that under conditions that excluded Ca++ in the bathing medium and EGTA, MEPP frequency depended on Mg++ concentration. These investigators suggested that Mg++ acted by a less specific mechanism than Ca++.

Similarly, Sr++ will restore the nerve impulse in the absence of Ca++ in the external bath (Dodge et al., 1969). Under these circumstances Ach is released as usual in the form of quanta but the Sr++ is less effective in bringing about this result than Ca++. The resulting quanta released in the presence of Sr++ have larger potentials apparently due to prolonged transmitter action or possibly, to postsynaptic effects of this cation. At higher Sr++ concentrations, transmission is blocked in some nerve fibers due to the failure of propagation of the nerve impulse. Other cations, with the exception of Ba++ (Elmqvist and Feldman, 1965), do not restore activity. Ba++ substitution for Ca++ yields an initial transient increase in MEPP frequency after which there is a decline similar to the MEPP frequency rate of Ca++ free solutions. (Laskowski & Thies, 1972). On the other hand, La+++ blocks transmission in the presence of Ca++ either by opposing Ca++ entry into the axon, by competing with Ca++ in the Ach release mechanism (Miledi, 1971) or by competitive binding at postsynaptic receptor sites. Mn++ blockade of synaptic transmission in frog NMJs appears to act at the presynaptic terminal where it interferes with transmitter release (Meiri and Rahamimoff, 1972).

The role of Na+ in the release of Ach from the nerve terminal has been demonstrated in experiments utilizing various cardiac glycosides, substances known to affect sodium transport. Greef and Westermann (1955) who studied the effects of g-strophanthin and Birks (1965) and Elmqvist and Feldman (1965) demonstrated that digitalis glycosides increased both spontaneous and induced Ach release. This is due either to mobilization of Ca++ (Govier and Holland, 1964; Elmqvist and Feldman, 1965) or to postsynaptic action of the cardiac glycosides (Gage, 1965). Digitalis and sodium azide also inhibit post-tetanic potentiation (Hubbard and Gage, 1964) possibly by interfering with post-tetanic hyperpolarization of NMJs (Hubbard and Schmidt, 1963).

Release of Ach in the Absence of Ca++

Situations where increased numbers of MEPPs can be recorded in Ca++ free media have also been reported. Black widow spider venom (see page 309) increases MEPP release as does certain alcohols (Gage, 1965; Okada, 1970). In the latter case, the Ca++-independent release system probably operates by a final pathway that is common to the normal secretion mechanism. These experiments have shown that the transfer of Ach to the synaptic gap does not require Ca++ whereas the coupling of nerve depolarization and Ach secretion does. Quastel et al. (1971) demonstrated that ethanol increased the frequency of MEPPs in an exponential fashion producing a 4 fold increment for each 0.40 M increase in ethanol concentration regardless of whether Ca++ was present. The ethanol effect was not opposed by Mg++. The authors concluded that Ca++ was not involved in the ethanol effect because they found no evidence of depletion of possible stores of bound Ca++ on repeated ethanol applications. Other substances that are effective in increasing MEPP frequency are propanol, butanol, chlorohydrate, pentobarbital, ether, carbon tetrachloride and chlorpromazine.

Experiments with diamide, a reagent that enters cells and oxidizes thiols, particularly increasing the quantity of glutathione disulphide from glutathione, have indicated that membrane dithiols may play a role in transmitter release. Werman et al. (1971) and Kosower and Werman (1971) have demonstrated a large increase in the release of transmitter when frog NMJs are treated with this reagent. A short time after exposure to 1.2×10^{-4}M diamide, there was marked increase in MEPP frequency and quantal content. Kosower and Werman (1971) hypothesized that calcium dithiolate formation in the presynaptic membrane regulates release of the Ach quanta.

Catecholamines also facilitate neuromuscular transmission. Norepinephrine increases transmitter release, epinephrine acts on both pre- and postsynaptic membranes whereas isoprenaline acts on the postsynaptic membrane. (Kuba, 1970).

With better understanding of the events leading to Ach release from terminal axons, new information has been obtained about unexpected actions of several drugs that affect cholinergic transmission. For example, several drugs best known for their actions at specific postsynaptic receptors have also been shown to act on presynaptic terminals affecting the quantal release of Ach. Among these are atropine which in relatively low concentration blocks the muscarinic actions of Ach and in higher concentration blocks the nicotinic receptors and tubocurarine best known for its competitive blocking action of the postsynaptic Ach receptors (Auerbach and Betz, 1971; Galindo, 1972). Atropine interferes with the Ach content of the quanta (Hubbard and Wilson, 1970) as well as the EPP equilibrium potential (Potapova, 1969). Hubbard and Wilson (1970) suggested that since atropine inhibits choline transport (Martin, 1969) it could interfere with the choline supplies required for Ach synthesis. On the other hand, epinephrine facilitates the release of Ach from nerve terminals (Bowman and Zaimis, 1958). This may be due to stimulation of cyclic AMP (adenosine 3':5' cyclic phosphate) production that occurs via activation of adenyl cyclase. Goldberg and Singer (1969) investigated the possibility that Ach release in NMJs is mediated by cyclic AMP. They studied the effect of dibutyryl cyclic AMP and various methyl xanthines on the amplitude of EPPs of single cells as well as the compound EPP in the presence of these inhibitors of cyclic AMP. They found that dibutyryl cyclic AMP, theophylline and caffeine increased EPP amplitude in isolated rat nerve-muscle preparations. Theophylline and dibutyryl cyclic AMP increased the frequency, but not the amplitude of spontaneous MEPPs and increased the number of Ach quanta in response to stimulation. These workers concluded that cyclic AMP plays a significant role in the release of Ach.

HISTOCHEMICAL DEMONSTRATION OF Ca++ RELEASE BY NEUROMUSCULAR JUNCTIONS

Histochemical staining methods utilizing alizarin have revealed sufficient Ca++ content in the subneural apparatus to make NMJs visible in the light microscope (Csillik and Savày, 1963; Nakamura et al., 1967). Liévremont et al. (1968) found maximum staining in the subneural apparatus 15-30 minutes after exposure to Ach. It is likely that the Ca++ is bound in the EL. (Savay and Csillik, 1963; Nakamura et al., 1967).

Ultrastructure Changes in Terminal Axons Produced by Divalent Cations

Heuser et al. (1971) demonstrated agglutination of synaptic vesicles within axons of frog NMJs exposed to isotonic CaCl . These changes correlated with a decrease in spontaneous Ach release. Mg++ did not produce agglutination of the vesicles. Although La+++ causes marked increase in release of transmitter, no fine structure changes were found in nerve terminals by Heuser and Miledi (1971). After prolong La+++ exposure, these investigators noted decreased MEPP frequency and depletion of synaptic vesicles. Unexpectedly, coated vesicles became more numerous.

The Postsynaptic Mechanism

In most general terms, Ach released spontaneously or in greater quantity following depolarization of the presynaptic terminal, diffuses across the synaptic space and is bound to specific postsynaptic receptor sites ("the receptive substance") of Langley (1909). Combination with the receptors in the postsynaptic membrane bring about changes in the resting conductance which alters the membrane potential to the point where a local reversal of polarity in sufficient degree leads to depolarization of the membrane and a propagated membrane potential. Before considering the details of current knowledge of the receptors and the mechanisms by which the potential changes come about, a brief review of the current understanding of the maintenance of membrane potentials is worthwhile.

Extensive study of bioelectric potentials at cell surfaces has led to the concept that alterations in permeability of the membranes to various ions are ultimately responsible for the electrical events that occur at the NMJ. Early studies by Dubois-Reymond (1843, 1849) and Overton (1895) indicated that generation of bioelectric currents was the result of cellular ionic concentration gradients. The resting potential is the potential difference between the external environment and the cytoplasm of the cell which in many neurons is approximately 70 mv. This is maintained by the greater concentration of K+ within the cytoplasm compared to the external K+ and the lesser quantity of Na+ within the cytoplasm compared to the external Na+. The resistance of the membrane can be measured by measurement of the voltage change in response to intracellular pulses of current recorded from a double electrode. If a constant current is applied across the membrane, it can be shown that voltage is not developed across it equally rapidly indicating a capacitative component of the membrane. The myofiber capacitance has two components: the surface membrane and the transverse tubular or "T" system (Falk and Fatt, 1960). The T system is the more important. Also, a length constant must be considered which is defined as the attenuation of the electric signal as a function of the distance traveled and the resistance of the nerve sheath and axoplasm. Thus, the electrotonic spread of the axon potential may be considered in terms of the cable characteristics of the nerve.

The first model used to explain membrane excitability was that of Bernstein (1868) who hypothesized that the outside of the resting cell membrane was positively charged with respect to the interior. During neural activity, the charges are neutralized and the membrane potential becomes zero. The distribution of the positive and negative charges are then restored to the resting state during the refractory period. (Fig. 79A).

In their classical study, Hodgkin and Huxley (1945) recorded potential changes across the membrane of the giant fiber of the first stellar nerve of the squid, *Loligo Forbesi*. A recording microelectrode within the axoplasm revealed that the membrane potential is *reversed* during excitation of the nerve and that the inside of the nerve becomes transiently positive during the passage of the nerve impulse (Fig. 79B).

In a later contribution, Hodgkin and Huxley (1952) examined the electrical behavior of the nerve "membrane" in greater detail. They pointed out that current can be carried through the membrane either by charging the membrane capacity or by movement of ions through the resistances in parallel with the capacity. The ionic current might be divided into components carried by Na+ and K+ (I_{Na}, I_K) and small leakage current (I_l) made up of Cl- and other ions. Each component of the ionic current developed is determined by the driving force measured as the electrical potential difference as well as the permeability coefficient that has the dimensions of conductance. Thus the sodium current equals the Na+ conductance multiplied by the difference between the membrane potential and the equilibrium potential for Na+. The experimental data suggested that the conductance for both Na+ and K+ are functions of time and the membrane potential. The effect of the membrane potential on permeability is that depolarization of the membrane causes a transient increase in Na+ conductance and a slower but maintained increase in K+ conductance. These changes are graded and can be reversed by repolarization of the membrane. Hodgkin and Huxley stressed the importance of the membrane potential rather than the membrane current in altering permeability, even though the thickness and composition of the membrane was unknown. They hypothe-

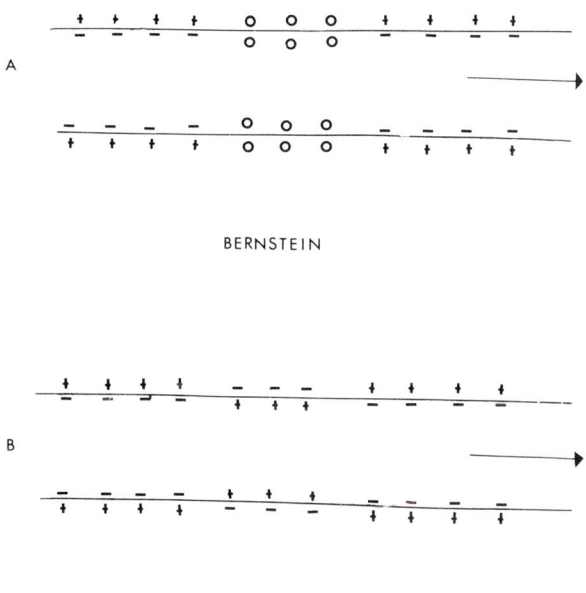

Figure 79. Diagram of the distribution of electrical charges in the classical Bernstein membrane model as compared to the Hodgkin-Huxley model. In the former *(A)* the resting membrane has positive charges on the outside and negative charges on the inside. At the time of stimulation and depolarization, the external and internal charge becomes zero, following which the original resting state is restored with the positive charges on the outside and the negative on the inside. The arrow indicates the direction of the current movement. In the Hodgkin-Huxley model *(B)* the resting state again shows negative charges on the inside and positive charges on the outside. At the time of stimulation, there is a reversal of charges, the outside becoming negative and the inside positive. After passage of impulse the resting state is again restored. (From Hodgkin and Huxley, 1952.)

sized that the relation of the membrane potential to permeability changes might arise from the effect of electrical field on the distribution or orientation of charged molecules having a dipole moment. Previous data (Hodgkin et al., 1949) had already indicated that sodium may not penetrate in the ionic form but in combination with lipid-soluble carrier molecules bearing large negative charges, that could bind with Na+. In this view, the action potential can be interpreted in the following way: the rising phase is due to the net increase of Na+ entry and the rate of rise of the spike and the extent of overshoot, is controlled by the size of the Na+ ratio, that is the momentary reversal of the internal negative environment of the resting cell to a positive potential at the peak of the voltage change. The declining phase of the action potential spike is due to the decline of the Na+ current and the increased K+ outflow. The after hyperpolarization of the membrane consists of a prolonged phase with rising K+ conductance.

In the central nervous system, if a nerve is stimulated and a microelectrode is used to record from the cell body on the other side of synapse, a potential change occurs across the membrane that increases and decays. This is the excitatory postsynaptic potential (EPSP) of Coombs et al. (1955). The delay between the arrival of the impulse and the development of postsynaptic depolarization is the "synaptic delay" characteristic of chemosynapses. The EPSP is characterized by spatial summation. In NMJs, the EPSP can be measured by the "voltage clamp" technique in which the membrane potential is held at a desired value and the varying currents required to maintain this value can be measured directly. The EPSP, or specifically, endplate potential (EPP) determined by this technique is about -20 to 0 mV. (Takeuchi and Takeuchi, 1960; Takeuchi, 1963). The propagated all or none action potential in the myofiber membrane is generated when a sufficient EPP is produced. This may occur when individual EPPs insufficient in themselves to depolarize the postsynaptic membrane may if close enough in time summate to produce an action potential.

STRUCTURAL CHARACTERISTICS
OF NEUROMUSCULAR JUNCTIONS:
RELATED TO THEIR ELECTRICAL PROPERTIES

As a result of their investigations of frog NMJ potentials with microelectrode techniques, Del Castillo and Katz (1956a) attempted to relate the observed electrical phenomena with the newly demonstrated fine structure anatomy of NMJs. They found that the point of maximum field strength was at the edge of the primary synaptic cleft and they concluded that their data could be best explained by assuming that the Ach receptors were buried in the "junctional folds" of the subneural apparatus (Fig. 80). Eccles and Jaeger (1958) noted that the fine structure of synapses in various sites including the CNS, retinal cells and NMJs was similar. Presynaptic and postsynaptic membranes each measured approximately 50 A in width and were separated by uniform 200 A gap filled with a material of low electron density. The synaptic cleft was presumed to be in direct communication with the extracellular space, at least in NMJs. The obvious characteristic of the NMJ synapse that differed from the central synapses, was the presence

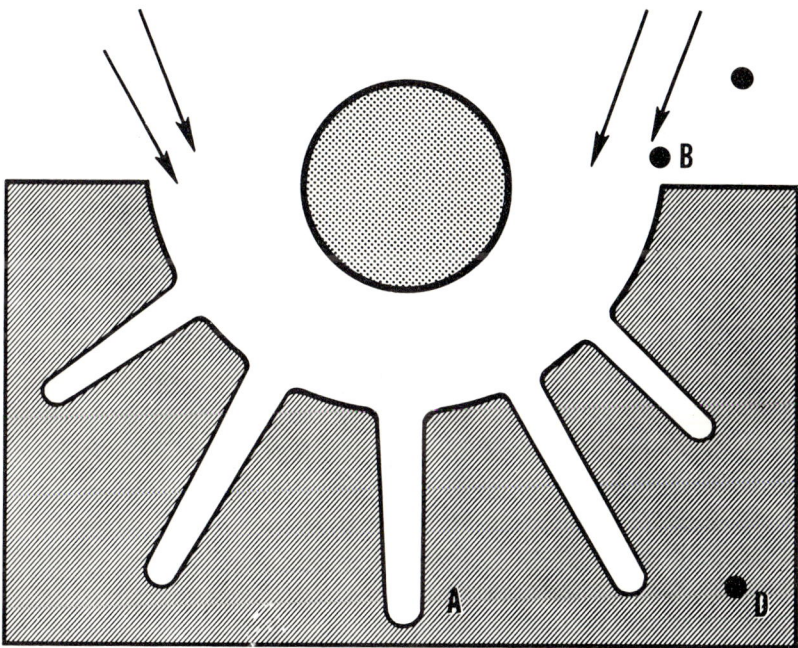

Figure 80. Diagram of electrode placement in the region of active spots within NMJs according to del Castillo and Katz, 1956. The point of greatest activity *(A)* might not actually be used for electrode placement, owing to the fact that damage would result to the preparation. Point *B* indicates the point of maximal current intensity actually recorded at the point of convergence of currents at the edge of the synaptic cleft. The unlabeled point indicates the indifferent electrode, and point *D* lies inside the muscle. External recording was between point *B* and the indifferent electrode, and internal recording was between the indifferent electrode and point *D*. (From del Castillo and Katz, 1956a.)

of the convolutions of the postsynaptic membrane, the so-called secondary synaptic clefts and the wider separation (500-700 A) compared to the 200 A gap of central synapses. They suggested that despite the width of the clefts, there is probably little resistance to the flow of the postsynaptic current due to the synaptic gap. Thus Ach is able to diffuse within the synaptic cleft and outward from the clefts without obstruction by diffusion barriers. The conditions for diffusion of the transmitter and the efficiency of the operation of the synaptic cleft in allowing large postsynaptic current flows requires that circular synaptic contacts be no more than a few microns in diameter and that strip contacts (such as the frog NMJ) measure not more than a few microns across. Therefore relatively large subneural areas are required to allow large currents to pass, and this is accomplished by the finger-like extensions of the secondary synaptic clefts. Secondary synaptic clefts are therefore regarded as a means of increasing the surface area that permits increasing the conductance of the subneural membrane. Del Castillo and Katz (1956a) also demonstrated that the Ach receptor sites must be situated on the external surface of the muscle cell membrane in a location where they are relatively inexcessible from the interior of the myofiber. For example, electrophoretic injection of Ach from a micro pipette effectively stimulates the membrane only when the tip of the pipette is on the outer surface of the NMJ facing the terminal axon. Equivalent doses of Ach were ineffective when the micro pipette was allowed to enter the myofiber.

A consideration of these proposed postsynaptic events raises the question of whether the quantity of Ach released per nerve impulse is sufficient to depolarize the postsynaptic membrane. From the known diameter and electrical characteristics of the muscle fibers and the spatial arrangement and time course of EPPs, Fatt and Katz (1951) calculated the magnitude of the current flow between the sarcoplasm and the external solution that corresponded to the potential change. These calculations revealed that even if the presynaptic nerve terminals contained isotonic univalent ions, the total quantity would be insufficient to generate more than a few EPPs. Thus it appeared that Ach must alter the postsynaptic membrane in such a way as to greatly increase its permeability to the various ions available in the external solution. Ach therefore appears to act much as a trigger similar to the regulating grid in the triode vaccum tube.

Subsequently, many investigators have demonstrated that several species of ions contribute to the current flow after increase in membrane permeability has resulted from Ach action (Takeuchi and Takeuchi, 1960). It is clear that the action of Ach does not depend entirely on Na+ in the extracellular solution (Fatt, 1950), although under normal conditions Na+ is very important. K+ can also contribute to the ion flow (Del Castillo and Katz, 1955) as can ammonium ion NH_4^+ (Furukawa et al., 1956).

Acetylcholine Receptor

The concept that there is a specific Ach receptor (AchR) was first suggested by Langley (1909) who attempted to explain the different responses of various tissues to Ach. Buchtal and Lindhard (1942) demonstrated that when Ach was applied to NMJs, propagated muscle contractions occurred that could be blocked by curare and by excessive concentrations of Ach. Curare appeared to interfere with the Ach mechanism at the level of the receptor because it did not seem to interfere with release of the neurohumor nor did it effect the electrical propagation of EPPs or muscle depolarization. The final step in the clarification of the exictatory process should be identification of the molecular substrate that is altered as a result of Ach binding. Considerable and significant progress toward this objective has been accomplished since the first edition of this monograph.

Localization of the Ach Receptor

Waser and Lüthi (1962) attempted to localize radioactive (C^{14}) curare in the subneural apparatus. Unfortunately their radioautographs are not of sufficient resolution to allow us to distinguish the precise site of curare binding. These investigators calculated that saturation of a mouse diaphragm NMJ occurred with $4 \times 10^6\text{-}10^7$ curarine molecules. Ehrenpreis (1962) used an immunohistochemical method to localize the protein with a high affinity for d-tubocurarine in both the innervated and non-innervated membrane of the electric eel electroplax. At the time, he believed that this protein was the Ach receptor, a view that he subsequently abandoned. A similar technique was used by Benda et al. (1970).

Attempts to demonstrate AchR sites using radioactive d-tubocurarine have revealed binding within the subneural apparatus and occasional "strands of radioactivity" that extended into the synaptic areas. Cohen et al. (1967) suggested a preterminal localization of the AchR. The low resolution obtained again does not permit more accurate localization. A polysaccharide toxin from snake venom, α-bungarotoxin binds to the region of AchR in the electroplax and NMJs and when labeled with ^{125}I can be used as a label for AchR. Using this procedure, Fambrough and Hartzell (1972) found that the number of AchR in rat diaphragm was proportional to rat myofiber size. Radioautography revealed that most of the radioactivity was confined to the NMJ. The mean number of AchR per NMJ was of the order $3.98 \pm 0.21 \times 10^7$ and the range was 1.14 to 8.70×10^7 sites per NMJ. (Figs. 81, 82). This useful method has also been employed by Berg et al. (1972) to localize AchR in mammalian muscle and by Clark et al. (1972) to study electroplax membranes.

Development of Ach Receptors

Diamond and Miledi (1962) demonstrated that immature myofibers are sensitive over their entire surface membrane and presumably have correspondingly diffuse Ach receptors. Following establishment of neuromuscular connections, the area of Ach sensitivity becomes more localized in the vicinity of the NMJs. Robbins and Yonezawa (1971b) demonstrated that developing myotubes in rat embryo spinal cord-muscle tissue cultures displayed Ach sensitivity over their entire surfaces before the earliest neural contacts. The earliest secretion of Ach occurred in the form of quanta as the NMJ developed but often the amount released was sufficient only to produce a subthreshold response. The quantal content increased with NMJ maturation, a phenomenon that roughly paralleled increased number of synaptic vesicles in the terminals.

Fambrough and Rash (1971; Rash and Fambrough, 1973) found that the development of Ach sensitivity during rat myogenesis correlated with the appearance of thick and thin myofilaments but preceded the formation of myofibrils. Development of Ach sensitivity was not dependent upon myotube fusion and there was no evidence that Ach receptors played a role in myogenesis since blockade of the receptors did not alter normal differentiation. Hartzell and Fambrough (1973) have used ^{125}I labelled α-bungarotoxin, a molecule that binds specifically to AchR to trace the development of AchR in cultured myoblasts. By means of

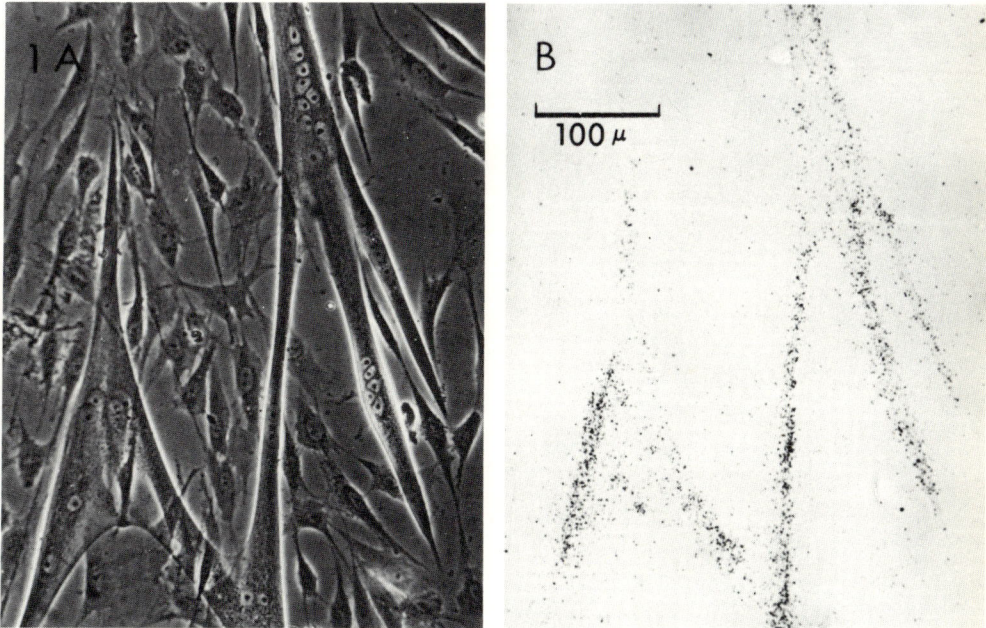

Figure 81. Autoradiograph of tissue cultured rat skeletal muscle labelled with $^{125}I\alpha$-bungarotoxin. A. phase contrast micrograph and B. bright field photomicrograph of silver grains produced by bound ^{125}I α-bungarotoxin indicating Ach receptor sites. From Hartzell, H.C. and Fambrough, D.M. *Developmental Biology* 30:153, 1973 by permission.

electrophysiological recording techniques, they found good correlation of sites of Ach sensitivity with sites of toxin binding. Binding sites were distributed in a non uniform fashion and electron microscopy did not reveal specialized structure in the membrane binding sites. (Fig. 81). Eventually, nearly all the toxin-binding receptor sites are limited to NMJs. In mature myotubes, the average receptor density was 1500-2000 receptors/m² (Fig. 82). The authors also found that inhibition of protein synthesis with cyclohexamide produced delayed incorporation of receptors into the membrane.

Changes in Ach Receptors in Denervated Muscle

Several investigators have studied the nature of the Ach receptors in denervated muscle. As will be discussed, (chapter 11) following denervation of some muscles, there is spread of the Ach receptors from the area containing the NMJs. A logical enquiry is does this spread of sensitivity imply synthesis of new receptors? Graff et al. (1965)

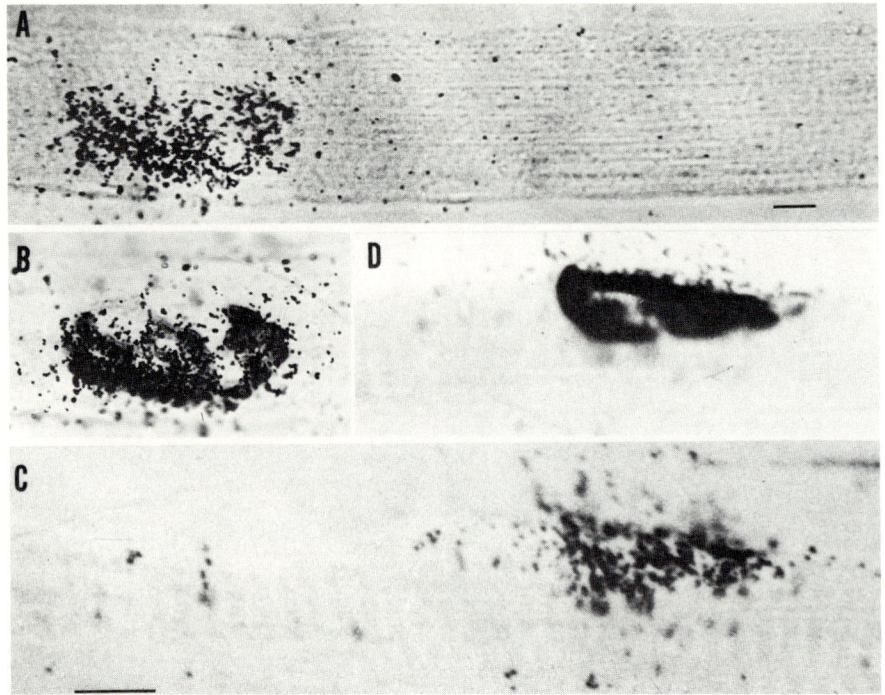

Figure 82. Radioautographs of rat diaphragm NMJ after incubation with [125]I α-bungarotoxin. A NMJ is illustrated *(A)* before and after *(B)* it was stained for AchE activity. Another NMJ is illustrated before *(C)* and after *(D)* staining for AchE. The bar indicates 10 M. From Fambrough, D.M. and Hartzell, H.C. Science 176:189-191, 1972. Copyright 1972 by The American Association for the Advancement of Science. By Permission.

found that denervation results in decreased muscle phospholipid content and increased uptake of P^{32} into phospholipids. Bunch et al. (1970) also reported an increased rate of incorporation of P^{32} and labeled glycerol into membrane components but did not correlate this data with the increase in the membrane area sensitive to Ach. Max et al. (1970) demonstrated an increase of hematoside, a major ganglioside of skeletal muscle, and *de novo* synthesis of this component as a response to denervation. Further studies are required to show whether this ganglioside is a specific component of the muscle membrane related to increased Ach sensitivity.

Fambrough (1970) concluded that genetically induced protein synthesis was responsible for formation of the Ach receptors and Grampp et al. (1972) demonstrated that inhibitors of protein synthesis such as actinomycin D and cycloheximide prevented the fall in resting potential, development of tetrodotoxin resistant action potentials and spread of Ach receptors that ordinarily occurs in denervated mouse muscle following denervation. Labelled α-bungarotoxin, possibly with HRP to permit more discrete localization in fine structure, will be a valuable tool for studying AchR alterations under a variety of experimental conditions.

Chemical Nature of the Ach Receptor

Chagas et al. (1956) and Chagas (1959, 1961) attempted to isolate AchR by precipitating it with curare or a curare-like molecule, gallamine from homogenates of the electric organ of the electric eel. He used the electric organ because of its functional similarity to NMJs and the relatively large amounts of tissue available for analysis. Chagas concluded that the receptor was associated with an acid mucopolysaccharide. Two fractions, Sf1 and Sf3 were isolated by DEAE chromatography. Sf1 appeared to be glycogen and Sf3, a mucopolysaccharide containing hyaluronic acid. Binding of gallamine, tubocurarine, dimethyl tubocurarine and succinylcholine were found to be strongly dependent on the ionic strength of the solutions. The Sf3 fraction behaved as a polyelectrolyte with cation exchange properties apparently due to the numerous carboxyl groups in the molecule. Hasson (1962) questioned the specificity of equilibrium dialysis used in these studies and the precipitation of components of the electric organ by quaternary ions as a reliable means of isolating AchR. For example, insulin and eel cholinesterase are also precipitated by tubocurarine. Trams and Lauter (1964) isolated a sialoprotein from the electric eel that had receptor-like properties but was not thought to be AchR whereas Milhaud et al. (1962) used C^{14} curare to isolate an acid mucopolysaccharide from eel electric organ. These investigators found competitive displacement of gallamine triiodoethylate by dimethylisochondodendrine and by other quaternary ammonium compounds. There was a correlation between the ability to displace curare in *in vitro* experiments with the electric potential produced *in vivo*. Later experience indicated that binding data alone was inadequate to identify the receptor (Chagas, 1961). Similar apparent initial success followed by reevaluation is associated with the work of Ehrenpreis and his associates. Ehrenpreis (1960a, b, 1961, 1963) described proteins isolated from eel electric organ that were initially thought to correspond to AchR. When ammonium sulfate fractionation was used to eliminate chondroitin sulfuric acids and nucleic acids from extracts of electric tissue, proteins were found that strongly bound curare. The two phenolic hydroxyl groups of curare were thought to form hydrogen bonds with the protein to form a complex that was soluble at pH 9. The molecular weight of the protein was approximately 100,000. Studies by Ahriens et al. (1962) also supported the concept of a proteinaceous Ach receptor and Belleau (1964) presented evidence that the AchR is a protein with AchE properties. Later Ehrenpreis withdrew his previous assertion that he had isolated the specific Ach receptor. The protein that he isolated was localized in both the innervated and non-innervated membranes of the electroplax and although this drug-binding protein may play a role in electrical activity of the electroplax, it is not the specific Ach receptor (Ehrenpreis, 1967). The controversy has continued between the Chagas group (Hassón-Voloch, 1968) who believe the Ach receptor is a polysaccharide and those who believe that AchR is a protein. Because of several recent experiments in which the molecular substratum of the receptor sites is altered by various reagents that react with proteins, AchR is more generally accepted to be a protein (Miledi et al., 1971) or a proteolipid (De Robertis, 1967). However, this does not rule out possible interaction with glycoproteins known to be in the immediate vicinity of the active sites. O'Brien et al. (1972) have concluded that the prospects are bright for isolation and characterization of AchR but that it has not yet been accomplished. More of a challenge, they suggest, will be explanation of the mechanism of Ach binding producing ion conductance. They speculate that AchR is a complex consisting of an Ach-recognizing molecule and an ionophore that can respond to Ach binding with conformational changes. More recently, α-bungarotoxin has been used to isolate detergent solubilized membrane fractions from electroplax (Schmidt and Raftery, 1973; Raftery, 1973). *Torpedo californica* yielded a major protein subunit with a molecular weight of $3.5\text{-}4.5 \times 10^4$ (get electrophoresis). Similar methods have been applied to mouse diaphragm (Berg et al., 1972) and frog sartorius muscle (Miledi and Potter, 1971). Recently, Fulpius and Klett (1973) have studied the properties of electric eel AchR obtained by affinity chromatography. They isolated a single protein species with a MW of approximately 50,000 that contains considerable cysteine but no tryptophane.

Albuquerque et al. (1973) have recently shown that there are at least two types of binding sites that participate in membrane excitation by Ach. They identified one site that is blocked by curare and bungarotoxin which they regard as AchR and a second site competitively blocked by bungarotoxin and the perhydroderivative of the frog poison histrionicotoxin, which is proposed as a part of the "ion conductance modulator" or ion-transporting molecule.

Other substances thought to have receptor properties include phosphatides from muscle (Woolley, 1959) and ribonucleoproteins (Namba and Grob, 1967). The latter authors demonstrated that tubocurarine precipitates from extracts of human muscle contained nucleoproteins but they concluded that this material was not the Ach receptor.

POSSIBLE IDENTITY OF ACETYLCHOLINESTERASE AND THE ACETYLCHOLINE RECEPTOR

Župančič (1953) suggested that since the molecular surface configurations of both AchE and AchR must be similar, and since both molecules must be spatially closely related in order to function, it is reasonable to suppose that both functions — stimulation and hydrolysis — are served by the same molecule. He suggested that Ach combines with AchE (the receptor), acts on it to produce depolarization), and is then hydrolyzed, leaving the active groups on AchE free to react again. To support this concept, this investigator cited the well known phenomenon of Ach stimulation at low concentrations and inhibition (block) at high concentrations which he believed is due to inhibition of AchE by high concentrations of Ach. However, in this view, it is combination of Ach with AchE that yields the stimulating effect, not the hydrolysis per se. Experimental evidence thought to support this concept was found in data showing that tubocurarine weakly inhibits AchE and shifts the optimal substrate concentration of Ach to higher values (Brzin and Župančič, 1956). The effect of tubocurarine with its quaternary nitrogen group is that it competes with the cationic head of Ach for anionic centers of the receptor AchE without blocking esterolytic sites. In his later publications, Ehrenpreis (1967) appears to return to the concept of Roepke (1937) and Župančič (1953) that AchR and AchE are identical. He suggested that the active site on the AchE molecule serves as the site of Ach binding on AchR and for other cholinergic compounds. Belleau also (1964) suggested that the muscarinic Ach receptor is acetylated AchE and in this form the normal reactivity of the esterasic sites is masked but retains its ability to form complexes. The acetylated form of the enzyme could be produced in specific regions of the sensitive membrane perhaps by the continuous quantal discharge of Ach.

However, the identity of AchE and AchR was rejected by many investigators who cited contrary evidence. Both Nachmansohn (1955, 1967) and Watkins (1965) considered that AchR was distinct from AchE despite the apparent similarity of the anionic and esterasic sites in these molecules. Changeux et al. (1967) concluded from their study of "affinity labeling" with p-trimethyl ammonium benzene diazonium fluoroborate (Tdf) that Tdf labels AchR sites that are topographically distinct from the esterasic site of AchE. In continuation of this work, Changeux et al. (1969) described two kinds of sites on the AchE molecule where Tdf might bind; the anionic site of the active center and the non-catalytic "peripheral anionic centers" that lie outside the active centers. Dithiothreitol (DTT), a reagent that breaks disulfide bonds, prevents the irreversible binding of Tdf to both AchE and AchR. Thus, both AchE and the AchR have disulphide bonds as important components of their structure and that they probably are closely related protein molecules but not necessarily identical.

In support of the concept that AchE and the AchR are chemically distinct, Karlin (1967) demonstrated that preincubation with p-chloromercuribenzoate (PCMB) or dithiothreitol had no significant effect on the K_m and V_{max} of AchE under experimental conditions similar to those that abolished the Ach response of the electroplax. Therefore, PCMB greatly interferes with the AchR function but not with AchE. Karlin concluded that these results were not consistent with the idea that the two functional sites, receptor and enzyme, could be separate but remain part of one protein molecule. Additional evidence that the active sites of AchE and AchR are not identical is found in the recent work of Bartels et al. (1970, 1971) who reported that a photochromic activator trans-3.3 ' bis [α-(trimethylammonium) methyl] azobenzene dibromide (Bis Q) that binds to AchR with great specificity only inhibits AchE 50% at equivalent concentrations. Furthermore, only the trans Bis Q binds to AchR but the cis form is equivalent to the trans form as an AchE inhibitor. These data are consistent with earlier observations that membrane AchE activity is absent in the extrajunctional area of myofiber membranes and that the extrajunctional membrane depolarization is not potentiated by edrophonium chloride (Tensilon).

In response to Karlin's (1967) demonstration of the distinctness of AchR and AchE by means of S-S reduction with dithiothreitol, Župančič (1969) claimed that parachloromercuribenzoate (PCMB) and dithiothreitol, are not specific for rabbit ileum cholinoreceptors, because PCMB blocked the action of Ach, acetyl-β-methylcholine, histamine and Ba++ irreversibly. This result may be due to possible differences in receptor sites in smooth muscle compared with either NMJs or the electroplax.

Recently Kato et al. (1970) used proton nuclear magnetic resonance technique to study the binding of atropine and eserine to AchE obtained from squid head ganglia. Normally eserine binds to the catalytic site of AchE and atropine has great affinity for the muscarinic site of AchR. The nuclear magnetic resonance data revealed a change in the line width of N methyl and phenyl groups of atropine and N methyl and C methyl groups of eserine as a result of binding to AchE. Experiments with other inhibitors led to the conclusion that there are at least two binding sites on AchE; an active center where eserine binds (the anionic or esterasic site) and an anionic site, where atropine binds that differs from the catalytic site.

It is clear that there are several properties of the AchE anionic site and that of AchR in the postsynaptic membrane (Belleau, 1964; Changeux, 1967, 1969) that are similar, but much of the available evidence indicates that they are not identical (Karlin, 1967; Bartels et al., 1971; De Robertis and Fizer de Plazas, 1970).

Molecular Interactions of Ach and AchR

We have now to consider how Ach is bound to AchR and current concepts of how this binding accomplishes the change in permeability characteristic of the postsynaptic membrane that is responsible for depolarization. Since the methylated quaternary ammonium "cationic head" of Ach is such a prominent feature of this molecule, much attention has been devoted to study of the nature and arrangement of anionic groups in AchR suitable for its binding. Welsh and Taub (1950) and Wilson (1952) demonstrated that the degree of methylation of quaternary ammonium ions is of considerable importance in the activity of Ach-like drugs because of the influence of variable chemical groups on binding. For example, Welsh and Taub (1950) found that at least two methyl groups on a quaternary nitrogen are required for a substance to have Ach-like activity when tested on the isolated clam heart preparation. Quaternary ammonium ions with three alkyl groups other than methyl show excitatory and Ach-blocking activity (Welsh and Taub, 1948) indicating that the catonic "head" rather than the "tail" is responsible for Ach-like action. Studies on a series of quaternary derivatives of pentanones and pentanols demonstrated that the carbonyl groups of Ach were also an important point of attachment, possibly by means of hydrogen bonding. Various evidence indicates that phospholipids with negative groups in AchR binding sites are the loci where the quaternary ammonium head of Ach is bound (Nastuk, 1967; Cavillito, 1967). In this view, the AchR contains a phospholipid-protein complex that could act as an ionic gate (Watkins, 1965; Ehrenpreis, 1967). Both UO++ and Ca++ compete with carbamylcholine for some common binding site that also is responsible for Ach binding and membrane depolarization (Liu and Nastuk, 1966; Nastuk and Liu, 1966).

Karlin and Bartels (1966) demonstrated that some component of AchR contains a disulfide bond that is essential for the depolarization of the electroplax by Ach. Reduction of these S-S groups by 1mM dithiothreitol and abolition of the depolarizing action of Ach on the electroplax could be reversed by oxidants such as 5.5' dithio bis (2 nitro benzoate), potassium ferricyanide or cysteine that restored the S-S groups.

That dithiothreitol was active in a specific AchR site was indicated by the change in specificity of the reduced receptor. For example, under these conditions, carbamylcholine became an inhibitor and hexamethionium, a normally competitive inhibitor, became an activator. They also found that quaternary ammonium alkylating or acylating reagents served as "affinity labels" for the reduced AchR binding sites by binding reversibly to negative sites on AchR and reacting covalently with adjacent -SH groups.

Bartels et al. (1970) investigated the action of cholinethiol, related quaternary ammonium thiols and bisquaternary ammonium disulfides on reduced AchR. They found that 1μ M cholinethiol reversed the dithiothreitol inhibited response of the electroplax to carbamylcholine and the disulfides of cholinethiol and homocholinethiol reversed the previously reduced AchR. These molecules also react with the normal receptor: the thiols are activators of AchR and the disulfides are competitive inhibitors (Mautner et al., 1966). Rang and Ritter (1971) have also shown the importance of disulfide bonds in AcR of chick muscle.

Changeux et al. (1967) used a tubocurarine analog, Tdf (p-trimethyl-ammonium) benzene diazonium fluoroborate, that had previously been used to label red cell AchE as an "affinity label" for AchR. This technique involves use of a reagent with a high affinity for binding to the specific AchR sites by means of irreversible covalent bonds with certain amino acid side chairs. They used Tdf which is a close analog of phenyltrimethylammonium ion, a potent activator of the AchR that also contains a reactive diazonium group which forms covalent bonds with histidine, lysine and tyrosine side chains.

Twenty minutes exposure of the electroplax membrane to 10^{-4}M Tdf irreversibly abolished its sensitivity to Ach and similar activators. D-tubocurarine and other specific inhibitors and activators protected the AchR from Tdf action and irreversible acylation of catalytic centers of AchE did not interfere with it. Tdf alone did not alter the resting potential or the membrane resistance of the electroplax membrane. Edwards et al. (1970) showed that water soluble carbodiimide which reacts with -COOH groups of sialic acid residues, phosphatidyl serine and membrane proteins and with phosphodiester groups of membrane phospholipids decreased the sensitivity of frog NMJs to applied Ach. They concluded that -COOH groups of sialic acid and phosphatidyl serine are essential in the AchR sites.

Bartels et al. (1971) described two photochromic activators of the postsynaptic membrane of the electric eel electroplax. Trans-3,3 prime-bis (α-trimethyl ammonium) methyl azobenzine dibromide is active in very low concentrations and only in the trans form. It thus becomes possible to regulate the membrane potential in the presence of this substance by the action of light.

The affinity labeling technique has also been used to estimate the average surface density of receptor binding sites in the electroplax membrane. Using dithiothreitol followed by tritiated 4-(N)maleimido)-α-benzyltrimethyl ammonium iodide, Karlin et al. (1971) calculated that the average surface density of receptor binding sites in the electroplax membrane of electrophorus is approximately 3,000 per μ m^2, a value of the order of 4-7 times as great as the number of AchE sites.

Additional data concerning the properties of AchR have been obtained by altering the dissociation of active groups in the molecule by altering the environmental pH. If the environmental pH is altered in the range pH 9-5.2, only pH values below 6 affected the action potential (Sokoll and Thesleff, 1968). They observed an increase in the level of depolarization at which the action potential was triggered, an effect similar to that produced by uranyl ions (0.2mM.). Under these conditions, the Ach sensitivity of the postsynaptic membrane was reduced 85%. The similarity of the effect of decreasing pH and of uranyl ions on the action potential and the Ach sensitivity of the postsynaptic membrane indicated that the binding sites on AchR for these two processes had a similar pK, possibly due to the presence of phosphate groups in the AchR molecules.

Recent studies by Eldefrawi et al. (1971) have indicated that phospholipoproteins are present in the AchR sites. Using the organophosphorus AchE inhibitor Tetram (0,0-diethyl s-diethylamino ethyl phosphorothiolate) to inhibit all AchE activity, without interference with nicotine or Ach binding by AchR, these investigators studied the binding of tritium acetate labeled Ach by particulate fractions of *Torpedo* electroplax. Two high affinity sites bound Ach reversibly and these could be blocked by nicotinic drugs. Pretreatment with trypsin, chymotrypsin and phospholipase C reduced the Ach binding 40, 48 and 66% respectively indicating that phospholipoproteins may be involved in the binding process. These enzymes also partially prevented binding of muscarone and nicotine. A high activity and a low activity site were identified. The authors speculated whether the two sites could be on the same or separate molecules or if the observed results were due to different configurations of an allosteric Ach molecule as had been suggested by Katz and Thesleff (1957), Karlin (1967) and Changeux et al. (1969). More recent progress in these studies have been published by Reiter et al. (1972), Lindstrom et al. (1972), O'Brien et al. (1972) and Edelstein (1972).

The polar heads of phospholipid or phospholipoprotein molecules within the bimolecular layer of the postsynaptic membrane could act as ion exchange sites to control the passive ionic transport involved in depolarization. Ing and Wright (1933) had previously suggested that ion exchange occurred when tubocurarine was bound by AchR and De Robertis et al. (1967) claimed specific binding of radioactive Ach to CNS proteolipids. Recent studies employing α-bungarotoxin (Clark et al, 1972) indicate that electroplax binding sites contain a membrane-bound phospholipoprotein or protein that contains exposed-SH groups.

Taylor et al. (1970) studied the interaction of several agonists and antagonists active at the NMJ from the point of view of considering these reactions as ion exchange processes. Unlike the classic treatment of drug receptor interactions based upon dissociation of molecules in solution, these investigators assumed that the drug interacted with receptors by exchanging cations present in the bathing solution, particularly K^+ and Ca^{++}. Nastuk (1967) had shown that divalent cations compete with Ach for binding at the Ach receptor and La^{+++} is known to reduce neural excitability (Blaustein and Goldman, 1968). Lambert and Parsons (1970) studied the relationship of divalent cations and the response of postsynaptic receptors to the activator carbamylcholine in frog sartorius muscle. Removal of divalent cations from the bathing medium reduced the receptor response to carbamylcholine whereas addition of Ca++ or Mg++ increased the response, Ca++ being more effective than Mg++. At higher levels of Ca++ and Mg++ concentrations, the NMJ responses to stimulation were reduced. On the other hand, La+++ increased the response of the receptors to both carbamylcholine and Ach. La+++ increased the change in conductance in the junction produced by carbamylcholine. Taylor et al. (1970) found that quaternary ammonium ions were displaced only when ions of similar charge were available. Data was obtained for tubocurarine and gallamine that yielded linear plots when the author's equations were applied. This permitted calculation of selectivity constants. The data was consistent with the concept that the same molecules that were responsible for the binding of decamethonium, tubocurarine and gallamine were also involved in depolarization. This obligatory exchange of cations at the time of binding of quaternary ammonium compounds is consistent with Ca++ displacement at the time of depolarization, the actions of uranyl and lanthum ions and possibly the morphological evidence for selective binding of metallic divalent cations. Although these investigators suggested that K+ was the naturally occurring exchanging cation, Ca++ was not ruled out. Since polyvalent cations such as Ca++, Sr++ and La+++ are bound by phospholipids, it is possible that Ca++ normally combined with the polar groups in the membrane could function as a gate to regulate the passage of sodium and potassium during depolarization of the membrane (Goldman, 1964).

The Nature of the Ach Receptor

The process of receptor action at the molecular level is complex and affected by many factors. Several hypothetical models have been suggested to explain the coupling between Ach binding to AchR and the subsequent membrane alteration that permits the large ion fluxes required to generate the EPP. Meyer (1937) suggested that changes in the intramolecular configuration of proteins might be the basis of permeability changes to ions during conduction, possibly resulting from rearrangement of acidic and basic groups within the molecules and Nachmanson has maintained for many years (1970) that Ach is bound to proteins within the membrane that undergo conformational changes leading to increased ionic permeability. AchE, also within the membrane, hydrolyzes the bound Ach and returns the system to its resting state in his hypothesis.

Belleau (1964) suggested that some of the difficulties encountered in much previous research were due to the failure to recognize multiple kinds of interaction between Ach and receptors. In one mode of interaction, Ach is bound to a portion of the cell surface that produces a specific conformational change whereas other molecules interact with hydrophobic groups in the periphery leading to nonspecific conformational changes. In the hypothesis offered by Watkins (1965), Ach-AchR interactions were thought to bring about depolarization on the basis of similar structure and charge distribution of the polar head portions of lipid and phospholipid molecules such as the phosphatidyl choline molecules with Ach. The postsynaptic membrane was conceived to have periodic interposed nonpolar lipid layers constituting restricted areas of increased vulnerability. Activators such as Ach would replace the polar head portion of the corresponding lipid by combination with the lipid protein complex thus bringing about alteration in permeability. In the Ach system, the receptor area would be characterized by electrostatic binding of the quaternary ammonium group of lecithin to various anionic side chains of the protein. Divalent metals would bridge between lipid phosphate and secondary anionic groups of proteins and there would be coordinated bonding between double bonded oxygen atoms of the phosphate groups and a peptide group in the protein chain. Ach would then compete with phosphatidyl choline for two of these sites producing a conformational change in the protein as it binds with the activator. This would weaken the bond to the divalent cation. This supposed phosphatidyl choline-protein complex could control regions of the membrane that would allow selective passage of Na+ and Ka+.

Data has also been obtained to indicate that there is cooperative binding at the AchR sites (Karlin, 1967; Changeux and Podleski, 1968). In studies of carbachol and decamethonium binding to the electroplax, a sigmoid-shaped response curve was found, strongly suggesting cooperativity. Thus it appeared that binding of an activator molecule to the AchR site facilitated the subsequent binding of the second and successive activator molecules. If the activators carbachol and decamethonium were used together, they found that one altered the shape of the dose response curve of the other. To explain the observed cooperativity, Changeux and Podleski (1968) suggested that allosteric transitions of the AchR (Monod et al., 1963, 1965) were responsible for the observed interaction between Ach and AchR. Two protomer states were suggested: 1) when the membrane was polarized and 2) when it was depolarized. The actual change in the membrane potential could be regulated by the proportion of the protomers that underwent transition to the depolarized state. Antagonism between various activators and inhibitors could be understood in terms of stabilization of either the polarized or depolarized protomer conformations. The observed cooperativity could be explained by the influence of bound activators in causing the appropriate transition in adjacent protomers.

In a different approach to the problem, Durell et al. (1969) hypothesized that Ach alters membrane permeability by facilitating enzymatic hydrolysis of one or more phospholipids present in the postsynaptic membranes. This concept is based on earlier work by Hokin and Hokin (1953) who demonstrated that Ach stimulates the incorporation of radioactive inorganic phosphate into the phospholipids, phosphatidyl inositol and phosphatidic acid. Uptake of P^{32} stimulated by Ach is maximal in the synaptosome fraction of brain homogenates and recent data on the action of Ach on the synthesis of phosphatidic acid and phosphatidyl inositol in these preparations indicate that Ach acts upon the hydrolysis of phosphoinositides and other phospholipids. Whereas Hokin and Hokin (1960, 1963) suggested that the phosphatidic acid cycle might be related to sodium secretion, Durell et al. (1969) has offered the hypothesis that membrane Na^+ and K^+ permeability are regulated by a mechanism involving phosphorylation of phosphatidyl inositol to phosphatidyl inositol phosphate (PIP) and phosphatidyl inositol diphosphate (PIPP). In this hypothesis, the breakdown of the phosphoinositides by phosphomonoesterases would be regulated by Ach. Durell proposed that the effects of Ach on membrane permeability are the consequence of Ach stimulation of phospholipid diesterase in the postsynaptic membrane. Hydrolysis by the enzyme would release phosphorylated molecules with anionic charges that might increase cation permeability and as a result, bring about depolarization. Since both PIP and PIPP are calcium chelators, this mechanism could also explain transient release of Ca^{++}. Both PIPP and PIP phosphodiesterases and monoesterases are activated by divalent cations and both phosphatidyl inositol kinase and PIP kinase are activated by Ach (Kai et al., 1966). Therefore Durell et al. (1969) suggested that Ach brings about depolarization of the postsynaptic membrane by means of direct and continuous effect on the rate of phosphodiesteratic cleavage of one or more phospholipids. Actual hydrolysis of a covalent bond would account for the permeability changes that occur during membrane depolarization.

Wei (1968, 1969) offered a generalized theory for chemosynaptic function based on the behavior of Ach dipoles. Multilayers of Ach dipoles lying in the synaptic cleft would permit ions to overcome the junctional barrier of the postsynaptic membrane and give rise to the bioelectric potential. However, Mourel and Galzigna (1971) found a discrepancy in the value of the dipole moment used by Wei and criticized the theory.

Hydrolysis of Ach by AchE

The final step in the series of events that occur during neuromuscular transmission is the restoration of the junction by hydrolysis of the secreted activator, Ach. This occurs extremely rapidly, mediated by AchE an enzyme with a remarkably rapid turnover number, approximately 2×10^7/min. at 25° (Nachmansohn, 1959). As discussed in chapter   the precise localization of this enzyme remains ellusive. The best histochemical data indicates that AchE is located in the postsynaptic membrane, possibly as discontinuous spots. AchE appears to be strongly bound to the subneural membranes since the activity withstands the procedures utilized in preparing empty sarcolemmal tubes and thiolacetic acid esterase activity can be demonstrated in isolated membranes from NMJ. The histochemical data to date has not been adequate to confirm Nachmansohn's suggestion (1970) that both the receptor and the AchE are present together in the membrane. Some recent data from our laboratory indicates that the enzyme may be located in the "cell coat" covering the external leaflet of the myofiber plasma membrane. Data indicating that NMJ AchE can be removed by collagenase without destroying the cell membrane (Hall and Kelly, 1971) also suggests that the enzyme is exposed on the outer surface of the membrane complex and is not an integral part of the membrane.

11

Denervation and Reinnervation of Neuromuscular Junctions

DENERVATION: PHYSIOLOGIC CONSIDERATIONS

Although paralysis, the consequence of motor nerve transection has long been recognized by clinicians and physiologists, modern electrophysiologic recording technique, particularly when correlated with morphologic studies, have revealed much new information about the workings of the neuromuscular unit. As a background to the morphological data with which this chapter is chiefly concerned, it is useful to briefly consider some of the current physiologic data.

Transection of the nerves of both fast and slow muscles of the rat is followed by a decrease in the muscle resting membrane potential (Albuquerque and McIsaac, 1969, 1970; Redfern and Theslett, 1971). At the same time, there is cessation of MEPPs and the development of extrajunctional Ach sensitivity (Chapter 10). Before the MEPPs disappeared, Albuquerque et al. (1971) observed an increase in MEPP frequency. This has been attributed to depolarization of the presynaptic nerve membrane (Birks et al., 1960). Albuquerque et al. (1971) identified four stages of denervation change in the NMJs: 1) partial depolarization of the postsynaptic membrane; 2) decrease of spontaneous MEPP release preceded by increased MEPP frequency in some fibers; 3) increased Ach sensitivity and 4) increased resistance of the postsynaptic membrane.

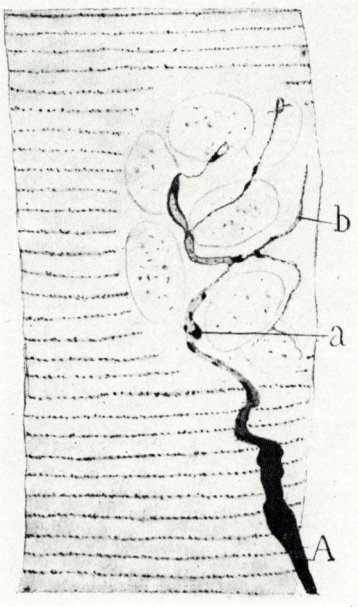

Figure 83. Drawing of a degenerating NMJ 9 hours after section of the sciatic nerve. Note the spotty deposits of silver at *(a)* and very fine, attenuated nerve fiber branches *(b)* in the terminal arborization. (After Tello, 1907.)

CLASSICAL MORPHOLOGIC INVESTIGATIONS

During the classical period, investigations of major significance were concerned with degeneration and reinnervation of NMJs after injury of the peripheral nerve. As early as 1907, Tello observed transient swelling and retraction of the terminal branches of the NMJ arborization soon after section of peripheral nerves (Fig. 83). Twelve to 14 hours after interruption of the nerve, the terminal arborizations were fragmented when examined after staining with silver. After a suitable period of time, when the axons had regenerated, Tello observed that the axons ran along the sheath of Henle-Key-Retzius and divided before reaching the muscle fiber. One of the resulting branches then reinnervated nearby NMJs (Fig. 84). Boeke (1935) summarized the available data on regeneration of NMJs using classical staining methods.

An exceedingly thorough investigation, outstanding in its clarity of presentation, was the work of Gutmann and Young (1944), who studied the reinnervation of rabbit muscle after various periods of atrophy. The NMJs were stained by the Bielschowsky silver method. Two kinds of experiments were performed. The peroneal nerve was

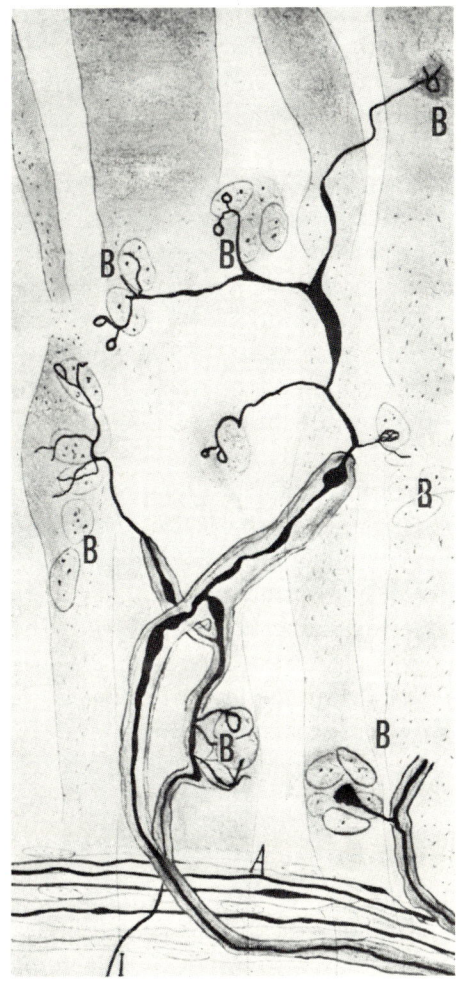

Figure 84. Drawing of various stages of NMJ regeneration demonstrated by silver staining. The nerve trunk is shown at *A* and NMJs at *B*. (After Tello, 1907.)

crushed a short distance from the muscle to obtain a brief period of denervation prior to reinnervation (approximately 18 days), and a similar experiment was performed wherein the nerve was crushed at a greater distance from the muscle so that the time of denervation was longer (35 to 42 days).

The second kind of experiment consisted of complete sectioning of the nerve. This provided a 17 day delay between denervation and the onset of reinnervation. In another experiment the method of delayed suture was used. In this procedure the tibial nerve was cut, and then after a suitable period of time, secondary cross suturing of the peroneal nerve to the tibial nerve stump was performed. This allowed longer periods of muscle atrophy before the arrival of the reinnervating nerve fibers. In all these experiments, the time required for return of direct excitability of the muscle and reflex excitability via the nerve was determined.

When the segment of crushed nerve was a short distance from the muscle fiber, wallerian degeneration occurred in the expected manner. A latent period of approximately five days was required before the regenerating axon tips began to move back along the neural sheath. The forward rate of advance was known to be 4.4 mm. per day according to previous work (Gutmann et al., 1942). Axon tips were first seen in the vicinity of NMJs 18 days after nerve crush. There was a delay of one to two days after the arrival of the nerve fibers before functional capability was restored. There was no evidence that the NMJs had undergone any significant morphologic alteration during the brief period of denervation. The soleplate sarcoplasm and nuclei appeared normal as did the Schwann cell nuclei. An observation of unknown significance was that the old NMJs stained unusually dark with silver at the time when the entering nerve fibers appeared. The first nerve fibers to approach the NMJs were very tenuous. Later the terminal axons appeared thickened at the point immediately before entering the old soleplate area. This appearance was interpreted by the authors as evidence of damming of axoplasmic flow. From this aggregated mass of axoplasm little branchlets appeared, which produced extensive ramifications ending in tapered tips or rings on the surface of the old soleplate.

Gutmann and Young (1944) were well aware that the ring form of terminal expansion might well be an artefact produced by fixation or silver staining, since spherical configurations of the terminal axons were never seen. They believed that the greatly expanded axoplasm in the terminal axon tip might show artefactual structure when fixed and stained in this manner.

A surprising aspect of these studies was the rapidity with which indirect stimulation reactivity and reflex reactivity returned, even though branches in the terminal arborizations were reduced in number and were morphologically abnormal.

An observation of considerable interest and importance in interpreting pathologic changes in NMJs was that all the axoplasm of the reinnervating fiber did not succeed in re-entering the old soleplate area. These "ultraterminal fibers," the authors stress, were not identical with the structures referred to by Hinsey (1934), who used the term to refer to side connections of nerve fibers extending between adjacent NMJs. In many cases, the fate of the new "ultraterminal fibers" was not clear. Some apparently stimulated the formation of new NMJs. None were seen in muscles after short periods of innervation. However, formation of new NMJs occurred in muscles subjected to long periods of denervation. Usually one fiber supplied an NMJ, but occasionally two were supplied by a single nerve fiber. It could not be established that the second nerve fiber was derived from a second neuron.

Another striking aspect of the reinnervation process was that during the outgrowth at the crushed end of the nerve fiber, many nerve filaments ran in the original endoneural tube that led back to the old NMJs, but only one nerve fiber usually arrived successfully. The others seemed to atrophy, although many persisted for months. After approximately 80 days, the number of branchlets within many terminal arborizations was normal. After 107 days, some "ultraterminal fibers" were still visible, and indeed some had become large and myelinated. However, morphologic abnormalities were still visible after 200 days.

When the nerve was crushed at a greater distance from the muscle, it required 35 to 42 days for the nerve fibers to reach the soleplate region. Although the muscle fibers appeared more atrophied than in the experiment of short duration of denervation, the soleplates persisted. Unlike experiments in which denervation was of short duration, after long periods of denervation, there was an abundance of nerve fibers that had gone astray, the so-called "escaped fibers." It seemed that for some reason it was more difficult for the reinnervating fibers to get into the old NMJ area. Only a part of the axon seemed to be able to get back to its old home. The rest of the axon passed on to make a new nerve fiber, which ran for a considerable distance between the muscle fibers. Schwann cells and fibrocytes were seen to invest these fibers. Many of the new nerve fibers terminated blindly in connective tissue, whereas others appeared to make new, exceedingly simple NMJs in the form of single endings without terminal ramifications on the end of nerve fibers which had "escaped" from old NMJs. This resulted in a series of interconnected NMJs that were never observed in normal muscle.

After this longer period of denervation, it required about 12 days for the newly reinnervated NMJs to become functional. Function returned despite the abnormal number of terminal branches in the arborizations and abnormal morphology of the NMJs. This particular point has great significance when it comes to attempting to correlate the pathologic abnormalities that occur in NMJs in various neuromuscular diseases. This subject will be discussed in greater detail in the chapter on the pathology of the NMJ (Chapter 14).

After function returned, it required many months before the NMJs were restored to their normal appearance. At the end of 200 days, many of the terminal arborizations still appeared abnormal, although there were fewer "ultraterminal fibers." Gutmann and Young believed that this indicated that the excess nerve fibers had been absorbed.

Nerve Section Experiments

In experiments in which the nerves were severed, return of function required more time and was less complete than in the nerve crush experiments. Furthermore, the morphologic restoration of the NMJs took longer, and indeed in many instances they were never fully restored. In the more acute experiments, there was a delay of 17 days between the arrival of the nerve fibers at the denervated NMJs and the onset of direct and indirect excitability. This may be compared with the approximately 6 days required after crush injury close to the muscle. A delay of 25 days before return of the fibers to the NMJ and reflex functioning was recorded after a good primary suture of the nerve. The delay after close crush injury was 11 days before return of reflex function, and after distant crush injury, 22 days. A histologic preparation made after 35 days, some 10 days after the calculated time for return of fibers to the NMJ regions, demonstrated thick nerve fibers and some nerve bundles, but only occasional endoneural tubes in each bundle contained a nerve fiber. This was unlike the pattern of regeneration observed after crush injury when nearly every endoneural tube contained nerve fibers. However, the morphology of individual NMJs was similar to that observed after crush injury and reinnervation. Many "escaped fibers" were present, and in the majority of the NMJs only a single fiber was seen entering the original soleplate area. This was not due to lack of opportunity, since some of the endoneural tubes contained more than one nerve fiber. The pattern of "escaped fibers" predominated; all the NMJs arose as collaterals composed of thick nerve fiber branches terminating in abnormally frequent knobs and endbulbs. Restoration of normal NMJs occurred some two months after reinnervation, as evidenced by further branching within the NMJ terminal arborization. Despite this, simple NMJs were still present and many "escaped fibers" and tangles of nerve fibers were observed; the latter were thought to be of sensory origin. The number of branches in the NMJs was still below normal four months after return of the nerve fibers to the junctional regions. Abnormalities in the number of branches in NMJs were still present after 10 months.

Delayed Suture Experiments

As might be expected, after delayed suture, when more severe muscle atrophy was allowed to occur, restoration of the function and morphologic structure of the NMJs was delayed still further. For example, after a three month period of muscle atrophy and biopsy two months after the calculated arrival of the nerve fibers, there was moderate muscle atrophy, but many intact NMJs were observed. Of these, many were reinnervated, but others showed adjacent nerve fibers without evidence of successful reinnervation. The proportion of the old NMJs reinnervated was greatly decreased, especially when the period of atrophy was allowed to lengthen prior to reinnervation. Even when nerve fibers lay close to NMJs, it appeared that they were unable to enter them; and when they were successful, only a few terminal nerve branches were present. As the period of atrophy was increased fewer and fewer of the returning nerve fibers found their old soleplate homes. All these reinnervated NMJs were very abnormal, with claw-like endings and other bizarre shapes.

After seven months of atrophy and two months after the arrival of the nerve fibers, there was little evidence of reinnervation of old NMJs, but a few feeble efforts toward forming NMJs were observed. By nine months no evidence of reinnervation could be found; the nerve fibers ended as knobs enmeshed in fibrous tissue. However, Gutmann and Young point out that since the muscle was functional, some of these abnormal nerve formations must have been physiologically if not morphologically adequate. Some of the NMJs demonstrated remarkable persistence in severely atrophic muscle that consisted of a few remaining threads of myofibers.

Apparently the reason for the failure to reinnervate old NMJs is the proliferation of fibrous tissue at the end of the old endoneural

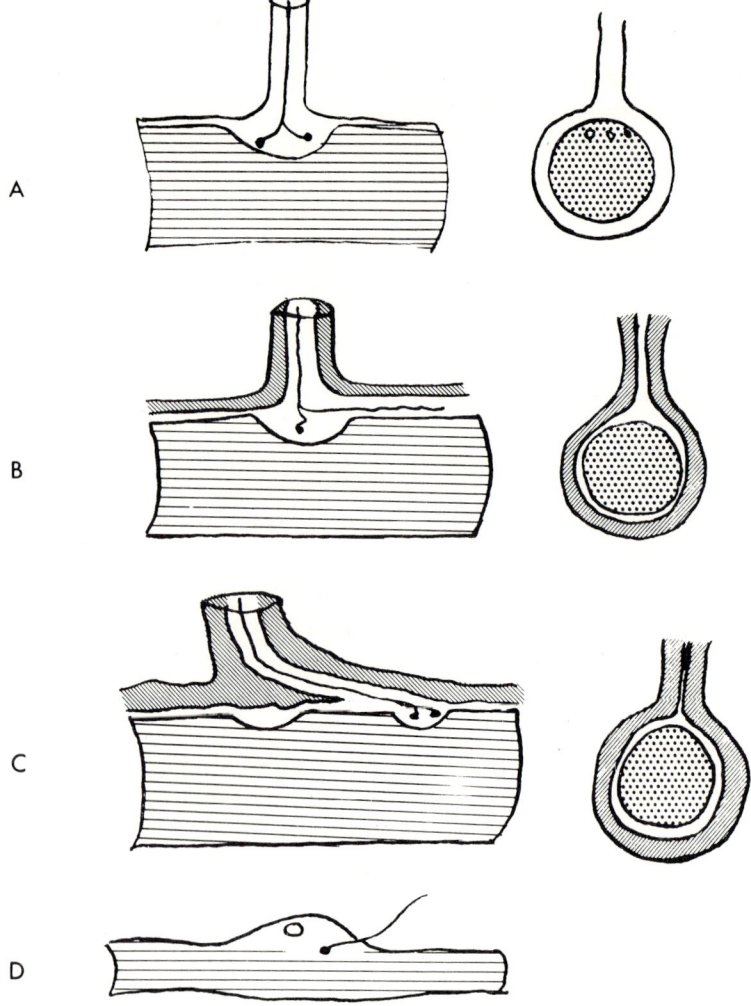

Figure 85. Diagrammatic summarization of the events occurring in reinnervation of atrophic muscle, after Gutmann and Young. The normal innervation site is illustrated at *A*. The terminal nerve branch is subdivided in the superficial Schwann and perineural sheaths indicated by the outer dark line. The myofilaments are represented by horizontal lines (left) and by dots (right). In diagram *B*, the perineural sheath is thick and fibrous, and an "escaped fiber" is shown lying beneath the fibrous connective tissue overlying the myofiber. The corresponding transverse section illustrates the thick and fibrous connective tissue layer and the narrowing of the pathway available for reinnervating nerve sprouts. At *C*, a late stage of this process is illustrated. There is severe thickening of the fibrous sheath and marked narrowing of the pathway available for the innervating fibers. Note that the original pathway to the old NMJ region is obstructed and that a new NMJ has been formed by the "escaped fiber". Diagram *D* illustrates a severely atrophic myofiber with an abortive attempt at reinnervation. (After Gutmann and Young, 1944.)

tube. After short periods of denervation, good restoration of structure and function occurred as the "axoplasmic stream" returned to its old haunts. As the time increased after denervation, newly formed fibrous tissue appeared to block the end of the Schwann cell tube, thus interfering with the outflow of returning axoplasm. Gutmann and Young suggested that the shape of the axoplasm, as revealed by silver-staining methods, indicated constriction of the end of the Schwann cell tube. This obstruction resulting from fibrous tissue is also responsible for the misdirection of the "escaped fibers." Figure 85 summarizes these observations diagramatically.

Experiments by Nathaniel (1962), Nathaniel and Pease (1963), Harkin (1966) and observations on hypertrophic neuritis (Zacks et al, 1968) strongly suggest that abnormal Schwann cells may lay down collagen. Thus if sufficiently delayed, the Schwann cells and perineural epithelial cells that guide the returning axons may ultimately interfere with reinnervation.

The work of Gutmann and Young (1944) also demonstrated that the "escaped fibers" may form new functional NMJs and that his occurs with decreasing frequency as the duration of atrophy increases. Also it was well demonstrated that previously innervated areas devoid of nerve fibers were capable of retaining the soleplate for very long periods of time after denervation (up to 17 months).

It is worthwhile to stress the fact that even though the pattern of branching of the terminal nerve arborization and the general form of the reconstituted NMJs were abnormal, frequently no functional abnormalities could be demonstrated in these muscles. If similar factors operate in abnormal NMJs observed in various neuromuscular diseases, prospects for correlating functional abnormalities with structural changes observed in biopsy specimens might seem to be unpromising. We must recall, however, that only one or at most two elements of NMJ structure are described in this kind of investigation: namely, the silver-stained appearance of terminal nerve branches and the disposition of the soleplate nuclei.

The studies of Gutmann and Young have revealed the pattern of reinnervation in rabbit muscles, have raised some basic questions concerning the form and function of abnormal NMJs, and have clearly established the clinical principle that the longer the period of muscle atrophy allowed, the poorer will be the innervation pattern and the ultimate functional capabilities of the reinnervated muscle. After a sufficient period of time, when muscle atrophy is severe, successful reinnervation appears impossible for the reasons discussed. Apparent also is the corollary: the less injury to the nerve, the better the reinnervation result.

Even under optimal conditions, there is poor or absent coordination of muscles reinnervated by cut and regenerated nerves in the higher vertebrates including man. Many of the questions concerning structural changes in denervated and reinnervated NMJs can only be answered by the increased resolution afforded by electron microscopy. Details of changes in the subneural apparatus and soleplate in denervated NMJs and the process of *de novo* NMJ formation are revealed by ultrastructure studies.

ELECTRON MICROSCOPY OF DENERVATED NEUROMUSCULAR JUNCTIONS

It was not long after the original description of the intricate fine structure of NMJs in several species that electron microscopic studies of denervation appeared. Such an early investigation was that of Reger (1959), who studied the early stages (one to five days post denervation) of NMJs in the rat gastrocnemius muscle. It should be noted that this early study utilized rather long osmium fixation (two hours) and employed methacrylate embedding without benefit of additives to reduce polymerization artefact ("explosion").

Twenty-four hours after denervation, the only change observed was decreased density in the axoplasm of the terminal axon branches. the synaptolemma (the axolemma plus the subsynaptic sarcolemma) and the subneural cytoplasm were normal. Forty-eight hours after denervation, the number of synaptic vesicles had decreased and there was retraction of the axolemma from the subneural membrane, which left clear, empty "retraction spaces." Some of these spaces contained material interpreted as axonal debris. Deep infolding of the axolemma appeared to occur concurrently with the retraction. Viewed with the experience gained in recent years, it seems likely that the "retraction spaces" illustrated by Reger were genuine but exaggerated by polymerization artefacts. The micrographs also show evidence of extraction of materials from both the axoplasm and the cytoplasm, probably owing to the relatively long periods of primary osmium fixation.

Seventy-two hours after denervation, some of the synaptic grooves contained partially "retracted" axon terminals which in some areas were still in synaptic contact with the sarcolemma. Others contained material interpreted as axonal debris. By 96 hours most of the terminal axon branches had degenerated completely, and where branches persisted, they were unremarkable except for decreased numbers of synaptic vesicles. The sarcolemma and sarcoplasm appeared normal. One hundred and twenty-four hours after denervation, practically all the terminal axon branches had "retracted" and degenerated, leaving Schwann cells lying directly on the sarcolemma.

An attempt to count synaptic vesicles per unit area of axoplasm during the process of degeneration was thought to indicate a significant decrease in number when the 24 to 48 hour experimental animals and the 96 to 120 hour animals were compared. Similarly, increase in the "retraction spaces" was thought to be statistically significant in the NMJs 48 to 120 hours after denervation. However, the author was disturbed by the wide range in size and number of vesicles and the wide range in width and degree of "retraction" of the axolemma, which led him seriously to consider the possibility that these apparent abnormalities were in part artefact.

Additional studies of degeneration of motor NMJs (frog) were made by Birks, et al. (1960), who correlated the neurophysiologic events occurring during denervation with fine structure changes revealed by electron microscopy. This investigation was chiefly concerned with the miniature endplate potentials (MEPPs), the spontaneous, randomly occurring subthreshold potentials that may be recorded with microelectrodes within NMJs. The authors divided the events that occurred following denervation into three periods; the first, or latent, period was characterized by no significant electrophysiologic changes. In the second, or "silent", period, instead of the expected gradual loss of endplate potentials, they found that three to four days after denervation, neuromuscular transmission ceased abruptly within a few hours and spontaneous activity stopped, probably owing to failure of transmitter release. Much to their surprise, the MEPPs recorded from regions of denervated NMJs resumed activity during the second week of denervation. These potentials differed in some respects from normal MEPPs. They were of low frequency and slower time course, and their amplitude was within the normal range but was of abnormal distribution. They were also less sensitive to various stimuli affecting the amplitude and rate of discharge. However, the abnormal MEPPs were claimed to be sufficiently similar to normal MEPPs to suggest that they also represented release of Ach quanta.

These investigators concluded that the resumption of the electrical activity was due to MEPPs similar to those normally found. The disappearance and resumption of the MEPPs during the first two weeks were unrelated to the chemical sensitivity of the muscle to Ach. The authors hypothesized that the wide margin (10 times) between the spontaneous and the maximal rates of Ach delivery capability of the nerve endings indicated that the limiting factor was the release and not the storage or Ach synthetic ability of the NMJs. The data also seemed to indicate that there was probably an increased turnover of Ach in the terminal axons, resulting in fewer and smaller Ach quanta.

As so frequently happens, the experimental evidence obtained from coincident electron microscopic studies led to results entirely different from those expected in the original hypothesis. During the latent period after denervation, no structural changes could be found by the authors. However, during the "silent period" that occurred 3 to 4 days after denervation, a plethora of anatomic changes appeared in the frog NMJs. Large mitochondria with fragmented inner structures and unusually dense matrix were observed. Many of the axon terminals were nearly devoid of synaptic vesicles. The clumped vesicles formed strange "honeycomb" structures in the axoplasm. Variable Schwann cell relationships were observed. No single anatomic abnormality could be correlated with the absence of MEPPs.

During the final stage, when MEPPs reappeared, the three cell components which are normally found in the junctional region had been reduced to two components; a Schwann cell and the underlying myofiber. The structure of the subneural clefts appeared normal even up to 130 days after denervation. Thus the Schwann cell lay in immediate proximity to the underlying muscle cell without the usual interposed terminal axon, as in the normal junction. The Schwann cell cytoplasm contained scattered fine filaments and granules, mitochondria, and vesicles of various size. The author stated that the contact of the Schwann cell with the muscle cell was indistinguishable from the normal contact of the nerve and muscle. They even refer to a "primary synaptic" space, and to "synaptic contact" of the myofiber with the Schwann cell: "It illustrates the extent of the synaptic contact with muscle fibers which the Schwan cell has established at this stage." This description seems somewhat prejudicial in referring to a contact between a Schwann cell and a muscle as a synaptic contact, for it implies that this abnormal arrangement amounts to actual innervation. As introduced by Sherrington (1897, 1906), "synapse" was used to "denote the nexus between neuron and neuron in the central nervous system and it has been extended to include connections between nerve endings and elements of the body they innervate." Even though "synapse" is primarily a physiologic term, the evidence does not warrant its use to describe the abnormal contact between the Schwann and muscle cells in denervated NMJs. Its use for this situation is surprising,: Birks et al. (1960) stated, "An obvious, though not inevitable, inference is that the source of renewed release and production of acetylcholine (or similarly acting substance) is inside the Schwann cell."

The authors also consider other possibilities to explain the restoration of MEPPs; namely, that Ach might be released from the muscle, that remnants of stored Ach may persist in the neighborhood, or possibly that sprouting from adjacent autonomic nerves not seen in the electron micrographs may provide a source of the Ach. If we accept the new concept that Schwann cells are capable of producing Ach and thus are responsible for generating MEPPs, a number of experiments and indeed new concepts of neuromuscular function are suggested.

Differences between denervated frog and rat NMJs have bee reported by Miledi and Slater (1963). These investigators found that unlike frog NMJs, which were covered with Schwann cell cytoplasm after degeneration of the terminal axons, rat NMJs were covered by collagen fibers in most cases. Correspondingly, there was no reappearance of MEPPs in the rat NMJs. This has been cited as additional support of the concept of Ach secretion by Schwann cells.

Bauer, Blumberg, and Zacks (1962) investigated the fine structure of denervated mouse NMJs two days to 11 weeks after denervation. Two days after denervation lamellar bodies, interpreted as degenerating myelin fragments, were found within Schwann cell cytoplasm and, surprisingly, in the soleplate sarcoplasm. These bodies were not seen in the later stages of degeneration. After seven days of denervation, retraction of degenerating axons was the major abnormality. The soleplate and the synaptic clefts were unaltered. Even after five weeks, the secondary synaptic clefts were still present. The opened directly onto the muscle surface, since the primary synaptic cleft was absent. In many NMJ areas the overlying Schwann cell cytoplasm was greatly thinned or absent entirely. The material remained within the secondary synaptic clefts and extended to the muscle surface as in normal NMJs. The soleplate nuclei, Golgi apparatus, mitochondria, endoplasmic reticulum, and granules were unaltered. The secondary clefts in some of the NMJs were few and wide. AchE activity demonstrated by the thiolacetic acid method persisted within the secondary synaptic clefts. After 11 weeks of denervation no NMJs could be found, with or without the aid of AchE staining.

Thus, the early stages of denervation of NMJs is characterized by loss of axons and reduction of the usual overlying covering of Schwann cells. The later stages demonstrated loss of the primary cleft and preservation of somewhat abnormal secondary clefts. AchE activity persisted until 11 weeks, when NMJs no longer could be found.

Electron micrographic examinations of frog NMJs following denervation have shown first a period during which nothing could be seen at the fine structure level, followed by a period in which several abnormalities, including "honeycomb" structures, swollen mitochondria, and dense mitochondrial matrix, were found. In the terminal phase, the terminal axon disappeared entirely and contact was made between the Schwann and muscle cells. "Honeycomb structures" are infrequent features in degenerating axons and are rarely observed in rodent NMJs.

Birks, Katz, and Miledi (1960) also confirmed the previous observation of Gutmann and Young (1944) that considerable restoration of structure occurred before the NMJs became functional.

In more recent correlated microphysiological and ultrastructure studies, Miledi and Slater (1968) studied denervation of the rat diaphragm. One day after nerve section, the axon had disintegrated and MEPPs had disappeared. Three weeks later, low frequency MEPPs appeared in 8 of 770 myofibers that were similar to normal. After long periods of denervation (more than three weeks) no MEPPs could be recorded and no cells were present over the old primary synaptic clefts of the denervated NMJs. This contrasts with the situation up to 3 weeks after operation where nucleated cells thought to be Schwann cells overlay the subneural apparatus. The authors concluded that the Schwann cells were the source of Ach packets, a concept presented in their previous studies (Katz and Miledi, 1959). Others have suggested that phagocytic incorporation of the remnants of degenerating axon terminals by adjacent Schwann cells permitted them to either acquire pre-existing Ach precursors or possibly the intact machinery for synthesizing Ach. From the morphologic point of view, the round profiles measuring 0.75-0.2 μ containing mitochondria but lacking EL illustrated in the work of Miledi and Slater (1968) could also be interpreted as Schwann cell processes or minute neurites that are characteristic of collateral nerve branches. Unless combined glutaraldehyde and osmium fixation is used, it is difficult to distinguish small (0.1-0.3 μ) immature axon branches from Schwann cell processes because both lack EL and contain small mitochondria and empty vesicles. The presence of collateral sprouts, which may form quite rapidly, could be detected by combined silver and cholinesterase staining techniques. To support the concept of Schwann cell release of Ach, Miledi and Slater cite the results of Mitchell and Silver (1963) who found the release of Ach from phrenic nerve-diaphragm preparations was reduced only 50% following denervation and thus suggests that the Schwann cells might have been the source of the transmitter. Miledi and Slater (1968) concluded that the Ach in the Schwann cells is probably newly acquired via phagocytosis rather than the result of acquisition of ribosomes capable of synthesizing Ach.

Nickel and Waser (1968) studied degeneration of mouse diaphragm NMJs for periods of 14 hours to 6 months after section of the phrenic nerve. As in previous experiments, the terminal axon, Schwann cell and muscle degenerated. During the initial 1-3 days, there was agglutination of synaptic vesicles, followed by fragmentation and ultimate lysis with apparent absorption by the adjacent Schwann cell. Nickel and Waser (1969) demonstrated zinc iodide osmium staining of synaptic vesicles in denervated mouse diaphragm NMJs. One day after nerve section, axon debris and vesicles containing zinc iodide osmium staining material was present within Schwann cells. Although it is well known that Schwann cells may be phagocytic, there is no conclusive evidence that associates vesicular Ach or the Ach-synthesizing system with the material that stains with zinc iodide osmium. Thus, this experiment does not necessarily support the hypothesis that Schwann cells may incorporate Ach or the Ach-synthesizing system and later release the neurotransmitter.

In studies of rat gastrocnemius muscle following sciatic nerve section, Song (1968) observed fine structure changes similar to those reported by others. Axon changes, loss of synaptic vesicles, breakdown of axoplasm and changes in the postsynaptic membrane were reported to occur by the 7th day. Ultrastructure changes characteristic of acute atrophy occurred in the myofibers.

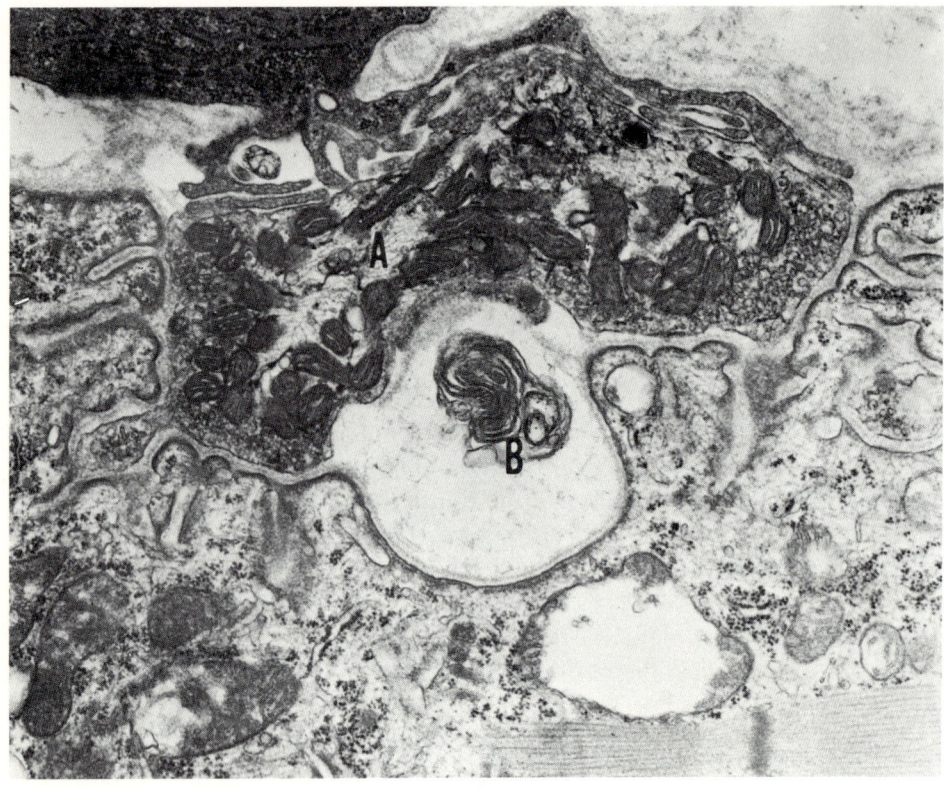

Figure 86. Electron micrograph of mouse neuromuscular junction 3 days after nerve section. Note the retraction of the axon *(A)* away from the subneural apparatus and the early changes in the secondary synaptic clefts. The large space contains a tangle of phospholipid membranes (myelin body) at *B* indicating degeneration. (X 25,000.)

In a combined histochemical and electron microscope study (Saito and Zacks, 1969) of denervation and reinnervation of mouse foot muscles after sectioning of the sciatic nerve, absence of axons was complete by the end of the first week. There was retraction of Schwann and perineural epithelial cells (Fig. 86) and degeneration of axoplasm indicated by fragmentation of organelles and formation of electron dense myelin bodies (Fig. 87). The primary synaptic cleft became shallow (Fig. 88, 89), the secondary synaptic clefts shorter and wider (Figs. 90, 91, 92) but EL demonstrated by ruthenium red (Fig. 93) in the subneural apparatus was unaltered. The characteristic subneural membrane thickening persisted and there were increased numbers of clustered ribosomes in the soleplate. Decreased numbers of coated vesicles were also noted in this area. Eventually, Schwann and perineural cell processes and collagen filaments covered the subneural apparatus (Figs. 89, 90, 92, 93).

The first evidence of spontaneous reinnervation of neuromuscular junctions occurred 4 weeks after nerve section. Regenerating axons returned to old subneural apparatuses which were recognized in the electron microscope by the criteria of shortened, widened secondary synaptic clefts and early formation of collagen fibrils over the subneural apparatus (Figs. 94-98). In the succeeding weeks, the primary synaptic cleft deepened and the secondary clefts became longer and narrower so that by 15 weeks they were barely indistinguishable from the control NMJs (Fig. 99).

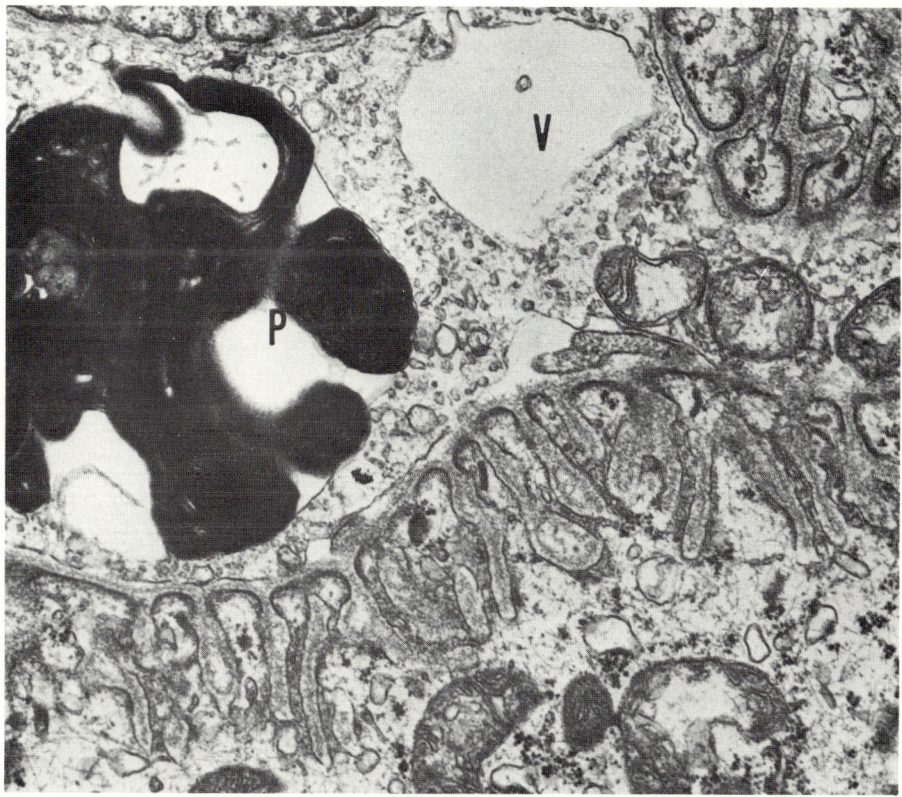

Figure 87. Electron micrograph showing more advanced stages of axon degeneration with large vacuoles *(V)* and masses of phospholipid membranes *(P)*. There are relatively few changes in the subneural apparatus. (X 24,600.)

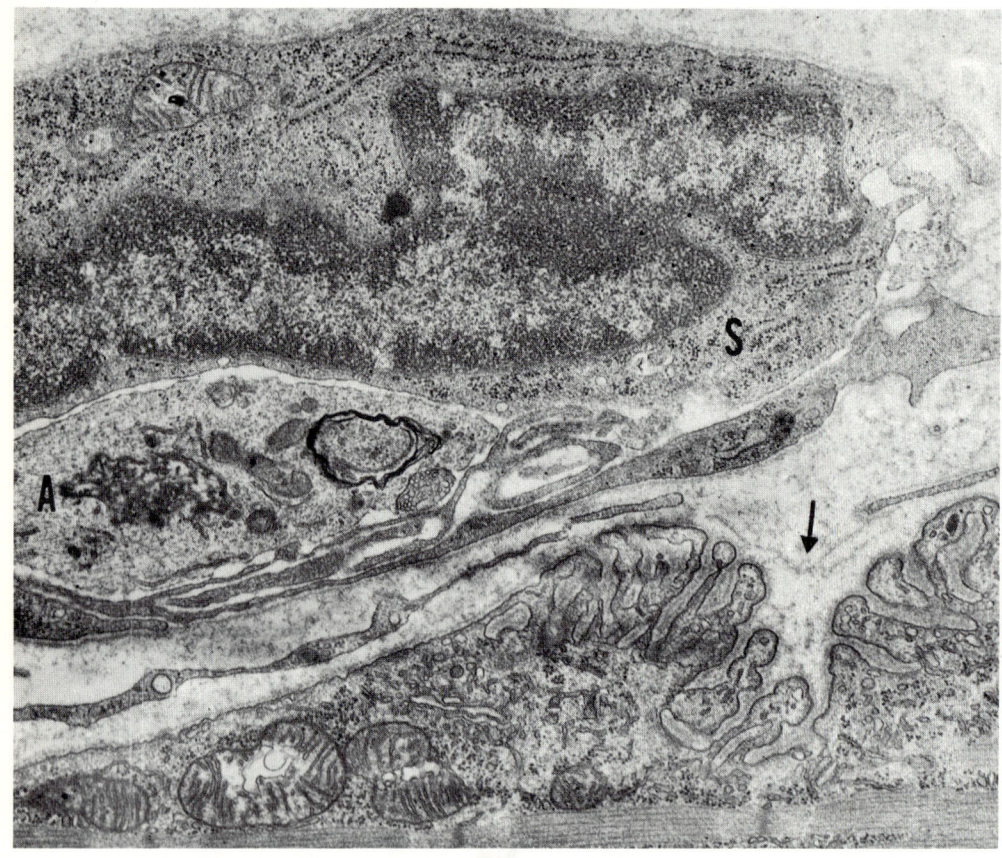

Figure 88. Electron micrograph of a later stage of a degenerating mouse NMJ showing the original innervation site devoid of axon (arrow) and early stages of the shortening and widening of the subneural apparatus that indicate denervation. Retrograde degenerative changes are visible in the axon *(A)* lying within the overlying Schwann cell *(S)*. (X 17,100.)

Denervation of En Grappe Neuromuscular Junctions

The fine structure changes in degenerating specialized junctions of extraocular muscle were studied by Teräväinen and Huikuri (1969). These investigators sectioned the rat oculomotor and trigeminal nerves and observed the fine structure changes in the two kinds of NMJs of the extraocular muscle from 10 hours to 10 days. Early changes (10-15 hours) occurred in NMJs arising from myelinated nerves (en plaque) and unmyelinated nerves (en grappe) following oculomotor nerve section. There was axoplasmic swelling, agglutination of synaptic vesicles and mitochondria and fragmentation of microtubules. By 24 hours, the terminal axons had separated from the postsynaptic membrane and hypertrophic teloglial cells had begun to ingest the axonal debris (42-48 hours) in both kinds of NMJs. Later, the relatively few clefts of the en grappe motor endings disappeared

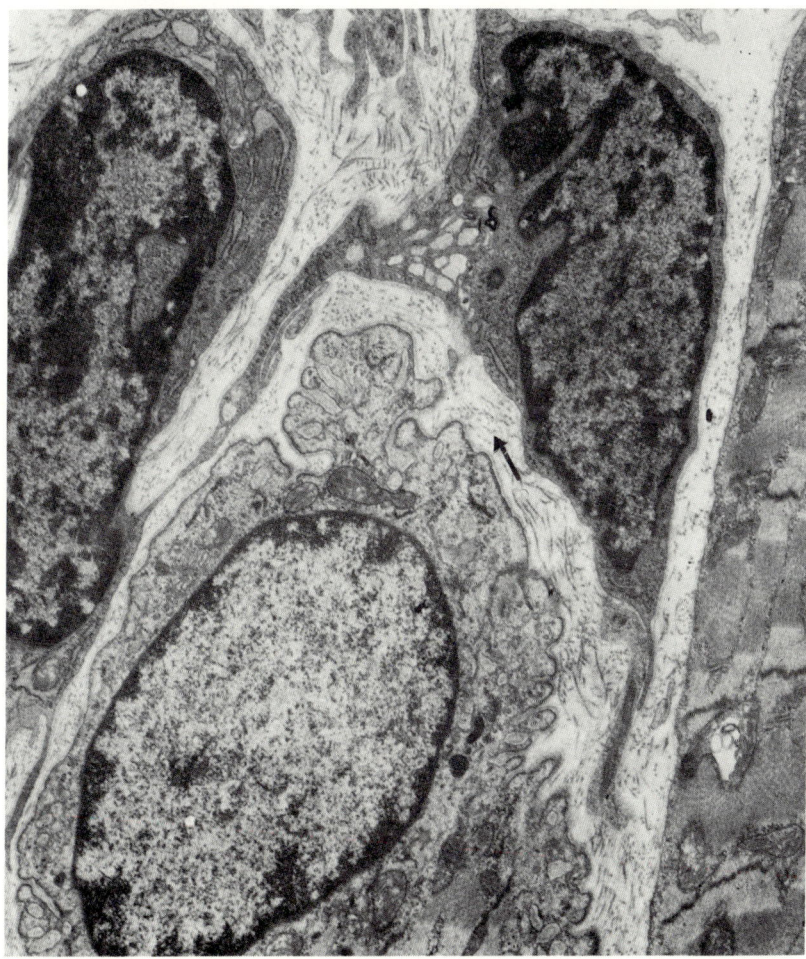

Figure 89. Electron micrograph of a denervated mouse neuromuscular junction showing changes in the subneural apparatus, absent axon and extension of collagen filaments (arrow) into the original innervation site. Note the persistence of the specialized thickening of the original synaptic membrane. (X 9,000.)

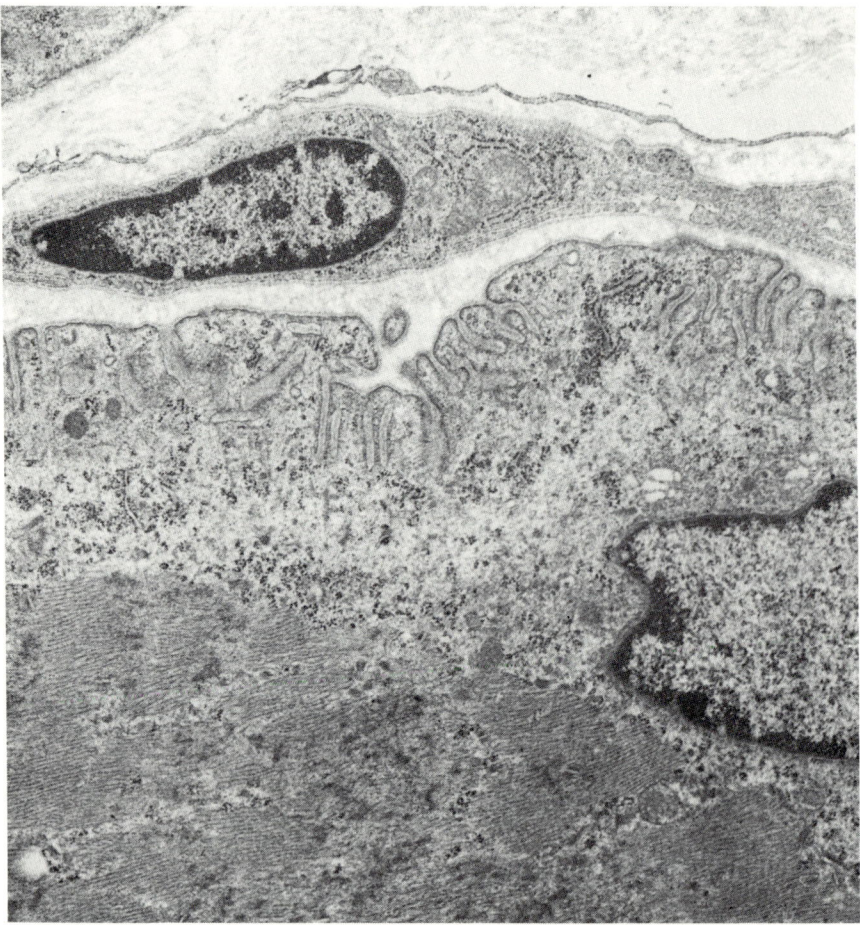

Figure 90. Electron micrograph illustrating a late stage in denervation of a mouse neuromuscular junction with absent axon, Schwann cell closely applied to the original innervation area and intervention of collagen filaments (white dots) in the original synaptic area. Degeneration is visible in the underlying myofiber. (X)13,200.)

whereas no changes were observed in the more complex subneural apparatus of the en plaque NMJs. However in the latter, there was an appreciable increase in the amount of ribosome-containing postsynaptic sarcoplasm. These experiments demonstrated that both kinds of motor endings arose from the oculomotor nerve. Previous experiments by Teräväinen (1968b) had demonstrated that the multiple endings on rat extraocular muscle are cholinergic. This view is in variance with that of Cheng et al. (1967); Cheng-Minoda et al. (1968) who claimed that only the myelinated nerve innervating en plaque NMJs arose from the oculomotor nerve.

Cholinesterase Activity in Denervated Neuromuscular Junctions

In a series of investigations beginning approximately in 1951, several investigators employed both histochemical and biochemical assay procedures to measure cholinesterase activity in NMJs after nerve degeneration. The results all showed persistence of the enzyme in the subneural apparatus long after degeneration of the nerve. These studies chiefly reported total esterase activity since it was assumed that AchE activity was responsible for the major esterase activity in NMJs (Kupfer, 1951; Bergner, 1957; Brzin and Zajicek, 1958; Bauer et al., 1962; Brzin and Majcentkacev, 1963; Csillik and Savdy, 1958; Gerebtzoff

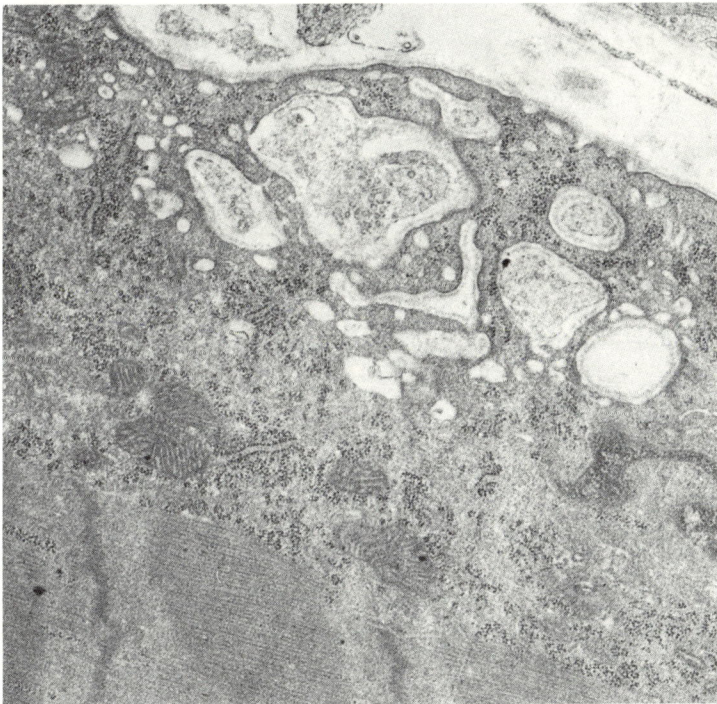

Figure 91. Electron micrograph of an atrophic mouse muscle following denervation. Note the wide distortion of the subneural apparatus. (X 17,100.)

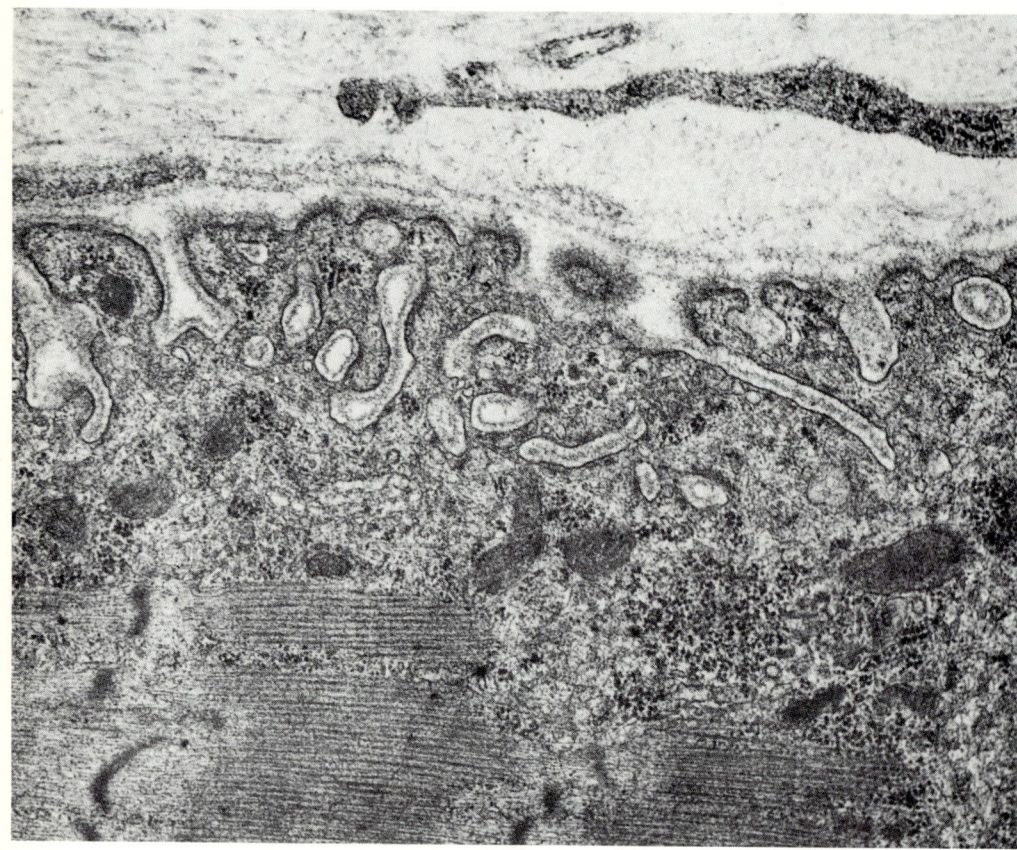

Figure 92. Electron micrograph showing a late stage of a denervated mouse muscle illustrating shortening and widening of the secondary synaptic clefts and ingrowth of collagen filaments in the original synaptic area. (X 24,600.)

and Vandermissen, 1956; Guth and Zalewski, 1963; Hines, 1960; Snell and McIntyre, 1956; Waser and Hadorn, 1961).

In a quantitative study of cholinesterase activity in denervated myofibers, Guth et al. (1964) used a microchemical method to follow activity of the soleplate and non soleplate enzymes. Following denervation, both soleplate and non soleplate cholinesterase activity decreased rapidly to a level of approximately 50% of normal by the first week following which there was little additional loss up to 7 weeks. The total protein content of the muscle declined to 50% of normal by 3 weeks. Thus it appeared that considerable cholinesterase activity was not associated with the soleplates and that denervation produced a rapid loss of the enzyme. These quantitative data contradict earlier histochemical observations that showed little cholinesterase activity outside of NMJs in normal muscle and little decrease in the enzyme following denervation. Since acetylthiocholine was used without inhibitors, both AchE and ChE were demonstrated. However, the work of the Finnish investigators and others have demonstrated that in addition to AchE, ChE and nsE are also present in NMJs (Eränkö et al., 1964; Härkönen, 1964; Kokko, 1965 and Eränkö and Terävainin, 1967). Few of the earlier investigators used inhibitors to distinguish the kinds of esterases demonstrated by the histochemical methods. Schwarzacher (1957) and Filogamo and Gabella (1966) used DFP to inhibit nonspecific ChE and Pearse (1960) and Holmsted and Sjoquist (1961) used butyrylcholine to distinguish ChE from AchE. Myelase

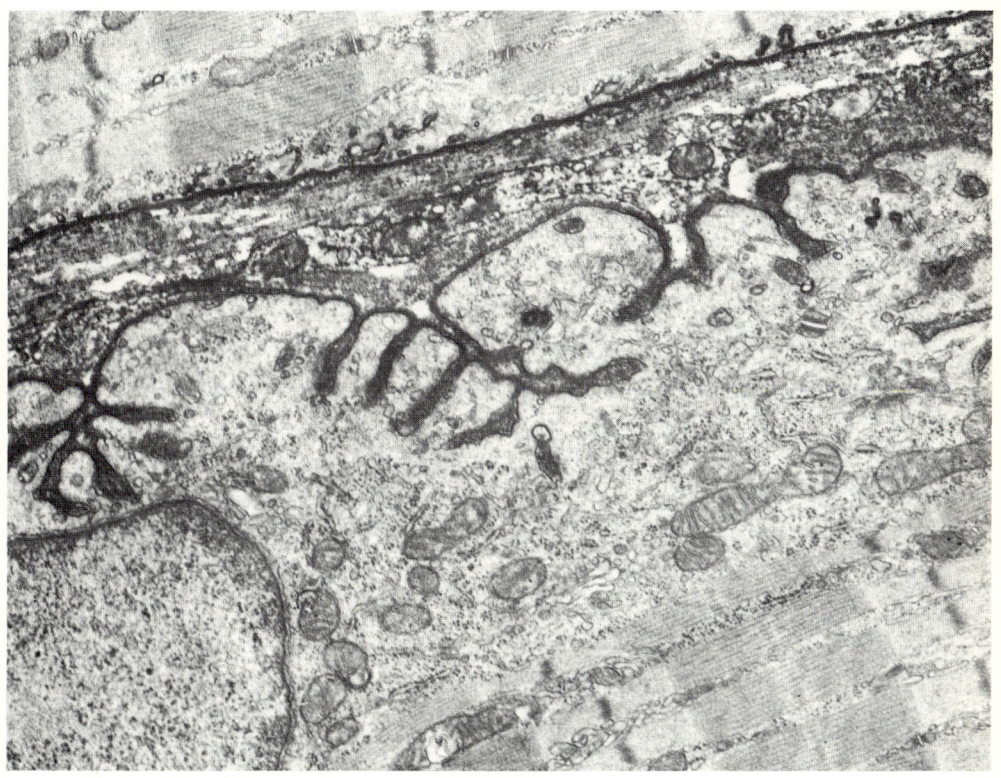

Figure 93. Electron micrograph of a denervated mouse neuromuscular junction illustrating persistence of the external lamina on the surface of the myofiber and within the subneural apparatus as demonstrated by ruthenium red staining. (X 17,100.)

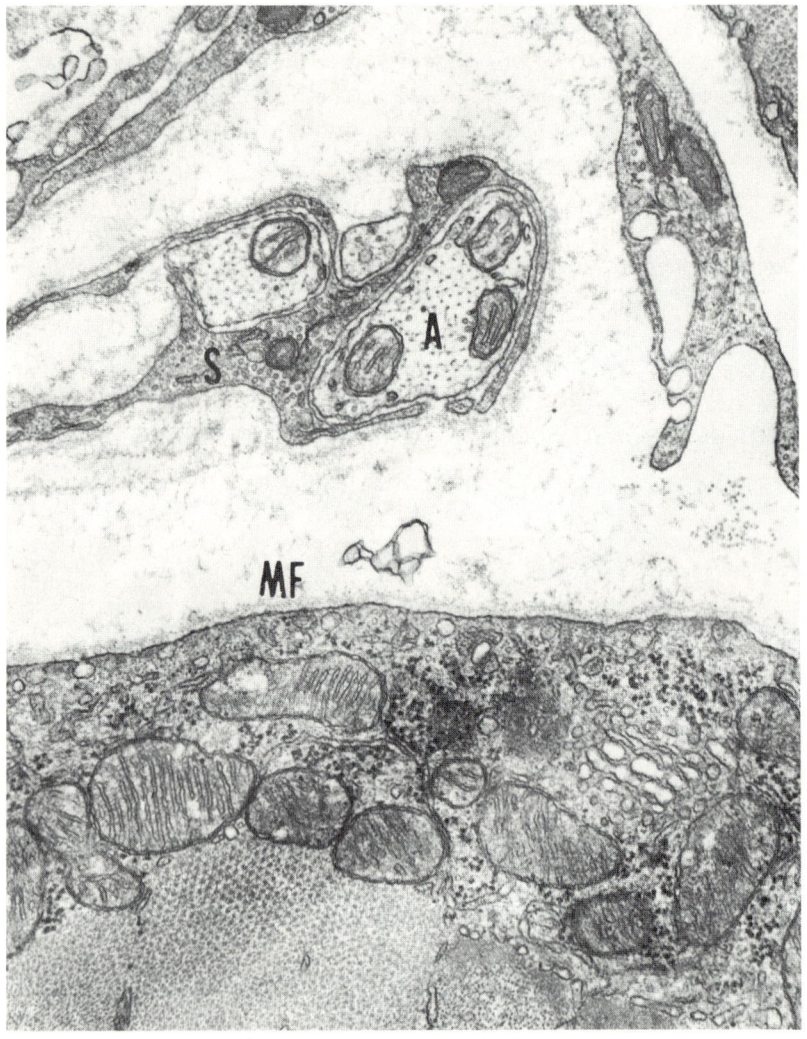

Figure 94. Electron micrograph illustrating an early stage in the reinnervation of denervated muscle. Axon sprouts *(A)* are loosely surrounded by Schwann cell cytoplasm *(S)* as they approach the myofiber surface *(MF)*. (X 37,500.)

Figure 96. Electron micrograph illustrating an early stage of reinnervation of a previously denervated NMJ. A small axon sprout *(A)* lies within Schwann cell *(S)* cytoplasm in close apposition to a subneural apparatus with short and wide synaptic clefts (arrow) that marks the site of a previously denervated NMJ. (X 24,600.)

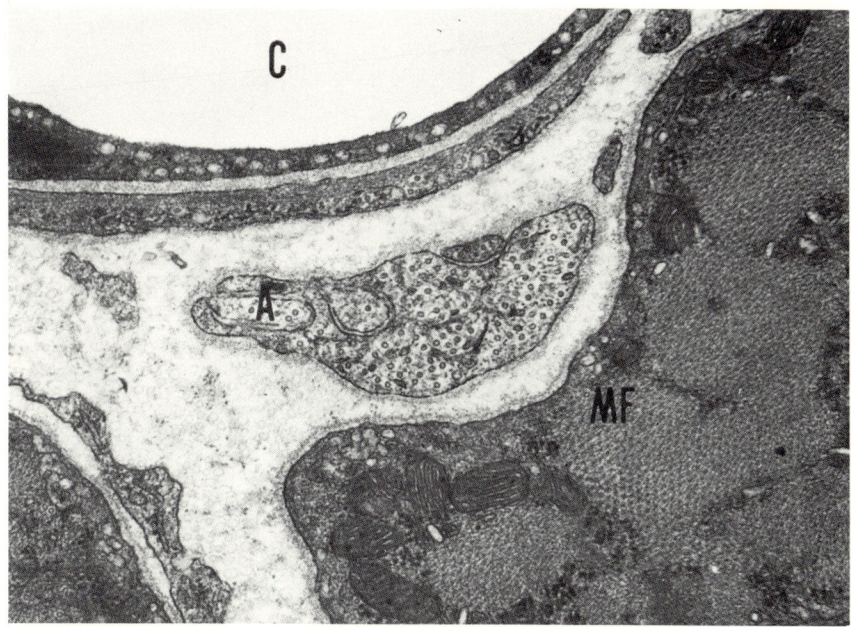

Figure 95. Electron micrograph showing axon sprouts *(A)* filled with small vesicles approaching the surface of a myofiber *(MF)*. A capillary *(C)* is present in the upper portion of the illustration. (X 37,500.)

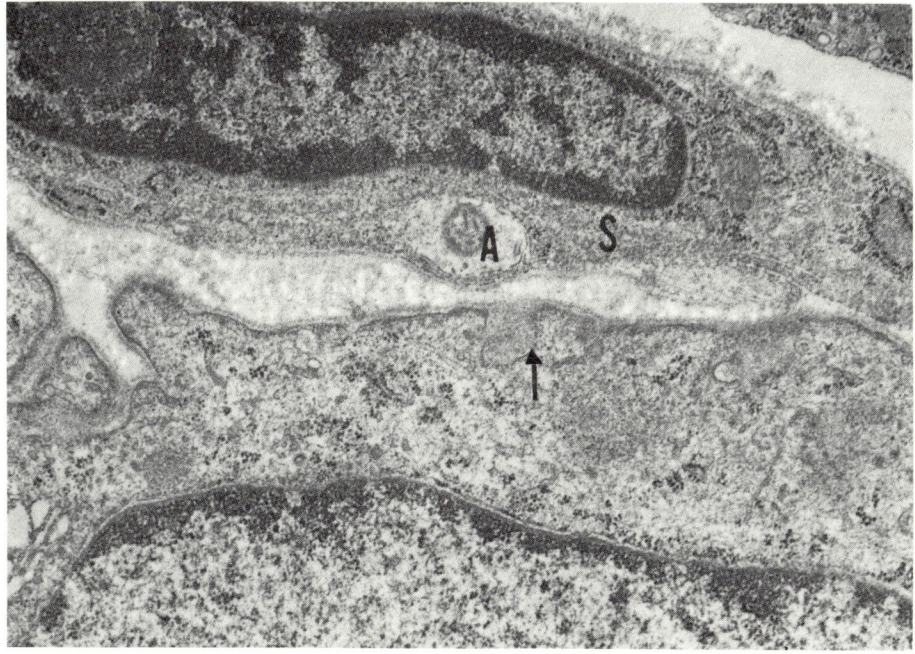

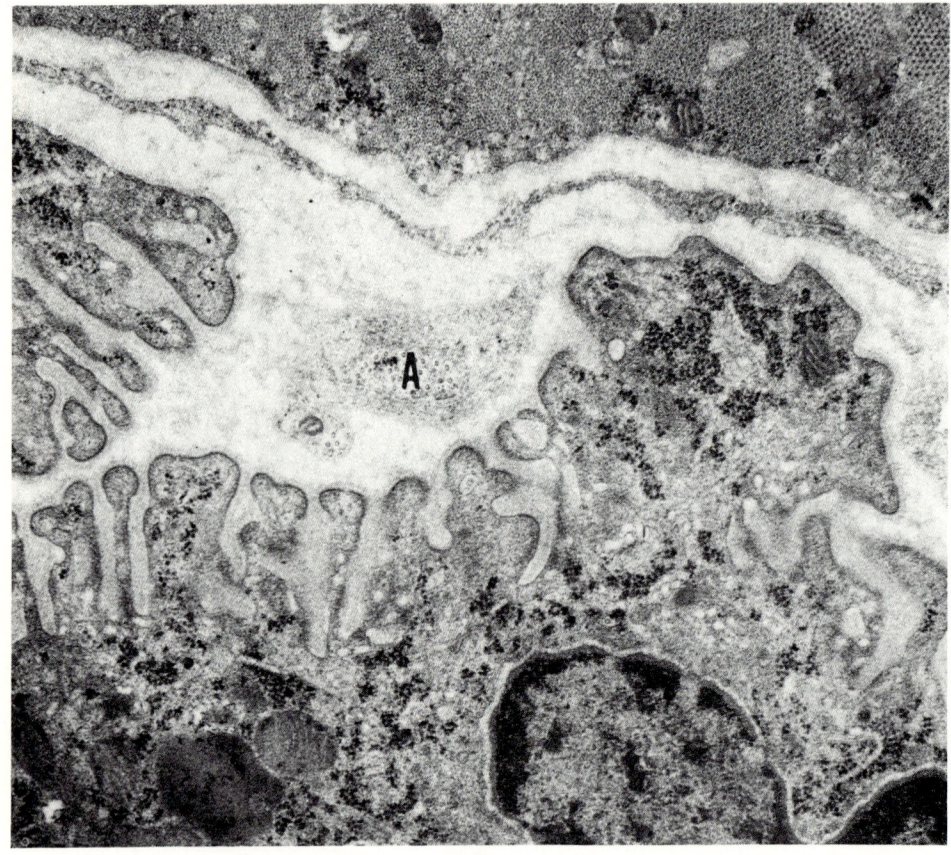

Figure 97. Electron micrograph of a previously denervated mouse NMJ during an early stage of reinnervation. A delicate axon sprout *(A)* lies in the vicinity of the previously denervated junction characterized by widened and shortened secondary synaptic clefts. (X 24,600.)

(N, M-bis 2-diethyaminoethyl) oxamide bis (2-chlorobenzylchloride) was used by Tuncbay (1964) to distinguish these two enzymes. Eränkö and Terävainen (1967) used isoOMPA as a specific inhibitor for ChE and 284C51 as a specific inhibitor for AchE as well as E600 to discriminate organophosphorus-resistent and -sensitive nsE. Using these inhibitors, Eränkö and Terävainen (1967) demonstrated that AchE activity in denervated rat muscle decreased gradually up to 8 months after nerve section whereas ChE also decreased in the subneural apparatus and teloglial cells during this interval. This contrasts with the normal absence of ChE in Schwann cells. No differences were found between experiments employing nerve crush and nerve section. During regeneration of the NMJs, the staining intensity of AchE and ChE as well as other esterases increased toward normal at approximately the same rate. However, as esterase activity recovered in the NMJs, the ChE in the Schwann cells decreased. Figures 100, and 101 illustrate changes in soleplate esterase activity of denervated and reinnervated mouse NMJs.

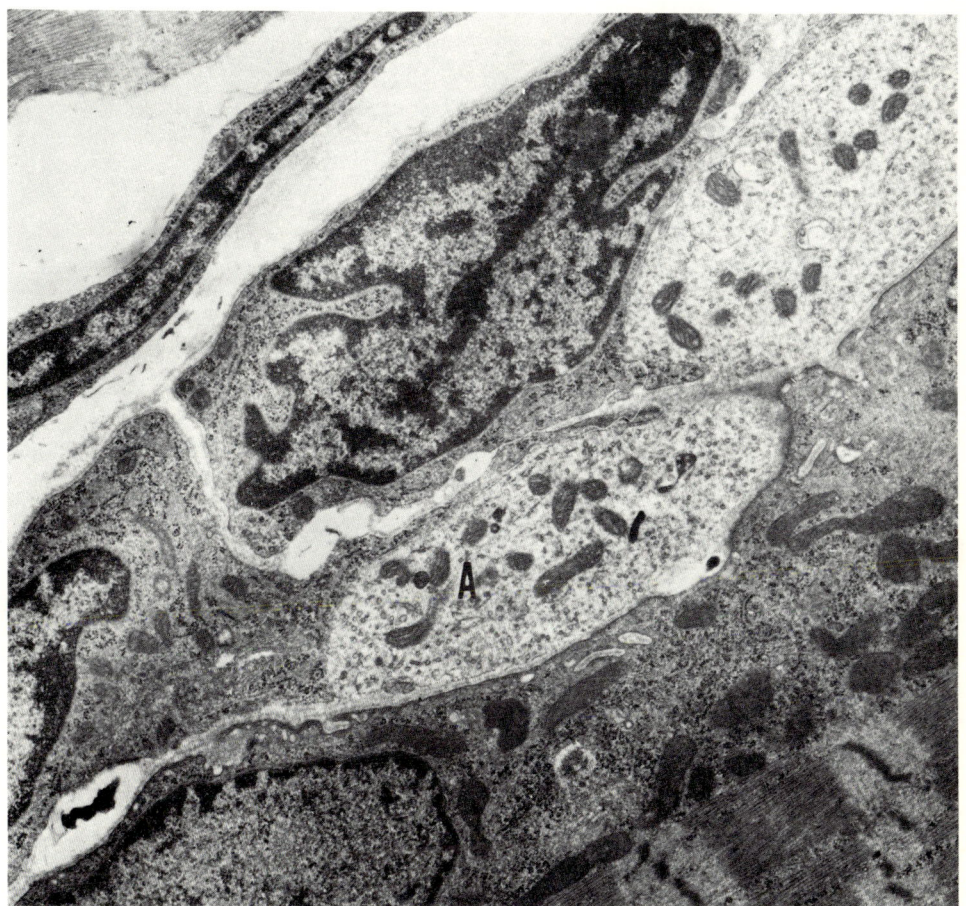

Figure 98. Electron micrograph illustrating an early stage in the reinnervation of a denervated muscle. Note the widened axon end bulb *(A)* filled with vesicles and mitochondria approaching a region of previous innervation. (X 30,000.)

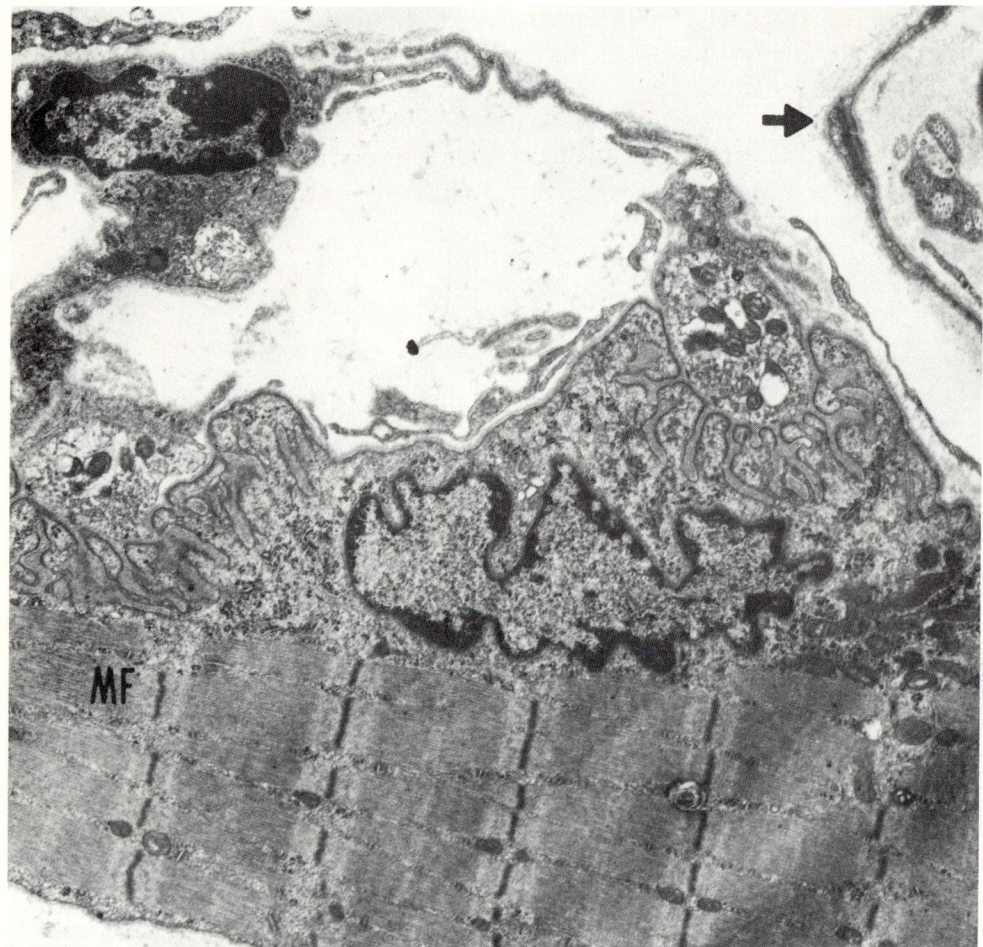

Figure 99. Electron micrograph illustrating a later stage of the reinnervation of a previously denervated muscle. Such an area may be recognized by the relatively atrophic appearance of the myofiber *(MF)* and the large surface depression in areas of relatively normal appearing neuromuscular junctions. A motor nerve containing small axon branches are visible (arrow) at the right of the illustration indicating the probable source of the reinnervating fibers. (X 24,600.)

Figure 100. Photomicrograph illustrating changes in denervated NMJs 6 weeks *(A, B, C and D)*, 8 weeks *(E)* and 30 weeks *(F)* after denervation. Although some of the NMJs appear essentially normal *(A)*, decreased stainable esterase activity and diffusion of the reaction product is visible in others *(B, C and especially in D)*. By 8 weeks, *(E)* the esterase activity is greatly reduced. By 30 weeks, regeneration and reinnervation have proceeded to nearly normal appearance of the subneural esterase content. (*A:* X 250, *B:* X 1,000, *C:* X 500, *D:* X 1,000, *E:* X 500, *F:* X 500.)

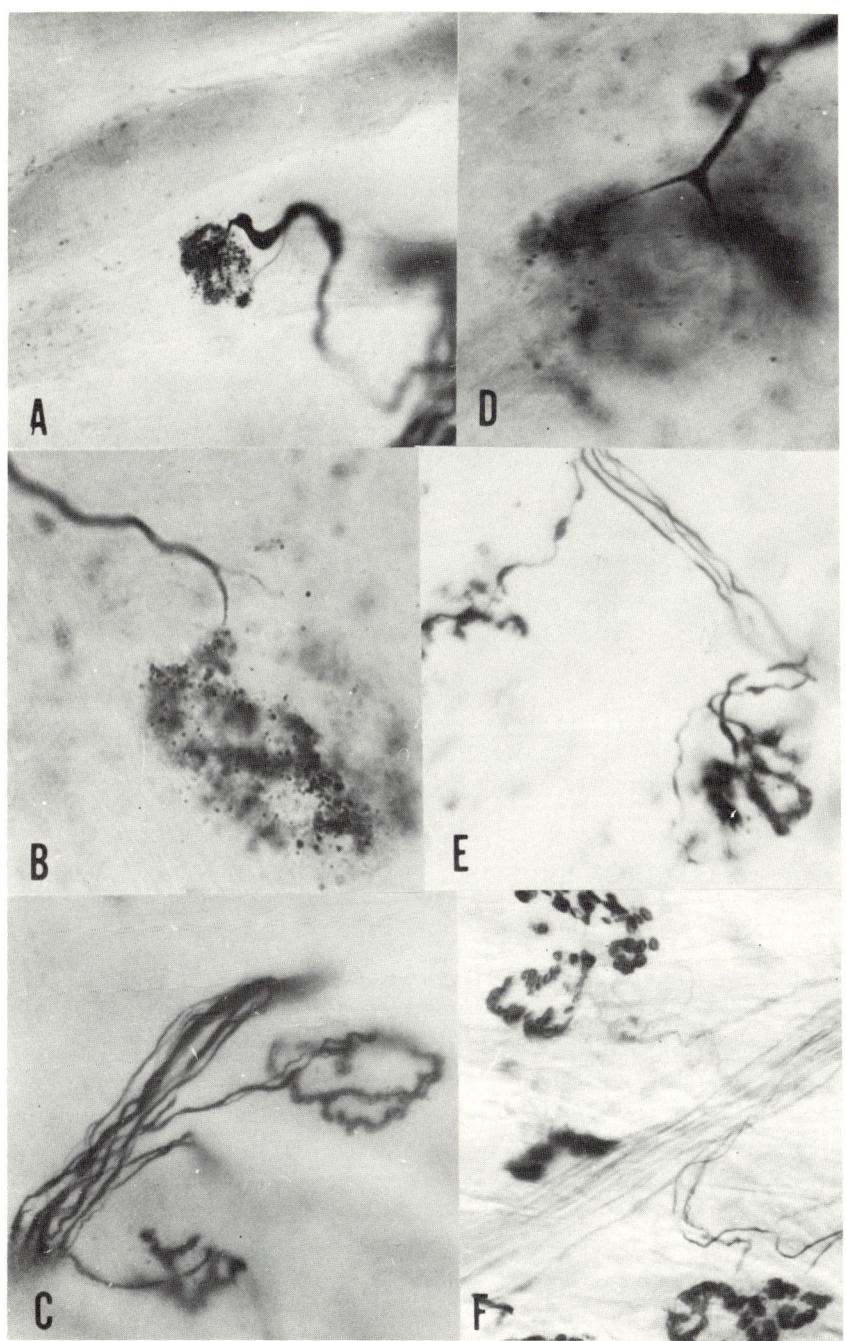

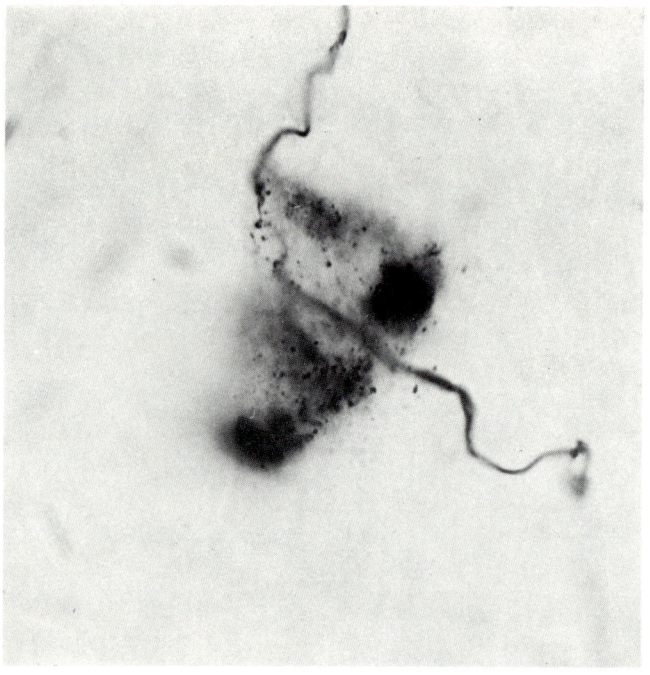

Figure 101. Photomicrograph illustrating a denervated mouse NMJ with decreased histochemical reaction product due to loss of esterase activity and a silver stained axon crossing through the area of innervation apparently representing a collateral branch en route to a possible new innervation site. (X 1,000.)

ELECTRON MICROSCOPIC HISTOCHEMISTRY

Bauer et al. (1962) found that esterase activity (thiolacetic acid method) persisted in the subneural apparatuses of denervated mouse NMJs for 11 weeks after denervation. At that time, of the original subneural apparatus only the secondary synaptic clefts remained. Unfortunately, this investigation did not include use of inhibitors or observations on the restoration of AchE activity in the NMJs during the process of reinnervation.

Csillik and Knyihar (1968) used electron microscopic methods to study esterase activity in NMJs following denervation of the rat diaphragm. Methods employed were the Koelle thiocholine, indoxyl acetate and the thiolacetic acid methods. Unfortunately, the inhibitors which most selectively distinguish the various kinds of esterases were not used. These investigators found that AchE was present in the pre- and postsynaptic membranes whereas ChE activity (indoxyl acetate method) was present in the subneural clefts. The thiolacetic acid method demonstrated the histochemical reaction product chiefly in the postsynaptic membrane. Eleven days after nerve section, few fragments of degenerating nerve remained and collagen had formed in the synaptic gutter. At this time, the nerve lacked esterase and cholinesterase activity but thiolacetic acid esterase activity was present. The authors suggested that this staining may have resulted from a proteolytic enzyme. They also observed slight reduction of enzyme activity in the postsynaptic membrane without apparent change in localization of AchE and NsE. The authors speculated that the membrane complex contains layers of esterolytic and proteolytic enzyme proteins and that the NsE is sandwiched between two layers of AchE activity. The absence of specific inhibition experiments make the identification of the enzymes doubtful solely on the basis of the histochemical staining reactions.

Lubinská and Zelená (1966) demonstrated that 2 weeks after denervation, new spots of cholinesterase activity appeared on the surface of the myofibers scattered at some distance from the NMJ area. These were not believed to be immature NMJs because total denervation did not permit such an early return of enzyme activity. The structures were raised and sharply outlined and occurred only at certain stages of development in young denervated muscle. The spots of enzyme activity were not found in embryonic muscle prior to innervation. The microscopic observations did not permit a decision whether the spots of enzyme activity lay within or on the myofibers. The authors suggested that these may represent Schwann cells that had acquired cholinesterase activity as suggested by Eränkö and Teräväinen (1967) because Schwann cells normally lack cholinesterase activity (Cavanagh et al., 1954) or they may be myofiber satellite cells.

Molecular Alterations in NMJs Caused by Denervation

Neither cytochemical nor ultrastructure methods have as yet detected changes in the molecular structure of EL or muscle cell membrane in denervated NMJs. Csillik et al. (1963) were unable to find changes in the micellar structure of the postsynaptic membrane by lead staining and polarization measurements and Saito and Zacks

(1969) found no change in lead or ruthenium red binding by EL in denervated NMJs.

Lunt et al. (1970) in a study of incorporation of leucine into proteopids of denervated muscle membranes showed an increased uptake of this amino acid compared to the controls. The change was most marked in the second proteolipid peak that showed a 5 fold increase in specific radioactivity. This is the peak that in previous experiments had been found to bind labelled Ach and methylhexamethonium. This investigator interpreted this as indicating an increase in turnover of particular receptor proteolipids following denervation. Hall (1973) using labelled α-bungarotoxin found that new Ach receptors induced by denervation had properties that differed from AchR in the junctional region. Less of toxin was greater from the new receptors. This work and studies by Hartzell and Fambrough (1973) indicate that AchR is synthesized within myofibers and is inserted into the membrane from within.

Time Required for Reinnervation

In an ingenious series of experiments, Fex and Thesleff (1967) took advantage of a previous observation of Aitkin (1950) that implantation of a foreign nerve into an *innervated* muscle led to growth of the neurofibers but *no* formation of NMJs. Functional innervation occurred only after denervation, local injury or botulinum intoxication. Since the time required to innervate previously denervated muscle is composed of two elements, the rate of growth of the axons and the time to form functional synapses, a technique was devised to interpose a delay between the implantation of a foreign nerve and denervation to allow growth of the nerve fibers but to delay formation of neuromuscular junctions until desired. This was accomplished in rats by implanting the deep peroneal nerve into the lateral head of the gastrocnemius muscle. After an interval of 2-12 weeks delay, the normal innervation (tibial nerve) was cut and the progress of formation of functional innervation was tested by electromyography. Fex and Thesleff (1967) confirmed the previous work of Aitkin (1950) that no new NMJs formed in a normally innervated muscle implanted with a foreign nerve. If the tibial nerve was cut at the time of implantation of the deep peroneal nerve, twitch responses to stimuli occurred after 12 days. If the tibial nerve was cut 2 or 12 weeks after implantation of the peroneal nerve, significant twitch tension was recorded as early as 2 days after tibial nerve section and strong twitches were obtained 10-15 days later. It appears that much of the delay before restoration of function during regeneration of axons is due to the growth of the axons rather than time required for establishing functional connections with the muscle. These studies also demonstrated that functional neuromuscular connections could form in 2 days and that the regenerating axons retained their potential for the reinnervation of muscle for considerable periods of time.

Reinnervation: The Problems of Guidance and Specificity

Two important and closely related problems, guidance of the regenerating axons and nerve specificity must be considered. The first question requiring explanation is the mechanism by which the returning axons find their original sites of innervation as suggested by some clinical experience and the experimental work of several investigators. Although this was not regarded as a serious problem by Dustin (1910), several of the early investigators (Forssman, 1898; Tello, 1907; Cajal, 1908) were much preoccupied by it. Dustin stated that "there is no reason to suppose that the outgrowing nerve fibers are in any way sorted or shunted into appropriate paths; similarly, there is no evidence of the attraction of any fiber back to its end organ. Thus many connections formed must be unsuitable ones, and it is to compensate for this that excessive innervation occurs at all stages of regeneration". However, many investigators believed that in order to obtain a given functional result resembling the original state prior to denervation, the original neurons must reinnervate the original innervation sites or changes in central connections must be made to achieve the same result. This question is of considerable clinical importance because, unlike reinnervation in certain lower vertebrates (newts, salamanders and certain fish), reinnervation in higher vertebrates including man leads to poor coordination and restoration of function.

If regenerating axons are destined to reach specific myofibers, how is this accomplished? Two hypotheses have been proposed to explain how regenerating axons are guided to their original sites of innervation; the chemotactic hypothesis and the concept of contact guidance.

Chemotactic Factors in Guidance. Cajal (1908) suggested that during the development of NMJs and during reinnervation of denervated NMJs, chemotropic factors were active in guiding the nerve fibers to their destinations but he did not rule out possible contact effects, which he called "tactile adhesions". The chemotropic concept was later extended to include the idea that the stimulus arose from degenerating Schwann cells. According to Cajal (1928), "the attractive substance elaborated by the embryonic connective cells and by the cell of Schwann of the peripheral stump — the apotrophic cells of Marinesco — have a generic character, acting without distinction on all sprouts, while the attractive substances given out by the spindles of Kűhne, motor endplates, cutaneous sensory structures, etc., have a specific character, acting only on certain functional categories of regenerated axons. These specific stimuli are both neurotropic and neurocladic and the final bundle of Meissner's corpuscle represent, in normal ontogeny as well as pathological regeneration, the last neurocladic effect of specific stimuli". He goes on to state that "once ontogenetic evolution is ended, the trophic sources appear to be especially localized in the cells of Schwann and the lemnoblasts of Lehhossék, in the substance of degenerated soleplates, in the satellite cells of the sensory ganglion cells, in the elements of the terminal sensory structures such as the sheaths of Kűhne, the cells of Meissner, etc., and finally in the embryonic connective tissue". Cajal hypothesized that "the orienting agent of the sprouts does not operate through attraction, as many have supposed, but by creating a region that is favorable, eminently trophic, and stimulative of the assimilation and growth of the newly formed axons". Various factors, including "active", "stimulating", "moderating", "indifferent", and "toxic", were thought to produce the final result. The active substances ("active enzymes") were thought to be secreted by Schwann cells.

Similar concepts were held by Forssman (1898) and Tello (1907, 1923). However, it is difficult to perceive how chemical attraction could operate over the considerable distance from nerve stump to denervated muscle. To avoid the difficulties of the chemotactic guidance theory, a hypothesis based on random nonspecific innervation or mechanical guidance is required. Since no evidence for the action of chemical influences acting over great distances was found, we must seek possible sources of guidance in the anatomic characteristics of regenerating nerves.

Mechanical Factors in Guidance

In vitro experiments by Weiss (1934) indicated that mechanical contact rather than chemical factors were important in the growth of nerve fibers in tissue culture. He observed that the tips of advancing axons had marked amoeboid activity in cultures of growing nerve explants. The axon tips extended pseudopods that were apparently selected for a particular direction of growth. The axon outgrowths from these explanted chick embryo spinal ganglia showed no chemotactic response to brain or other tissue extracts. If a barrier was placed in the path of the developing nerve fibers, a complex tangle or plexus was formed at the site of obstruction. As a result of these *in vitro* experiments, Weiss concluded that the axonal pseudopods grew along phase boundaries. He was able to show that branching occurred in two ways: terminal bifurcation and collateral sprouting. Terminal bifurcation was thought to be dependent on the "ultrastructure" of the medium because nerve branching was increased in disoriented media and reduced in oriented media. Weiss (1941, 1950) favored the mechanical guidance (contact guidance) hypothesis because the chemotactic hypothesis required a constant source of chemical diffusion with a steady concentration gradient. There would have to be selective sensitivity of the growing nerve fibers to this hypothetical chemical, and the nerve fibers would have to be capable of orienting themselves along the lines of the concentration gradient. This hypothesis also requires the presence of a stagnant, homogeneous medium in which the concentration gradient could remain stationary during the whole process of oriented growth. However, it certainly is not clear why the outflowing axoplasm, once having reached the innervation site, stops and branches to form a terminal arborization. In a review of the accumulated data, Young (1942) concluded that there is no chemotactic factor operating during reinnervation. Hoffman and Springell (1951) were unsuccessful in finding a chemotactic factor that might be of clinical use in facilitating reinnervation after peripheral nerve injuries. More recently, evidence for the existence of uncharacterized factors that stimulate nerve growth has been demonstrated in specialized circumstances (Levi-Montalcini and Angelletti, 1961) but these substances are not known to affect the terminal innervation.

In addition to the *in vitro* experiments demonstrating mechanical factors in guidance of axons, several *in vivo* experiments have been performed. The careful work of Gutmann and Young (1944) demonstrated that in the early stages at least, guidance of the regenerating axons to the original soleplate regions is largely accomplished by preservation of the endoneural tube composed of the Schwann cell and Key-Retzius sheaths.

This was confirmed by the work of Shanthaveerappa and Bourne (1964) who emphasized the importance of the Henle sheath (perineural epithelium) in forming a guide for the return of regenerating axons to sites of previous innervation. In histochemical and electron microscopic studies, they demonstrated that the perineural epithelial cells, though reduced to an extremely thin layer of cytoplasm, did not degenerate after nerve section. The specific histochemical characteristics of these cells, including the presence of ATPase, acid phsophatase, alkaline phosphatase, glucose-1-phosphatase, glucose-6-phosphatase and succinic dehydrogenase also were not altered by denervation. Shanthaveerappa and Bourne (1962b, 1964) had previously claimed that the perisynaptic cells surrounding the NMJ are a continuation of the perineural epithelium rather than of Schwann cells. More recent work by Saito and Zacks (1968) confirmed the presence of perineural epithelium close to the axon terminal and demonstrated that a layer of Schwann cell cytoplasm within the perineural sheath extends to cover the junctional folds of the subneural apparatus. However, neither cell layer fuses with the "sarcolemma" as originally suggested by these investigators. Thus, following degeneration of the sectioned axon, the Schwann tube composed of Schwann cell cytoplasm and remarkably resistant basement lamina reinforced by the perineural epithelial cells forms a conduit that extends to within 1μ of the original soleplate areas and permits return of the appropriate regenerating axon. If reinnervation is delayed, fibrous tissue derived from fibrocytes and Schwann cells may obstruct the Schwann tubes and the old soleplate areas (Fig. 85). Under these circumstances ultraterminal and collateral sprouting may give rise to new NMJs.

Selective Reinnervation

Several investigators have performed *in vivo* experiments to evaluate the accuracy of reinnervation to determine if the returning axons were capable of finding their original innervation sites. If specific axons could be shown to find their way unerringly to their old innervation sites, this would be evidence for a more complex guidance mechanism. To investigate possible selectivity of reinnervation, Elsberg (1917) resutured a sectioned peripheral nerve supplying a given muscle and simultaneously sutured another nerve into the muscle that ordinarily did not innervate it. In other experiments he inserted both nerves directly into the muscle. His results indicated that the original nerve reinnervated the muscle to a greater degree than the foreign nerve thus suggesting selective reinnervation. This kind of experiment was criticized by Weiss and Hoag (1946), who pointed out that the two groups of nerve fibers in Elsberg's experiment did not have equal opportunity to innervate the muscle. The original nerve had the advantage of the original intramuscular Schwann tube system.

A later study by Weiss and Taylor (1944) employed a forked artery to reveal possible trophic influences on the guidance of regenerating nerves. The regenerating nerve trunk was given the opportunity to follow one limb of the forked artery to the distal nerve stump or the other limb which led to a blind channel or a tendon. No evidence of selectivity appeared. Nerve fibers traveled in both channels. Additional experiments by Weiss and Hoag (1946) led to similar conclusions. In these experiments the proximal stumps of sectioned peroneal and tibial nerves were allowed to competitively reinnervate tibial muscle. When the peroneal and tibial nerves were placed in the two limbs of a forked artery and regeneration was allowed to proceed to the distal nerve stump, isometric tension recordings from the triceps surae showed that for the most part the original (tibial) and foreign nerve (peroneal) reinnervated the muscles equally. In some experiments, more innervation was received from the tibial nerve. Therefore it appeared that the first nerve to arrive interfered with the nerve fibers that arrived subsequently.

Bernstein and Guth (1961) performed a somewhat different experiment. In adult rats, L4 contributes a greater proportion of innervating fibers to the plantaris muscle than to the soleus. Recording of tensions of these two muscles on stimulation of the fourth and fifth lumbar nerves normally produces a characteristic tension ratio. Therefore an experiment was designed in which the plantaris/soleus tension ratio after reinnervation was used as an indication of the specificity of reinnervation and the effectiveness of possible guidance factors. For if the normal L4/L5 tension ratio for the plantaris and soleus muscles was restored following nerve degeneration and regeneration, good evidence of selective innervation would be obtained. Bernstein and Guth (1961) found that the relative preference of L4 fibers for the plantaris muscle was not restored, and therefore there was no evidence of selectivity. This lack of specificity was observed even after crush injuries, when surviving endoneural tubes were available to guide the nerve fibers directly to their NMJs, as suggested by earlier workers. As we have seen, even when the endoneural tubes remain, Gutmann and Young (1944) had shown that "escaped fibers" were present, and Edds (1950) showed that collateral sprouting occurred. Therefore the endoneural tubes did not serve as a foolproof guidance pathway. This observation may help to explain the lack of specificity observed. Where overlap occurred, probably due to collateral branching, innervation by an axon from a foreign neuron may have induced new properties in the reinnervated myofiber (see Chapter 12 for a discussion of trophic effects demonstrated in cross innervation experiments).

Another observation resulting from these experiments was the finding of a 10 per cent tension overlap in the innervation of the normal plantaris muscle and a 40 per cent overlap in the normal soleus muscle. This indicated an increased number of dually innervated NMJs after regeneration, which was more pronounced in the soleus than in the plantaris muscles. These experiments indicate that there is little selectivity for reinnervation of denervated NMJs acting at a distance, although this does not rule out all possibility of locally acting chemotropic factors.

Not only is there evidence for nonspecificity of reinnervation of particular muscles but there is also some evidence of nonspecificity of reinnervation of the kind of nerve (motor of sensory).

In a series of interesting experiments by Weiss (1935), experimental innervation of muscles by the central ends of afferent nerves was accomplished and the establishment of a "one neuron connection" between receptor and motor effector organ was produced. The central end of the ninth or tenth dorsal root was disconnected from the spinal cord and inserted into denervated muscle which had previously been transplanted to the back of adult toads. Thus a direct connection between the peripheral sense organs and the muscle fibers was achieved by forming a single sensory neuron motor effector connection. This eliminated the central nervous system entirely as an intermediate between receptor and effector.

In five of 12 experiments, the dorsal root fibers formed functional connections with muscle fibers. Electrical stimulation of the *sensory* nerves produced prompt muscular contractions. However, mechanical stimulation of the sense organs failed to produce muscular contraction. Histologic studies revealed extensive branching of the reinnervating nerve fibers, but typical NMJs were never seen. The authors concluded that these experiments demonstrated absence of absolute selectivity of nerve fibers in their connections with particular peripheral organs. Only a "relative predilection" seemed to be present. Thus Weiss concluded that the pathway of outgrowing nerve fibers is largely determined by mechanical factors.

The bulk of available evidence indicates that the mechanical guidance afforded by the persisting Schwann tubes is the means by which the regenerating axons return to the general vicinity, if not the actual site, of the previously denervated original soleplates (Koenig, 1970, 1971; Koenig and Pecot-Dechavassine, 1971). Therefore if retrograde degeneration of a bundle of axons extends only to the previous node, it is likely that considerable dislocation of individual axons with respect to each other occurs, particularly as they reach critical branch points in the Schwann tubes. Partial compensation for these errors may be effected by ultraterminal branching from intact NMJs and collateral sprouting. Many of the inappropriate regenerating axons probably degenerate and others, once establishing neuromuscular connections, alter both the biochemical and physiologic properties of the reinnervated myofibers (Chapter 12). New NMJs may form either by ultraterminal sprouting or by means of *de novo* formation of NMJs by regenerating axons.

An unsolved problem concerns the stimulus for ultraterminal branching and the regulation of axonal elongation both in the ultraterminal sprouts and in the regenerating axons once they have reestablished contact with the old soleplates. Despite this data, there are instances in both the central and peripheral nervous systems where selective innervation apparently occurs. For example, Sperry (1963) ingeniously demonstrated that nerve fibers arising from different parts of a fish retina preferentially selected separate central pathways as they grew into the brain, and that ultimately they connected with apparently specific, predetermined "target zones" in the midbrain tectum. In the case of peripheral nerve, there is evidence that a sensory nerve can stimulate denervated skeletal muscle without NMJs present (Bowden and Gutmann, 1944) but Zelewski (1970) has clearly demonstrated that only the original or a foreign motor nerve can produce functional reinnervation of skeletal myofibers.

Several hypotheses have been offered to explain why reinnervation in certain lower vertebrates leads to a better functional result than in mammals including man. Weiss's (1928) "resonance" theory with its analogy to radio-frequency selectivity was not supported by electrophysiological measurements and the more credible idea of Sperry (1941) that suggested neuronal membrane changes that would encourage specific synaptic interactions was less easily subjected to test. Other experiments demonstrated that the synaptic connections of motor neurons in the spinal cord did not change easily. These results were in general supported by detailed investigations by Eccles et al. (1960). Mark (1969) has suggested that the more successful reinnervation patterns that occur in lizards and teleost fish is a consequence of the multiple innervation that occurs in these animals. For example, a myofiber normally innervated by a single en plaque NMJ would receive any motor axon after denervation whereas in multiply innervated muscles persisting partial innervation may play a role in selecting amongst regenerating axons. Conservation of synaptic organization of the spinal neurons in these animals seems comparable to that of the higher vertebrates. Marotte and Mark (1970) have obtained evidence indicating that there is apparently selectivity or competition between the axons of regenerating nerves for innervation sites. These investigators used rotation of the carp eye by the extraocular muscles as an experimental system to analyze the effect of cross innervation of the muscles with foreign nerves. Reinnervation of the superior oblique muscle by its own nerve restored counter rotation of the eye whereas cross innervation of the muscle by the inferior oblique nerve produced reversed counter rotation in the head down position. When the regenerating superior oblique nerve established neuromuscular connections with the superior oblique muscle that had previously been cross innervated, the authors observed that the correct action of the superior oblique muscle was restored indicating that reinnervation by the appropriate nerve in some way inhibited innervation by the inappropriate inferior oblique nerve. The appearance of the NMJs was not evaluated in detail since no ultrastructure studies were made. Also, Hoh (1971) obtained evidence for selective reinnervation of fast twitch muscle by low threshold nerve fibers and slow graded response myofibers by high threshold nerve fibers in the toad.

Collateral Reinnervation and Hyperneurotization

We must now consider another important phenomenon that tends further to complicate the pattern of restoration of innervation after denervation.

Exner (1885) first discovered that rapid recovery of muscle function occurred following nerve injury long before reinnervation could have taken place by means of regeneration. He found that both the superior and medial laryngeal nerves must be cut to obtain degeneration of the rabbit cricothyroid muscle. In 1945, Heines et al. demonstrated that partially denervated rat and cat gastrocnemius muscle rapidly recovered isometric twitch tension after operation. Similarly, Van Harreveld (1945, 1952) and Weiss and Edds (1946) found rapid recovery of muscle strength despite the lack of regeneration of previously severed axons. This restoration of strength is explained by the occurrence of reinnervation by means of axon sprouts arising from adjacent persisting axons. These appeared as early as the second week after denervation (Edds, 1950; Hoffman, 1950; Van Harreveld, 1952; Morris, 1953; Wohlfart, 1958). Edds (1950) and Hoffman (1950) described collateral reinnervation in partially devervated muscle. These investigators demonstrated that collateral sprouting of intact nerve fibers occurred as a response to adjacent degenerating nerve fibers. Collateral and ultraterminal outgrowths from the surviving motor nerve fibers reinnervated the old denervated soleplates. This usually occurred before the return of the interrupted nerve fiber to the muscles.

Two kinds of abnormal axonal sprouting of nerve fibers have been described. The first, collateral sprouting, consists of new growth of axon processes arising at nodes of Ranvier in adjacent uninvolved nerve fibers which grow into the Schwann tubes previously emptied by retrograde degeneration. Weiss and Edds (1946) had previously concluded that collateral reinnervation must occur by indirect means. Collateral sprouts may appear as early as 4-5 days after partial denervation and axon sprouts are extremely numerous in the earliest weeks. Hatsuyama (1964) described numerous collaterals at 6 weeks in the rat leg following incomplete denervation.

Causey and Hoffman (1955) demonstrated that collaterals form along the whole neuron distant from the injury, not only near the innervated muscle. The terminal branches however are the main source of collaterals. Wohlfart (1957, 1958) suggested that muscular recovery in experimental mouse encephalomyelitis is largely due to this mechanism. However, since the collaterals are extremely fine, they can not be demonstrated easily by conventional staining and optical microscopy. In the light microscope, the collaterals are in the range of $0.5\,\mu$ or less whereas in the electron microscope sprouts as small as $0.1\,\mu$ may be recognized. The sprouts arise at the nodes of Ranvier and run within the remaining Schwann tubes. Saito (1967) produced partial denervation by cutting the ventral roots and posterior ganglia of the dorsal roots of dog intercostal nerves. This produced partial denervation because approximately 4% of the nerve fibers in the ventral root for a given segment are contained in the intercostal nerve of the adjacent lower segment. Collaterals appeared 50 to 70 days after operation.

Weiss and Edds (1946) believed that the stimulus for axonal sprouting was some material released from the degenerating nerve fibers or NMJs. Hoffman and Springell (1951) and Hoffman (1958) have unsuccessfully attempted to influence this collateral outgrowth experimentally. It is obvious that if the mechanism of the stimulus for axonal sprouting were better understood, this information might be of great clinical value. Evidence for peripheral sprouting in man will be considered in more detail when pathologic changes in NMJs in muscle disease are considered.

Coërs (1955b) suggested that this kind of sprouting is an attempt to compensate for the absent axons and in this way is analogous to muscular hypertrophy. Sprouting results in increasing the terminal innervation ratio as the motor unit is extended. Collateral sprouting and reinnervation occurs in chronic muscle disease including motor neuron disease, spinal root compression, chronic neuropathies and following recovery from acute poliomyelitis (Coërs and Woolf, 1954) and some cases of polyneuritis. Another kind of sprouting, so called "ultraterminal sprouting" or "neurocladism" occurs within the terminal arborization of the NMJ. This consists of increased numbers of axon branches arising from terminal axons that extend to adjacent myofibers and form new, adjacent NMJs. Ultraterminal sprouting increases the size of junctional areas as if to compensate for NMJ dysfunction. It occurs in primary muscular or neuromuscular diseases such as polymyositis, myotonic dystrophy and myasthenia gravis (Coërs, 1955b; Coërs and Desmedt, 1959; MacDermot, 1960, 1961). NMJs in myasthenia gravis are also said to have elongated and branch-

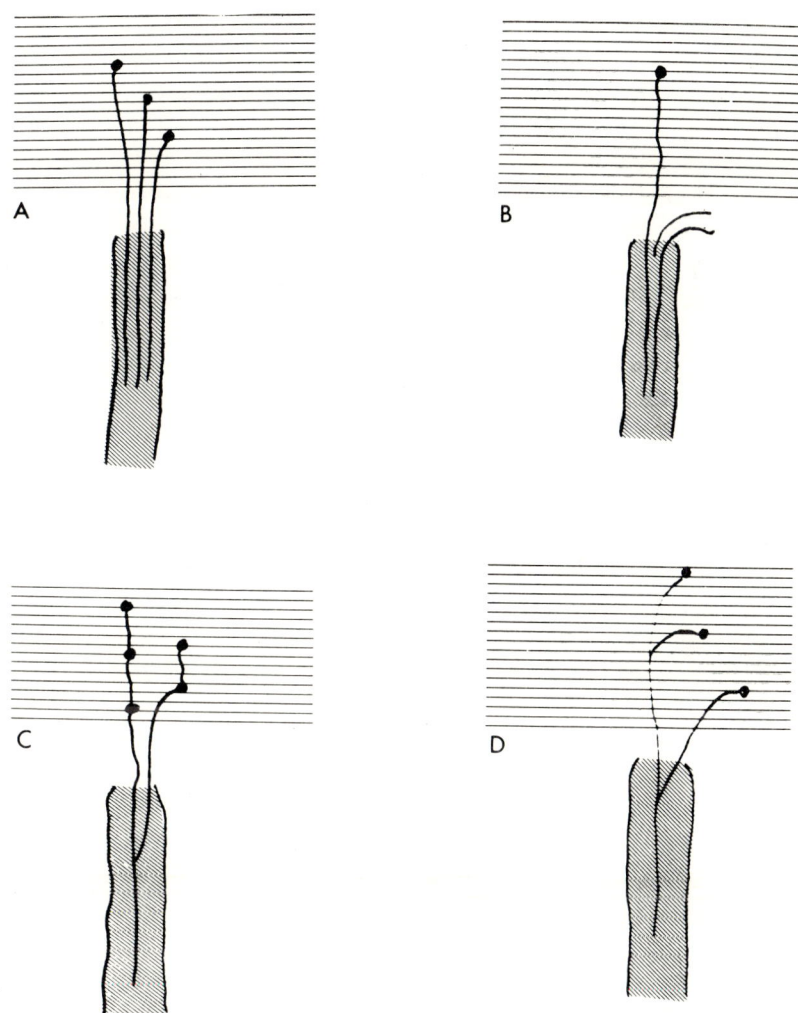

Figure 102. Diagram showing the probable mechanism of collateral sprouting and reinnervation. Diagram *A* shows normal arrangement of terminal innervation. One nerve fiber terminates usually on but one myofiber, yielding a terminal innervation ratio of 1. In diagram *B*, all but one nerve fiber has degenerated. Two degenerated nerve fibers are shown without connection to the muscle. In diagram C, nerve fibers are shown without connection to the muscle. In diagram C, nerve sprouts are seen arising from the intact axon at the node of Ranvier. Although most of these sprouts are very fine and ultimately degenerate, some (indicated in the diagram) grow down the old Schwann sheath and successfully reinnervate denervated myofibers. Diagram *D* shows the final stage of reinnervation. One nerve fiber now innervates several myofibers which increases the terminal innervation ratio. There is also a coincident change in the innervation pattern. (After Coërs and Woolf, 1959.)

ing terminal axons. Furthermore, abnormalities in terminal arborization demonstrated by methylene blue staining has also been reported in diabetes mellitis, alcoholism (Coërs and Hildebrand, 1965), renal insufficiency (Coërs et al., 1965) and in malnutrition (Hildebrand and Coërs, 1967).

With respect to identification of myofibers undergoing collateral reinnervation, Morris (1970) has observed that histochemically intermediate myofibers were associated with collateral reinnervation in a series of patients with various neuromuscular diseases. He suggested that the intermediate fibers were an early stage prior to the formation of definitive kinds of myofibers under the influence of the reinnervating nerve branches.

Hyperneurotization

Hyperneurotization, the presence of more than one axon in a given soleplate, results when a denervated soleplate is reinnervated by collateral branches from an adjacent, intact axon (Hoffman, 1950; Edds, 1950; Hoffman, 1953) followed by delayed reinnervation of the same soleplate by the regenerating original axon. The result is a doubly innervated NMJ. Figs. 102, and 103 illustrate this process.

The stimulus for collateral sprouting is unknown. Peterfi and Kapel (1928) suggested that local "irritation" of the nerve fiber caused collateral branching. However, hyperneurotization following partial denervation may play a significant role in maintaining neuromuscular function in injured and diseased muscle.

Collateral Sprouting as a NMJ Replacement Mechanism

Barker and Ip (1965, 1966) suggested that the terminal axon arborization is a dynamic structure that is subject to normal replacement, possibly through the mechanism of collateral ultraterminal sprouting. These investigators demonstrated axon sprouting in normal cat and rabbit muscle. Using a silver method, the hind limb muscles demonstrated an incidence of collateral sprouting of approximately 30.4% in the cat and 34% in the rabbit. If small accessory NMJs observed in this study were interpreted as newly formed NMJs, the incidence increased to 33.9% and 38.3% respectively. Of the motor

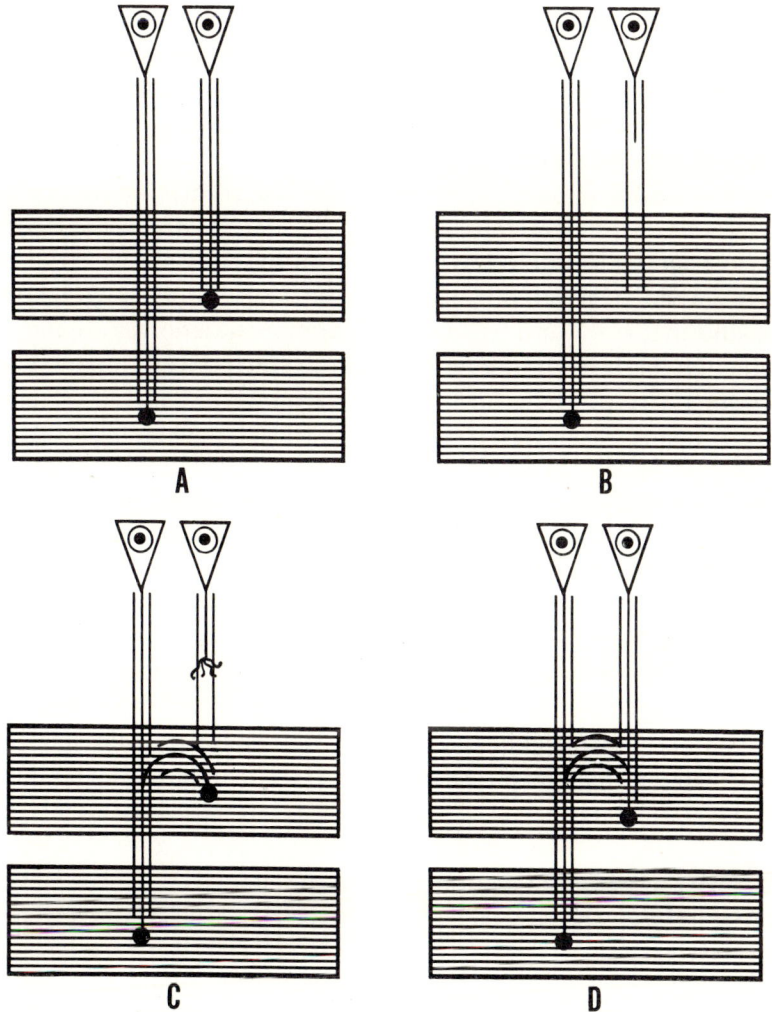

Figure 103. Diagrams illustrating the process of hyperneurotization: in diagram A, two neurons send axons to innervate upper and lower myofibers. In diagram B, the axons supplying the upper myofiber have been sectioned and degeneration of the axon has occurred. Note that the Schwann cell "sheath" remains. In diagram C, a new fiber has arisen from a node of Ranvier in the axon supplying the lower myofiber. The new nerve fiber extends to the upper myofiber, forming a new site of innervation. At the same time, as indicated by the multiple filament processes at the end of the injured neuron, regeneration has begun, leading to elongation of the axon. In D, the process of hyperneurotization is complete: a nerve fiber branch from the original, uninjured axon innervates the upper myofiber. In addition, the axon from the now regenerated neuron, which originally supplied the upper myofiber, has grown down to doubly innervate the NMJ of the upper myofiber. (After Hoffman, 1951.)

axons, approximately 8% had sprouts or as many as 19.4% if collaterals with so-called "accessory endings" were included. They concluded that this evidence of normal replacement of NMJs which normally degenerate and that formation of an axon sprout and a new NMJ adjacent to an old NMJ was a means of "rejuvenating" the original subneural apparatus. However, in our studies of mouse intercostal and diaphragm muscle in which sections from thousands of blocks have been studied in the electron microscope, we have never encountered degenerating or immature neuromuscular junctions of the kind that are found following experimental denervation and reimplantation of foreign nerves. Certainly, the concept that collateral sprouting is responsible for the peculiar motor endings in extraocular muscle seems erroneous. It is not surprising that a significant number of collaterals are found since random study of muscle detects many pathologic changes which result from "wear and tear". In such muscles one might expect reinnervation. One would expect to overlook such focal myofiber injury in the usual ultramicroscopic studies because of limited sampling. However, it is premature to conclude that normal replacement of "senescent" NMJs occurs or that "rejuvenation" is ever required. Since the subneural apparatus persists in degenerating NMJs it might be expected that such structures might be seen occasionally in normal human muscle, if they were at all common. There is no fine structure evidence to support this hypothesis.

De Novo Formation of Neuromuscular Junctions During Reinnervation

Although investigators of the collateral sprouting phenomenon generally stated that old soleplates were reinnervated by the collaterals (Hoffman, 1950), several investigators using methylene blue staining recognized formation of new NMJs on ultraterminal sprouts arising from terminal axons in diseased muscle (Coërs, 1955b; Coërs and Desmedt, 1959).

Histochemical studies of cholinesterase activity also revealed small or abnormally shaped subneural apparatuses that appeared to be in immature NMJs (Csillik and Savày, 1958). Miledi (1962, 1963), Koenig (1963) and Guth and Zalewski (1963) demonstrated that nerves implanted into denervated muscle or muscle deprived of original NMJs formed new NMJs containing cholinesterase. Although Guth and Zalewski (1963) found that 38% of the myofibers had double innervation after implantation of a foreign nerve, it was not clear if the original NMJs had been reinnervated. Shulka and Aitkin (1963) and Waggener and Boggs (1967) concluded that regenerating axons preferred to reinnervate original soleplates but Gwyn and Aitkin (1966) obtained evidence that there was no preference for the original areas of innervation and that NMJs could form *de novo*.

In addition to showing that *de novo* formation of NMJs occurred in reinnervated muscle, Guth et al. (1966) found that development of new NMJs following implantation of a foreign nerve affected the AchE activity in persisting denervated soleplates. In these experiments with rats, cholinesterase activity was measured in denervated sternomastoid muscles and in denervated muscles with implanted hypoglossal nerves 1 to 8 weeks after operation. In the initial post operative week, all the experimental muscles lost 60% of their cholinesterase activity. Cholinesterase activity in the denervated muscle fell an additional 10% by 10 weeks after operation whereas in the muscle that had been denervated and had received a foreign nerve, cholinesterase activity increased after the second week and had twice the activity of the denervated muscle by 8 weeks after operation. This occurred while the original soleplates remained without reinnervation. It appears that a close anatomic relationship between the nerve and the subneural apparatus of the NMJ is not necessary for neural regulation of cholinesterase activity in the soleplate.

Because silver and methylene blue staining methods do not reliably stain all the axon filaments and because AchE histochemical methods may reveal the site of the enzyme activity but not the underlying structure, reliable recognition of newly formed NMJs requires ultramicroscopy. Electron microscopic criteria may be used to distinguish old from recently formed NMJs. In a study of *de novo* formation of mouse NMJs, Saito and Zacks (1969) used two kinds of preparations. In the first, the anterior tibial muscle was denervated and its nerve was immediately reimplanted into the muscle in the vicinity of its original site of entry. In the second kind of experiment, the anterior tibial nerve was sectioned and turned back and ligatured so that it could not reinnervate the muscle. Then the nerve to the posterior peroneal muscle was removed from its normal site of innervation and implanted into the anterior tibial muscle at the end opposite to its normal site of innervation. Reinnervation was followed by the combined AchE-silver impregnation method of Namba et al. (1967) and by electron microscopy. Frozen sections and whole mounts of the leg muscles were stained for esterase activity. Other mice similarly treated were perfused with glutaraldehyde and the muscles were prepared for electron microscopy. At varying periods after denervation and self-reinnervation, the stages of degeneration of the terminal axon and alterations in the subneural apparatus were studied.

In the mice where regeneration was allowed to occur without interference, there was no change in the subneural apparatus during the initial period when the axon was degenerating. In the succeeding days and weeks, the primary synaptic cleft became more shallow and the secondary synaptic clefts became shorter and wider. The external

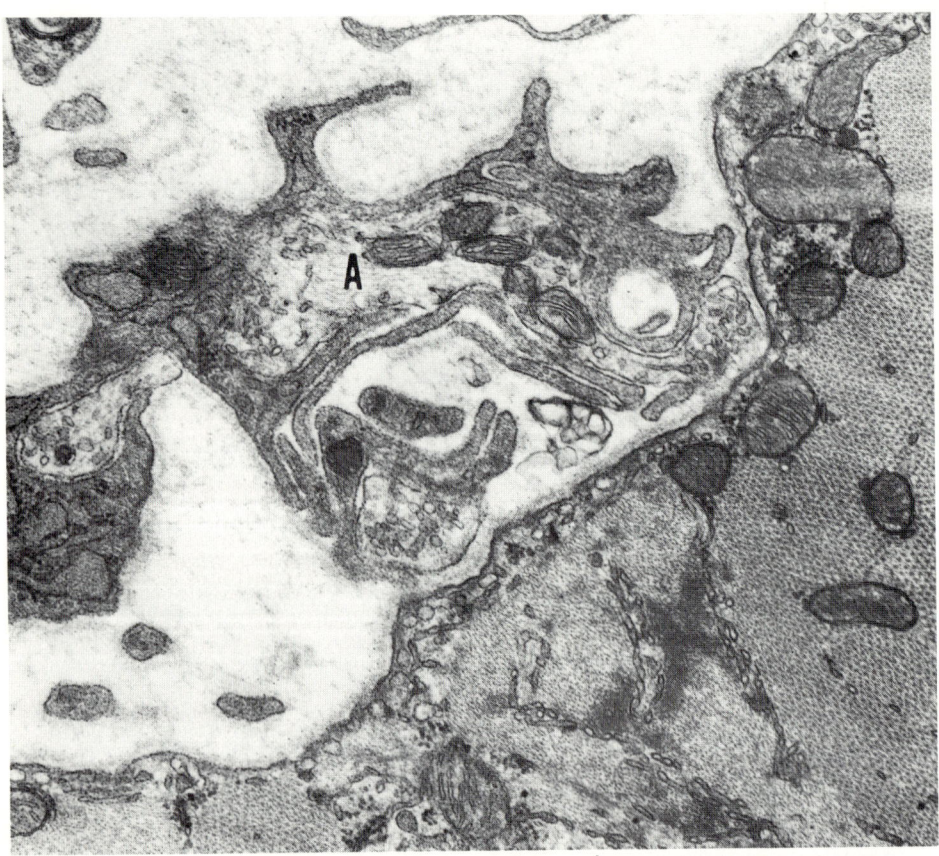

Figure 104. Electron micrograph illustrating minute axon processes *(A)* surrounded by a small amount of Schwann cell cytoplasm approaching the surface of the myofiber. Focal thickening of the myofiber plasma membrane is visible at this stage of *de novo* formation of a NMJ. (X 54,000.)

lamina persisted as did the area of subneural membrane thickening. In the early stages of degeneration, Schwann cell cytoplasm was found lying in the primary synaptic cleft whereas in later stages, cells laying down collagen were a prominent feature. These may represent altered Schwann cells or fibroblasts. Eventually, the primary synaptic cleft was covered by collagenous fibrils making future access of regenerating axons to the junctional region more difficult. In the reinnervated myofibers, the first indication of reinnervation was the presence of aggregates of small (0.1-0.5 A) axon sprouts lying within Schwann cell cytoplasm (Figs. 94-96). On subsequent days, these sprouts became more closely applied to the old subneural apparatus. Simultaneously, the primary synaptic cleft became deeper and eventually the secondary synaptic clefts elongated and reverted to their normal appearance. All the NMJs observed in the simple reinnervation experiments were of this kind. There was no evidence of new NMJ formation such as that observed as a result of reinnervation by a foreign nerve.

In the mice receiving foreign nerves in the opposite, normally non-innervated end of the muscle, a new innervation band was demonstrated histochemically at 6 to 8 weeks after operation. The original mid-zonal innervation band could still be detected histochemically by the persistence of cholinesterase activity. In the electron microscope, 3 kinds of NMJ structure was found. The first had atrophic subneural apparatuses with shallow primary and secondary synaptic clefts partially covered by collagen fibrils. Neither Schwann cells nor axons were found in the vicinity of the subneural apparatus. The second kind of NMJ was characterized by focal thickening of the myofiber cell membrane and the presence of a few small pit-like structures indenting the membrane associated with overlying minute axon sprouts containing synaptic vesicles (Figs. 104-106). The small v-shaped pits were interpreted as presumptive secondary synaptic clefts. Unlike the situation in embryonic muscle where presumptive secondary clefts appear similar, external lamina covered the cell membrane in sites of new NMJ formation. The third kind of NMJ observed appeared essentially normal with normal shape and size of terminal axons and subneural apparatus. A majority of these were probably due to reinnervation of previously denervated NMJs although advanced maturation of NMJs formed *de novo* could not be excluded. The earliest changes of *de novo* NMJ formation consist of thickening of the muscle surface membrane and the development of shallow pits, an appearance closely resembling the formation of embryonic NMJs in the chick (Hirano, 1966) and the rat

(Kelly and Zacks, 1968) (Fig. 25) or regenerating newt NMJs (Lentz, 1969). The only major difference between NMJ formation in embryos compared with *de novo* innervation of denervated adult myofibers was the absence of EL covering the embryonic myotubes. With EL absent, intermediate junctions between axons and myotubes were noted before

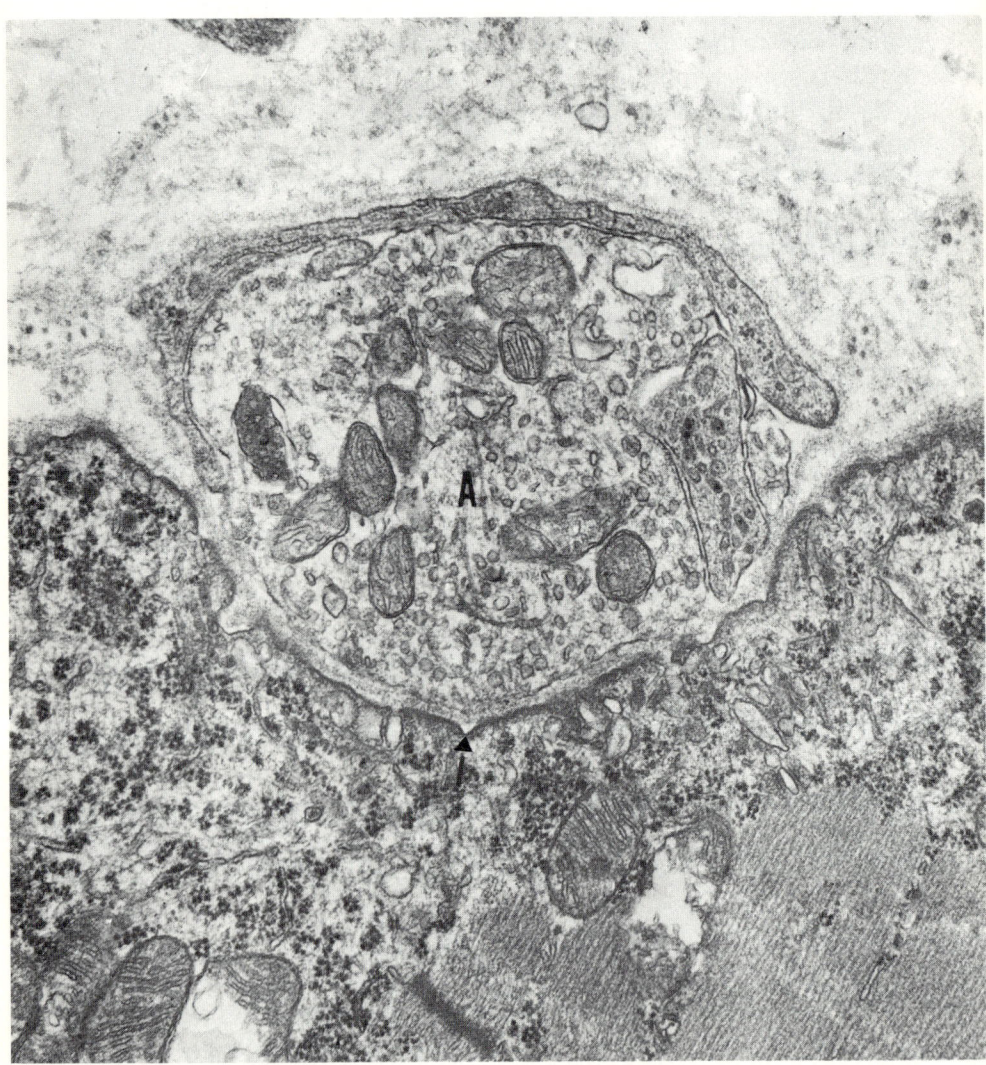

Figure 105. Electron micrograph illustrating an early stage of *de novo* formation of a neuromuscular junction. The terminal axon bulb *(A)* is separated by external lamina from the focally thickened postsynaptic membrane from which short pits (arrow) indent the underlying sarcoplasm. These are forerunners of the subneural apparatus. (X 54,000.)

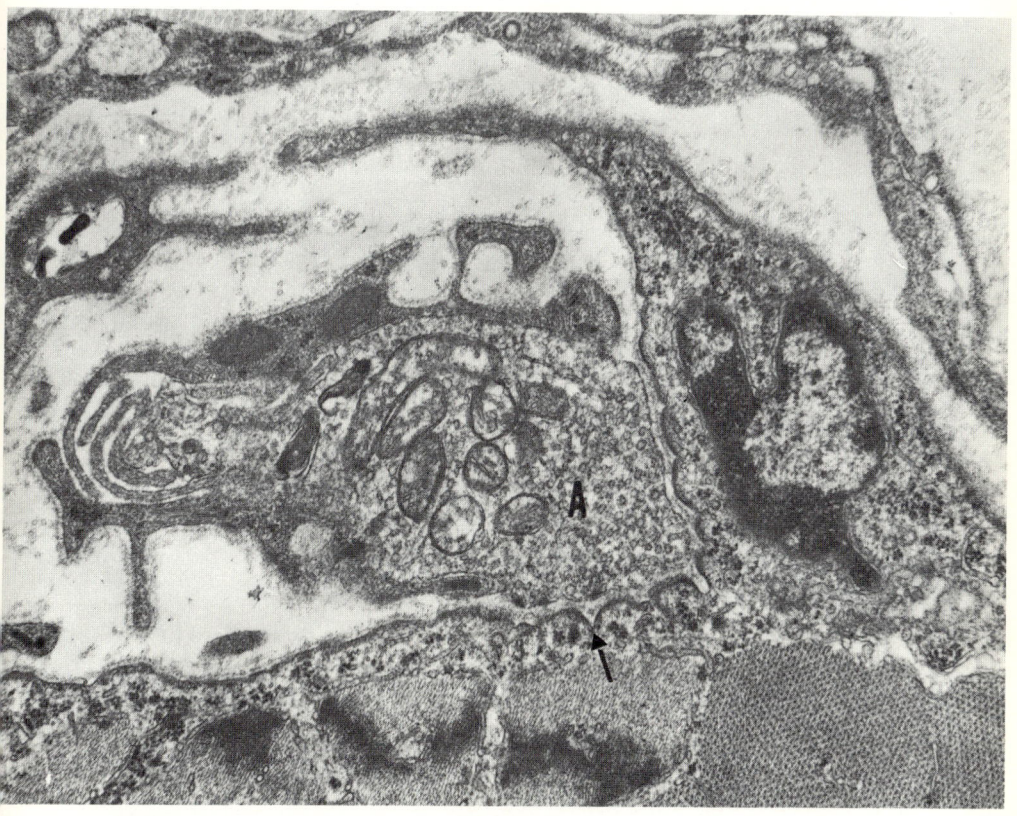

Figure 106. Electron micrograph illustrating the process of *de novo* formation of a NMJ. Note the terminal axon *(A)* lying in close apposition to the focally thickened myofiber plasma membrane from which short pit-like structures, the forerunners of the subneural apparatus protrude into the underlying sarcoplasm (arrow). (X 37,500.)

definitive NMJ formation occurred. This did not occur in adult reinnervation because of the persistence of the EL.

Koenig (1970a) also demonstrated preferred reinnervation of old subneural apparatuses. In correlated electrophysiological studies MEPPs could be recorded from reinnervated NMJs 10 days after nerve section, at a time that preceded the restoration of normal fine structure relationships between the terminal axons and subneural apparatus. In studies of newly formed NMJs, MEPPs were recorded 19 days after nerve section, before normal NMJ structure had been established (Koenig, 1971).

12

Nonexcitatory Aspects of Innervation Trophic Effects of Axons

That withering of skeletal muscles follows nerve injury has been known to medicine for many centuries. Interest in the consequences of nerve injuries has characteristically been stimulated by the plight of the survivors of periodic wars. As a result of study of these patients and experimental animals, it has long been recognized that motor innervation controls more than the excitability of skeletal muscle. Included in these influences are prevention of muscle atrophy, regulation of synthesis of specific and metabolically active proteins, intracellular electrolytes, speed of contraction as well as induction of NMJs in embryos and adults and regeneration of amphibian limbs. These numerous effects have been ascribed to "trophic" influences or "nonexcitatory functions of the peripheral nerves" since the mechanism is obscure. Guth (1968) has defined as "trophic" the functions of the nerve that affect metabolism of the muscle cell. In recent years, an extensive literature has accumulated concerning impulse transmission, release of Ach, details of membrane depolarization including MEPPs and the mechanism of muscular excitation-contraction coupling, but relatively few studies have been made on the non-excitatory aspects of innervation. However, there is sufficient data to indicate that motor nerves synthesize, transport and secrete substances that affect the growth, metabolism and function of myofibers.

Physiologic Results of Denervation

Since 1868 it has been known that when peripheral nerves are completely sectioned, as in gunshot wounds or other traumatic injuries, the muscles innervated by the nerve fibers traveling in that nerve not only lose their ability to contract on stimulation of the nerve but in time lose their ability to respond to direct stimulation of the muscle as well.

The profound effect of denervation on the electrical characteristics of the denervated muscle was known by 1868 when Erb described the "reaction of degeneration". With partial or complete denervation, stimulation of the nerve reveals increased excitability to faradic current two to three days after nerve injury, followed by a decrease in excitability to faradic and galvanic stimulation. Extinction of electrical response occurs in seven to 12 days. When stimulated at the motor point, decreased excitability to faradic stimulation and extinction of response occur by the second week. There is also decreased excitability to galvanic stimulation during the first week, followed by increased excitability and change of the response from a twitch on make and break current to a sluggish, sustained contraction, which can be elicited for months associated with gradually decreasing excitability. The final result is irreversible muscle contracture. With total denervation, atrophy and ultimate nearly total disappearance of the muscle occurs.

Histopathology of Denervation Atrophy

Ricker and Ellenbeck (1899) found decrease of muscle substance as early as the third day after denervation; it proceeded rapidly during the first few weeks after denervation and then slowed appreciably and Knowlton and Hines (1936) found that 79 per cent of the muscle mass in the rat was lost 42 days after denervation. Tower (1935, 1937) recognized the rapid and profound loss of protein that occurred in denervated muscles of some laboratory animals. The gross appearance of atrophic muscle in less well advanced stages is characterized by pale myofibers that are abnormally inexcitable and in advanced stages, the myofibers may be completely replaced by fatty and fibrous connective tissue.

Microscopically, a characteristic sequence of events occurs. Boeke (1916) described atrophy and eventual disappearance of telodendrial nuclei and increase in number of the outlying "sohlenkerne" in NMJs and loss of myofibers. Tower (1939) described rounding up of subsarcolemmal nuclei and dispersion of them throughout the denervated muscle fibers by the second week. The chromatin in the nuclei and nucleoli was diminished. Toward the end of the first month, the muscle cell nuclei became vesicular and apparently increased in number, forming clusters and chains. However, when counted, the apparent "increase" in the number of nuclei appeared to be due to condensation and redistribution of nuclei already present. Cells undergoing mitotic division were never observed. The characteristic striations of skeletal muscle persisted for long periods of time — up to a year in some cases. Actual degeneration of muscle fibers was a late phenomenon, and was characterized by swelling and vacuolization of the entire muscle fiber, granular change in the myofibrils, nuclear swelling, and final disintegration, leaving fragmented debris. The sarcolemma became thickened and phagocytic cells appeared. The final stage, which required several years to complete, was replacement of the muscle cells by a mass of fibrous tissue indistinguishable from the perimysial connective tissue present normally around the muscle cell. Tower suggested that the apparent proliferation of myofiber nuclei in denervated muscle cells was the result of loss of some specific "trophic" substance.

In the current era of electron microscopy, several investigators have considerably extended our knowledge of the changes that occur in the microscopic organelles and myofilaments of skeletal muscle during denervation atrophy (Pellegrino and Franzini, 1963; Wechsler and Hager, 1961).

Species Differences

An interesting aspect of denervation atrophy that must be considered is that there is marked species differences in the muscle response to nerve section. Tower (1935) noted that rabbit muscles did not lose mass following denervation as did the rat and mouse. Miledi and Slater (1968) commented on the slow atrophy of denervated frog muscles when compared to the rat and even muscle segments remaining after excision of their innervated portions atrophied slowly (Katz and Miledi, 1964). Furthermore, some muscles undergo *hypertrophy* for a period of time after denervation before atrophy occurs. The hemidiaphragm of mouse, rat and rabbit show a temporary hypertrophy of the order of 25-27% following denervation following which the muscles lose weight and atrophy (Steward and Martin, 1956). These muscles had increased protein content and little change in the water content during their hypertrophic stage. Similar changes also occur in birds (Hikida and Bock, 1972). Several hypotheses have been offered to explain hypertrophy following denervation including mechanical as well as "trophic" factors. Following denervation of the diaphragm, the RNA content increases as does the uptake of thymidine (Manchester and Harris, 1968) and there is increased uptake of radioactive acetate into neutral lipids but decreased production of carbon^{14} carbon dioxide suggesting abnormal mitochondrial function.

Not only are there species differences in the muscle response to denervation, but there are differences between different kinds of muscle, "fast" and "slow", in a given species. For example, in the chick the denervated anterior latissimus dorsi muscle becomes hypertrophic following denervation unlike the fast posterior latissimus dorsi which undergoes the usual kind of atrophy. There is decrease in ATP, phosphocreatine and total creatine concentrations one week after denervation in this muscle and there is less noncollagen nitrogen and 15% decrease in weight. During the same interval and up to 3 weeks after denervation, the slow anterior latissimus dorsi muscle shows no decrease in ATP or phophocreatine content (Malvey et al., 1971). Hajek et al. (1966) have found that there is a pronounced increase in sarcoplasmic proteolytic activity in the atrophic posterior latissimus dorsi muscle, which is lacking in the hypertrophied anterior latissimus dorsi muscle. That these differences do not constitute a general rule for slow and fast muscles is shown by recent studies of enzymes and protein content of denervated rat muscle. Both the extensor digitorum longus and soleus muscles decreased in weight and protein content to an approximately equal degree following denervation and there were no differences in the activities of acid and alkaline cathepsins, acid or neutral ribonucleases and acid α-glucosidase in both muscles. Creatine kinase and AMP deminase were somewhat more decreased in the extensor digitorum longus than in the soleus muscle (Goldspink et al., 1971). Denervation produces major changes in Ca++ transport in the sarcoplasmic reticulum. It is in this system where changes in the speed of contraction may occur under conditions of denervation (Margreth et al, 1972).

Many experiments were performed by several investigators to determine how innervation prevented muscle atrophy. Obvious consequences of denervation, including the observed hyperexcitability of the muscle and its shortening and lack of normal contractility were considered as possible causes of muscle atrophy.

Tower (1939) raised the question whether the atrophy and acute degenerative and fibrous tissue changes might all result from exhaustion of the denervated muscle by the endless fibrillation that occurs following denervation. This fibrillation, which may represent the combination of earlier changes in excitability and contractility reported for denervated muscle, might explain all the phenomena of denervation. The flaccidity of the muscle might also be the cause of the abnormal arrangement of nuclei which could result from relaxation of normal muscle tension.

Tower emphasized the fact that trophic activity implies nutritional control of the muscle by the innervating nerve fiber. In a special sense, she considered that denervation could cause nutritional depletion due to the endless fibrillation of denervated muscle. This constant muscular activity might deplete the stores of phosphocreatine and other metabolities necessary for maintenance of muscle function. After considering the various aspects of this problem, she concluded that fibrillation activity alone could not account for the several properties of denervated muscle. She suggested that normal motor innervation provides a "conditioning influence" that is essential for maintaining the normal properties of muscle fibers. This factor acts to maintain the "dominance of the rapid mode of response over the slow mode of respouse with suppression of spontaneous contraction" (see Margreth et al, 1972). It was for later investigators to discover the basis of denervation hyperexcitability.

To examine the possiblity that inactivity following denervation was responsible for the histological changes in the myofibers, Tower compared denervation atrophy with changes occurring as the result of other kinds of atrophy. Tower (1937) devised a preparation in which the spinal cord was isolated by transection above and below the lumbosacral enlargement and the dorsal roots were sectioned. Animals prepared in this way had myofiber atrophy with fibrosis and nuclear destruction that resembled the atrophy following nerve section. She observed that only the intial nuclear proliferation that occurred in denervated muscles failed to occur in the isolated spinal cord preparations.

Myofiber inactivity can also be produced by cutting the tendons that keep the muscle stretched at normal resting length. After varying intervals of time tenotomized muscles respond abnormally (Fischer and Ramsey, 1945) and there is loss of muscle mass. There have been many reports of biochemical (Davenport and Ranson, 1930; Gutmann and Vrbová, 1952) and morphologic changes (Davenport and Ranson, 1930; McMinn and Vrbová, 1967; Walker, 1965; Shafiq et al., 1969) following tenotomy. Myofiber atrophy caused by tenotomy is more severe in the soleus, a slow muscle (Eccles, 1944; McMinn and Vrbová, 1967) than in the gastrocnemius, a fast nuscle (Walker, 1965). Although comparative data on the effects of denervation or tenotomy on the fine structure of atrophic muscles has not appeared, review of published data for some animals indicates that both peripheral loss of myofilaments (Wechsler and Hager, 1961) and central degeneration occurs (Shafiq et al., 1969).

The importance of the length at which the muscle is maintained on the subsequent changes have been demonstrated in denervated chicken muscles (Jirmanová and Zelená, 1970). The slow anterior latissimus dorsi muscle that normally hypertrophies after denervation, undergoes atrophy if its tendon is also cut. There was little effect of tenotomy on the atrophy of denervated fast posterior latissimus dorsi muscle.

There is also evidence that there is sensory feedback from tenotomized skeletal muscles that affects myofiber atrophy. Hník et al (1963) and Hník (1964) observed that tenotomized muscles that were allowed to relax, continued to produce sensory outflow without spindle activity. When atrophy in rat muscles following tenotomy was compared with muscles that were deafferented by cutting the dorsal roots and tenotomized, the former preparations demonstrated greater muscle atrophy than the latter (Hník, 1964). This suggested that possible metabolic stimulation of sensory nerves associated with the atrophic myofibers and central responses to this stimulation retarded muscle atrophy. If the muscle is reinnervated before irreversible changes have occurred, the integrity of the muscle fiber can be restored and the neuromuscular unit may function normally again. Thus it is clear that motor nerves play a major role in the control the structure and functional capabilities of the muscles they innervate.

Biochemical Changes in Denervated Muscle

The influence of the motor nerve on the muscle it innervates is dramatically revealed by the profound biochemical changes that occur in denervated muscle (Knowlton and Hines, 1934; Chor et al., 1937; Samuels, 1957, 1961, 1963). Nearly all aspects of the myofiber are affected. Changes in structural proteins (Fischer and Ramsey, 1944; Stewart, 1955), enzymes (Michelazzi et al., 1957; Carafoli et al., 1962, 1964; Brody, 1965; Dawson & Kaplan, 1965; Bárány and Close, 1971), amino acid transport (Diehl and Jones, 1966) and electrolytes (Harris and Nicholls, 1956; Kernan, 1965; Hoh and Salafsky, 1971) have been reported. Following denervation, there is decrease in oxygen consumption (Schmidt, 1952) and reduction in cytochrome oxidase activity (Hearn, 1959) and succinic dehydrogenase activity (Hogan et al., 1965).

Numerous investigators have described increased glycogen content following denervation whereas others have observed decreased glycogen content. Domonkos and Heiner (1965) found differences in the glycogen content of tetanic and tonic muscles of the adult rabbit and after denervation there was an initial phase in which the glycogen content of the tonic muscle decreased for a few days followed by a second phase in which there was increase in the glycogen content. On the other hand, the glycogen content of the tetanic muscle increased in the initial phase and decreased in the later phase. Both immobilization and denervation produced practically the same effect on the glycogen content and metabolism in the two kinds of muscle. Changes in muscular glycogen synthesis in denervated muscle was described by Canal & Frattola (1966). There is also evidence that specific isozymes are regulated by the motor nerve. This is illustrated by the reversion of LDH isozyme pattern of denervated adult guinea pig muscles to the newborn state (Brody, 1965). Dawson et al. (1964) found that in rabbit soleus muscle, the H form of LDH increased more rapidly during the early weeks of life than the M form. Following nerve section, there was greater loss of the H than the M isozyme.

These are but a few examples from the extensive literature describing biochemical changes in denervated muscle. This data supports the concept of neural control of skeletal muscle and metabolism. However, Guth and Wells (1972) have emphasized that the functional demands of the muscle must also be considered. The proteins of muscles whose synergists have been excised, also changed. The influence of normally innervated myofibers can also be transferred to denervated myofibers by means of union of intact with previously isolated myofibers (Hall-Craggs, 1971).

Histochemical Demonstration of Enzyme Changes in Denervated Muscle

In addition to the classical biochemical studies of the composition and metabolic activity of denervated skeletal muscle, the trophic influence of motor nerves on the enzyme content of myofibers is illustrated by numerous histochemical investigations. Hogenhuis and Engle (1965) demonstrated that marked changes in enzyme activity occurred in denervated guinea pig muscle. During the first week after denervation, both glycogen content and phosphorylase activity decreased and both were absent by the third week. However, myofibril A band ATPase activity was barely affected by 11 weeks although there had been a slight decline at the fifth week. The activity of oxidative enzymes, DPN linked α-glycerophosphate dehydrogenase and succinic dehydrogenase decreased from the first week and were absent by the 11th week. DPN linked lactic dehydrogenase and DPNH dehydrogenase activity were also severely reduced but still present at 11 weeks. In contrast to the effects of denervation, tenotomy produced slight and temporary decrease in glycogen but the oxidative enzymes were unaffected.

Histochemical Typing of Myofibers

It is generally recognized that histochemical staining methods show various kinds of myofibers within red and white mammalian muscles. Most white muscles contain three fiber types and red muscles one or two. However species variations frustrate a uniform classification system. In general, fast twitch muscle contains high glycolytic enzyme activity and myosin ATPase whereas slow twitch muscle contains lower glycolytic activity and less ATPase activity (Guth, 1968; Yellin and Guth, 1970). Within a given fast or slow muscle, individual motor units have different contraction speed and different enzyme patterns. There is a reciprocal relationship between oxidative and glycolytic enzyme activity in individual fibers (Dubowitz and Pearse, 1960). According to this early classification, type I fibers have have high oxidative activity, low glycolytic activity and type II fibers have high glycolytic activity and low oxidative enzyme activity. Engle (1962) pointed out the value of the ATPase reaction in the study of abnormal muscle. He demonstrated that type I myofibers contain low myosin ATPase activity whereas type II fibers had high activity. The irregular arrangement of myofibers of different histochemical staining characteristics within a muscle is responsible for the characteristic "checkerboard" pattern.

Several investigators have now demonstrated from 3 to 8 separate histochemical kinds of myofibers. However, most histochemical studies of human muscle demonstrate two basic kinds of myofibers rather than three. Stein and Padykula (1962) described A, B, C fibers using criteria of sarcoplasmic dehydrogenase and ATPase histochemistry in rat muscles. Many investigators now agree that the histochemical characteristics of a myofiber are determined by the kind of innervating nerve fiber but accurate correlation of structure and function requires study of individual myofibers rather than reliance on histochemical staining alone (Henneman and Olson, 1965).

Changes in the "checkerboard" pattern may be used as an indicator to study the effects of denervation, self reinnervation and crossed reinnervation. Karpati and Engle (1968) found that suprasegmental denervation produced different alterations of myofiber histochemical staining than did simple denervation. They studied the gastrocenmius (white muscle) and soleus (red muscle) of adult and newborn guinea pigs after cordotomy. Both myofiber types underwent moderate atrophy in the adult gastrocnemius muscle whereas lesser degrees of atrophy occurred after immobilization by skeletal fixation. Denervation produced preferential atrophy of type II myofibers. In the newborn guinea pig soleus, the myofiber histochemical pattern was mixed with approximately 50% type I and type II myofibers whereas by the age of 6 weeks, there were only type I fibers. If cordotomy was performed in the neonate, sciatic nerve section or skeletal fixation interfered with the conversion of the mixed type I and II myofiber pattern to the uniform type I pattern with the result that at 6 weeks of age, the animals retained a mixed myofiber pattern. In the adult soleus muscle 30 days after cordotomy, there were 30% type II fibers whereas after skeletal fixation, only 5% were of this type. Furthermore, section of the sciatic nerve in the adult guinea pig led to the appearance of type II myofibers from 3-6 months. Of great interest was the fact that oxidative enzymes and amylophosphorylase failed to decrease in the muscle following cordotomy unlike the loss of these enzymes that invariably followed denervation. Explanation for the failure of the soleus mixed pattern to proceed to a uniform type I pattern following neonatal denervation was not explained by these experiments.

This data suggested that the motor nerve controlled the enzyme activities of individual myofibers and thus the histochemical properties of the different kinds of myofibers. Buller et al. (1959, 1960) demonstrated physiologic interconversion of fast and slow myofibers following cross innervation and histochemical studies by several investigators revealed changes in the histochemical properties of the cross innervated muscles. Dubowitz and Newman (1967) reported that cross innervation of the slow soleus with a fast nerve in kittens, cats and rabbits led to enzyme patterns similar to the fast flexor digitorum muscle and implantation of the soleus nerve into flexor hallucis longus produced enzyme patterns characteristic of the soleus muscle. The change of histochemical myofiber types from slow to fast muscle occurred less consistently. Dubowitz was unable to demonstrate significant changes in ATPase activity of fast and slow muscles after cross innervation. Confirmation of Dubowitz's histochemical studies was provided by Karpati and Engle (1967) who studied albino guinea pigs. These investigators implanted the common peroneal nerve into the denervated soleus muscle and compared the results of histochemical staining for several enzymes with muscle changes caused by crush and complete nerve section. A proportion of type I fibers (40%) in the original soleus muscle were converted to type II as a result of foreign nerve innervation in a period of approximately 6 months after operation. Further confirmation was obtained by Romanul and Van de Muelen (1967) who studied cross innervation in cats and rats. In these experiments the soleus muscle was used as an example of a slow muscle and the flexor digitorum longus or flexor hallucis longus were used for fast muscle. Following cross innervation, the muscles showed alternation in the speed of contraction and enzymatic characteristics of the myofibers. The soleus muscle, with high oxidative activity and low glycolytic activity, was converted into a muscle with low oxidative high glycolytic activity and the converse occurred in the flexor digitorum longus and flexor hallucis longus. On the other hand, muscles reinnervated with their own nerves showed no change in the contraction speed or the proportion of myofibers of the appropriate enzymatic types. Buller et al. (1969) demonstrated that after cross innervation, myofibrillar ATPase of the fast flexor digitorum longus of the cat decreased to become approximately similar to the enzyme activity of the normal slow soleus muscle. Under normal circumstances, the myofibrils of normal fast twitch muscle hydrolyze ATP at a greater rate than the myofibrils of slow twitch muscle. Ogata et al. (1968) observed that following cross innervation of the external digitorum brevis nerve and the soleus, a tendency toward grouping of myofibers of a single histochemical variety occurred in contrast with the usual "checkerboard" mosaic of red, white and intermediate myofibers in normal skeletal muscle. However in the soleus, which is normally a red muscle containing the intermediate type of myofibers, 3 kinds of myofibers including white appeared. Criteria for identifying the kinds of myofibers used included the presence of mitochondria at the I band in the subsarcolemmal region and chain aggregates of interfibrillar mitochondria. Guth et al. (1968) also found that cross innervation of slow muscle of adult rats and cats resulted in the development of histochemical and electrophoretic aspects of fast muscle but that complete conversion did not occur. Cross innervation of white fast muscles showed little histochemical or quantitative evidence of conversion. The electrophoretic pattern obtained from the rostral part of the cross innervated medial gastrocnemius muscle (white) was converted to a pattern similar to red muscle. These authors suggested that the failure of cross innervated white muscle to be converted indicates that the slow red muscle represents a less differentiated state.

Specific innervation also appears to control and activity and kind of isoenzyme present in skeletal muscles. Muscle (M) LDH is the predominant form in white skeletal muscle and the heart (H) type in cardiac muscle. Guth et al. (1968) demonstrated that implantation of a "slow" nerve into a "fast" muscle caused a change from the normally predominant muscle LDH isozyme to the cardiac or H variety of the enzyme. When adult guinea pig soleus muscle which normally contains faster migrating LDH isozymes (H type) is denervated, the slow moving or M isozyme is found. This pattern is regarded as less well differentiated because it resembles the LDH isozyme activity of immature soleus muscle (Brody, 1965). ATPase activity of contractile proteins are also under neural control. Bárány and Close (1971) found that ATPase activity of "fast" muscle reinnervated by a "slow" nerve decreased to the activity of slow muscle (soleus) and that ATPase activity of soleus muscle reinnervated by a "fast" nerve approached that of normally innervated fast muscle. Similarly, cross innervation of cat soleus and flexor digitorum longus muscles produces altered myoglobin content in these muscles (McPherson and Tokunagu, 1967). This kind of neural influence is also reflected in the overall pattern of muscle patterns. Guth and Watson (1967) using gel electrophoresis, demonstrated that denervation of fast myofibers yielded a protein pattern more characteristic of slow soleus muscle whereas denervation of the soleus muscle failed to change the protein electrophoretic pattern. When the denervated soleus muscle was reinnervated with a fast nerve, the protein pattern changed to that of a typically fast muscle (Plantaris).

In a later investigation of cross innervation in rats and cats, Guth et al. (1968) studied enzyme histochemistry, biochemistry and soluble proteins six months after operation. The cross innervated slow muscle incompletely acquired the electrophoretic and histochemical properties of fast muscle. The cross innervated white fast muscle demonstrated little histochemical evidence of conversion. However, the rostral portion of the cross innervated medial gastrocnemius muscle acquired the electrophoretic pattern similar to red muscle.

The content of intracellular ions and small molecules is also altered by cross union. For example, the glycogen and potassium content of fast muscle is greater than in slow muscle (Drahota and Gutmann, 1963) whereas soleus muscle reinnervated with a "fast" nerve produces an increase in both glycogen and potassium. Small ions as well as complex proteins including those with enzymatic activity are apparently regulated by some factor from the nerve. For example, denervated frog muscles take up appreciably less potassium per gram of muscle from the external solution during the first hour than do innervated muscles (Harris and Nicholls, 1956) and Kernan (1965) found that in rats, innervation appeared to promote sodium excretion from previously loaded muscle and prevented or diminished hydration of the muscles. In cross innervation experiments, Hoh and Salafsky (1971) demonstrated that the potassium content of cross innervated "fast" rat extensor digitorum longus muscle was reduced and the potassium content was increased in cross innervated "slow" soleus muscle. Muscle weight and other electrolytes did not change appreciably in cross innervated soleus muscle whereas cross innervated extensor digitorum longus muscle lost half its mass and had increased sodium chloride and water content. With respect to Ca^{++}, Margreth et al (1972) found that denervation of slow muscle produced increased Ca^{++} transport rates and specific activities of Mg^{++} activated Ca^{++} stimulated ATP-ase. Denervated fast muscle demonstrated slight decrease in ATP-ase-linked Ca^{++} transport.

These several experiments clearly indicate that not only does the motor nerve regulate many aspects of myofiber metabolism, but it does so in highly specific ways. Vrbová (1963) suggested that the pattern of nerve impulses from a peripheral nerve determines the contractile characteristics of the muscle it innervates with respect to "slow" and "fast" responses, but, the histochemical data suggests that each neuron is capable of regulating specific enzyme characteristics in the myofiber it innervates and that motor units are histochemically homogenous.

Influence of Innervation on Cholinesterase Activity

The presence of proteins with cholinesterase activity within the NMJ is also dependent on innervation. Much of this data has been obtained by histochemical methods during the development of NMJs. It has been shown that cholinesterase activity in NMJs appears in specific junctional loci only after the arrival of the motor nerve (Mumenthaler and Engle, 1961) and there also is evidence that nonjunctional (sarcoplasmic) cholinesterase activity is neurally regulated (Kovacs et al., 1961).

Evidence for the dependence of junctional cholinesterase activity on innervation has been obtained by many studies of denervation in adult animals. Guth et al. (1964) demonstrated a 70% decrease in nonsoleplate cholinesterase activity by the third day after denervation and 50% reduction in soleplate enzyme activity in rat sternomastoid muscle. Similar results were obtained by Brzin and Majcentkacev (1963) using a microgasometric method and by Eränkö and Teräväinen (1967b) who used histochemical methods.

Quantitative measures of AchE activity were found to correlate poorly with the histochemical data that demonstrated gradual loss of cholinesterase activity in the 10-45 days after denervation (Savày and Csillik, 1956) and apparent rapid restoration of enzyme activity after reinnervation. This data indicates an abrupt decline of enzyme activity (approximately 50%) in the 3 days after denervation followed by an interval of slow restoration of cholinesterase activity. Unfortunately no attempt was made to distinguish between AchE and ChE in these studies. Discrepancies in the histochemical data are due to the use of thiolacetic acid as substrate in the histochemical studies rather than the more specific substrate acetylthiocholine, which was used in the direct chemical determinations.

Regulation of cholinesterase activity in muscle by nerve was studied by Guth and Brown (1965a, b) in denervation and tenotomy experiments. With denervation, there was greater loss of cholinesterase activity than of total protein whereas after tenotomy, the cholinesterase level remained the same but the total protein decreased. Quantitative methods for cholinesterase activity were used as well as thiolacetic acid histochemistry. Following crush injury of the nerve supplying the sternomastoid muscle, the background and soleplate cholinesterase activity declined 68% of normal in 1 week after operation and by 6 weeks, was restored to 93% of normal. The approximate ratio of background cholinesterase to soleplate enzyme appeared constant at 1, 3 and 6 weeks indicating a simultaneous rate of reappearance of the enzyme activity at both sites. Since histologic evidence suggested reinnervation was complete at 2 weeks, increase in cholinesterase activity after that time was interpreted as due to a slow synthetic rate. This contrasts sharply with the rapid (40%) loss of enzyme activity 3 days after denervation.

Although immobilization of striated muscle also affects the cholinesterase activity of the soleplate and myofibers, Guth (1969) demonstrated that cholinesterase activity decreased more in denervation atrophy than in disuse atrophy. In these experiments, Guth prevented shortening of the rat soleus muscle by mechanical fixation and compared the loss of protein and changes in cholinesterase activity in the muscles with muscles which had been denervated by transection of the sciatic nerve. In muscles that had been immobilized and denervated, the protein loss was 31.7% compared to 19.9% for muscles that had been immobilized alone. Correspondingly, immobilization and denervation yielded a loss of 35.6% of the sarcoplasmic cholinesterase activity and 53.4% in the soleplate enzyme activity compared to 22.4% and 8.7% in the immobilized muscle respectively. The data does not clarify the question of whether the sarcoplasmic cholinesterase is regulated by the nerve but clearly indicates that the nerve does specifically regulate the cholinesterase activity in the soleplate.

There also appears to be a neural influence affecting the quantity of cholinesterase activity in muscle. For example, rat muscle which normally undergoes a 50% reduction in the myofiber cholinesterase activity following nerve section, loses only 25% of cholinesterase activity if only half of the nerve supply is cut (Guth and Brown, 1965b). As residual nerves and collateral fibers reinnervate the muscle, the cholinesterase activity increases toward normal. Thus the activity of cholinesterase is apparently proportional to the number of the innervating nerve fibers. This is reminiscent of the situation where the sum of all kinds of nerve fibers is an important factor in lizard limb regeneration and is suggestive of the presence of a trophic factor. Under conditions of hyperneurotization produced by partial denervation and regeneration, the cholinesterase activity in the dually innervated soleplates never becomes greater than normal (Guth and Brown, 1965b) indicating an interplay between nerve and muscle which in some way determines the enzymatic activity of the muscle. Furthermore, restoration of cholinesterase activity in nerve and muscle following reinnervation occurs simultaneously. The regenerating axon sprouts influence the cholinesterase activity in the underlying myofiber and this influence extends over considerable distance. It has been shown by Guth et al. (1966) that if a nerve is implanted in one end of a denervated myofiber at some distance from the original soleplates, the new NMJs form with appropriate cholinesterase activity in the subneural apparatus and cholinesterase activity is restored in the original soleplate areas as well as in the sarcoplasm. Several other lines of evidence indicate that nerve must be present for the restoration of cholinesterase activity. When the enzyme is irreversibly blocked by DFP, restoration of cholinesterase activity occurs only in the normally innervated soleplates but not in the previously denervated soleplates (Filogamo and Gabella, 1966). Maintenance of Ach in the environment of denervated soleplates by continuous infusion has no effect on the resynthesis of cholinesterase (Rose and Glow, 1967) and block of Ach secretion by means of botulinum toxin does not cause loss of cholinesterase activity (Stromblad, 1960).

Experiments by Zelená (1965) have also demonstrated that the cholinesterase activity of the musculotendinous junction is regulated by the motor innervation. This effect is also dependent upon the time of innervation during development (Lubinská and Zelená, 1967).

Although the foregoing evidence suggests that we must look for trophic molecules that can specifically alter protein synthesis, Ach, the normally secreted neurohumoral substance has been considered as a likely prospect for the trophic substance. The hyperirritability of denervated muscle was well known and early investigators hypothesized that the muscle atrophy that occurred after nerve section was the result of lack of neural stimulation or excessive irritability and fasciculations (Tower, 1937). Several early experiments demonstrated that neuromuscular transmission fails before neural conduction and that this failure is correlated with the Ach content of the nerve (Lissák et al., 1939) and that transmission fails in recently transected nerves before changes can be demonstrated in axon excitability (Luco and

Ezaguirre, 1955; Novak and Salafsky, 1967). Furthermore muscular atrophy and hyperexcitability do not occur in nerve crush injuries (Denny-Brown and Brenner, 1944) or in tourniquet paralysis (Moldaver, 1954). All these data could equally be explained by trophic action of Ach or other unidentified substances. In the Denny-Brown and Brenner (1944) experiments, Ach synthesis may have proceeded in some surviving axons and secretion of trophic materials could equally be explained by trophic action of Ach or other unidentified substances. In the Denny-Brown and Brenner (1944) experiments, Ach synthesis may have proceeded in some surviving axons and secretion of trophic materials could have continued despite regeneration of many of the injured axons. More recent evidence that neural conduction is not required for the trophic influence of motor nerves is the demonstration that in the rabbit, peripheral nerves blocked to electrical silence by lidocaine maintain normal excitability in the innervated muscle (Robert and Oester, 1970). However, this could not be confirmed in rat muscles. Lomo and Rosenthal (1972) found atrophy in rat muscles similar to that produced by denervation after blocking the nerve with anesthetics or diphtheria toxin.

Experimental evidence supporting the hypothesis that Ach is a trophic substance is found in the experiments utilizing botulinum toxin and the data indicating that Ach secretion influences the number, location and kind of postsynaptic Ach receptors. Since botulinum toxin prevents Ach release (page 293) muscle atrophy with preservation of normal NMJ structure in chronic botulinum intoxication has been cited as evidence for the trophic action of Ach. Josefsson and Thesleff (1961), Drachman (1964, 1967), Jirmanová et al. (1964), Duchen and Strich (1968) and Drachman and Romanul (1970) found that the toxin produced enzymatic histochemical changes in rat muscles identical to those produced by denervation. In this experiment, muscle bulk decreased as well as the activities of several enzymes including phosphorylase, esterase, cytochrome oxidase and several dehydrogenases.

Also cited as evidence of the trophic action of Ach, but not necessarily responsible for prevention of muscular atrophy, is the role that the neurohumor plays in maintaining the normal Ach sensitivity of the myofiber membrane. Axelsson and Thesleff (1959) demonstrated that following denervation, the entire myofiber membrane became sensitive to Ach in addition to the sensitive areas in or adjacent to the NMJs. Thesleff (1961) explained the "supersensitivity" of denervated muscle as the result of the decreased reduction of effective membrane resistance caused by the increased area of Ach sensitivity. Isolated frog sartorius muscle exposed to diffusely applied Ach had a reduction of membrane potential from -90 to -20 mV. Without removal of Ach, depolarization subsided spontaneously and the membrane potential was restored to its original value. During the period of depolarization, neuromuscular block developed and persisted despite repolarization of the membrane to the normal level. The muscle was unresponsive as long as Ach was present in the muscle bath, and chemosensitivity of the junctional areas was restored only after prolonged washing. Thesleff therefore concluded that Ach, whether applied or released by stimulation, reversibly reduces the chemosensitivity of the Ach receptors and that this "desensitization" is probably related to the action of the motor nerve that controls the size of the receptor area on the myofiber. In experiments employing iontophoretically injected Ach from micropipettes and microelectrode recordings, Thesleff found that he could produce transient membrane depolarization when Ach was added to the region containing NMJs. In innervated muscle, Ach depolarized only at the NMJ region in a small zone less than a millimeter in length, whereas following degeneration of the motor nerve, the entire muscle membrane became sensitive to injected Ach. This phenomenon was observed five days after denervation in the cat and two to three days after denervation in the rat. This increase in the chemosensitive area of the muscle began at the NMJ and spread toward each end of the muscle fiber. One to two weeks after denervation, the entire muscle became as sensitive to Ach as the NMJ was originally. Therefore, there is not a true "supersensitivity" of the NMJ receptors during denervation but a spread of the excitable area (Axelsson and Thesleff, 1959).

The new Ach receptors had properties in common with the normally innervated NMJs. They responded to Ach, carbamylcholine, and tubocurarine. However, cholinesterase inhibitors did not potentiate in chronically denervated muscle, as they do in normal NMJs. Thesleff concluded that conversion of the muscle membrane to an Ach-sensitive surface was due to influences exerted by normal innervation, a view supported by observations that spread of Ach sensitivity also occurred in chronic botulinum intoxication (Thesleff, 1959). Furthermore, in experiments where motor neurons were isolated in spinal cord segments to abolish neural transmitter release while preserving spontaneous transmitter release, Thesleff found that the increased area of muscle membrane sensitivity did not occur. Therefore, continuous subthreshold transmitter release was sufficient to maintain the chemosensitivity of the normal endplate area (Johns and Thesleff, 1951). Thesleff suggested that the atrophic changes in muscle fibers following denervation are related to changes in chemosensitivity of the muscle membrane.

Miledi (1960 a) found that with increased amounts of Ach, a larger (approximately 500μ) area could be shown to be Ach-sensitive. This suggested that these were extrajunctional Ach receptors. Miledi agreed that the maximum sensitivity occurred over the NMJs where MEPPs could be recorded and that a marked decrease in sensitivity occurred on either side of the innervation zone beyond a distance of 200μ . At 400μ away from the NMJ, little response could be obtained, indicating few receptors. These changes occurred even if the muscle was removed and maintained *in vitro*. The NMJs retained their Ach sensitivity and the remainder of the muscle showed increased Ach sensitivity (Harris and Miledi, 1966).

Attempts to locate the indicated extrajunctional receptors by means of labelled ^{14}C curare (Waser and Hadorn, 1961) revealed binding in both the innervated and denervated soleplates but not at new sites distant from the junctional regions in the denervated muscle.

Probable structural changes in the junctional receptors following denervation are suggested by experiments by Rohr-Hadorn (1961) who denervated mouse diaphragm by section of the phrenic nerve and studied the binding of ^{14}C curarine 2 to 120 days after nerve section. Up to 60 days after operation, degenerating NMJs showed increased binding of radioactive curarine and similar increased binding occurred in regenerating junctions up to 45 days. In later stages of NMJ degeneration, radioactive curarine binding decreased toward zero in the period beyond 60 days. In the regenerating NMJs, normal fixation of curarine occurred in the period beyond 45 days to 120 days. No evidence was available to indicate whether uncovering of binding sites occurred or whether some substance from the innervating axon affected the receptor.

Hartzell and Fambrough (1972, 1973) used ^{125} iodine-labelled α-bungarotoxin to study the location of acetylcholine receptors in rat diaphragm muscle and the time course of changes in the receptors after denervation. In normally innervated myofibers, bungarotoxin binding indicating AchR sites, occurred primarily within NMJs. Two to three days after denervation, there was an approximately linear increase was observed until 45 days. The change in extrajunctional AchR density was correlated with increased extrajunctional Ach sensitivity.

Ach also regulates Ach sensitivity throughout the whole extent of the myofiber. In partially denervated frog sartorius muscle (which has two innervation sites) the remaining innervated NMJs develop increased Ach sensitivity (Frank and Inoue, 1966). These investigators found that the size of MEPPs at the innervated NMJs was 2 or 3 times as large as normal, indicating that there was an increase in Ach sensitivity in the partially denervated muscle, possibly due to changes in the postsynaptic membrane. Thus changes in response to Ach are not limited merely to the spread of sensitivity in skeletal muscles but may, in dually innervated muscles, produce increased sensitivity in the surviving NMJs.

Because the properties of the Ach receptor and the AchE molecule are parallel in many respects, it is not surprising that some investigators have considered that AchE activity might affect the Ach sensitivity of the muscle membrane. However, it has been shown that changes in AchE activity do not parallel the changes in Ach sensitivity following denervation. Guth et al. (1964) demonstrated that cholinesterase activity declined 60-75% within 3 days after which there was little change in soleplate and nonsoleplate areas. Furthermore, there was no evidence of centrifugal spread of cholinesterase activity from the soleplate region. In animals subjected to spinal cord section, cholinesterase activity declined but little change in Ach sensitivity occurred (Johns and Thesleff, 1961; Guth et al., 1967).

The influence of innervation on the development of Ach receptors in embryonic muscle has also been cited as an example of the trophic action of Ach (Guth, 1968). Diamond and Miledi (1959, 1962) demonstrated that immature, non-innervated myofibers are diffusely sensitive to Ach and that when innervation takes place, Ach sensitivity becomes more or less confined to the region of the NMJs. Similar restriction of Ach sensitivity on innervation has been observed in nerve-muscle explants (Kano and Shimada, 1971). Restriction of Ach sensitivity to NMJ areas following innervation is most marked in "fast" muscles (Miledi and Zelená, 1966). However, this data does not exclude other hypotheses.

Contrary to Drachman's view (1967) that Ach is the trophic substance, Guth (1968) concluded that neither Ach nor membrane depolarization are responsible for the maintenance of Ach sensitivity of the postsynaptic membrane. He pointed out that in the animals with transected spinal cords, the spread of Ach-sensitivity occurred to a lesser degree than in denervated myofibers and that during reinnervation of frog muscle, both MEPPs and Ach sensitivity are restored to normal before impulse transmission is re-established. Guth concluded that the MEPPs, reflecting quantal secretion of Ach, were related to the restriction of Ach sensitivity rather than to greater quantities of impulse released Ach that took place on excitation. Correlated physiologic and ultrastructure data obtained by Birks et al. (1960) also demonstrated that the spread of Ach sensitivity in frog muscle appeared at a time when the MEPPs had vanished following denervation and that *in vitro*, denervated frog muscle developed increased sensitivity to Ach even though this substance was present in the bathing medium (Miledi, 1960b). Evidence contrary to the Thesleff concept of Ach regulation of membrane Ach sensitivity was also obtained by Miledi (1960b) who demonstrated that both innervated and denervated soleplates had similar numbers of MEPPs following iontophoretic injection of Ach despite the fact that supersensitivity of the denervated membrane was present. Furthermore, denervated NMJs were more sensitive to diffusely applied Ach than the innervated NMJs. In some way, the nerve appeared to restrain myofiber chemosensitivity without involvement of Ach. Solandt et al. (1943) had previously shown that immobilization does not prevent the spread of Ach sensitivity.

Further evidence that Ach alone can not be responsible for the multiplicity of axonal influences on skeletal muscle is obtained when a foreign cholinergic nerve is implanted into a skeletal muscle. When frog vagus nerve is implanted into the sartorius muscle, the fine structure of the myofiber is preserved, and they retained normal electrical and mechanical properties but there was no postsynaptic AchE activity and no *de novo* NMJ induction (Landmesser, 1972). These results point to the probability that several trophic substances are involved.

Rejection of Superinnervation

The nearly universal tendancy for vertebrate myofibers to have single innervation has been cited as evidence for the regulatory properties of motor nerves. With few exceptions, the presence of an NMJ on a myofiber prevents the acceptance by that myofiber of additional innervation (Steindler, 1916; Elsberg, 1917). Where dual innervation does occur in vertebrates, muscles such as extraocular muscles, en grappe NMJs are associated with the en plaque NMJs. Van Harreveld and Tachibana (1961) demonstrated that the cricothyroid muscle lacks dual innervation despite previous claims to the contrary. However dual innervation occurs in the human vocalis muscle and the frog sartorius (Miledi, 1960b). In situations where more than one en plaque NMJ can be demonstrated on a single myofiber, it is usually the result of degeneration followed by collateral reinnervation arising from either adjacent nodes of Ranvier or from adjacent NMJs (Brown and Matthews, 1960). Attempts to experimentally induce additional NMJs are unsuccessful unless the influence of the existing innervation is blocked in some way or the muscle is injured.

Acceptance by denervated muscle of its own implanted nerve or a foreign nerve was reported by Gutmann and Young (1944); Bowden and Gutmann (1944); Aitken (1950); Hoffman (1951); Csillik and Saváy (1958); Guth and Zalewski (1963); Miledi (1962); Koenig (1963) and Saito and Zacks (1969). Guth and Zalewski (1963) implanted hypoglassal nerve in denervated sternomastoid muscle of the rat and demonstrated two NMJs on many myofibers by means of cholinesterase staining. These were the originally denervated soleplates and newly formed NMJs.

Miledi (1963) demonstrated that a foreign nerve would not be accepted by an innervated myofiber unless the myofiber had first been denervated or injured. Under these conditions, foreign nerves would be accepted and new functional connections were established. He also showed that any part of a nerve-free myofiber could be innervated and that the resulting innervation exerted its usual inhibitory influence on additional innervation at a distance from the NMJs. Histochemical methods were used to demonstrate that new NMJs formed in frog sartorius muscle under these conditions. They were also shown to be functional. Thus, local myofiber injury as well as denervation overcame the resistance of the myofiber to innervation by foreign nerves. Katz and Miledi (1964) suggested that the resistance of the myofiber membrane to additional innervation is related to the spread of Ach sensitivity that follows denervation. For example, Ach sensitivity increases in the denervated segment of frog sartorius muscle which also accepts foreign innervation whereas the innervated sartorius muscle segment only accepts a nerve in the injured area where Ach sensitivity has also increased.

Gwyn and Aitkin (1966) implanted the common peroneal nerve into the proximal NMJ-free region of the anterior tibial muscle of the rat following excision of the original NMJ region. They found that new NMJs formed as evidenced by cholinesterase staining. Both *de novo* formation of NMJs as well as reinnervation of the original NMJs occurred. If the common peroneal nerve was placed on the surface of the muscle with minimal injury, new NMJs were also formed. There appears to be no relationship to myofibril atrophy per se since new NMJs fail to form following implantation of a foreign nerve into atrophic muscle resulting from tenotomy (Aitkin, 1950). The experimental strategy of partial denervation with resultant collateral reinnervation producing dual innervation indicates that this is sufficient injury to the muscle membrane to reduce its resistance to multiple innervation. Experiments in which multiple innervation was produced in soleus muscle by partial denervation (crush injury) were performed by Gutmann and Hazlíková (1967). Their data suggests that reinnervated muscle, similar to traumatized muscle, is less resistant to hyperneurotization. Experiments by Thesleff (1960) and Fex et al. (1966) also demonstrated that botulinum toxin, which is thought to prevent relase of Ach from the presynaptic terminal, suppressed the resistance of myofibers to multiple innervation. These results point to regulation of NMJ formation by influences exerted by the terminal nerve, but not necessarily to Ach. The mechanism for rejection of foreign super innervation remains obscure.

Induction of Neuromuscular Junctions

From the data obtained in studies of embryogenesis of NMJs in cultured explants and of new soleplate formation in reinnervated adult myofibers, it is clear that the axon is capable of inducing the characteristic membrane changes that constitute a NMJ if the myofiber is prepared to accept new innervation. In this sense, some "trophic" influence from the nerve is capable of bringing about profound specialization in the structure of the myofiber membrane. Early students of NMJ formation had called attention to the apparent aggregation of soleplate nuclei as the nerve approached the future region of innervation and more recent investigations including ultrastructure studies have revealed the morphological changes in the postsynaptic membrane that occur as the axon approaches what eventually constitutes the neuromuscular synapse (chapter 2). Since the myotube is sensitive to Ach before synaptic contact is made and depolarization of the myotube membrane can occur before definitive NMJs are formed, these observations do not help us to decide whether depolarization per se, Ach, or some other nerve substance secreted by the axon induces the membrane changes characteristic of NMJs. Since the fine structure of the subneural apparatus is apparently correlated with the speed of contraction of the myofibers, it is unlikely that a molecule as simple as Ach could regulate the formation of this structure.

There is also convincing evidence that the appearance of esterases in developing NMJs is dependent on the arrival of the innervating axons. Using manometric and histochemical methods, Kupfer and Koelle (1951) demonstrated that AchE appeared in significant amounts in rat forelimb muscles at approximately the sixteenth day of prenatal life, when movement is known to begin but no motor nerve endings are present (Straus and Weddell, 1940). Since NMJs of normal structure and cholinesterase staining characteristics do not appear until the twenty-first to twenty-second day of prenatal life, early cholinesterase activity was thought chiefly to be associated with the specialized muscle nuclei of the soleplate. Straus and Weddell suggested that cholinesterase activity might constitute a trophic influence on the nerves innervating the muscles. Filogamo and Gabella (1967) demonstrated that early nerve-induced cholinesterase activity could be demonstrated in myofibers followed by decrease in the activity of the enzyme as differentiation and growth proceeded in non-junctional portions of the myofiber. Eventually, the characteristic pattern of enzyme activity appeared in the subneural apparatus. Changes in the chick cholinesterase-active proteins during development has also been studied by electrophoretic methods (Maynard, 1966). He observed a marked decrease in cholinesterase activity in developing chick breast muscle at the 10-20 day stage at the time that soleplate enzyme activity was increasing. Nachmansohn (1939) also found that there is a marked decrease in total cholinesterase activity of developing skeletal muscle on a weight basis as the enzyme activity becomes more localized in the NMJs. In the post natal growth period, rat NMJ cholinesterase activity remains constant.

Lubinská and Zelená (1966) have reported a peculiar observation in their histochemical studies of cholinesterase activity in denervated neonatal rat muscle. These investigators found focal, 26-40μ long areas of cholinesterase activity that changed to small foci scattered on the muscle surface membrane within 17 days of denervation in normal neonatal rats. It was not possible to determine whether these were separate cells or part of the myofiber since this study was limited to optical microscopy.

Neural Regulation of the Speed of Muscle Contraction

As we have discussed in chapter 10, differences in the speed of contraction as well as other parameters such as the rate of motor cell discharge, required frequency for tetanus and nerve conduction velocity are recognized in various kinds of mammalian muscle (Eccles, 1963). It is convenient to refer to "fast" and "slow" muscles, a designation based on one major difference, the time required for contraction after stimulation. Slow muscle appears to be the less differentiated state since immature muscles usually fall in this category and there is little to suggest that the changes in the speed of contraction between future "slow" and "fast" twitch muscles are related to the conduction velocity of their nerves since this does not change appreciably after birth (Ridge, 1967).

The work of several investigators has revealed that the intrinsic properties of motor nerves directly regulate the mechanical behavior of the myofibers they innervate. Denervated "fast" muscle is markedly slowed (Eccles et al., 1962) and "slow" muscle responds with reduced contraction time (Buller et al., 1960). In a classic physiologic study, Buller et al. (1960) demonstrated that muscular contraction speed could be altered by cross innervation. Subsequent studies by Close (1964, 1965, 1969) and Miledi and Orkand (1966) confirmed these observations. These investigators found that if the motor nerve supplying a fast muscle was implanted into a slow muscle and vice versa, the properties of the reinnervated muscle was altered to conform to the properties of the innervating nerve, that is, the fast myofiber became slow or slower in its rate of contraction and the slow myofiber became faster. As we have discussed, this kind of cross innervation experiment also produces marked changes in the histochemical ("checkerboard") pattern of the myofibers.

More complex experimental results from cross innervation have been reported by other investigators. Hník et al. (1967) studied the multiply innervated anterior latissimus dorsi and focally innervated posterior latissimus dorsi muscle of chicks 2-18 months after cross union. The specificity of nerve affecting NMJ formation and muscle characteristics was strikingly confirmed in these studies in which the fast posterior latissimus dorsi muscle reinnervated by a slow muscle nerve formed en grappe NMJs and responded to single nerve volleys with local potentials only whereas the control posterior latissimus dorsi muscle reinnervated by its original nerve formed en plaque NMJs and responded to single nerve volleys by a synchronous succession of action potentials similar to the normal muscle. Thus the morphologic structure as well as the histochemical and physiologic properties of the muscle were altered. When the slow anterior latissimus dorsi muscle was innervated with a fast nerve, there was little change in the electromyogram and type of innervation with the exception that propagated action potentials to single nerve volleys occurred. When the anterior latissimus dorsi of young chickens was reinnervated with implanted fast muscle nerve and the regenerating original nerve, two kinds of innervation occurred. En plaque NMJs formed in the vicinity of the implant and en grappe NMJs appeared in areas supplied by the anterior latissimus dorsi nerve. The contraction velocity was not substantially changed in posterior latissimus dorsi and anterior latissimus dorsi muscles after cross union. It is notable that there was no change in the fine structure of the myofibers in the extrajunctional regions.

Using acetylthiocholine staining for cholinesterases and electron microscopy to demonstrate NMJs, major changes in the character of NMJs after cross union occurred but there were no major changes in the speed of contraction or the ultrastructure of myofibers. In the chicken, innervation by slow nerve yielded en grappe NMJs and fast nerve, en plaque NMJs. Cholinesterase activity associated with the NMJs that formed in the slow multiterminal kind of innervation was always less intense than in the fast en plaque junctions.

Other investigators, Koenig (1963), and Gutmann and Hazlikova (1967) have found that en grappe NMJs are formed in mammalian muscles following implantation of a twitch nerve. Thus the en grappe kind of NMJ by itself is not a reliable criterion for recognizing fast and slow muscle. Miledi and Orkand (1966) also reported that the ultrastructure of slow frog muscle was not altered by innervation by a twitch nerve. Hrík et al. (1967) concluded that the speed of contraction of the anterior and posterior latissimus dorsi muscles is practically unaltered by cross union. Thus the transformation of contractile properties appears limited in chickens. Koenig (1970 b) also demonstrated that structural changes occur in chicken muscle NMJs following cross innervation. NMJs that were formed in the slow anterior latissimus dorsi supplied with the nerve from the fast posterior latissimus dorsi contained strong AchE activity and the subneural apparatus consisted of interconnected gutters in a limited region near the nerve. Their morphology suggested that the slow muscle fibers had received focal innervation similar to fast muscle. Multiple innervation was found in some myofibers of previously fast muscle that had been supplied with the slow nerve. These new NMJs consisted of clusters of very small synaptic areas with weak AchE activity as determined histochemically. These NMJs were similar to those present in normally multi-innervated, slow chick muscle.

Recent physiologic studies of the responses of cross innervated muscles have demonstrated that the interconversion of fast to slow and visa versa is not as complete as originally believed. If only the speed of isometric contraction is studied many interesting data are overlooked.

Buller et al. (1968) demonstrated that the physiologic responses of cross innervated slow muscle never became comparable to normal fast muscle. In experiments where slow cat muscle (soleus) was innervated by a fast nerve and a fast muscle (flexor hallucis longus) by a slow nerve, these investigators observed that the fast twitch muscles became comparable to normal slow muscle in their response to stimulation, but that slow muscle innervated with a fast nerve never responded as rapidly as a normal fast muscle. These responses persisted for years. If the muscles were cooled 10° (38-28°C.), the time to peak tension was reduced in both fast and slow normal muscle but the maximum twitch tension of fast muscle increased 25% and the twitch tension of slow muscle decreased 20%. In cross innervated muscle, the maximum twitch tension of the cross innervated fast muscle was decreased approximately 11% as the temperature was lowered from 38 to 28°C. and the maximum twitch tension of the cross innervated slow muscle was reduced 7%. Therefore, the previously cross innervated slow muscle never really approximated the normal fast muscle following cross innervation.

More recently, Close (1969) found that the maximum speed of shortening of whole muscle fibers was the same for cross innervated soleus, cross innervated extensor digitorum longus and normally innervated extensor digitorum longus muscles and similarly with cross innervated soleus, and normally innervated soleus muscles. However when isometric twitch contraction time was measured, there was incomplete transformation of fast extensor digitorum longus muscle to slow muscle when the soleus nerve was implanted and similarly there was incomplete transformation of the slow soleus muscle that received the fast extensor digitorum nerve. Close suggested that this data indicated that the neural influence had a direct effect on the myofibrils and that changes in speed of contraction resembled those that normally occurred during myofiber development (Close, 1964). It is clear that when the total performance of the muscle is considered rather than only its twitch properties, the responses of these muscles are found to be more complex. Such indices as tetanus to twitch ratios and total tension developed indicate that there is more complete conversion of "fast" muscle to "slow" muscle the less differentiated form than in the reverse circumstances. There is evidence that fast skeletal muscle differentiation is independent of nerve impulses since it occurs normally in kittens despite isolation of the muscle by the Tower procedure (Buller et al., 1960). Yet, even under these circumstances myoneural contact is required. If the peripheral nerve is cut, the muscle becomes slower (Eccles et al., 1962). On the other hand, slow muscle becomes faster when it is isolated from nerve impulses (Buller et al., 1960). These experiments suggest that nerve influences play a greater role in the regulation of contraction time in slow muscle, but how this regulation is mediated remains obscure.

Another possibly related phenomenon is the differences in the distribution of Ach sensitive areas, presumably due to the presence of Ach receptors between slow and fast muscles. Miledi and Zelená (1966) demonstrated that the membrane of slow rat muscle was sensitive over its entire surface unlike the fast muscle which was Ach-sensitive only in innervated areas. Maximal Ach-sensitivity in the slow muscle occurred in the junctional areas. Recently, Albuquerque and McIssac (1970) studied the Ach sensitivity and electrical characteristics of denervated muscle up to 45 days after denervation. The rat fast external digitorum longus and the slow soleus muscles were studied. Twenty to 24 hours after denervation, miniature endplate potentials were lost and after 24 hours, extrajunctional Ach sensitivity appeared in the external digitorum longus muscle and increased in the soleus. By 48 hours, Ach sensitivity in the musculotendinous junction of the external digitorum longus muscle appeared but it was not found in most myofibers midway between the NMJs and the musculotendinous junction. On the other hand, Ach sensitivity increased generally along the myofibers of the soleus muscle. Ach sensitivity did not develop centrifugally and did not become greater than in the sensitivity of the NMJ region. Ach sensitivity appeared before a change in membrane resistance could be measured. Thus, there is a distinctive difference between fast and slow muscle in the kind and development of Ach sensitivity resulting from denervation. Ach sensitive sites in fast muscle were restricted to the NMJ area whereas in a slow muscle, the Ach sensitive sites were found along the entire membrane surface of the myofiber. This extends the earlier work of Albuquerque and McIssac (1969), Thesleff (1968) and Miledi and Zelená (1966). In experiments with cross innervated muscles, Miledi et al. (1968) found that cross innervated soleus muscle, which normally has widely dispersed Ach receptors, became more like the fast extensor digitorum longus muscle in which the Ach receptors are closely associated with the innervated area. When the soleus muscle was reinnervated by its own nerve, the usual pattern of diffuse Ach sensitivity was found, indicating that the changes observed were not the result of the process of degeneration and regeneration of NMJs.

How the nerve regulates the speed of muscular contraction is obscure. Elul et al. (1968) suggested that some neural factor regulated calcium receptors in the myofiber membrane and Howell et al. (1966) and Streter (1970) demonstrated increased leakiness of the sarcoplasmic reticulum membranes in denervated skeletal muscle. Streter (1970) demonstrated that denervation produces a transient increase in calcium uptake by frog sarcoplasmic reticulum in the presence of oxalate that reverts to normal or below normal by 6 weeks after nerve section. During the same period, there is a concomitant slow increase in ATPase activity of the calcium-independent component. Denervation effected both red and white muscles but the changes in the red myofibers were less intense and were confined to ATPase activity. Barany and Close (1971) concluded that the actin and magnesium activated ATPase activity of myosin and magnesium activated ATPase activity of actomyosin correlated best with the intrinsic speed of muscle shortening. Data obtained by Margreth et al, (1972) suggests that slow muscle is capable of Ca^{++} transport mechanisms characteristic of fast muscle that are repressed under normal circumstances.

Changes in these proteins by neural influence thus requires that the nerve is capable of influencing the gene expression of the myofiber. The nerves appear to initiate but do not maintain the specific proteins associated with myosin (Guth et al., 1971).

The Influence of Nerves on Limb Regeneration

Although this phenomenon is restructed to a small number of infrahuman species (urodele amphibia, larvae of anurans, fish, and certain parts of lizards) and is not entirely restricted to motor innervation, the influence of nerves on regeneration is an exceedingly interesting phenomenon that may contribute significant insights into the "trophic" influence of nerve fibers.

In 1823 Todd observed that if the sciatic nerve was cut at the time of amputation of a salamander limb, the stump below the site of nerve section became necrotic. However, if the nerve was cut after regeneration of the limb had begun, regeneration stopped and the stump degenerated. Therefore, innervation was essential for regeneration. Similar data were obtained by Schotté and Butler (1944) and Singer (1949). However, Yntema (1949) observed that larval limbs that developed without innervation did not require innervation for regeneration. If nerve fibers were supplied to these limbs, regeneration of supernumerary structures occurred. Singer (1959) pointed out that the control of regeneration effected by nerve fibers was especially remarkable when one considered how difficult it was to influence this process. In the usual case, section of the nerve trunk or application of colchicine prevented the normal sequence of regeneration (Singer et al., 1956). We shall describe the series of events that occur in limb degeneration and regeneration as they occur in the urodele.

On the first day after amputation, the wound is re-epithelialized and an inflammatory reaction begins. This reaction is characterized by the presence of phagocytes, which remove debris, and the formation of scar tissue. Following this stage, there is dissolution of the fibrotic wound tissue and adjacent tissues including muscle, tendon, and connective tissue. This stage has been called "dedifferentiation." The covering epithelium also thickens at this stage. Cells of regeneration, the socalled "blastemal cells," form the blastema, which is an accumulation of mesenchymal cells of uncertain origin. As they aggregate they form "the early regenerate bud," which grows rapidly. Breakdown of the pre-existing tissue components slows and eventually stops. The final phase consists of differentiation of new tissue structures. In the normal process of regeneration, nerve fibers are seen in the wound in all phases except during the first few days after nerve section, and are related to the regenerating tissues (Singer, 1949). The innervation is very rich, especially in the blastema and epidermis. The nerve fibers are present in the form of individual strands or as bundles that have naked endings. The number of nerve fibers decreases as regeneration proceeds.

Denervation at various periods during the normal course of regeneration produces interesting results. If the nerve is cut at the time of amputation, no regeneration occurs. The epidermis recovers the wound and phagocytes remove tissue debris, but no degeneration of adjacent tissue occurs and the epidermis does not thicken. Very few blastemal cells can be found. Whatever regeneration does occur is limited to the area of the wound and includes connective tissue, muscle, and tendon regrowth. It is clear, therefore, that what is suppressed by denervation is the formation of the blastema. This suggests that organ formation but not tissue regrowth is dependent on innervation. The nerve must be responsible for providing some organizing factor.

In larval urodeles, the effects of denervation are more extensive. Initial wound healing occurs, followed by extensive destruction of all tissue elements. The mesenchymal cells appear, but instead of accumulating, are destroyed. The stump continues to dedifferentiate and resorption occurs. Entry of nerve fibers at this stage can halt resorption and initiate regeneration. If the stump is denervated later during the time of blastema formation, regeneration stops and no more growth occurs. A marked decrease in the mitotic rate, after a transient increase, can be shown in such denervated blastemas (Singer and Craven, 1948).

We can therefore conclude that the nerve is required throughout the early postamputation period and until the time when the blastema has begun to grow rapidly. Denervation after the blastema has formed results in a small limb with differentiated tissues. Axial elongation occurs, but increase in volume does not. Thus, beyond a certain stage of development, the nerve is no longer required for regeneration. The nerve is needed for the "normal process of dedifferentiation" (Schotté and Butler, 1944), which includes the appearance and accumulation of mesenchymal cells, cell division, and possibly tissue breakdown.

Factors in the Control of Limb Regeneration

The mechanism of the nerve influence on regeneration is unknown. Several possibilities have been considered. For example, there might be selective migration of cells along the neural pathway. Polarized growth of nerve fibers might orient the ground substance of the stump thus be a factor in distal cell migration. The nerve itself might contribute cellular elements such as connective tissue and Schwann cell components. However, we must not forget that the axon must be present for regeneration; the sheath alone is not sufficient. Because of the inherent difficulties in these suggestions, a widely held concept is that some chemical material secreted by the innervating nerve fibers is responsible. Studies by Schotté (1926) and Needham (1952) support this view.

Welsh (1946) observed that atropine interrupts regeneration in the flatworm *Planaria*, and pilocarpine enhances it. He considered the possibility that the Ach mechanism was involved in this trophic activity.

However, the influence of nerve on regeneration seems unrealted to impulse conduction. Reflex connections or other types of connections with the central nervous system are not required for the trophic action. *Sensory* nerves separated from their connections with the central nervous system alone can evoke growth (Singer, 1943). Furthermore, sensory fibers contain little if any Ach, yet are effective. We must still account for the fact that substances that interfere with the Ach mechanism also block regeneration for a few days, after which it resumes spontaneously. If exposure to atropine is repeated, regeneration stops again. Procaine and tetraethylammonium are similarly effective. Eserine pilocarpine, and methacholine, are incapable of maintaining growth of denervated limbs.

Further data concerning the possible role of Ach in regeneration were provided by Singer (1959), who found substantial amounts of Ach in normal and regenerating tissues of the newt forelimb. A few days after amputation, but before the appearance of mesenchymal cells, the Ach content was similar to that of the normal tissue. However, during the time when the nerve exerted its greatest influence upon growth, the Ach content was found to be greater than in normal limb tissue. As differentiation proceeded, the Ach content decreased and eventually reached the level of the normal tissue.

Another interesting aspect of this problem is that a critical number of nerve fibers are required for regeneration (Singer, 1959). Apparently the ratio of nerve fibers to limb mass is important, since regeneration occurs in the larval frog but not in the adult (Singer, 1954). The sum of these experiments indicate that the Ach mechanism may be involved in the process of growth and redifferentiation of the amputation stump.

However, other interpretations are possible. Since the mechanism that controls regeneration is unknown, various substances (atropine, procaine, and tetraethylammonium) that do interfere with regeneration may act in other ways unrelated to the normal Ach mechanism. These may be involved in the process of growth and redifferentiation of the amputation stump. Even though classic Ach-blocking agents interfere with regeneration (Singer et al., 1960), it was concluded that these substances most likely acted as general tissue "poisons" rather than as specific blocking agents. Although Welsh (1948) suggested that Ach might function as a coenzyme in its action on growth or by altering cellular permeability (Welsh and Taub, 1948) and Gerard (1950) suggested that Ach may play some role in oxidative metabolism, it is difficult to imagine how Ach could act as the trophic factor that regulates limb regeneration. Singer and his colleagues considered the role of AchE activity as a possible factor in regeneration. Singer et al. (1960) found that AchE activity in the regenerating forelimb of *Triturus* was low during the early phases of development and increased with the greatest rate of change during the regenerative stage preceding muscle differentiation. The enzyme activity leveled off at this point and returned to normal as regeneration was completed. This variation in AchE activity correlated well with the changes in Ach levels during regeneration. Ach content was high during regeneration and fell to normal as cholinesterase activity increased. Unfortunately these data do not clarify the role of the Ach mechanism in regeneration. The histochemical data reported by Singer et al. (1960) showed that the major part of the AchE activity was present in the muscles. The illustrations provided show a rather diffuse reaction without staining of identifiable NMJs. Ultrastructure studies (Bryant et al., 1971) have shown that the nerve is important in maintaining large numbers of blastema cells.

The dependence of muscle fibers on innervation in all animals tested, and the more specific and circumscribed dependence of certain animals on innervation for regeneration of missing limbs, has been demonstrated. The basic mechanism of both phenomena is unknown. The conduction and transmission functions of the nerve do not seem to be the major factors, but there is evidence suggesting the action of some neurohumoral substance secreted by nerves.

Neural Regulation of Skeletal Muscle: Speculations

These several aspects of neural influence on skeletal muscle ranging from changes in a wide variety of myofiber constituents to changes in membrane excitability can most easily be explained by secretion of some regulatory substances by the nerve in addition to Ach, the normal transmitter. It is unlikely that Ach could regulate protein synthesis in the muscle. Guth et al. (1967) suggested that the nerve secretes messenger nucleic acids or derepressor agents to regulate protein synthesis in the innervated muscle. Fambrough (1970) demonstrated that inhibitors of RNA and protein synthesis interfere with development of Ach receptors. A possible mediator is RNA which Miani et al. (1970) claimed is transported down axons. Thus regulation of protein synthesis in the muscle, probably mediated by sarcoplasmic ribosomes may be responsible for the changes in membrane receptors as well as many metabolic activities of the myofibers. We have demonstrated abnormal myofiber protein synthesis in a genetically determined myopathy in mice that appears to be related to some factor in nervous tissue (Zacks and Sheff, 1972), Lentz (1972) has demonstrated that less degeneration occurs in newt NMJs cultured in the presence of sensory ganglia and Singer and Caston (1972) have found that nerve influences macromolecular synthesis and turnover in regenerating newt limbs. Harris and Thesleff (1972) found that denervation of rat muscle is delayed if the nerve is cut at a distance from the muscle. Despite this data indicating action of a trophic substance other than Ach, the Ach hypothesis is invoked by Giacobini (1972) to interpret development of choline acetylase activity in chick embryos and by Drachman and Witzke (1972) who found that the spread of Ach sensitivity in denervated rat diaphragm was reduced if the denervated muscle was stimulated electrically.

A reasonable hypothesis is that the trophic substances are synthesized in the nerve cell and carried via axonal transport to the innervated muscle. In recent years, evidence for neurosecretion by terminal axons and evidence for bidirectional axonal flow has curiously supported the original theory of Emmert (1836) concerning circulation of material from brain to muscle. Torrey (1934) demonstrated that catfish taste buds degenerate more rapidly if the nerve is cut close to the taste organs suggesting that the short stump contains less of a peripherally migrating substance. Similar experiments have been performed on the neuromuscular system. Gutmann et al. (1955) demonstrated that if the nerve is cut near the muscle, soleplate breakdown is more rapid. This work was confirmed by Harris and Thesleff (1972). The small distal stump had a disproportionate loss of glycogen (Gutmann et al., 1955) and a greater loss of acetylcholine transferase (Emmelin et al., 1966) as well as greater Ach hypersensitivity (Emmelin and Malm, 1965).

Axonal Flow

Considerable data indicates that a variety of substances pass up as well as down motor axons. Movement of materials from the nerve cell body to the periphery and return may be the mechanism by which the neuron regulates the action of the muscle with respect to properties not dependent on Ach depolarization.

In 1953, Hughes demonstrated bidirectional flow in axons in tissue culture and Weiss et al. (1962) and Kreutzberg (1963) obtained indirect evidence of axonal flow by ligating axons. Barondes (1964) studied subcellular fractions of mouse brain after exposure to radioleucine ^{14}C and found that specific activity increased 5 times in soluble protein after 2-130 hours indicating axoplasmic flow. Lubinska (1964) had previously shown centrifugal migration of organelles and macromolecules in nerve fibers. Korr et al. (1967) demonstrated that substances labelled with ^{32}P and ^{14}C amino acids applied to the hypoglossal nuclei of rabbits traveled down the hypoglossal nerve and entered the muscle cells of the tongue after several days. Blockage of one nerve caused unilateral radioactive labelling of the tongue. The substances moved at a rate of 5-5.5mm. a day. The radioactive tracer was found in the axons and the nerve sheaths. This study showed that labelled materials apparently crossed the NMJ from the terminal axon to enter the myofiber. Kerkut et al. (1967) obtained evidence for centripetal flow in axons by means of radioautographs from the hypoglossal nerve 1 hour to 4 days after injection. No radioactivity could be demonstrated in the nerve less than 6 hours after injection whereas after 6-12 hours, all the branches were radioactive. The radioactive material reached as high as the carotid bifurcation on the third day and ligation experiments showed accumulation of the label within the nerve. These results are compatible with either of two hypotheses: 1) that the labelled amino acid ascended the axon and became incorporated into protein or 2) ascent of labelled protein synthesized in either the muscle or the axon. When radioleucine was injected into the central nervous system, it appeared rapidly in nerve endings following a delay due to transport of the soluble protein via the axon. After 1 hour, particulate but not soluble protein was present. Droz and Barondes (1969) used radioautography to demonstrate the localization of radioactivity from tritiated L leucine and DL lysine. Cycloheximide, an inhibitor of protein synthesis, decreased incorporation of the labelled amino acids indicating that synthesis of new protein had occurred either in mitochondria or endoplasmic reticulum. These investigators found that new protein appeared very rapidly following injection of the radioactive amino acids.

With respect to the possible kinds of trophic materials other than Ach that might travel in peripheral axons innervating skeletal muscle, Samuels et al. (1951) described a peripherally moving "phosphoprotein" or "phosphoinositide" which he extracted from nerve with ethanol-ether. In a later study, Samuels and Gorevic (1968) claimed that injection of a brain proteolipid extract would retard denervation atrophy. Heller and Hesse (1964) described a rapidly diffusible substance, possibly thiamin, that was released by rat nerves and recently, Musick and Hubbard (1972) have described the release of protein from nerve terminals which they suggested may have trophic activity.

Further research is required to isolate and characterize regulatory materials from nerve.

13

Effects of Toxins on Neuromuscular Junctions

A large variety of naturally occurring and synthetic substances affect the function and in some instances, the morphology of neuromuscular junctions. Some of these toxins are economically important whereas others, particularly naturally occurring neurotoxins are of medical importance or are valuable tools for the experimental study of neuromuscular function.

Curare

Since the remarkable effects of calabash curare on neuromuscular transmission was known before 1900 (Claude Bernard, 1857), it is not surprising that early students of the NMJ sought morphologic abnormalities in NMJs from poisoned animals. All these studies by necessity were limited by the then available staining methods.

As early as 1860, Kűhne reported that the appearance of reptilian NMJs was more distinct after curare poisoning. In 1886, Miura claimed to find atrophy of NMJs in lizards 40 days after curare poisoning. Herzen and Odier (1904) reported that the interdigitations of the terminal arborization in frog NMJs appeared irregular after curare poisoning. Rojas et al. (1939), using gold-staining and silver-staining methods, reported that curare poisoning in lizards produced enlarged

NMJs containing hypolemmal axons of increased prominence. However, Carey et al. (1944a) reported that curare produced shrunken NMJs with increased numbers of Kűhne granules. On the other hand, Dublin (1944), using a gold-staining method, found no alteration in rabbit NMJs, and King (1945) found no changes in rat NMJs. More recently, Harris (1954) found no change in soleplate diameter measured after gold or histochemical staining for esterases in muscles blocked by curare (intercostrin).

Anticholinesterase Toxins

Chemistry and Physiology of Organophosphorous Insecticides.

The organophosphorous compounds in common use include malathion (0,0-dimethyl S-1, 2-dicarbethyoxyethyl phosphorodithionate), tetra ethylpyrophosphate, parathion (dimethyl paranitrophenyl thiophosphate), and hexaethytetraphosphate. Other potent organophosphorous compounds include DFP (di-isopropyl fluorophosphate) sarin (isopropyl methyl phosphonofluoridate) and tabun (ethyl phosphorodimethyllamide cyanidate). All these compounds are potent cholinesterase inhibitors. Some of these substances, especially DFP, are known to act on other enzymes as well. All these substances inhibit AchE by essentially irreversible phosphorylation of the esteratic sites on the enzyme. This chemical combination can be overcome only by regeneration of the enzyme over a period of time, or by competively removing the phosphate group with 2-PAM and 3-PAM (Wilson, 1951; Wilson and Ginsburg, 1955). The physiologic results of AchE inhibition are identical with those of excessive Ach accumulation. Normally, AchE in NMJs and ganglionic synapses destroy Ach following stimulation, thereby allowing the repolarization of the synapses. When AchE is inhibited, Ach accumulates, producing marked parasympathetic symptoms and muscular paralysis.

Accidental and Suicidal Poisoning with Organophosphorous Insecticides

Since the development of potent organophosphorous compounds in 1940 by the Germans for use as chemical warfare agents and insecticides, there have been increasing numbers of accidental and suicidal poisonings by these agents. Abrams and co-workers (1950) reported 198 cases of poisoning with HETP, TEPP, and parathion. Of these cases seven instances of fatal parathion poisoning are recorded. Toivonen et al. (1959), reported 286 fatal cases in Finland in the period 1952-57. Of this number, homicide accounted for seven cases, suicide for 237, and accidental poisoning for the remaining 42. Thirteen suicidal cases of parathion poisoning were reported from Denmark for the year 1956, and four additional cases of parathion poisoning and one of methyl parathion poisoning were collected by Petty (1958b) in the American Southwest.

Petty (1958a) reported the first case of fatal organophosphorous poisoning, which was proven by AchE determinations and histochemical staining of NMJs and Grob et al. (1950) reported a case of parathion poisoning that was proven by recovery of parathion from the tissues at autopsy.

Since the physiologic abnormality is excessive accumulation of the normal transmitter, Ach, the clinical symptoms and signs are of excessive parasympathetic stimulation. After absorption of these organophosphorous inhibitors through the lungs, skin or gastrointestinal tract clinical symptoms include headache, giddiness, blurred vision, muscle weakness, nausea, intestinal cramps, diarrhea, chest discomfort, and nervousness. Clinical signs include sweating, miosis, tearing, salivation, pulmonary edema, papilledema, twitching, cyanosis, convulsions, and coma.

Petty (1958b) has also described residual paralysis apparently due to peripheral nerve injury following recovery from accidental poisoning in two cases. Similarly, Bidstrup et al. (1953) have reported delayed paralysis following mipafox poisoning and Namba et al. (1971) have reviewed acute and chronic aspects of organophosphate insecticide poisoning.

A typical case history and autopsy findings (Zacks and Blumberg, 1961) are as follows:

Case Report. J.S., a 48 year old male crop duster, was completing a dusting operation, when his aircraft collided with a high tension wire. The patient was treated at the site of the accident with an intramuscular injection and then taken to the hospital.

Physical examination revealed fractures of both legs and right arm. The patient was in acute distress, with respirations of 28 per minute. He was oriented and alert. He was then taken to surgery for repair of the fractures. One and one-half hours after arrival he lapsed into shock and then into coma. Morphine sulfate (1/6 grain) and atropine (1/150 grain) had previously been given. Because of suspected brain injury, three burr holes were made. No abnormality was found. The patient died 11 hours after admission.

At autopsy the pupils were constricted. Subendocardial petechiae were present in the left ventricle. The heart was of normal weight. The lungs weighed 1700 gms, and were filled with frothy, bloody fluid. The liver weighed 2450 gms, and was congested. The small intestine showed patchy areas of redness. Slight subarachnoid hemorrhage was present on the surface and base of the brain.

Toxicology. Parathion in tissues was determined by the method of Averell and Norris (1948). The Table tabulates the parathion content of various organs from this patient.

Table 1.   PARATHION CONTENT OF ORGANS OF PATIENT IN REPORTED CASE

TISSUE	PARATHION CONTENT
Liver	0.4 mg. per 100 gm. wet tissue
Kidneys	0.3 mg.
Brain	0.25 mg.
Lung	0.2 mg.
Heart blood	0.05 mg.
Stomach	1.40 per 100 mg. (1.7 mg. in total of 120 gm.)

Postmortem AchE determination by the Michel method (1949) on a sample of frozen hemolyzed blood showed a 0.10Δ pH (normal: $0.65\text{-}1.00\Delta$ pH).

Histochemical Observations. Blocks of frozen intercostal muscle were cut in a cryostat at -40°C. and stained by the method of Raven et al. (1953). After 30 minutes of incubation in the histochemical reagents, no detectable staining of NMJs was observed.

Control rat intercostal muscle showed NMJ staining within 15 minutes. Other samples of the patient's intercostal muscle were stained by the modified Koelle method (1951), which showed slight AchE activity after 25 minutes of incubation. Pretreatment with 2-PAM reversed the inhibition of NMJ staining.

Toxicologic Identification of Organophosphorous Insecticides. The diagnosis of poisoning can be established by measuring the serum

ChE and red cell AchE activity by the Michel method (1949). Chemical methods are available for identification of various agents in urine and gastric contents.

Histochemical Demonstration of Cholinesterase Inhibition. Several methods are available for demonstrating cholinesterase activity in recently fixed or fresh frozen tissue (see appendix). These methods serve as an important adjunct to toxicologic examination for the detection of enzyme inhibition in the blood and tissues because they demonstrate the abnormality at the physiologic site of action (Bergner and Durlacher, 1951). The enzyme is surprisingly stable in human NMJs, surviving in bodies after 120 days of water immersion or 150 days after embalming. A particularly useful proof that AchE inhibition was due to anticholinesterase poisoning is demonstration of restoration of AchE staining following incubation in 2-PAM which reactivates the enzyme by dephosphorylation (Bergner, 1959). Similar results have been reported by Jonecko (1963, 1965a, b) and Fischer (1968) for various organophosphorous inhibitors. Demonstration of AchE inhibition in NMJs and the finding of organophosphorous compounds in the body, coupled with the unusual clinical pattern, gives strong evidence of fatal poisoning by these agents.

Experimental Attempts to Produce Morphologic Alterations in NMJs with Anticholinesterases

Several attempts were made to alter the structure of NMJs by inhibiting cholinesterases. Carey (1944a) reported that morphologic changes occurred in NMJs stained by the gold method after inhibition of cholinesterase by physostigmine. However, Harris (1954), who studied the effects of DFP and TEPA, and Denz (1951), who studied the effect of a powerful phosphate ester inhibitor (E 605), were unable to confirm these observations. Attempts to demonstrate AchE in NMJs after exposure to cholinesterase inhibitors resulted either in no staining at all, or in less severely inhibited NMJs, greatly prolonged incubation time to produce a visible pigment deposition. Often partially inhibited NMJs had irregular, discontinuous staining of the subneural apparatus. One must be particularly careful not to interpret changes in the pattern of cholinesterase staining as an indication of structural abnormalities in the synaptic clefts. This particular objection is seen in the early work of Coërs and Woolf (1959), who studied AchE-staining characteristics of NMJs in various neuromuscular diseases. The fact that the microscopic outline of the subneural apparatus as demonstrated by AchE staining is altered is certainly not equivalent to a demonstration that the structure of the subneural apparatus is altered correspondingly. Thus it would seem that histochemical demonstration of AchE activity should be used for studying the enzyme in experimentally or pathologically altered NMJs, and that no interpretations regarding structure should be made from such data.

The increased resolution of the electron microscope is required before statements can be made about the morphologic status of the subneural apparatus in neuromuscular disease. Thus it is not surprising that powerful cholinesterase inhibitors, such as the irreversible inhibitors DFP and TEPA, should not produce anatomic abnormalities in NMJs stained with the gold method, when studied by optical microscopy. In addition to ChE inhibition, Preusser (1967) described degenerative changes in the fine structure of NMJs and myofibers after intraperitoneal injection of Soman (methylpinacolyloxy-phosphonylfluoride) which has similar anticholinesterase action as DFP, Tabun, E600 and Sarin. There was destruction of the sarcolemma within the subneural apparatus and in the myofibers, mitochondrial swelling, destruction of cristae and formation of myelin figures occurred. Muscle striations disappeared and the orientation of myofilaments was lost. Electron micrographs obtained by this investigator show a kind of spheromembranous degeneration but changes in the subneural apparatus of the NMJs were not evident in the micrographs.

In addition to toxic cholinesterase inhibitors, other manmade neuromuscular toxins include industrial chemicals or drugs used in the therapy of various disease. Substances of this kind include lead, triaryl phosphate, isoniazid, vincristine, various barbiturates (Westmoreland, 1971), di-nitro-phenol (Iwasaki, 1964) (DNP) and various antibiotics (Brazil and Corrado, 1957; Elmqvist and Josefsson, 1962; Brazil and Prado-Franceschi, 1969). Only toxins that are known to produce major structural changes in the neuromuscular apparatus will be described.

Lead Poisoning

De Villaverdes (1926) found no degeneration of the "periterminal network" in NMJs from cases of lead poisoning. In our laboratory, Dr. Henry Schutta has found myelin-like bodies in intercostal NMJs from rats chronically poisoned with lead acetate.

Isoniazid

Isoniazid (isonicotinic acid hydrazide) produces degeneration of peripheral nerves in both man and experimental animals (Schlaepfer and Hager, 1964). Hildebrand et al. (1968) found that rats fed 90 mg. of INH via gastric tube for 3 to 13 days developed nerve damage associated with reduction of the mean maximum afferent conduction velocity. The percentage of damaged nerve fibers increased from 10% at 3 days to 32% after 7 days and there was extensive fragmentation of axons in the intramuscular nerves and collateral sprouting was observed. Rats given INH for 13 days and examined 1-28 days later, had significant reduction of maximum motor conduction velocity and 76% incidence of damaged nerve fibers. By 37 days after completion of the 13 day course of INH, there were many damaged nerve fibers, evidence of atrophy of large groups of myofibers but all physiologic parameters were within normal limits. This recovery resulted from reinnervation of the myofibers by means of collateral branching. Schröder (1970) described the fine structure changes that occur in

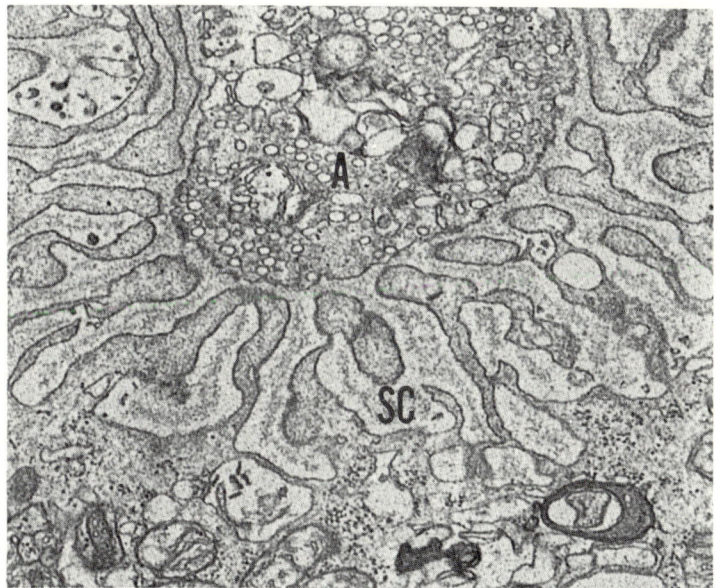

Figure 107. Electron micrograph of a NMJ from vincristine treated rat soleus muscle. The terminal axon *(A)* contains large vesicles and there is irregular infolding and invagination of synaptic clefts *(SC).* (X 20,100.) (From Anderson, P.J. et al., *J. Neuropath. & Exp. Neurol.* 26:15, 1967.)

isoniazid neuropathy that included striking proliferation of the smooth endoplasmic reticulum within Schwann cells and a variety of abnormal structures within regenerating Schwann cells. He also called attention to leakage of red cells from capillaries, which does not occur in Wallerian degeneration.

Vincristine Neuromyopathy

Peripheral neuromyopathy resulting from treatment with vincristine sulfate has been described in patients and produced experimentally in rats (Slotwiner et al., 1966; Anderson et al., 1967). These investigators found no abnormalities in peripheral and terminal nerve fibers but there were changes in the NMJs consisting of distortion, increased complexity and widening of secondary synaptic clefts in the subneural apparatus (Fig. 107). The terminal axon contained swollen synaptic vesicles and cisternal structures. Sarcoplasm underlying the subneural apparatus contained spheromembranous bodies. The myofibrils were fragmented and there were many spheromembranous bodies, which were intepreted as the result of a form of autophagy.

Tri-Ortho-Cresyl Phosphate Poisoning

Cavanagh (1954) observed that the neuropathy caused by accidental ingestion of tri-ortho-cresyl phosphate produced changes in distal axons, the "dying back" phenomenon described by Mott (1896). Prineas (1969a) described the ultrastructure changes in this process of distal axonal destruction (Fig. 108).

Steroid Neuromyopathy

Clinical experience with ACTH and cortisone therapy includes myasthenic and non-myasthenic patients that experience increased muscular weakness (Grob and Harvey, 1952; Sprague et al., 1950). Although several studies have shown evidence of myofiber necrosis (Hagstrom et al., 1961), there is also evidence of involvement of NMJs. Tuncbay et al. (1965) described diffusion of esterases and elongation and "fragmentation" of the subneural apparatus in NMJs from rabbits

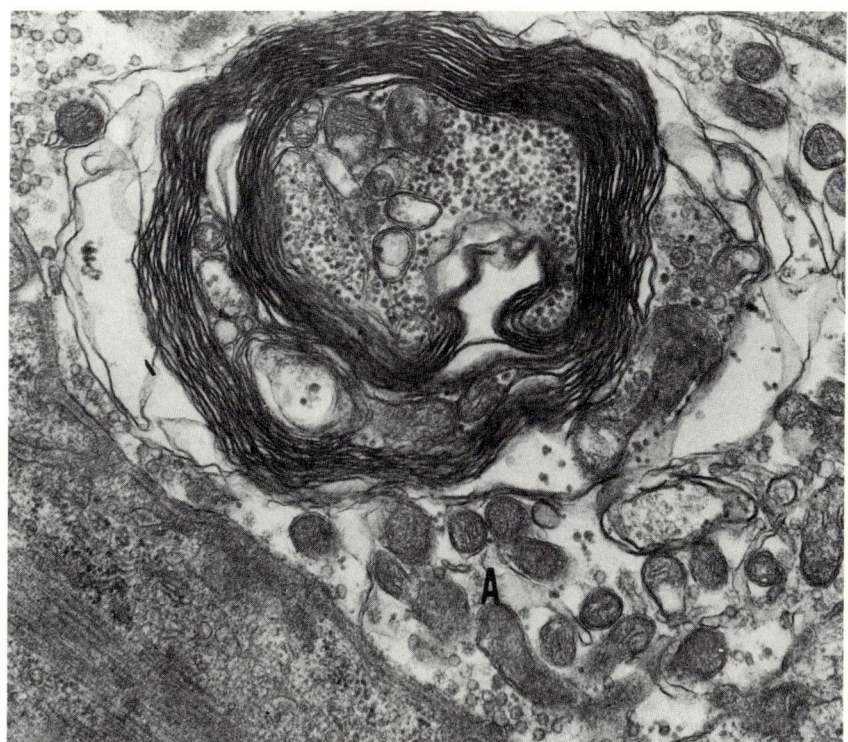

Figure 108. Electron micrograph illustrating NMJ in interosseous muscle 26 days after tri-ortho-cresyl phosphate intoxication. The terminal axon *(A)* contains a large lamellated body *(L)* enclosing degenerating mitochondria and electron dense granules. (X 22,000.) (From Prineas, J., *Arch. Neurol. 21;* 1969.)

injected with large doses of cortisone acetate. Silver-stained terminal axons were thickened and had club-shaped swellings of the terminal expansions.

NATURALLY OCCURRING NEUROMUSCULAR TOXINS

In addition to the neuromuscular toxins of plant or synthetic origin, a great variety of living organisms produce various neurotoxins active at the neuromuscular junction. Bacterial toxins, particularly originating in a small group of obligatory anaerobes will be considered before discussing the great variety of important neuromuscular toxins of animal origin.

Bacterial Toxins

A form of polyneuritis produced by diphtheria exotoxin, is particularly damaging to peripheral nerves. Local and distant paralysis and sensory loss constitute the major signs and symptoms.

The pathology of diphtheritic polyneuritis studied by optical microscopy is not distinctive. There is demyelination, proliferation of Schwann cells, and phagocytosis of the resulting debris. In an electron microscope investigation, Webster et al. (1961) demonstrated early lesions in the Schwann cell membrane and destruction of myelin.

Few descriptions of NMJ changes in diphtheria are available. In a histochemical study by Knyazeva (1962), there was decrease in ChE and increase in AchE activity in guinea pig NMJs three days after intoxication. By the thirty-second day after intoxication, AchE activity was elevated when compared to the control animals, but the subneural apparatus appeared indistinct. Concurrently, proliferation of soleplate nuclei occurred between the fourteenth and the thirty-fifth day after injection of the toxin. Knyazeva (1962) concluded that these observations could be best explained by alteration in the pH optimum or other characteristics of the NMJ esterases.

Botulinus Toxin

Botulinus toxin in its purified form is the most toxic biologic substance known. The estimated lethal human oral dose is approximately 0.5-5.0 micrograms (Lamanna and Carr, 1967; Zacks et al., 1968), a quantity so small that it is below the threshold of the most sensitive of taste receptors. The site and mode of action of the toxin has been studied extensively since Van Ermengem's discovery (1896) that it is produced by the growth of *Clostridium botulinum.*

A series of later investigations, primarily physiologic in nature, by Edmunds and Long (1923), Dickson and Shevky (1923a, b), Schübel (1922), Burgen et al. (1949), Brooks (1956), and Guyton and MacDonald (1947) have indicated that the site of action of botulinus toxin is at the NMJ. All the physiologic effects produced by the toxin can be explained by blocking of somatic and parasympathetic motor nerves. Investigations by Guyton and MacDonald (1947) and Bishop and Bronfenbrenner (1936) have shown that both the peripheral nerve and underlying muscle respond normally when the NMJ is blocked.

The Mode of Action of Botulinus Toxin. The nature of the Ach mechanism suggests several possible sites for the action of botulinus toxin. Torda and Wolff (1947) suggested that botulinus toxin blocks Ach synthesis in brain. This has not been confirmed by other investigators (Burgen et al., 1949). Another possibility, that changes in membrane permeability within NMJs results from botulinus poisoning, has not been investigated in detail. The large size of the botulinus toxin molecule (approximately 100 A) suggests that this substance probably acts at the surfaces of the cells rather than by penetrating cell membranes. Although at first compared to curare poisoning, the apparent curare-like activity of botulinus toxin has not been confirmed by experimentation. Unlike curare poisoning, botulinus intoxication is not reversed by physostigmine or KCl. There is normal tetanic response of the botulinus-poisoned muscle, which does not occur in curare poisoning. The botulinus-poisoned muscle responds normally to direct stimulation by Ach, whereas the curare-blocked muscle does not. The botulinus-poisoned muscle also lacks the supernormal phase that is commonly seen in curarized muscle.

Brooks (1956) demonstrated that the toxin does not interfere with impulse conduction in motor nerves. Burgen et al. (1949) concluded that the toxin either interferes with Ach synthesis or its release from the presynaptic terminal. Studies by Burgen et al. (1947) and Simpson (1968) showed that Ach synthesis and storage were normal. Despite observations by Fex et al. (1966) that suggested that the toxin also acts, possibly directly, on the postsynaptic side of the synapse to influence reinnervation, the overwhelming evidence that the toxin acts on the presynaptic terminal is the more rapid restoration of neuromuscular function that occurs as a result of nerve crush injury. Nerve injury stimulates the formation of new, functional terminals (Thesleff et al., 1964). Similar results were obtained by Duchen (1970) who used cholinesterase staining to demonstrate reinnervation of the old subneural apparatuses. Without nerve injury to stimulate regeneration and new NMJ formation, the partial recovery that occurs in botulinus poisoned muscle is largely due to axonal sprouting.

Although Brooks (1956) and Thesleff (1960) reported that both EPPs and MEPPs are abolished by the toxin, Harris and Miledi (1971) reported that MEPPs did not disappear completely but persisted in many NMJs at reduced frequency during intoxication. These investigators demonstrated that nerve impulses invaded the axon terminals but failed to evoke normal release of transmitter. Of greater interest was the finding that tetanic nerve stimulation evoked large amplitude MEPPs of increased frequency. These data suggest that the toxin does not affect spontaneous and evoked release of transmitter in the same way but that in some fashion, the toxin affected the coupling between depolarization of the presynaptic terminal and transmitter release (Harris and Miledi, 1971). Simpson (1971) however has concluded that the toxin does not appear to act on the depolarization-repolarization cycle because nerve terminals are impervious to the toxin unless Ca++ is present. Simpson suggested that a two step process consisting of initial binding of the toxin to the terminal and secondary blockage occurs as some molecular grouping that ordinarily is not exposed to the toxin becomes available during Ach release.

Localization of Botulinum Toxin Binding Sites

Localization of Ferritin-Labeled Botulinus Toxin in NMJs.

In order to learn more about the site of action of botulinus toxin in the NMJs, a series of experiments with ferritin-labeled botulinus toxin were performed (Zacks et al., 1962). These studies utilized ferritin, which was coupled to the toxin protein to provide a characteristic electron-dense label, which is visible in electron micrographs (Farrant, 1954; Smith et al., 1960). Partially purified botulinum B toxin was coupled to purified horse spleen ferritin by the method of Smith et al. (1960). When the mice injected with toxin or ferritin-labeled toxin showed evidence of hind leg and respiratory paralysis, usually after two and a half to three hours, the animals sacrificed and tissue was taken for examination in the electron microscope. No significant abnormalities in NMJs of acutely poisoned mice were observed and no changes were recognized in the primary or secondary synaptic clefts, nor were there changes in the synaptic vesicles or mitochondria. The Schwann cells also appeared normal. Normal fine structure in NMJs after acute botulinus intoxication was also described by Thesleff (1960).

NMJs from mice injected with ferritin-labeled botulinus toxin showed numerous scattered particles of uniform size and shape, which, when measured, were consistent with the 50 to 55 A diameter reported for ferritin micelles (Farrant, 1954; Kerr and Muir, 1960).

These particles had the sharp edges and square shape typical of ferritin particles observed in methacrylate or Epon embeddings. Numerous ferritin particles were present in the external lamina on the Schwann cell surface. However, the majority of the particles lay within the primary and secondary synaptic clefts. In many cases, ferritin particles were lined up in rows separated by distances approximately two to six times their diameters. For the most part, the particles lay within the midportions of the primary and secondary synaptic clefts rather than closely attached to the muscle surface membrane of the clefts. Rare ferritin particles were found within axoplasm.

NMJs from animals injected with ferritin alone and sacrificed three hours after injection showed a striking absence of ferritin particles in the vicinity or within the structure of NMJs. Occasional ferritin particles were observed in these NMJs, but these lacked the distribution pattern observed in the NMJs of mice poisoned with ferritin-labeled toxin. More ferritin particles were observed in these preparations, however, than in the neuromuscular junctions from mice injected with ferritin only.

These control experiments demonstrated that the localization of ferritin was not due to unbound free ferritin particles, and specificity of the binding was suggested by the failure of ferritin-labeled serum albumin to be localized in the NMJ regions. Since we may suppose that there was a comparable amount of ferritin isothiocyanate not bound to protein in the experiments with ferritin-labeled botulinus toxin and serum albumin, it is unlikely that the ferritin localization obtained with ferritin-labeled toxin was due to ferritin-isothiocyanate.

The results obtained in this investigation indicated that botulinus B toxin was selectively bound in the external lamina that coats the Schwann cell and muscle surface membranes and extends into the primary and secondary synaptic clefts of mouse NMJs. The control experiments showed that this was not a spurious localization of ferritin particles. Later studies (Zacks et al., 1968) employing fluorescein-labelled botulinum A toxin also suggested a postsynaptic localization but binding to terminal axons could not be excluded with the resolution available in fluorescence microscopy. The earlier experiments with ferritin labelled toxin do not coincide with much of the physiologic data cited above and thus must be questioned. However, nonspecific ferritin binding such as that which occurs in skeletal muscle does not appear to be the cause of the discrepancy. It is likely that the toxin is bound by the terminal axons, a reaction that may be facilitated by the large numbers of anionic groups in the toxin molecule (Buehler et al., 1947) and in the external lamina. However, the latency of botulinus intoxication and its Q10 (Duff et al., 1957) is more compatible with the hypothesis that a chemical reaction occurs between the toxin and the axon plasma membrane or its glycoprotein cell coat.

The remarkable toxicity of botulinum toxin and the observation that the lethal dose is poorly related to body mass can be partially explained by the remarkable specificity of binding of the toxin. *In vitro* studies with flourescein labeled toxin or indirectly with flourescein labeled antibodies showed remarkable selectivity for NMJs (Zacks et al., 1968). There was no *in vitro* staining of cardiac muscle, lung, spleen, liver and kidney. Only NMJs and skeletal muscle sarcoplasm bound the toxin (Zacks et al., 1968).

To explain the similar lethal doses in small and large animals, the following considerations apply. If one NMJ per myofiber in twitch muscles is assumed and the soleplate size is directly related to the diameter of the myofiber rather than its volume or length, then the number of NMJs in the mouse should be less by 1-2 orders of magnitude than the ratio of the body weights of mouse to man. Calculations of this kind suggest the minimum oral dose of botulinum toxin for man is approximately 5×10^{-9} to 5×10^{-8} grams.

STRUCTURAL CHANGES IN NMJs POISONED BY BOTULINUS TOXIN

Classical Staining Methods

Guyton and MacDonald (1957), who used a gold-staining method, reported that they were unable to demonstrate definite changes in NMJs poisoned by botulinus toxin. It appeared to them that some abnormalities were present in the earlier stages of intoxication. However, no effort was made to assess the normal variations in NMJ morphology in their material. Indeed, these investigators were somewhat surprised that in the presence of such severe incapacitation of transmission, lasting more than six months, so few changes could be found in the NMJs. Another investigation reporting similar results was that of Davenport et al. (1929). Tyler (1963) also failed to find abnormal NMJ structure or alterations of cholinesterase activity in a human case of botulism studied by silver and histochemical-staining methods. The toxin also does not cause neural degeneration (Thesleff, 1960; Duchen and Strich, 1967, 1968) in acutely poisoned animals. Abnormalities in NMJ demonstrated by intravital methylene blue staining consist of abnormal axon sprouting, a change interpreted as an attempt to compensate for functional denervation.

Electron microscopic studies of acutely poisoned NMJs have also shown no morphologic abnormalities (Thesleff, 1960; Zacks and Blumberg, 1962). However, despite the structural integrity of NMJs following poisoning, the underlying muscle gradually atrophies (Jirmanova et al., 1964; Drachman, 1964, 1967; Duchen and Strich, 1968). With doses of 0.1-0.4 micrograms of A toxin, Duchen and Strich (1968) produced local paralysis and atrophy in mouse gastrocnemius and hamstring muscles. There was no histologic evidence of degeneration of either the nerve or NMJs but silver staining revealed sprouting from terminal nerve fibers and staining for AchE revealed elongation and abnormal configurations of the soleplates. Nine months after intoxication, the pattern of innervation still appeared abnormal. The authors hypothesized that terminal sprouting is a response to blocked transmission.

Hoffman et al. (1964) demonstrated that the effect of botulinum toxin was similar to denervation in that poisoned muscle with completely blocked neuromuscular transmission would accept foreign innervation as if the muscle had been physically denervated by nerve section. Demonstration of reinnervation was achieved by electrical stimulation and recording as well as morphologic demonstration of new zones of AchE in the subneural apparatus.

Thesleff et al. (1964) had also shown that muscles paralyzed by botulinum toxin recover function more rapidly if the nerves innervating the muscle fibers are crushed and then allowed to regenerate. After sublethal quantity of type A toxin was injected into the legs of mice, paralysis developed within 24 hours. In another group of animals, the right sciatic nerve was crushed and in another group the nerve was exposed but not injured. The crushed nerve fibers degenerated distal to the injury and within 10 days regenerating axons reinnervated the original soleplates. The muscles recovered more rapidly when the nerve was crushed than if the nerve was not disturbed after the injection of the toxin. Degenerated axons lacked terminal axon sprouts of the kind that appeared in poisoned muscles with intact nerves. As the regenerating axons arrived in the muscles, new NMJs were formed. These results indicate that the toxin irreversibly alters some component within the terminal axon, a conclusion in concert with the known physiological data. Thus, newly formed axons from regenerating nerve fibers without toxin bound to their surface or axoplasmic organelles, are capable of re-establishing neuromuscular transmission. These experiments indicate that the demonstrated botulinum toxin binding to external lamina or muscle cell membrane may interfere with Ach secretion by interacting with some membrane components. Experiments utilizing flourescene-labeled toxin and antitoxin also demonstrated binding in the region of the soleplate but whether the binding occurred in terminal axon arborization or within the external lamina could not be determined because of insufficient resolution.

A series of experiments utilizing botulinum toxin as a tool to study the "trophic" actions of motor innervation have revealed many unexpected consequences of botulinum intoxication. For example, increased sensitivity to Ach develops in the postsynaptic membrane of botulinum poisoned muscles (Thesleff, 1960; Josefesson and Thesleff, 1961) similar to the denervation sensitivity that occurs following nerve section. Unlike the situation in which reinnervation of previously denervated muscle leads to reversal of muscle atrophy, the hyperneurotized botulinum poisoned muscles (Fex et al., 1966) continued to be severely atrophic. Duchen and Strich (1968) and Watson (1969) found extensive sprouting of axons from the terminal motor axon after local injection of botulinum toxin, a response similar to that which occurs following nerve section. The axonal sprouting was also associated with increased ribosomal RNA synthesis.

Although it is generally accepted that axonal sprouting is an attempt to compensate for a NMJ functional deficiency, the stimulus for this response is obscure. Recently, Duchen (1970) studied the effect of botulinum toxin on cholinesterase activity and axonal sprouting in fast and slow muscles. Both soleus and gastrocnemius muscles of the mouse were paralyzed within 24 hours of injection of the toxin. The slow soleus muscle atrophied faster than the fast gastrocnemius. Using a modified Koelle histochemical method, Duchen (1970) demonstrated sprouting of terminal axons in the soleus muscle by the 6th to 7th day which progressed for several weeks. Notable myofiber atrophy in the soleus occurred in 3 to 4 weeks. In the gastrocnemius muscle, atrophy continued for 6 weeks or more and the muscle eventually became more atrophic than the soleus muscle. Axon sprouting in the gastrocnemius occurred only after 3 to 4 weeks and was maximal at 6-8 weeks. After recovery from the effects of the toxin, stimulation of both the original and the new motor nerve evoked twitch responses in the muscle. However, stimulation of both nerves simultaneously did not augment muscle tension. Botulinum toxin apparently suppressed the influence of the original NMJs that prevents acceptance of additional innervation despite the morphologic integrity of the NMJs, thus confirming the observations of Thesleff et al. (1964).

Cholinesterase activity appeared in both muscles, but at different rates. NsChE was found along the nerve sprouts rather than AchE and as new NMJs formed, they contained less cholinesterase activity than normal. Since the neural mechanism that controls the muscle speed of contraction is unknown, it is difficult to interpret the significance of the observed altered NsChE activity and the degree of axon sprouting occured.

In ultrastructure studies of slow and fast mouse myofibers locally poisoned with small doses of botulinum A toxin, Duchen (1971a) observed myofiber atrophy in both kinds of muscle. Lysosomes and multivesicular bodies, evidence of degeneration, were present in both the soleus and gastrocnemius muscles 18-24 days after poisoning The soleus myofibers recovered their normal size and had increased glycogen content by 4-6 weeks but the gastrocnemius myofibers became more severely atrophic. Recovery of this muscle did not begin until the 5th-6th week. More rapid recovery of the soleus muscle fibers coincided with more rapid axonal sprouting (4 days) whereas the gastrocnemius muscle remained longer without reinnervation (4 weeks). However, many other factors could explain these differences including the metabolic differences in the two kinds of myofibers. In a parallel description of fine structure changes in the NMJs, Duchen (1971b) reported that axon sprouts were enclosed in Schwann cells and early nerve-muscle contacts ellicited no postsynaptic membrane modifications for the first few weeks. Later, subneural clefts were formed. After 4 months or longer, the

NMJs on soleus myofibers resembled normal junctions but were scattered along the myofibers and often lacked associated soleplate nuclei. Some NMJs in gastrocnemius muscles were normal but several junctions with abnormal subneural apparatus were observed.

Several of the illustrations presented of "new" nerve muscle junctions in soleus muscle after 14 days and gastrocnemius muscle after 24 days show large terminal axons overlying deep irregular primary clefts often containing widened and shallow secondary synaptic clefts. These NMJs resemble previously denervated soleplates in the process of reinnervation (Saito and Zacks, 1969), and especially in the gastrocnemius muscle, may represent a similar process in the botulinum toxin poisoned muscle. Certainly illustrations of NMJs in the soleus and gastrocnemius at 7 weeks strongly suggest what we have come to recognize as *de novo* formation of NMJs. Recovery of muscle function and structure that occurs after several months is clearly the result of new innervation from the sprouting of motor nerve fibers at their terminals and probably is due to reinnervation of some previously denervated NMJs.

Rand and Whaler (1965) have also described impairment of sympathetic transmission by botulinum toxin.

Tetanus Toxin

Over the long history of investigation of tetanus intoxication, the primary emphasis of clinical and laboratory investigations has been on the central nervous system. Much of the controversy that occurred resulted from the use of impure and poorly standardized preparations of the toxin by various investigators.

Several investigations concerning the purification and mode of action of tetanus toxin were published before the turn of the century and in the years immediately following 1900. Classical studies were published on the action of tetanus toxin (Meyer and Ransom, 1903), purification (Madsen, 1899), and binding of tetanus toxin by various tissues (Landsteiner and Botteri, 1906). Investigations by Morax and Marie (1903) and Meyer and Ransom (1903) led to the Marie-Meyer Theory, which stated that tetanus toxin entered the central nervous system by centripetal migration within the nerve trunks. A contrary view of hematogenous dissemination was defended by Abel et al. (1938). However, this problem is not immediately germane to the question of possible effects of tetanus toxin on NMJs.

Harvey (1939) reported that he had produced transient local tetanus by intramuscular injections of 1/50th to 1/100th of a cat lethal dose. Electrical activity was recorded by concentric needle electrodes. He reported that electrical activity, voluntary movement and clonus of the dorsal flexor of the foot were present before evidense of muscular rigidity occurred. Following section of the motor nerve, there was slight decrease in muscular rigidity that was followed by complete relaxation after a period of 3-5 days. Harvey interpreted this delay as the time required to complete degeneration of the NMJs. He also stated that muscular rigidity did not occur if denervated muscles were injected with toxin but there was gradual loss of muscular response to maximal stimulation of the motor nerve approximately 5 days after local injection of the toxin. Harvey concluded that the toxin acted at the NMJs. His EMG data that indicated oscillatory potentials and outbursts of electrical activity as well as spontaneous twitches were not confirmed by other investigators (Schaeffer, 1944; Perdrup, 1946; Wright, 1955).

Ambache (1948) also showed depression of Ach action at cholinergic nerve endings during tetanus intoxication. In these experiments, tetanus toxin was injected into rabbit eyes, with the result that mydriasis without reactivity to light occurred. Since the pupil responded to Ach and carbachol with miosis, it was evident that the toxin effect was not due to direct action on the sphincter pupillae muscle. Mydriatic response to tetanus toxin still occurred despite ablation of the sympathetic ganglia and postsynaptic fibers, indicating that the toxin effect was not due to sympathetic overstimulation. However, the normally occurring miosis, which was produced by stimulation of oculomotor nerve, was prevented by tetanus toxin. Ambache (1948) concluded that there was paralysis of cholinergic transmission in tetanus-intoxicated eyes which could be partially antagonized by eserine. This indicated a decrease in the available Ach in the poisoned iris. Genuit and Labenz (1941) have claimed that tetanus toxin was a potent AchE inhibitor, but this could not be confirmed by Schaefer (1944) or Ammon (1943).

More recently, Mackereth and Scott (1954) recorded *in situ* local electrical activity from the rat diaphragm following injection of tetanus toxin. In *in vivo* experiments, the diaphragm produced continuous irregular potentials superimposed upon the respiratory potentials whereas *in vitro* there were no spontaneous action potentials nor repetitive firing response to single stimuli in the poisoned nerve-muscle preparations. Also, there were no differences in curare sensitivity between the control and the intoxicated muscle. Therefore, these findings failed to confirm Harvey's observations that toxin acted peripherally at the NMJ. Kobinger et al. (1956) studied the release of potassium from cat skeletal in which local tetanus had been established. Ach was injected interarterially and change in the release of potassium was measured. Thirteen to 21 days after intoxication the pattern of potassium release resembled that which occurs following denervation.

Brooks et al. (1957) concluded from their study of several forms of spinal inhibitory mechanisms in cats that tetanus toxin, like strychnine, increases polysynaptic reflexes. Of the five forms of spinal inhibition investigated, all were diminished and eventually abolished by tetanus toxin, regardless of the site of injection. These investigators concluded that tetanus toxin exerted its effect near synaptic junctions between specific interneurons of the inhibitory pathway and the motor neuron.

Stevenson (1958) suggested that tetanus toxin is irreversibly fixed at cholinergic endings or possibly in the terminal unmyelinated fibers proximal to the region where Ach is released. He stated that there appeared to be a diminution in the production of Ach *in vivo*, although the toxin did not seem to depress the acetylation of choline. Furthermore, Prabhu and Oester (1962), using EMG techniques, studied local tetanus in rabbit muscle and recorded polyphasic potentials, positive sharp waves and fibrillation potentials 5-8 days after tetanus intoxication. These potentials in the interval of 10-35 days after intoxication also resembled the potentials recorded from chronically denervated muscle. These investigators concluded that their findings could only be explained by action of the toxin at the level of the muscle as well as in the central nervous system.

Studies by Feigen et al. (1963) and Parsons et al. (1966) demonstrated that impure tetanus toxin increased the frequency of random discharges of MEPPs recorded from tetanus intoxicated isolated nerve-muscle preparations. They concluded that the toxin produced depolarization of the presynaptic terminal, which did not occur when calcium was excluded from the bathing medium. They observed that depolarization by potassium blocked or reversed the peripheral effects of tetanus toxin suggesting that the toxin probably acted by lowering the presynaptic resting potential. Stirnemann and Bronnimann (1957) and Kaeser et al. (1968) also reported toxin action on NMJs. Large doses of tetanus toxin produced progressive decrease in the amplitude of the mechanical response of tetanus intoxicated rat phrenic nerve-diaphragm preparations stimulated indirectly, an effect which could be blocked by pretreatment with tetanus antitoxin. In situ injections of toxin produced fatigue of muscular contractions during low frequency stimulation and tetanic fusion occurred at lower stimulation frequencies than in controls (Muchnick and Rubenstein, 1967). These investigators concluded that tetanus toxin has direct local action on skeletal muscle and that central stimulation is necessary to make this evident in whole animal experiments. We concur with the view that the rigidity of muscle produced by local or systemic tetanus intoxication is the result of a combined lesion in the central nervous system involving blocked inhibitory synapses on central neurons as well as hyperexcitable phenomena in the peripheral musculature (Zacks and Sheff, 1970). Diamond and Mellanby (1971) studied the effect of tetanus toxin on central and peripheral sites of action of tetanus toxin in goldfish. Electrophysiologic investigation of the Mauthner cells revealed no effect on either collateral inhibition or crossed 8th nerve inhibition but local injection of the toxin into pectoral muscles produced paralysis that was ascribed to block of neuromuscular transmission. Mellanby (1971) and Mellanby and Thompson (1972) concluded that the site of action was the presynaptic terminal. This subject has recently been reviewed by Kryzhanovsky (1973) who agrees that the site of action of the toxin is presynaptic.

Morphologic Aspects of Tetanus Intoxication

Kura and Kamesawa (1928) claimed to find an abnormally coarse outline of the hypolemmal axons, thickening of the nerve fibers, and irregularity of silver staining in NMJs of animals poisoned with tetanus toxin. Some doubt was cast on these findings by similar changes that they claimed also occurred in beriberi, as reported from the same laboratory by Tsunoda (1928).

Electron Microscopic Studies In a study of muscle and the central nervous system of mice acutely poisoned with purified tetanus toxin, Zacks and Sheff (1964) encountered an entirely unexpected finding in both muscle and brain mitochondria. Numerous round or oval electron-dense granules were found within the mitochondrial profiles in sections of mouse intercostal muscles from animals poisoned with crude or purified tetanus toxin. These granules were present in mitochondria that lay beneath the muscle cell membrane, between individual myofibrils, and in the vicinity of NMJs.

The dense granules in many respects resembled the infrequent mitochondrial dense granules found in normal muscle. However, unlike the normal dense granules, which measure approximately 200 × 200 A and contain three to four round electron-dense subunits, the abnormal, or for convenience, "tetanus dense granules" ranged in size from 200 × 150 A to 500 × 300 A and contained up to six recognizable subunits. Of these subunits, many were comparable in size (approximately 60 to 70 A) to the subunits of normal dense granules. The subunits were embedded in a matrix of moderate electron density, but no limiting membrane was present. The dense granules were never found outside the mitochondrial profiles.

A maximum of three dense granules were seen in normal intercostal muscle mitochondrial profiles, and many mitochondrial profiles contained no dense granules. After tetanus intoxication nearly every mitochondrial profile contained at least one or two dense granules and many had 20 or more. The majority of the dense granules were found in the mitochondrial matrix. After lead staining (pH 12) the dense granules appeared even more dense. Slightly swollen mitochondria were observed in some of the muscle and brain sections. Other components of the muscle fine structure, including the sarcoplasm, myofibrils, and sarcoplasmic reticulum, were unaltered. NMJs demonstrated normal architecture of both primary and secondary clefts. No abnormalities were observed in the synaptic vesicles.

Muscle mitochondria from animals protected with tetanus antitoxin and subsequently challenged with toxin showed slight increase in number of dense granules when compared with the number found in the normal mitochondrial profiles. No abnormal dense granules were seen in antitoxin-protected animals.

When the incidence of dense granules in normal intercostal muscle mitochondrial profiles was determined, it was found that 6.9 per cent of interstitial mitochondria and 14.3 per cent of subsarcolemmal mitochondria contained at least one dense granule, whereas after tetanus poisoning 58.7 per cent of interfilbrillar mitochondria and 72.8 per cent of subsarcolemmal mitochondria in intercostal muscle contained one or more dense granules. Muscles from animals protected with tetanus antitoxin and subsequently challenged with tetanus toxin demonstrated incidences of 21.5 and 19.5 per cent respectively.

The discovery by Price and Nishi (1961) of dramatic mitochondrial abnormalities in renal tubular mitochondria chronically poisoned with tetanus toxin, and the dense-granule changes in acutely poisoned mitochondria suggest that the mitochondria both in the central nervous system and in muscle may be a major site of toxin action. That the latter phenomenon is not specific for tetanus intoxication is indicated by the observation of Andersson-Cedergren (1959), who found increased numbers of large intramitochondrial dense granules in the muscles of "occasional" mice. However, in a previous study of more than 50 mouse intercostal muscle samples (Zacks and Blumberg, 1961a), increased numbers of intramitochondrial dense granules were never observed.

When the incidence of dense granules in mitochondria was analyzed by the chi square test, the observed increase in dense granules in muscle from poisoned animals was found to be significant, with $p < 0.001$. Comparison of the incidence of mitochondrial dense granules in poisoned mice with antitoxin-protected mice demonstrated a statistically significant difference ($p < 0.001$). These tests further indicate that the increased numbers of dense granules in poisoned mice was not a sampling artefact. Furthermore, the dense granules did not resemble the intramitochondrial iron aggregates reported by Bessis and Breton-Gorius (1959).

The increase in mitochondrial dense granules is now regarded as a secondary phenomenon related to calcium accumulation since there are no primary abnormalities in mitochondrial oxidative phosphorylation produced by purified toxin *in vitro* (Zacks and Sheff, 1971). The original findings of abnormal oxidative phosphorylation (Sheff et al., 1963b) were found to be due to a bacterial oxidase in impure toxin preparations.

Modern electron microscopic studies of mice acutely or chronically poisoned with purified tetanus neurotoxin have failed to show fine structure abnormalities in terminal axons. However, Duchen et al. (1972) has claimed that 1 week after sublethal doses of toxin were injected into mice hind limbs, axonal sprouting and new NMJ formation occurred on slow soleus muscle but not on fast extensor digitorum longus muscles. This correlated with the selective effect of the toxin on slow muscles reported by Duchen et al. (1972b). The soleus muscle showed Z line disruption and disorganized myofilaments but no data concerning the fine structure of NMJs was included in this brief report (Duchen et al., 1972a).

We have been unable to localize labeled tetanus toxin in the region of NMJs either by optical (fluorescence) or electron microscopic methods (horseradish peroxidase-labelled tetanus antitoxin). The toxin binds at the junction of the sarcoplasmic reticulum and the T system and localizes within the terminal sacs of the sarcoplasmic reticulum (Zacks and Sheff, 1968).

Agostini and Noetzel (1969) confirmed the absence of morphologic abnormalities in human NMJs in patients with severe tetanus intoxication. However, the soleplates contained vesicles measuring up to 2μ in diameter that appeared to contain moderately large calcium aggregates. Similar calcific aggregates were observed by Weller and McArdle (1971) in myofibers from patients with periodic paralysis. They suggested that abnormal accumulations of electrolytes occurred in the sarcoplasmic reticulum since there was no evidence of mitochondrial involvement.

Agostini and Noetzel (1969) also described degenerative changes in the myofibers in non-innervated areas of muscle. This evidence of muscle injury corresponds with the electromyographic and biochemical observations of Eyrich et al. (1967) who found myopathic changes in patients with tetanus intoxication. In an earlier study, Zacks et al. (1966) found changes in intramitochondrial dense granules in muscle biopsy specimens from five tetanus intoxicated patients but no myofibrillar changes. Unlike the cases reported by Agostini and Noetzel (1969), muscle relaxants had not been used. Zacks and Sheff (1970) suggested that the toxin has no specific action on the NMJ although the postsynaptic membrane like the remainder of the myofiber membrane appeared to bind the toxin and they concluded that the toxin may produce abnormal excitation relaxation coupling in the myofibers as well as a lesion of the inhibitory synapses in the spinal cord. However, Francois (1970) found no difference in the transport capacity and membrane permeability of isolated vesicles from the sarcoplasmic reticulum of rabbit white muscle incubated *in vitro* with tetanus toxin. There was no effect on the rapid, magnesium-dependent ATP-driven calcium transport system *in vitro*.

The data obtained by several groups of investigators has not resolved the question of possible primary action of tetanus toxin on the NMJ. Although some of the disagreement is probably due to the use of impure toxin, it is possible that tetanus toxin may bind to either the pre- or postsynaptic membranes to produce abnormal electrolyte flux despite our failure to demonstrate it in these locations by labeling techniques (Zacks and Sheff, 1970).

Animal Toxins Active at Neuromuscular Junctions

A second group of toxins of natural origin is composed of numerous and varied substances, chiefly proteins, polypeptides or steroids, as well as smaller ions, that are produced by protista, various marine invertebrates, many arthropods, snakes, and amphibians. In some cases, isolation and purification of the active materials have been performed and electrophysiologic data has been obtained to indicate uniquivocal action at the pre- or postsynaptic membranes of the NMJ. In a few cases, histochemical and ultrastructure studies have also been made that characterize the site of action of the toxin. Several toxins have become valuable tools for the study of neuromuscular function.

PROTOZOAN TOXINS

Saxitoxin

Paralytic shell fish intoxication is due to the ingestion of shell fish or fish containing the protozoan, *Gonyaulax catenella*. This organism in large numbers is responsible for the "red tide." Symptoms of saxitoxin intoxication include numbness of the lips, tongue and finger tips followed by numbness of the legs, arms and neck and general muscular incoordination. Dizziness, weakness, drowsiness, headache, have also been described prior to the development of respiratory paralysis within 2-12 hours; recovery may occur in 24 hours. Only symptomatic treatment and artificial respiration are available therapy for poisoned individuals.

Saxitoxin has been purified and has the molecular formula $C_{10}H_{17}O_7N_4 \cdot 2HCl$ (Schantz, 1971). It produces muscular weakness due to a rapidly developing noncompetitive neuromuscular block that is not antagonized by increasing the rate of stimulation or use of anticholinesterases. However, unlike depolarizing molecules such as hexamethonium, saxitoxin does not produce initial muscular stimulation. The block appears to occur at the level of the motor axons or skeletal muscle membrane but not in the NMJs (Kao, 1967). The mechanism of saxitoxin blockade is its apparent interference with the membrane channels for the initial peak transient inward current mediated by sodium ions. The effects of the toxin are easily reversed by washing indicating loose binding. Saxitoxin slightly reduces MEPP amplitude after long exposure (Nishiyama, 1968; Katz & Miledi, 1969), possibly by interfering with transmitter release or alteration of the postsynaptic membrane.

Invertebrate Toxins

As reviewed by Welsh (1964), several marine invertebrates contain complex mixtures of biologically active substances including those which act at the NMJ. However, substances such as serotonin, histamine and tetramethylammonium hydroxide (tetramine) common in these species are chiefly pain producing components and not true neurotoxins in the sense of producing significant interference with neuromuscular function. Coelenterate toxin obtained from sea anemones and the jelly fish is heat labile, digested by proteolytic enzymes and non-dialyzable. It produces irreversible depolarization in the isolated crayfish nerve-muscle preparation apparently by altering the selective permeability of the crayfish NMJ. Physalia toxin with similar properties contains 9 chromatographically demonstrable peptides (Lane and Dodge, 1958). A purified steroid glycoside toxin possessing marked cytotoxic effects has been obtained from the sea cucumber. This material called Holothurin A, produces irreversible block at frog sciatic nerve nodes of Ranvier and irreversible destruction of the twitch response in rat phrenic-nerve diaphragm preparations when stimulated directly or indirectly (Thron et al., 1964). These investigators demonstrated that a small amount of physostigmine (10^{-10} to $10^{-9}M$) protects the neuromuscular junctions of the rat phrenic nerve diaphragm preparations from the action of the toxin. This protection disappears when the level of physostigmine is raised beyond 7×10^{-9}M. Since the toxin has saponin properties and will hemolyse red cells, it is possible that similar action occurs at the junctional membranes.

Octopus toxin produces depolarization followed by flaccid paralysis. It is a non-acetone soluble, heat labile, non-dialyzable substance that is also destroyed by proteolytic enzymes. Ghiretti (1960) has called this material "cephalotoxin". A low molecular weight, water soluble toxin, "maculotoxin" that blocks action potentials in toad myofibers has been extracted from octopus salivary glands by Dulhunty and Gage (1971). This substance appears to block neuromuscular transmission by interfering with action potentials in the nerve terminals; there being no postsynaptic action. Gastropod venoms from various cone molluscs also act on NMJs or directly on muscle.

Insect Toxins

Among the insects, the toxin in wasp venom that paralyses its prey and permits them to survive though completely paralysed is apparently a protein (Beard, 1960). Similar protein toxins are present in arthropods.

Venoms of various arthropods including the black widow spider, tarantula and scorpion contain protein substances which cause neuromuscular malfunction. The scorpion contains a substance thought to interfere with Ach production.

Black Widow Spider Venom

Frog and toad nerve muscle preparations are affected by black widow spider venom and it produces blockade of the rat nerve-diaphragm preparation. Longenecker et al. (1970) investigated the action of black widow spider venom on single NMJs in frog sartorius muscle. They found that the MEPP frequency rose after an initial period of lag and then declined to low levels over a period of about 5 minutes. MEPP amplitude remained about the same throughout the experiment and the toxin produced no change in the myofiber membrane potential. These investigators concluded that the venom acted on the presynaptic terminal producing release of transmitter independent of calcium concentration and depolarization of the nerve terminal. Preparations of this type prepared for electron microscopy revealed nearly complete obliteration of the synaptic vesicles in the terminal axon (Fig. 109) (Clark et al., 1970, 1972; Okamoto et al., 1971).

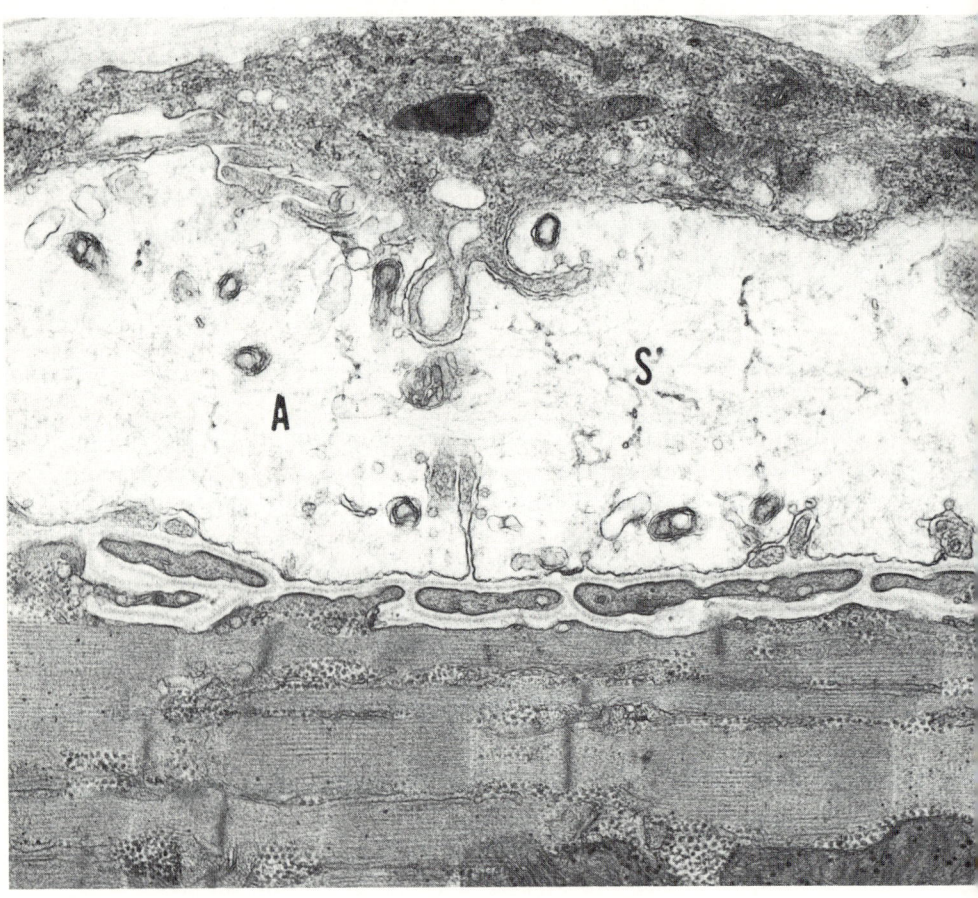

Figure 109. Electron micrograph illustrating a longitudinal section through a frog NMJ 30 minutes after the onset of the MEPP avalanche caused by black widow spider toxin. The presynaptic membrane has returned to its original position opposite the postsynaptic membrane but the axon *(A)* is devoid of synaptic vesicles. Elements of the smooth endoplasmic reticulum are prominent *(S)*. (X 22,300.) (From Clark, A.W., *Nature* 225, 1970).

Tick Paralysis

A disease apparently due to intoxication with a natural neurotoxin is tick paralysis (Ross, 1926). Although we are unable to provide data on the morphology of NMJs in this syndrome, we include it in our discussion because the available evidence strongly suggests that it primarily affects NMJs.

This interesting acute ascending motor paralysis following the bite of various ticks of the *Dermacentor* and *Ixodes* species occurs in both eastern and western portions of the United States and in Europe, South Africa, and Australia. Symmetrical flaccid paralysis usually begins in the lower extremities and ascends to invade the upper extremities and respiratory muscles. There is rapid recovery of muscle strength following removal of the tick from the skin. During the paralysis, the subject does not respond to neostigmine, which tends to exclude the curariform type of block. A mortality rate of approximately 12% was reported by the U.S. Department of HEW (1965). Electromyograph recordings reveal the absence of synaptic potentials at the NMJs and the absence of Ach in the effluent of perfused muscles. These experiments have led to the conclusion that the toxin blocks the liberation of Ach (Emmons and McLennan, 1959; Murnaghan, 1958, 1960). A toxin has been isolated by Kaire (1966).

One aspect of tick paralysis that differs from myasthenia gravis (see discussion pg. 346) is the change in muscle potential that occurs on successive stimuli. In tick paralysis, there is no decrease in the endplate potential as a response to low frequency stimulation such as occurs in myasthenia gravis. Emmons and McLennan (1959) concluded that the toxin reduces excitability of all excitable tissues and Esplin et al., (1960) found evidence of toxin action on central reflex activity. Also Lagos and Thies (1969) found evidence of central action.

Unlike the tick toxin, scorpion venom has both excitatory and inhibitory actions. Although there is evidence that the toxin may act on muscle (Zlotkin and Shulov, 1969), Katz and Edwards (1972) have demonstrated that the toxin acts on motor nerve terminals, probably affecting their $Na+$ permeability. The effect of scorpion venom on the fine structure of frog sartorius muscle has been studied by Yarom and Meiri (1972).

Fish Toxins

A toxin similar to saxitoxin is tetrodotoxin, which is found in s several organs of the puffer fish and in some newts. Its molecular weight is 319.3 and its formula is $C_{11}H_{17}N_3O_8$. The toxin has an interesting structure with a guanidinium group and a hemi lactal configuration (Camougis et al., 1967). Unlike saxitoxin, which has a minimal effect, tetrodotoxin has no effect on NMJs. Similar to saxitoxin in its action, it interferes with the inward flow of sodium through the nerve membrane producing block of the peak transient inward current (Dettbarn, 1971).

Amphibian Toxins

The toxic skin secretions from certain frogs were used by Columbian Indians to prepare poison darts. This material's toxicity is due to its blockade of neuromuscular transmission and its action on muscle. Four substances have been obtained and found to be steroidal alkaloids with the formula of $C_{24}H_{35}NO_5$ (batrachotoxin A). The toxin blocks the twitch response of myofibers stimulated indirectly via the nerve and at the same time there is gradual decline of the response of the muscle to direct stimulation. There is irreversible depolarization of the nerve membrane eventually leading to reversal of its polarity. Tetrodotoxin restores the depolarization produced by batrachotoxin and reduction of the sodium content of the external medium produces hyperpolarization of the batrachotoxin-poisoned membrane. All these changes occur however without change in the resting membrane potential in the absence of sodium in the external bath. Narahashi et al. (1971) concluded that batrachotoxin causes a specific increase of sodium permeability and depolarization of electrically excitable membranes of both nerve and muscle. The toxin is thought to bind irreversibly to membrane proteins and sulphydryl groups are believed to play a role in the toxin's action (Albuquerque et al., 1971; Warnick et al., 1971). Presynaptic block is the cause of transmission failure because the postsynaptic membrane responds with normal sensitivity to Ach added to the vicinity of the NMJs (Albuquerque et al., 1971). The toxin causes swelling of terminal axons and aggregates of tightly packed swollen synaptic vesicles (Fig. 110).

In further studies of the action of batrachotoxin on striated muscle (Albuquerque, 1972), it was demonstrated that there are two phases of muscle contracture and damage of the sarcoplasmic reticulum and cisternae in mammalian muscles, whereas in the frog, there was only one phase of contracture when the muscle was stimulated. The sarcoplasmic reticulum of frog muscle was unaffected. Also, the toxin had no destructive effect on the NMJ of the frog *Phyllobates aurotaenia*, the animal which produces the toxin. Caffeine insensitivity of rat muscle after batrachotoxin poisoning is due to destruction of the SR whereas frog (*R. pipiens*) muscle remains sensitive to caffeine. Albuquerque suggests that the toxin acts on a SH-containing protein in the membrane "sodium channel".

Other studies (Albuquerque et al., 1973a, b) demonstrated that *P. aurotaenia*, the frog that produces the toxin suffers no NMJ struc-

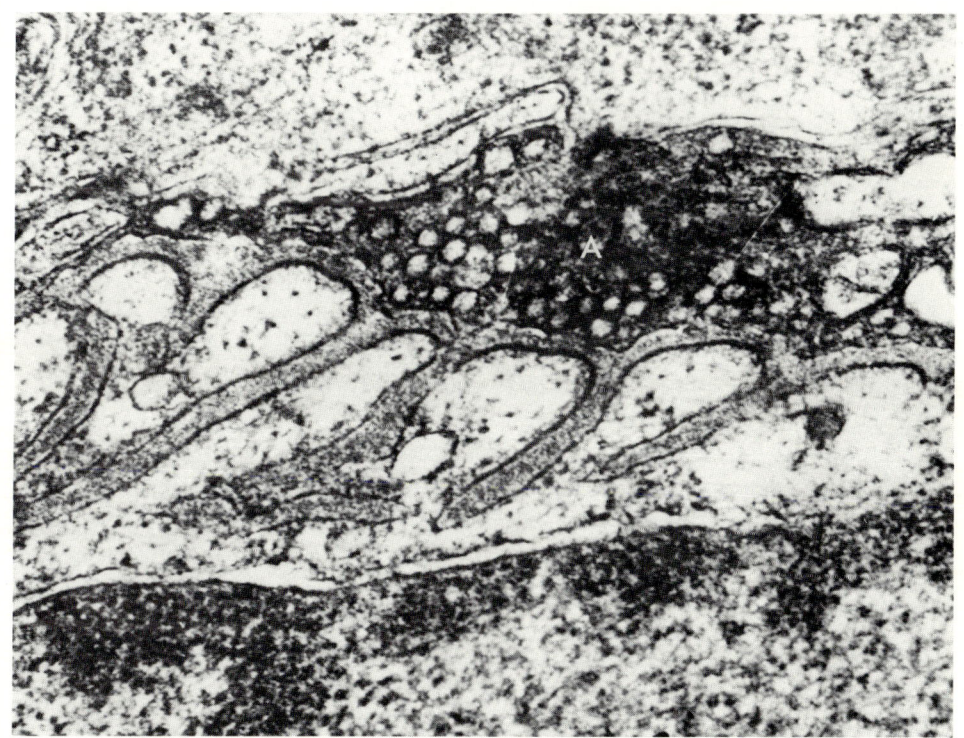

Figure 110. Electron micrograph of a neuromuscular junction from rat diaphragm muscle after incubation for 60 minutes in batrachotoxin. The terminal axon *(A)* is electron dense and contains tightly packed swollen synaptic vesicles. (X 45,000.) (From Albuquerque et al., *J. Pharmacol. & Exp. Therap.* 176:511, 1971.)

tural damage from batrachotoxin whereas the NMJs of *R. pipiens* are damaged.

Snake Toxins

The venoms of various snakes contain numerous neurotoxins as well as other toxic substances. In addition to the phospholipases that are responsible for hemolysis and interference with mitochondrial metabolism, certain elapid (cobras, coral snakes and kraits) toxins contain proteins or polypeptides that are active at the NMJ. Because of this mixture of substances, the clinical symptoms may be exceedingly varied. Venoms may be classified into three groups: neurotoxic, hemotoxic, and depressant (Braganca, 1955). Venoms from the colubrid class of snakes, which includes the Indian cobra *(Naja haje)* produce the most striking neurotoxic effects. Individuals unfortunate enough to be bitten by these snakes usually die as a result of paralysis of respiratory muscles. This effect so resembled curare poisoning, which we recall was brought to the attention of the scientific community by the work of Claude Bernard and others, that many early investigators (Brunton and Fayrer, 1873) suggested that the venoms acted in a similar way. Houssay and Pavé (1922) found that the curare-like activity of snake venoms roughly paralleled their toxicity when tested on the frog. Kellaway (1932, 1937) concluded that nearly all snake venoms contain curare-like activity. Thus it became generally accepted that death from venom poisoning was due to paralysis of the peripheral motor innervation rather than action on the central respiratory center (Kellaway et al., 1932). When solutions containing 2 to 5 mg. per cc. of copperhead, death adder, or cobra venoms were applied to the floor of the fourth ventricle, slowing of respirations to six or seven per minute resulted, and spasmodic respirations with prolonged inspiratory phase were observed. In a few experiments respiration ceased completely. A similar result was obtained when procaine (9 mg. per cc.) was applied to the same region. These investigators therefore concluded that the action of the venoms in this location might be an indirect effect due to vasoconstriction. However, Kellaway (1937) pointed out that the colubrid neurotoxins were unlike curare in that their effects were irreversible except with antivenin. Furthermore, there was no antagonism by eserine (Cushney and Yagi, 1918). Kellaway (1932) was unable to reverse the paralysis produced by the Australian tiger snake and copperhead venom even by giving massive doses of specific antivenin.

The problem of the site of action of snake venoms is further complicated by the observations of Houssay et al. (1922), which indicated that direct excitability is altered in frog muscle preparations exposed to various snake venoms. These changes parallel the hemolytic action of the same toxins on dog red cells. Kellaway and Holden (1932) confirmed the direct action of several venoms on muscle.

Although of interest that AchE is present in the venom of *Naja tripudians* and other snakes (Iyengar et al., 1938), it does not seem likely that the presence of the enzyme is responsible for its neurotoxic effects. For example, AchE is absent in the venom of *Crotalus terrificus*, that has marked neurotoxic activity. Ghosh et al. (1941) demonstrated that AchE activity is distinct from the neurotoxic principle in venom by heating the venom to destroy AchE activity and showing that the venom retained its neurotoxic properties.

More informative data concerning the effects of venoms on tissue metabolism was contributed by Chain (1939), who observed that venom from the black tiger snake inhibits dehydrogenases which use DPN as an electron carrier. The toxic effect was thought to be due to the diphosphopyridine nucleotidase which was present in the toxin. Ghosh and Chatterjee (1948) found that venom of cobras and of several vipers inhibited oxidation of glucose, pyruvate, and succinate in pigeon brain minces. This appeared to be due to inhibition of the cytochrome oxidase system. Studies by Chatterjee (1949) contributed more information concerning the effects of pH, temperature, and ultraviolet light on the stability of the inhibitor of cytochrome oxidase in cobra venom. Other studies by Fleckenstein et al. (1950) further contributed to information on dehydrogenase inhibition produced by snake venoms. Braganca (1955) found that the heated venom that retained its toxicity in mice was free of all enzymatic activity with the exception of lecithinase. She suggested that the action of heated venom is due to enzymatic attack on phospholipids in brain (Braganca and Quastel, 1952). Since the heated toxin appears to selectively attack respiratory enzymes that are associated with cellular particles, it is likely that at least part of the mechanism of action of these venoms is due to the attack of lecithinase on the phospholipids in mitochondrial membranes.

In support of this concept, Gautrelet and Corteggiani (1938) showed that low concentrations of cobra venom could release Ach from its bound complex in rat brain. Braganca and Quastel (1952) also found that Ach is freed from brain by heated cobra venom. However, heated cobra venom does not inhibit acetylation of choline by brain extracts in the presence of ATP. This suggests that the activating action observed with heated venom does not depend upon direct action of the choline acetylase system.

The neurotoxin, "cobrotoxin or A toxin", is the most important of the various components of cobra venom. It is responsible for respiratory paralysis. This toxin combines strongly with the Ach receptor of the NMJ producing a nondepolarizing block. The EPP are depressed without changing the resting potential, action potential or nerve spike. The response to repetitive stimulation is similar to that of curarized muscle in that both the EPP amplitude and its time course are prolonged by neostigmine (Lee, 1971). However, high concentrations of cobra venom depress the response of directly stimulated muscles. The release of Ach is unaffected.

The bulk of the evidence indicates specific, irreversible combination of the toxin with AchR. Lester (1970, 1972) has shown that a peptide fraction of cobra venom produces a reversible, curare-like block of frog NMJs. Cobra neurotoxin is a basic polypeptide with a molecular weight of 7000. It contains 4 disulfide groups that are essential for toxicity. Structure-function relationships of *Naja haje* neurotoxins have recently been reported by Chicheportiche et al. (1972).

The banded krait *(Bungarus multicinctus)* possesses a doubly potent mixture of neurotoxins, α and β-bungarotoxins. The α toxin produces nondepolarizing block by acting on the postsynaptic membrane whereas the β form acts presynaptically by preventing the release of Ach from the motor nerve endings without affecting the postsynaptic membrane (Chang and Lee, 1963). β-bungarotoxin eliminates MEPPs after an initial period of increased frequency (Chang and Lee, 1966). The effect is similar to combined curare and botulinum poisoning. The immunochemical characteristics of α-bungarotoxin have been studied by Clark et al. (1972a, b).

In studies of the action of 3 varieties of sea snake venom (erabutoxins) on rat nerve diaphragm preparations, Cheymol et al. (1967) found nearly irreversible blockade of the specific Ach receptors of the postsynaptic membrane in a manner otherwise resembling the action of curare and cobra venom.

Crotoxin

Nondepolarizing blockage of NMJs is produced by crotoxin, a component of rattlesnake venom. This material is tightly fixed to NMJ receptors but has no effect on ganglionic synapses (Brazil, 1966). There have been no attempts to localize the sites of binding nor have ultrastructure studies been done.

Morphology of NMJs Poisoned by Snake Venom. *Classical Staining Methods.* No studies of morphologic changes in NMJs stained by classical methods were found in literature.

Electron Microscopic Studies. Because of the data indicating an attack by the phospholipases of snake venom on phospholipid-containing membranes, it was of interest to study the effect of cobra venom on the fine structure of NMJs. In unpublished experiments by Zacks and Sheff, white mice were injected via the intraperitoneal route with cobra venom *(Naja haje)* in concentrations of 0.3 to 9 micrograms per gram. The mice were sacrificed a short time before their expected time of death as previously determined by a series of dose-response experiments.

No alterations were found in the axolemma or muscle surface membrane either at the surface or within the secondary synaptic clefts. Furthermore, no decrease in the number of synaptic vesicles was found. Even when very low toxin concentrations were used and the mice survived for several hours, no abnormalities of fine structure were observed. Subsequent studies have shown that *Naja haje* toxin acts on the postsynaptic receptors rather than the terminal axon. Now that purified venom neurotoxins are available, it is practical to localize their binding sites with fluorochrome labeled antibodies or for ultrastructure investigations, horseradish peroxidase labeled antibodies. Tiru-Chelvan (1972) found that fluorescein-labelled antivenin demonstrated localization of *Bothrops* neurotoxin in the medulla and cervical cord whereas *Crotalis* venom a hemolytic toxin, also was localized in renal tubules and in the walls of blood vessels.

Chen and Lee (1970) found that α toxin which acts on the postsynaptic membrane has no effect on the ultrastructure of mouse NMJs whereas β toxin, which acts presynaptically depleted the synaptic vesicles. By 2 hours, there was nearly complete depletion of synaptic vesicles and swelling of mitochondria. Furthermore, there were numerous indentations of the axolemma which they interpreted as sites of opening of synaptic vesicles.

14

The Pathology of Neuromuscular Junctions

This chapter is concerned with the available data on pathologic alterations in NMJs produced by age, and by a variety of neuromuscular diseases occurring naturally in man and laboratory animals.

Before considering the pathology of these diseases, it is useful to consider morphologic changes in NMJs reported to occur under a variety of conditions to compare with the changes caused by disease. Carey recognized the variability of neuromuscular relationships which he believed resulted from ameboid motion of the NMJs. In a series of more than 13 contributions in 8 years, Carey reported on alleged ameboid motion and evidence of neurosecretion in gold stained NMJs under a wide variety of experimental conditions, including carbon dioxide (1941a, b), electric shock (1942), curare, quinine, and Ach (19441), DDT (1946), lactic acid (1944), traumatic shock (1945), thermal shock (1946), nerve section (1946), and disuse atrophy (1948). This series of reports included many unusual views on the structure and implied physiologic function of NMJs. As has been pointed out by several critics (Harris, 1954; Denz, 1951), two main objections to this work may be made: first, the method of staining is notoriously uncertain and poorly controlled; and secondly, the normal range of NMJ variation was not adequately controlled nor was any correlation made with the muscle fiber diameter. A discussion of these limitations is particularly well stated in a report by Denz (1951). Denz concluded that methods of staining with gold, silver, and methylene blue are inadequate to study morphologic changes in NMJs caused by drugs.

Even if the alleged structural changes in NMJs described by Carey are accepted as unreliable findings, many of his inferences concerning physiologic function, such as increasing the junctional area to increase synaptic contact and therefore functional activity have found some support in subsequent work. This early work suggested that structural changes may well occur in NMJs particularly within the terminal nerve branches and postsynaptic apparatus under various chemical and physical stresses, although these are undoubtedly not demonstrable by means of conventional optical microscopy. We know that the terminal nerve branches, at least during embryogenesis and regeneration of NMJs, possess a considerable degree of plasticity. It is possible that these branches may also respond to transient physical and chemical stimuli. If some of Carey's experiments were repeated with the aid of electron microscopy, some of the changes originally claimed by Carey, using insufficient methodology, might be found. Thus, perhaps, this experimental approach should not be considered a closed chapter. More recent attempts to produce morphologic alterations in NMJ structure by various means, but still using classical staining methods, have been reported.

Cole (1957) induced atrophy in rat muscles by pinning the leg to produce immobilization and followed the changes in the NMJs at 7, 14, 21 and 28 day intervals. After 7 days of immobilization, the NMJs were said to be enlarged. However, they decreased in size from the fourteenth to the twenty-first day. At 28 days, the NMJs and the myofibers appeared larger than the controls. There was no evidence of degeneration. The occasional swelling or shrinkage that occurred in NMJs was attributed to changes in the myofiber.

In an attempt to clarify the obscure neuromuscular dysfunction following cold injury (Senay et al., 1956; Sayen et al., 1960), Sayen (1962) stained NMJs by the gold chloride method in rabbit leg muscles exposed to cold water for varying periods of time. This investigator found many variations in the size and shape of NMJs in the control preparations. However, in the animals subjected to cold injury, there was alteration in the ratio of the number of NMJs to the number of terminal axons (EP : TA). Immediately after immersion, no changes in this ratio were detected, whereas after 24 hours, the ratio became small owing to decreased numbers of stained NMJs. By 168 hours after immersion the normal ratio was restored. Previously chilled muscles showed evidence of "collateral regenerative formations". Illustrations provided in this report show staining of peripheral axons but no visible stain within the terminal arborizations.

Sayen did not use other staining methods to clarify the fate of the apparently missing NMJs. She did not indicate a preference for the two obvious alternatives: (1) that the NMJs had been destroyed, or (2) that they were grossly intact but had lost their aurophilia. The former possibility seems more likely in view of the evidence of collateral branching. Apparently the terminal axons were injured since the subneural apparatus persists for long periods of time following denervation. It is also possible that the aurophilia of the external lamina or postsynaptic membrane was destroyed in a fashion analogous to the loss of lead staining caused by freezing (Savay and Csillik, 1948). We may speculate that gold is bound to the same structure as lead in the unfixed NMJ and that the phenomenon of nostaining with gold after cold injury is due to similar alteration at the binding sites.

Age Changes in Neuromuscular Junctions

Also important in consideration of morphologic changes in NMJs caused by disease are the alterations in structure that result from normal aging. Using histochemical staining for soleplate AchE activity, Gutmann and Hanzlíková (1965) studied NMJs in extensor digitorum and soleus muscles of rats 10 days to 24 months of age.

They found irregular innervation patterns in the muscles of the aged rats that they attributed to random degeneration and regeneration of NMJs. AchE staining of the soleplates in aged rat muscles was irregular, possibly due to decline in the availability of "trophic factors" that regulate this enzyme activity (see page 260). Barker and Ip (1965, 1966) also concluded that NMJs had a limited life span and that during the life of the animal there is a continuous replacement of NMJs. The mechanism for this rejuvenation includes formation of new terminal branches which enter previously established soleplate areas or the formation of new NMJs adjacent to the old by means of collateral sprouting.

In a quantitative study of NMJs in cat peroneus digiti quinti and soleus muscles, Tuffery (1971) found significant changes in the NMJs from old cats These NMJs were more complex in the sense that there were increased numbers of myelinated branches arising from terminal axons. Although the young peroneus digiti quinti muscles had more complex NMJs than the soleus muscle, this difference was accentuated in the older muscles. Extremely abnormal NMJs with axonal swellings were occasionally observed in the muscles of the older cats. Tuffery (1971) concluded that there is no causal relationship between growth and degeneration and that when NMJ degeneration occurs, there is a corresponding loss of myofibers. Increased complexity of NMJs in his view is an attempt to compensate for an increasing muscle workload or possibly the result of a decrease in the "trophic" activity of the neuron. Gutmann et al. (1971), using the electron microscope, were unable to find morphologic evidence of denervation in NMJs from aged rats although muscle atrophy was present. Changes in synaptic vesicles, neurotubules, external lamina and junctional clefts were observed and electrophysiological measurements revealed slowing of many parameters of myofiber contraction.

Pathologic Changes in Human Neuromuscular Junctions

It is surprising perhaps, in view of the thoroughness of the early studies of NMJ structure, that human NMJ pathology was largely neglected until recently. Only occasional attempts were made to find abnormalities in diseases thought to be of neuromuscular origin (Woolard, 1926; Chor, 1933; Falin and Kanarejkin, 1940). This neglect probably stemmed from the relatively late development of neurophysiologic methods adequate for the localization of neuromuscular dysfunction within NMJs. In addition, available staining methods were capricious and not well suited to the study of human biopsy material. NMJs were difficult to locate until improved methods utilizing methylene blue for finding them were developed (Coërs, 1952a, 1953b). Because of the marked variation in myofiber cross section area and proportional synaptic area in normal muscle biopsy specimens as well as the normal occurrence of collateral branching in 7-18% of the specimens, considerable caution must be used in interpreting the significance of innervation abnormalities revealed by methylene blue staining (Reske-Nielsen et al., 1970).

As reviewed in chapter 11, considerable emphasis was given to the study of the course of peripheral nerve regeneration and reinnervation of NMJs because of the practical clinical implications of this process. Neurosurgeons have long been interested in the proper repair of pe-

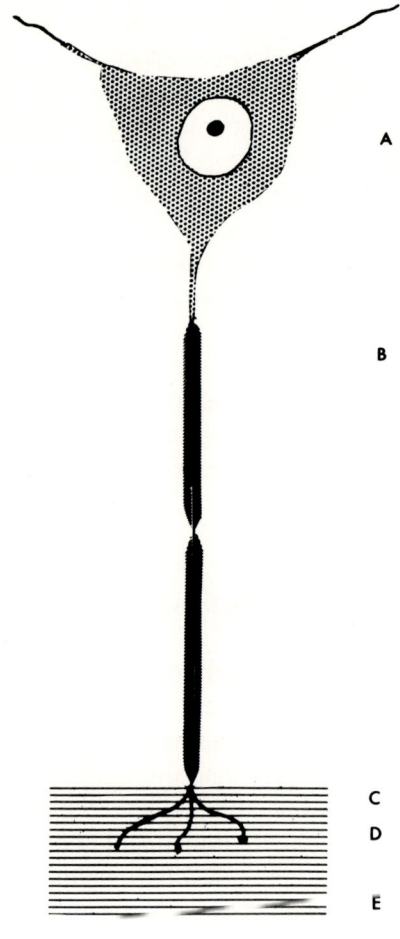

Figure 111. Diagram of the motor neuron innervating an underlying myofiber. The various possible sites of pathology are indicated by the letters *A* through *E*. *A* represents the cell body, *B* the axon, *C* the subterminal nerve fibers, *D* the neuromuscular junction and *E* the underlying myofiber.

ripheral nerve injuries and the results that might be expected under various conditions. The importance of early suture and the role of fibrosis and atrophy on functional reestablishment of NMJs were greatly clarified by the studies of Gutmann et al. (1942), Gutmann and Young (1944), and Hoffman (1950, 1951).

Classification of Diseases of the Motor Unit

Diseases of the motor unit may be simply classified by considering where disease might affect the various portions of the intact motor neuron and its processes. These levels may be divided into the cell body (soma), the axon with its associated myelin covering, the terminal branches of the axon, and the terminal arborization. The postsynaptic component represented by the subneural apparatus must also be included as a possible site for disease. Furthermore, primary muscle disease may also produce secondary changes in NMJs, a phenomenon that must be considered when we try to relate anatomic and physiologic abnormalities in NMJ structure to various disease entities. Thus disease affecting one or more of these elements of the lower motor neuron unit may be expressed in pathologic changes in NMJs. Figure 111 illustrates these levels of possible pathologic abnormality.

Diseases Affecting the Neuron Cell Body

Diseases affecting the cell body of the lower motor neuron may be inflammatory, such as poliomyelitis, or may be of "degenerative" nature of unknown etiology, such as amyotrophic lateral sclerosis, progressive muscular atrophy, and Werdnig-Hoffmann disease.

Numerous disease processes affect the terminal axon and surrounding Schwann cell and Key-Retzius sheaths. Penetrating wounds may sever nerves, producing wallerian degeneration and subsequent muscle atrophy. Mechanical pressure on nerve roots resulting from various causes, several inflammatory diseases caused by bacteria and viruses, and numerous metabolic abnormalities are encountered at this level. In addition, there are several poorly understood disease processes yielding demyelination and ultimate destruction of axons. All these diseases may ultimately interfere with neuromuscular function. Other disease processes appear chiefly to involve the terminal nerve branches.

Diseases Directly Affecting Neuromuscular Junctions

At the NMJ level, studies of fine structure anatomy suggest that some diseases involve the presynaptic as well as the postsynaptic membranes. Diseases believed to involve the NMJ directly include myasthenia gravis and possibly amyotonia congenita. Neurotoxins such as botulinus toxin, various snake venoms, and spider venom also act at the NMJ.

Diseases Affecting Muscle Fibers

Diseases primarily involving the myofibers include inflammatory states caused by various organisms, familial periodic paralysis, and a group of dystrophic diseases characterized in some cases by myotonia. It seems likely that nondystrophic myotonia and idiopathic myoglobinuria should also be classified as primary diseases of muscle on the basis of present knowledge.

Principle Pathologic Changes in Neuromuscular Junctions

Regardless of the nature of the underlying pathologic process, the pathologic changes that can be recognized in conventionally stained NMJs are relatively few when examined in the optical microscope. The principal pathologic changes revealed by gold, silver, methylene blue, and histochemical staining consist of variation in size of soleplates, "degenerative" changes in the nerve fibers and endings, and reactive sprouting. In a few neuromuscular diseases, ultrastructure data is also available.

Changes in Size of Neuromuscular Junctions

As reported by several investigators, the dimensions of NMJs (greatest dimensions of the soleplate) vary with the size of the innervated myofiber (Coërs, 1955a, b; Harris, 1954). Thus on hypertrophied muscle fibers it is not surprising to find unusually large and complicated soleplates. Large soleplates also occur on spastic muscles (chronic degeneration of the lower motor neuron) and in myotonia congenita. Unusually small NMJs are present in muscular dystrophy and denervation atrophy and probably represent newly formed NMJs.

Degenerative and Reactive Changes

Evidence of "degeneration" of NMJs has been confined to various abnormalities in the terminal arborization within the soleplate. Variations in pattern and diameter of the nerve fibrils such as unusual thickness, thinness, beading, and so forth have been reported in various neuromuscular diseases (Woolf, 1959). For example, in the acute lesions of poliomyelitis, swelling of axon branches can be observed in the terminal arborization after staining with methylene blue. Later the arborization is fragmented and the axonic debris is removed.

In peripheral neuritis, however, few abnormalities can be identified in either the nerve or the NMJs. As pointed out by Coërs and Woolf (1959) degenerative changes are most easily observed when the disease process is slow, as in diabetic neuropathy. In this condition the earliest change consists of swelling of the terminal nerve fibers, which may have a foamy appearance in methylene blue-stained preparations. NMJ degeneration is often, but not always, accompanied by swelling of terminal nerve fibers. Coërs and Woolf (1959) also observed that the subneural apparatus may show corresponding changes, consisting of a single large unit with well preserved subneural lamellas. In the last stages of degeneration, after the soleplates lose their connections with the terminal nerve fiber, the soleplates may disintegrate or persist for variable periods of time.

Degeneration of the nerve fibers may produce several patterns. Typical wallerian degeneration is seen in several acute neuromuscular diseases leading to peripheral nerve destruction. In chronic diseases affecting the peripheral nerve, degenerative changes are most often seen in the subterminal nerve fibers, rather than in the intramuscular nerve trunks (Coërs and Woolf, 1959).

More recently, ultrastructure studies of denervation and reinnervation of NMJs in experimental animals have suggested morphologic criteria for recognizing atrophic, reinnervated and newly formed NMJs (pg. 245).

Sprouting of Nerve Fibers

The phenomenon of reactive sprouting is believed to have considerable importance in the evolution of pathologic processes involving NMJs. According to Coërs and Woolf (1959), degeneration of nerve fibers and NMJs in human neuromuscular diseases is rarely seen without some evidence of axonal sprouting. These axons arise from injured nerve trunks and adjacent intact nerve fibers. In the early stages, regardless of the nature of the neuromuscular disease, the patterns of nerve fiber sprouting appear quite similar. Multiple filaments arising from the parent ultraterminal or subterminal nerve fibers each terminate in a small, pyramidal growth cone. Because of multiple sprouts, a single axon may give rise to large numbers of collaterals. When the collaterals form NMJs, there is an increase in the number of myofibers innervated by a single neuron. Axonal sprouting is particularly prominent when the nerve cell body is minimally and chronically injured by disease. Microscopic identification of one subterminal fiber innervating three or more muscle fibers is regarded as diagnostic of previous degeneration and reinnervation by Coërs and Woolf (1959) because only 10 per cent of normal NMJs have subterminal fiber innervation of more than one muscle fiber.

Collateral sprouting of intact nerve fibers as a response to degeneration of adjacent nerve fibers was demonstrated by Edds (1950) and Hoffman (1950) in partially denervated muscle. They observed collateral outgrowths from surviving motor nerve fibers and NMJs, which reinnervated persisting denervated NMJs. This was usually completed before the interrupted nerve fiber could regenerate back to the muscle. The result was hyperneurotization — two axons supplying in a single NMJ. Weiss and Edds (1946) had previously deduced that such reinnervation occurred by indirect means and believed that the stimulus for axonal sprouting might be some material released from degenerating nerve fibers or soleplates.

Causey and Hoffman (1955) demonstrated that ultramicroscopic sprouts (0.1μ) develop within 24 to 48 hours of the onset of degeneration of adjacent nerve fibers. Some sprouting appears to occur even in normal soleplates free of evidence of degeneration, especially in subjects recovering from poliomyelitis or peripheral neuritis. This phenomenon is related to the extensive axon sprouting and branching that occurs in experimental denervation. When skeletal muscle degenerates, as in myotonic dystrophy and thyrotoxic myopathy, axonal sprouting may be extensive. The sprouts arise from the distal part of the subterminal nerve fibers, and anastomoses between sprouts are frequent. Occasionally there are many more sprouts than original nerve fibers, a situation that gives rise to multiple NMJs on individual muscle fibers. The process producing such a tangle is termed "neurocladism". When muscle atrophy rather than degeneration occurs, axon sprouting tends to be inconspicuous, though some beaded nerve fibers can be found in methylene blue stained preparations. In simple muscle atrophy no sprouts appear, and simplification and reduction in size of soleplates and number of nerve fibers are the rule.

The phenomenon of reinnervation via lateral sprouting observed by Gutmann and Young (1944), Bowden (1954), and Coërs and Woolf (1959) in human biopsy specimens appears to be an important mechanism operating to restore normal function in patients with neuromuscular disease.

The work of Coërs and Woolf summarized in their monograph (1959) represents the most extensive studies of human neuromuscular diseases employing methylene blue and cholinesterase staining. We shall frequently refer to the publications of these investigators in the following description of NMJ abnormalities in specific human neuromuscular diseases. We must bear in mind, however, that these techniques show only a limited aspect of the complex NMJ structure. We agree with Coërs and Woolf that the changes shown by methylene blue staining are not entirely specific but nonetheless may be of value in diagnosis and prognosis of neuromuscular disease. For example, an increased functional terminal innervation ratio indicates neural degeneration but may be associated with myositis. Prognosis should be good when methylene blue staining shows continuity of axons in NMJs even in the presence of complete paralysis, especially if clinical indications suggest that the active disease process may be limited such as in poliomyelitis and the Guillain-Barré syndrome. On the other hand, if the nerve bundles lack nerve fibers, it is less likely that restoration of function will be accomplished. Coërs and Woolf (1959) point out that a single biopsy specimen cannot serve as a basis for predicting the future course of the disease with certainty. One can only determine the likely course of the disease process and gain some insight into the likelihood of eventual functional recovery if the disease appears clinically arrested. Collateral sprouting, which is capable of producing functional reinnervation of muscle fibers, is an important mechanism that helps explain rapid clinical recovery after severe partial denervation (Hoffman, 1950) and the late appearance of muscle weakness in peripheral neuritis and root compression syndromes. This mechanism also helps explain the electromyographic findings of polyphasic potentials in these conditions.

DISEASES OF THE MOTOR NERVE CELL BODY

Poliomyelitis

Acute polimyelitis is now known to be a disease primarily affecting the lower motor neuron cell body, caused by one of three types of neurotropic viruses. Soon after infection the virus produces injury or total destruction of scattered anterior horn cells within the spinal cord. Before the pathogenesis of poliomyelitis was understood, Chor (1933) found extensive injury of nerve fibers and NMJs after staining with a silver method. Carey (1943a) and Carey et al. (1944b), using a gold-staining method, reported abnormalities in monkey NMJs after experimental poliomyelitis infection. Dublin et al. (1944) found that changes in human muscle, consisting of degenerated nerve fibers, soleplates, and muscle fibers, were proportional to the degree of paralysis suffered by the patient. The irregular distribution of the muscular lesions corresponded to the irregularity of the injured neurons within the spinal cord. No evidence of regeneration of nerve fibers was found. These investigators concluded that both peripheral nerve fibers and changes were the result of disease of the nerve cell bodies. Methylene blue staining of muscle biopsies performed two months after the onset of poliomyelitis showed in some cases that no motor nerve fibers or soleplates could be found, whereas sensory and intrafusal nerve fibers were preserved (Coërs and Woolf, 1959). The AchE activity was still detectable in the subneural apparatuses in the early cases, but the subneural "cups" were poorly stained. Return of muscle power was apparently due to collateral reinnervation. Silver-stained soleplates, five to six months after acute onset of poliomyelitis, contained broad, swollen axons that were interpreted as possibly of sensory origin. The terminal innervation ratio was increased. As many as eight NMJs were formed by one nerve fiber during the process of collateral reinnervation.

MOTOR NEURON DISEASE

Amyotrophic Lateral Sclerosis, Progressive Muscular Atrophy, and Infantile Forms of Muscle Atrophy

These motor neuron diseases of unknown etiology have many features in common.

Amyotrophic lateral sclerosis is characterized by progressive wasting of muscles, particularly in the upper arms. Other muscles innervated by motor neurons in the medulla are also affected. Symptoms of pyramidal degeneration are prominent clinical features. Disease patterns characterized primarily by lower motor neuron disease (Aran, 1850; Duchenne, 1853) were separated by Charcot and Joffroy (1869) from disease patterns that also included pyramidal signs and symptoms. The former group were classified as "progressive muscular dystrophy" and the latter as "amyotrophic lateral sclerosis." Usually mixtures of both types are encountered clinically. Similar disease entities in infants are spinal muscular atrophy (Werdnig, 1891; Hoffman, 1893) and "amyotonia congenita" (Oppenheim, 1900). More chronic forms of degeneration of anterior horn neurons occur in the syndrome of Kugelberg and Welander (1956) where there is childhood onset and slow progression. Inheritance by a non sex linked recessive gene has also been demonstrated. All of these lesions lead to loss of motor innervation with consequent denervation atrophy of the affected muscles. In addition to muscular atrophy, the muscles of these patients frequently have myopathic features including variation in myofiber diameter, central location of sarcolemmal nuclei, muscle giant cells, necrosis and regeneration. Although these syndromes differ in age of onset, familial tendencies, and rate of progression, they are all characterized by primary degeneration of motor neurons. It might be expected, therefore, that NMJ lesions should be present.

Wohlfart (1955, 1957) described swelling and metachromatic degeneration of neural growth cones in amyotrophic lateral sclerosis. He believed that the growth cones degenerated into amyloid bodies. Pommé and Noël (1934) observed decreased numbers of soleplate granules ("telosomes") in NMJs from patients suffering from progressive muscular atrophy. Coërs and Woolf (1959) described the results of a series of 36 biopsies from patients with motor neuron disease stained by the methylene blue method. They found that in rapidly progressive cases of amyotrophic lateral sclerosis, the NMJ abnormalities resembled abnormalities seen in Werdnig-Hoffmann disease. Fine, beaded branched fibers were present in the intramuscular nerve trunks, and little evidence of distal sprouting was found. Biopsies from patients with less rapidly progressive disease demonstrated muscle fiber hypertrophy, large complex soleplates, and collateral reinnervation. Pearce and Harriman (1966) also used the intravital methylene blue technic to study terminal axons in patients with chronic spinal muscular atrophy.

There was histologic evidence of branching of subterminal axons and collateral innervation suggesting repair of previous denervation. Although no ultrastructure studies of terminal innervation in this disease have come to my attention, one would expect that the kind of changes following nerve section should be found.

An Animal Model of Motor Neuron Disease

Evidence of a hereditary motor neuron disease resembling human motor neuron disease has been described in the "Wobbler" mouse (wr). This disease, which arose from a spontaneous mutation, is transmitted by a single autosomal recessive gene (Falconer, 1956). The mice have progressive muscular weakness and atrophy and histological preparations from brain and skeletal muscle reveal evidence of degeneration of motor neurons in the brain stem and spinal cord and motor denervation of skeletal muscle (Duchen and Strich, 1968). Andrews and Maxwell (1967) described many vesicles in the cytoplasm of ventral horn cells in the "Wobbler" mouse which in some cases, nearly replaced the cytoplasm. They suggested that a primary degeneration of the neuron causes the clinical syndrome.

Dying Back Neuropathy

The phenomenon of "dying back" (Greenfield, 1964) refers to the form of degeneration of neurons that is first manifested by alterations in the distal portion of the axon. This phenomenon was first described by Mott (1896). Distal degeneration of long axons occurs in metabolic deficiencies such as thiamin deficiency and in tri-ortho-cresyl-phosphate (TOCP) and acrylamide polyneuropathy as well as an obscure entity, distal neuronitis (Bauwens, 1955, 1957). Cavanagh (1954) found that the distal extremities of nerve fibers were first attacked in TOCP poisoning.

The "dying back" phenomenon in Werdnig-Hoffmann disease is characterized by normal-appearing nerve fibers in the larger intramuscular bundles. However, the smaller nerve fibers are beaded and form complex tangles of beaded fibers, some of which may in turn give rise to small, single terminal expansions on narrow muscle fibers (Woolf and Till, 1955). Small and poorly developed NMJs were also observed on normal-sized myofibers. When the disease process begins *in utero,* there is failure of innervation and the muscle fibers fail to develop normally. When the disease develops later, the pattern of denervation characterized by muscle atrophy is seen. Collateral reinnervation occurs, especially in cases with muscle hypertrophy.

Histochemical staining for AchE activity revealed occasional normal-appearing subneural apparatuses. The common appearance, however, was that of simplified soleplates with relatively low AchE activity, as indicated by the necessity for prolonged incubation with the histochemical reagents. In an ultrastructure study of TOCP neuropathy, Prineas (1969a) demonstrated accumulation of abnormal membrane bound vesicles and tubules within the axoplasm of small motor nerve terminals in the foot muscles of cats as well as in the spinal gray matter approximately a week before the onset of neurologic signs. At the time when neurological injury became clinically evident, large concentrically laminated osmiophilic bodies were found in the terminal axon expansions within NMJs (Fig. 108) as well as in synaptic knobs on spinal cord anterior horn neurons. Prineas concluded that the fine structure changes in the NMJs did not resemble the changes that occur following nerve transection. The mechanism of this form of peripheral axonal degeneration is not clear, but in general abnormal synthetic processes in the neuron cell body were thought to be responsible for the transport, via the nerve fiber, of abnormal products to the axon terminal.

In experimental acrylamide intoxication in cats, the dying-back phenomena first occurs in terminal axons and is characterized by marked increase in the number of neurofilaments. Prineas (1969b) concluded that the changes in subcellular organelles preceding degeneration of the distal axon branches differs in acrylamide neuropathy from the changes observed in TOCP polyneuropathy.

Similar changes in the terminal axon expansions occur in experimental thiamine deficiency in rats. Prineas (1970) demonstrated occasional degenerating terminal axon expansions within NMJs containing accumulations of mitochondria, dense and laminated bodies and membrane bound sacs. Severe degeneration of the NMJs was associated with nearby multivesicular bodies but myelin debris was rarely observed. Abnormalities in the intramuscular nerve branches were found in the muscles of nearly all of the thiamine deficient animals consisting of nonspecific degeneration of myelin and alterations of the axoplasm. The axoplasm contained accumulations of flattened membrane bound sacs and decreased numbers of neurotubules and neurofilaments.

Coërs and Woolf (1959) concluded that the appearance of the NMJs in various neuromuscular diseases stained by the methylene blue method varies with the tempo of development of the disease. When rapid, the changes observed in the terminal axons are similar to those that occur in Werdnig-Hoffmann disease; namely fine, beaded, branched axons and little distal sprouting. In less rapidly progressive disease, hypertrophy of myofibers occurs with formation of large complex soleplates accompanied by collateral branching arising from adjacent less affected or unaffected nerve fibers.

Peroneal Muscular Atrophy

This disease, first described by Charcot and Marie (1886), is characterized by muscular atrophy affecting the small muscles of both hands and feet. Lesions are found in the motor nerves (a condition called interstitial neuritis by Buzzard and Greenfield, 1921). Although degeneration of anterior horn cells also occurs, it is not entirely clear which is the initial lesion.

NMJ pathology in this disease is similar to that of amyotrophic lateral sclerosis.

Upper Motor Neuron Disease

Few observations on the pathology of NMJs in upper motor neuron disease and parkinsonism have been made. Coërs and Woolf (1959) suggested that hemiparesis with increased muscle tone tends to encourage great increase of peripheral nerve sprouting. This is expressed as repeated branching of the subterminal fibers on multiple well formed or small NMJs. Occasional spherical, palestained swellings were observed on the terminal axons, indicating possible degeneration. ChE activity was demonstrated in the enlarged subneural apparatuses. These changes were interpreted as being due to repeated trauma to hypertonic muscle fibers. Similar changes were seen in a case of parkinsonism. Terminal sprouting occurring in these diseases, unlike that seen in diseases of the lower motor neuron, produced large and multiple NMJs, which did not increase the functional terminal innervation ratio.

Neuromuscular Junction Pathology
in Diseases of Peripheral Nerve

The clinical forms of neuritis are legion and the corresponding pathology is complex and controversial. If we limit our consideration toperipheral neuritis, a term often used to refer to polyneuritis, we encounter bacterial, toxic, metabolic, ischemic, and a poorly understood group of miscellaneous entities. Clinical signs and symptoms in acute febrile polyneuritis include paresthesias and weakness, which begin at the periphery and spread proximally, accompanied by flaccid paralysis and sensory and reflex loss. Toxic, alcoholic, diabetic, and other disease entities show differing patterns. It is therefore not surprising that studies of NMJs in these conditions are few. In many of these disease entities it is not clear whether the cell body, the peripheral nerve, or the nerve terminal is the primary site of the disease process. As we have seen, secondary changes in NMJs may be expected when other portions of the neuron are diseased. In some cases of neuritis it is the axons that appear to be primarily affected, whereas in others it is the myelin sheath. Because the neural bundle is a complex structure of many cells, it is possible that various forms of neuritis may affect different portions selectively. When complete paralysis is present clinically, histologic examination of biopsy specimens often reveals no trace of the NMJs. Frequently even axonic debris is absent. In other cases the subterminal nerve fibers appear to degenerate. They are characterized by finely beaded neural sprouts ending in abnormal terminal arborizations. However, some cases of neuritis show normal nerve fibers and NMJs, whereas in others only axons are swollen and pale-staining. In many cases of peripheral neuritis described by Coërs and Woolf (1959), occasional NMJs were swollen, with swelling confined to a single portion of the terminal expansion, or several portions of the terminal arborization fused together to form a blob. During recovery from neuritis, collateral reinnervation was very pronounced in some cases. Even years after complete recovery from peripheral neuritis, coarsely beaded nerve fibers lying parallel to atrophic muscle fibers gave rise to short, poorly formed collateral sprouts that ended in poorly formed NMJs.

Some viruses show marked selectivity for different components of the neuron. Coxsackie virus A spares nerve fibers and attacks striated muscle, whereas the B virus spares skeletal muscle and attacks the nerve fibers and NMJs (Sanz Ibáñez, 1951).

"Amyotonia Congenita"

Several entities are probably included in the clinical diagnosis of "amyotonia congenita". In some, the cause of muscular weakness appears to be a form of polyneuritis (Debré and Thieffry, 1951; Chambers and MacDermot, 1957) whereas in others the lesion appears to lie in the neuromuscular apparatus. Coërs and Woolf (1959) examined muscle biopsies from two children who clinically presented as examples of "amyotonia congenita". In the younger child they found loss of muscle fibers as well as some normal, some very elaborate, and some poorly formed NMJs. In the older child, single axons innervated several muscle fibers, providing evidence of previous denervation and subsequent reinnervation. These investigators also described NMJ changes in these cases were quite variable; some demonstrated excessive branching of the intramuscular nerve fibers, and others had normal subneural apparatuses, as demonstrated by AchE staining. Other findings in these cases were small NMJs, loss of myelinated fibers, and degenerative shrinking of NMJs with fine ultraterminal sprouts and anastomoses of distal parts of the subterminal nerve fibers.

Alcoholic polyneuritis and vitamin B deficiency disease produced loss of axons but little evidence of reinnervation in some cases (Coërs and Woolf, 1959), whereas other biopsy specimens demonstrated complex terminal arborizations and "ribbon-like" axon swellings.

B_{12} Deficiency Polyneuritis

In subacute combined degeneration due to deficiency of vitamin B_{12}, degeneration of sensory nerves (Greenfield and Carmichael, 1935) and motor nerves (Woolf, 1956) has been described. Changes in the motor nerve endings observed by Coërs and Woolf (1959) also occur in pernicious anemia and other diseases with low serum levels of vitamin B_{12}. In these cases the intramuscular nerve fibers have a peculiar series of regularly spaced fusiform swellings that are lightly stained by methylene blue. Occasionally axons that stained dark blue were observed within the swellings. Spherical axon swellings and fusion of swellings on the terminal arborizations were also observed. Some subterminal nerve fibers had finely beaded sprouts and balloon-shaped NMJs. Collateral branching with formation of double NMJs also ofcurred. Occasionally the material in the axon swellings was metachromatic.

Friede (1963) reported the formation of axonal swellings indistinguishable from similar swellings in pathologic nerve as a result of the application of longitudinal electric current to fresh nerve. The axonal swellings produced in this way contained accumulations of mitochondria, proteins, and ribonucleic acid. There was also an increase in oxidative enzyme activity. Somewhat similar changes in the central nervous system of rats kept on a diet deficient in vitamin E have been reported by Lampert et al. (1964). Electron microscopy revealed axon enlargements filled with numerous, frequently abnormal mitochondria and electron-dense bodies of uncertain nature. These observations suggest that there early signs of axon injury may also be responsible for the axon swellings observed in vitamin B_{12} deficiency.

Diabetic Neuropathy and Myopathy

Diabetic polyneuritis, which occurs in middle aged and elderly diabetics, is characterized by loss of tendon reflexes and vibration sense in the lower extremities. Symptoms include cramps, aching, burning, and numbness in the legs. Paralysis is rare but does occur (Greenfield et al., 1960). Pathologic findings include include diffuse and patchy degeneration of peripheral nerves and thickening of small intraneural vessels (Woltman and Wilder, 1929). The concept that small vessel abnormalities are responsible for diabetic neuropathy has been supported by electron microscopic studies, which have demonstrated more or less generalized widening of capillary basement lamina in many tissues of diabetic subjects (Aagenaes and Moe, 1961; Bergstrand and Bucht, 1957; Zacks et al., 1962). It is possible that vascular changes in the vasa nervorum are responsible for the changes in the peripheral nerves of diabetics (Blumenthal, 1963). Capillary disease may interfere with the normal nutritional exchange in peripheral nerves and thereby produce the pathologic abnormalities observed.

Woolf and Malins (1957) employed the methylene blue staining technique to study muscles from diabetic patients. Of this group, some patients had signs and symptoms of typical diabetic neuropathy, whereas other patients were free of symptoms and had only electromyographic evidence of partial denervation. Characteristic abnormalities in the NMJs were found in these diabetic patients. The earliest changes in NMJs consisted of swelling and pale staining of the terminal nerve arborizations. Eventually all the arborizations tended to fuse together to form balloon-shaped masses (Woolf, 1955). It was surprising that a large number of NMJs simultaneously showed this change at a time when the proximal nerve fibers were unaffected. There was little evidence of sprouting or subterminal nerve fiber formation. In preparations stained by the Koelle AchE method, no decrease in number of stainable subneural apparatuses were observed. However, there were decreased numbers of subunits in individual NMJs, some of which seemed abnormally large and possibly were formed by fusion of several subunits. It appeared that only the neural part of the NMJ was affected while the subneural portion was intact, at least by optical microscopic criteria.

A later stage appeared to be NMJ degeneration and subsequent nerve fiber degeneration. Occasionally irregular swollen and pale-stained axons with a few small sprouts were observed. The authors point out that occasional spherical axonic swellings were seen that closely resembled those seen in vitamin B_{12} deficiency and other peripheral neuritides. It was suggested by these workers that diabetes mellitus may primarily affect the anterior horn cell, but demonstration of segmental demyelination in diabetic neuropathy suggests that abnormalities in Schwann cells may be of greater importance in the pathogenesis of this lesion.

Abnormally large or small expansion of the terminal arborizations was described by Coërs and Hildebrand (1965) as an early change that could be recognized in NMJs in diabetic muscle biopsy specimens stained by the methylene blue method. Later, collateral sprouting from subterminal axons and isolated atrophy of myofibers occurred. In late stages, group atrophy of myofibers could be found. The neuromuscular abnormalities in experimental alloxan hyperglycemia were studied in rats by Hildebrand et al. (1968). They found significant reduction in the mean afferent conduction velocity of the nerves after 4 months of hyperglycemia but no decrease in the mean maximum efferent conduction velocity of the nerves after 4 to 6 months of hyperglycemia. The morphology of the NMJs was studied by a modified gold chloride technique. The authors found abnormal collateral and ultraterminal branching of the motor nerve fibers in approximately half of the animals and there was occasional hyperneurotization. There was also segmental demyelination of peripheral nerve fibers after 4 months and demyelination adjacent to the nodes of Ranvier after 3 months of hyperglycemia. No degeneration of the intramuscular axons was observed. The authors concluded that slight neuromuscular changes result from prolonged alloxan-induced hyperglycemia and the defect in neural transmission results from segmental demyelination. This deficit was mostly compensated by distal sprouting of the motor nerve fibers.

Ultrastructure studies of diabetic muscle reveal a variety of nonspecific myopathic changes sufficient to warrant the term diabetic myopathy (Bloodworth and Epstein, 1967).

Norris (1966) demonstrated abnormal neuromuscular transmission in 4 patients with thyroid disease consisting of generalized muscle weakness and easy fatigability. EMG studies revealed abnormal decrease of muscle action potentials evoked by stimulation in 3 patients with myxedema that was improved by anticholinesterase medication. There were no histologic studies of the NMJs or the affected muscles.

Carcinomatous Neuromyopathy

Denny-Brown (1948) described sensory neuropathy in two patients with bronchogenic carcinoma. Since that report, there have been several reports of involvement of peripheral nerve and muscle in patients with malignant disease. The term "carcinomatous neuromyopathy" was introduced by Brain and Henson (1958) to describe this group of neurologic disorders that are not due to direct metastasis of tumor cells. Thus diseases of the central nervous system as well as peripheral nerves are included. Patients with this syndrome have proximal weakness and muscle wasting as well as loss of tendon reflexes. Shy and Silverstein (1965) perferred the term "neuromyopathy" to describe a syndrome restricted to abnormalities of the peripheral nerve and muscle.

Eaton and Lambert (1957) described a syndrome in patients with malignancies that had features resembling myasthenia gravis (myasthenic syndrome). All these syndromes occur primarily in men with bronchogenic carcinoma. Hildebrand and Coërs (1967) studied clinical, electromyographic and histological aspects of this syndrome in 46 patients with lung, gastrointestinal, breast, ovarian and uterine tumors. The only common EMG change found was post tetanic facilitation in 4 patients that occurred in weak and wasted muscles. There was no significant reduction of conduction velocity in the peripheral nerves of any of the patients. However, histological evidence of increased collateral branching of motor nerve fibers was found. The common appearance of the myofibers was uniform atrophy and in 19 of the 46 cases there was abnormal variation in myofiber size. Small myofibers in groups occurred in only 2 cases. Thus, evidence of collateral branching suggested partial denervation. The authors suggested that nutritional factors must be considered in the etiology of carcinomatous neuromyopathy. Muscle biopsies stained with methylene blue (Woolf, 1957; Bickerstaff and Woolf, 1958) in rare instances showed fusion of terminal arborizations, and more commonly, fusiform swellings on the subterminal nerve fibers in carcinomatous neuropathy. Some cases had large axonic swellings similar to those observed in vitamin B_{12} deficiency. Collateral reinnervation was also noted in these cases. The fine structure of NMJs in the Eaton-Lambert syndrome was studied by Fukuhara et al., (1972). They described demyelination and remyelination of intramuscular nerves, atrophy of terminal axons, increased numbers of elongated and widened secondary synaptic clefts and megaconial mitochondria in the myofibers. The changes in the subneural apparatus are unlike the changes that occur in myasthenia gravis (see pg. 358).

An investigation of three patients with carcinomatous neuropathy by Awad (1968) yielded similar morphologic findings. Methylene blue staining revealed axonal swellings, axon fragmentation and axon fusion as well as active collateral sprouting and new NMJ formation. The myofibers were small or medium sized and some were necrotic. Santa et al. (1972) studied the fine structure of intercostal NMJs from patients with the myasthenic syndrome which may occur in patients with bronchogenic carcinoma. They found marked increase in the area of the subneural clefts (see also Fukuhara et al., 1972) and the ratio of postsynaptic to presynaptic membrane length. There was no increase in the numbers of synaptic vesicles. These changes in NMJ fine structure differed from those which occur in myasthenia gravis. Correlated electrophysiologic studies in these patients confirmed the low quantum content of the endplate potential reported by Elmqvist and Lambert (1968).

Inflammatory, immune and metabolic mechanisms have been considered as possible causes of this syndrome but there is no evidence to choose one or another of these hypotheses.

"Distal Neuronitis"

A syndrome thought to be due to a lesion of the terminal axon branches before they enter NMJs was called "distal neuronitis" by Bauwens (1955). This syndrome is characterized by electromyographic evidence of both neuropathic and myopathic degeneration. Bauwens concluded that the lesions must involve the lower motor neuron at a point distal to the site of branching of the nerve fiber in the muscle. Guy et al. (1950) reported similar features in a case of dermatomyositis. Bauwens (1955) suggested that this disease may result from degeneration of terminal axon branches in polyneuritis and neuromyositis. Similar electromyographic findings were obtained by Richardson (1956), who was able to demonstrate neuropathic and myopathic tracings by moving the recording electrode to various sites in muscles affected by myositis. Biopsy specimens stained with methylene blue (Toussaint et al., 1959) revealed degenerative swelling of the subterminal nerve fibers and collateral reinnervation. These investigators suggest that degeneration of the subterminal nerve fibers is the source of the fibrillation potentials and potentials of short duration and low voltage recorded from myositic muscles, whereas the polyphasic potentials of long duration recorded from other parts of the same muscle are due to collateral reinnervation. Bauwens (1957) found that this syndrome also occurred in motor neuron disease when "dying back" from the NMJs occurred.

Spinal Nerve Compression

In cases of spinal nerve compression either by prolapse of intervertebral discs or spinal tumor, the NMJs have well developed collateral reinnervation and increase in the functional terminal innervation ratio. These cases are the naturally occurring parallel of experimental compression injuries. The NMJs stained by methylene blue show increased variation in size and complexity. Finely beaded nerve fibers are less prominent than in NMJs from patients with lower motor neuron disease, although occasional swollen terminal arborizations occur (Coërs and Woolf, 1959).

Diseases Primarily Affecting Neuromuscular Junctions

The point has previously been stressed that in many instances it is not possible to decide which level of the motor neuron is affected by various disease processes. We must rely on clinical and electrophysiologic data to make tentative classifications to serve as the basis for future research.

Before describing what we believe to be the best example of primary NMJ disease, a few isolated reports of NMJ disease not previously discussed in detail are presented. It is uncertain whether these reported abnormalities are primary NMJ lesions or the result of other lesions of the neuron. These conditions include metabolic diseases (vitamin E deficiency), a group of hypotonic diseases ("amyotonia congenita"), and a group of vague diseases characterized by paralysis.

Nutritional and Metabolic Disease Affecting Neuromuscular Junctions

Although Woolard (1926-27) reported abnormalities in rat NMJs revealed by gold and methylene blue staining in experimental beriberi, similar changes were observed after short periods of starvation (in less time than that needed to produce beriberi). Thus the specificity of these results may be challenged. Tsunoda (1928) claimed that in experimental beriberi, pigeon NMJs had irregular outlines and Hines et al. (1943) found no evidence of functional degeneration in acute or prolonged inanition in rats or guinea pigs. Rogers et al. (1931) reported that the finest ramifications of the hypolemmal axons were preserved on muscle fibers that had been completely transformed by hyaline necrosis in experimental nutritional (vitamin E deficiency) "muscular dystrophy" of guinea pigs.

"Amyotonia Congenita"

This congenital disease syndrome, first described by Oppenheim (1900), is usually present at birth and is characterized by marked hypotonicity of all the muscles. There is no paralysis, however. Deep tendon reflexes are absent, and usually the muscles will respond only to galvanic stimulation. More recent studies by Brandt (1950) and Walton

(1956) indicate that amyotonia congenita should be regarded as a syndrome caused by various lesions rather than as a specific entity. In a follow-up of 109 cases, Walton (1956) found that 67 cases ultimately proved to be spinal muscular atrophy, three cases proved to be progressive muscular dystrophy, 20 were due to "cerebral palsy", and the remainder represented a mixed collection of scurvy, spinal ganglioneuroma, arachnodactyly, neuropathy and so forth. This group of cases also included a particularly interesting instance of "benign congenital myopathy with myasthenic features" (Walton et al., 1956). Consequently, description of NMJ abnormalities in the "amyotonia congenita" syndrome must be carefully evaluated in terms of the ultimate diagnosis. Coërs and Pelc (1954) demonstrated simplified NMJs consisting of single globular or elongated masses of axonplasm after methylene blue staining in a case of "amyotonia congenita". Normal terminal arborizations were rare, although the subterminal nerve fibers were normal except for slight beading. Histochemical staining for AchE demonstrated very simple subneural apparatuses in this case. These investigators concluded that although this appearance could be the result of delayed maturation of NMJs, it was more likely to be an example of incomplete regeneration following an unknown degenerative process limited to the terminal axon tips and therefore not associated with axon sprouting or collateral reinnervation. These NMJs appeared similar to those described by Woolf and Till (1955) in a case of Werdnig-Hoffmann disease.

As suggested by Walton (1956), many cases of "amyotonia congenita" ultimately must be classified as spinal muscular atrophy (Werdnig-Hoffmann).

Another case reported by Coërs and Woolf (1959) was that of a 14 month old child with hypotonia who failed to react to electrical stimuli and who showed extremely simple subneural apparatuses and terminal arborizations in methylene blue stained NMJs. Some of the terminal arborizations were present as single ballooned masses of axoplasm. A third case of "amyotonia congenita" had normal motor and sensory innervation, although some smaller than usual subneural apparatuses were demonstrated by histochemical staining. These investigators also described the presence of normal NMJs in three cases of infantile hypotonia associated with mental deficiency or mongolism. No ultrasturcture studies were made in these cases.

Myasthenia Gravis

This fascinating disease, described first by Willis (1672) and then in greater detail by Jolly (1895) and Oppenheim (1887), is characterized by weakness and fatigue of voluntary muscles. Clinical aspects and detailed consideration of the voluminous data concerning the pathophysiology of this disease are well discussed in reviews by Osserman (1958), Viets (1961), and Desmedt (1962a) and in a recent conference volume edited by Fields (1971). For the sake of brevity we can state that the bulk of the evidence indicates a primary defect in the Ach secretion mechanism of the NMJ. This conclusion has been reached as a result of the therapeutic action of various drugs active at the NMJ (Walker, 1934; Aranow et al., 1957) and electromyographic findings of Grob et al. (1956), Grob and Johns (1961) and Desmedt (1961).

Myasthenia Gravis: NMJ Physiology

Despite the extensive data on normal NMJ function that is available, the nature of the lesion in myasthenia gravis has remained obscure. In recent years, refinement of techniques, particularly the use of intracellular microelectrodes had clarified many aspects of the myasthenia gravis problem. The major possible sites of the myasthenic defect are synthesis, packaging and release of Ach from the axon terminal, increased AchE activity, blockade by a circulating blocking agent or abnormal Ach receptors in the postsynaptic membrane. More recently, many investigators have been concerned with immunological aspects of the disease. Hypotheses concerning abnormalities in AchE activity and the presence of a circulating blocking substance seem less promising than possible abnormalities in the pre- or postsynaptic membranes. In the 1959 symposium (Viets, 1961) on myasthenia gravis, much of the discussion was concerned with whether the myasthenic defect was presynaptic in the axon terminal or postsynaptic in the membrane receptors. Although some microelectrode studies favored the former interpretation, data suggesting abnormal receptor action based upon depolarizing compounds responsible for desensitization of receptors led to an emphasis on the postsynaptic membrane.

Grob et al. (1966) studied the effect of intraarterial administration of Ach to patients with generalized myasthenia gravis who responded to anticholinesterase medication. They found that in these patients, the "prompt" depolarizing effect was less severe and that there was a greater "late" depressant effect on the junctions than in normal subjects. The "late" depressant effect of Ach was described as having properties of competitive block with repeated Ach administration or prolonged stimulation. Reversibility of the block by Ach or neostigmine was reduced and the block was changed from the kind that interferred with the depolarizing action of Ach and could be reversed by Ach (competitive block) to a kind of block that inhibited the action of Ach but could not be reversed by Ach. It was also of interest that myasthenic patients who had upper motor neuron disease had great increase in the "prompt" depressant action of Ach in the affected muscles suggesting a change from competitive to depolarizing block. Foldes (1969) suggested that possible alteration of the receptors by a depolarizing agent could explain the myasthenic defect and Grob and Johns (1961) hypothesized that abnormal forms of the receptor substance responding abnormally to normally released Ach caused the block. Choline, the normal product of Ach hydrolysis was also considered as a possible blocking agent.

Desmedt (1956, 1959) was among the first to suggest that there was a presynaptic defect in myasthenia gravis because the post-tetanic variations in the degree of neuromuscular block could not be explained by a postsynaptic defect. He suggested that Ach synthesis in the terminal axon might be impaired or possibly a circulating substance similar to hemicholinium might interfere with Ach synthesis. In a study of endplate potentials from muscle biopsy specimens obtained from myasthenic patients, Dahlbeck et al. (1961) concluded that the block arose in the presynaptic terminal and that the sensitivity of the postsynaptic membrane to Ach was normal. In a more extensive study employing muscle biopsy specimens from myasthenic patients, Elmqvist et al. (1964) made valuable observations on endplate potentials in a group of 8 patients. Despite the fact that cholinesterase medication had been continued and that the muscles studied were not clinically involved, all the biopsy specimens from the patients showed a striking defect in neuromuscular transmission. The characteristic abnormality was a significant reduction in the size of Ach quanta as measured by the resultant junctional depolarization. These investigators concluded that this defect is the sole cause of the neuromuscular block that occurs *in vitro* and seems sufficient to account for the muscle weakness that occurred in patients. Depolarization of NMJs produced by carbachol or decamethonium in specimens of myasthenic muscle studied *in vitro* could not be distinguished from normal muscle and a small depression of MEPP amplitude by antagonists used to inhibit postsynaptic sensitivity occurred with a marked decrease of the carbachol response. This indicated that the postsynaptic membrane Ach receptors of the myasthenic NMJ are normal.

These experiments have ruled out several possible functional abnormalities that were previously considered as the cause of the transmission block in myasthenia gravis. For example, demonstration of a normal quantum content of the endplate potentials obtained following stimulation at several frequencies eliminates the previous hypothesis that Ach quanta in the storage site are deficient. This data also indicates that liberation of the Ach quanta is normal. Since there was no restoration of quantal size following application of cholinesterase inhibitors, the possible role of increased AchE activity is also ruled out. Maintenance of normal Ach diffusion is also suggested since the recorded endplate potentials had a normal time course. Elmqvist et al. (1964) also provided evidence that there is no major limitation of the ability of the presynaptic terminal to synthesize Ach. Unlike the normal NMJ treated with hemicholinium, no changes in size of the Ach quanta occurred with either stimulation or rest. The authors concluded that the myasthenic transmission defect is due to a deficiency of Ach in the quanta within the presynaptic terminal resulting from a probable defect of Ach packaging or binding. The possibility of a "false" or abnormal transmitter however, has not been ruled out. Elmqvist et al. (1964) cite the possibility that triethylcholine could be acetylated and the resulting molecule dealt with inappropriately by the receptors (Bowman and Rand, 1961).

Two model systems can be compared with the myasthenic phenomenon. For example, in low calcium, high magnesium solution (de Castillo and Katz, 1956b) or after intoxication with botulinum poison (Brooks, 1956) Ach release is prevented. Thus when the terminals are stimulated, they release a small amount of the neurohumor. Successive stimulation causes little depression because there is little drain on the store of Ach. Repetitive stimulation increases the response of the NMJ as a result of post-activation potentiation of the release mechanism. This kind of reaction is different from that which occurs in myasthenia gravis where after an initial large response, the response diminishes with additional stimulation. However, when prevention of choline uptake and Ach synthesis by terminal axons is brought about by exposure to hemicholinium and the nerve is repetitively stimulated, the result is normal release of Ach but deficient resynthesis. In such a preparation, the number of quanta of Ach is reduced as the Ach is released from a deficient store. Following hemicholinium poisoning, studies of prolonged stimulation reveal an initial small and transient facilitation followed by a prolonged phase of exhaustion. This type of defect is similar to that observed in myasthenia gravis and thus indicates a defect in Ach synthesis. Elmqvist et al. (1964) concluded that the myasthenic defect was located in the presynaptic terminal and involved reduction of quantum content possibly due to some abnormality in the sites where Ach was packaged. Desmedt (1966) suggested that the abnormalities described by Elmqvist et al. (1964) might indicate a preclinical stage of the defect since they also occurred in unaffected muscles. Intracellular recording from NMJs obtained from patients with severe myasthenia by Knickenberg et al. (1971) demonstrated that the number of Ach quanta released by a single nerve action potential was normal but that the effectiveness of a single quantum was reduced.

Data that might be interpreted as supporting the concept of a postsynaptic defect in myasthenia gravis is the work of Churchill-Davidson and Wise (1963) who demonstrated that NMJs in apparently normal newborn infants possess physiologic characteristics similar to myasthenic junctions. The infants are remarkably resistant to high doses of depolarizing drugs such as succinylcholine, and fasciculation does not occur after injections of this drug. Furthermore, electrophysiologic studies have revealed that the infants, like myasthenic patients, respond to repetitive stimulation of the motor nerve with decrease in successive muscle responses. Post-tetanic facilitation and tolerance to decamethonium (C_{10}) are also found in newborn infants, phenomena which disappear by the age of six months. It is possible that the postsynaptic membrane of NMJs in newborn infants has not attained the degree of molecular orientation of the receptor regions characteristic of the adult or that there is immaturity of Ach synthetic or packaging mechanism in the terminal axon.

Recently, Takamori and Gutmann (1971) described a 29 year old woman with typical myasthenia gravis who had periodic episodes of increased weakness that were characterized by interesting electrophysiologic abnormalities. The authors found that single evoked potentials had abnormally low amplitude, there was marked facilitation of single evoked potentials after a brief tetanus, facilitation of the second of a pair of evoked potentials at short intervals between stimuli occured, and there was alteration of these responses immediately following parenteral injection of calcium gluconate. These findings support the hypothesis that the myasthenic defect lies in the presynaptic release of Ach. During repetitive nerve stimulation, the amplitude of a train of evoked muscle action potentials decreased rather than increased, indicating that the kind of defect in the release of Ach resembles that which occurs in the Eaton-Lambert syndrome and in calcium deficiency (Elmqvist and Lambert, 1968). It is not clear how this data may be related to the evidence for reduced Ach quantum size in myasthenic NMJs (Thesleff, 1966).

The Role of Magnesium and Calcium on the Release of Acetylcholine in Myasthenia Gravis

The concentration of calcium and magnesium affects the size of Ach quantal release from stimulated nerve terminals. A low calcium, high magnesium environment results in reduced Ach release per nerve impulse with resulting decrease in size of the MEPPs. As the extracellular calcium concentration increases, there is increased release of Ach from the terminals whereas magnesium acts in the opposite direction. It appears that both calcium and magnesium compete for some specific molecule in the presynaptic membrane and that only the calcium complex with this molecule can be dissociated by the nerve impulse. Thus the activated complex in turn might release Ach. On the other hand, Hubbard et al. (1967) suggested that depolarization and calcium effects occur in different parts of the release process. However, there are significant differences between magnesium induced neuromuscular block and the characteristic myasthenic defect. Magnesium excess prevents the release of Ach whereas in myasthenia gravis, Ach quantum size is affected. Several investigators (Desmedt et al., 1965 and Kornfeld et al., 1969) have attempted to enhance the effect of anticholinesterase medication by calcium gluconate injections. These investigators found that calcium was useful in therapy only when sufficient response could not be obtained with the usual anticholinesterase medications.

Ach Synthesis in Myasthenia Gravis

Interesting data on Ach synthesis in a myasthenia gravis patient has been presented by Rosenberg et al., 1971; Gentner and Rosenberg,

1972. These investigators found that there was decrease of choline-O-acetyltransferase in myasthenic muscle compared to normal muscle and the AchE activity of impaired muscle samples was also reduced. Analysis of substrate concentration curves for acetyl coenzyme A and choline-O-acetyltransferase revealed decrease in the rate of Ach formation when the normal and the myasthenic muscle were compared. The authors suggested that this data could be explained by possible inhibition of substrate binding to the acetyltransferase due to some component in the muscle, a "false" transmitter, or abnormal discharge of the synaptic vesicles.

Immunological Abnormalities in Myasthenia Gravis

In the decade 1961 to 1971, major research efforts by several investigators were devoted to investigating immunological abnormalities in myasthenic patients. Nastuk et al. (1960) demonstrated that serum compliment activity in myasthenic patients was often abnormal and Simpson (1960) suggested on clinical grounds that myasthenia gravis might be an "autoimmune" disease. Considerable interest developed when Strauss et al. (1960) found muscle-binding, compliment-fixing serum globulin in the serum of some patients with myasthenia gravis. These antibodies were found to bind to myofiber striations in experimental animals, normal humans, and myasthenic patients but not particularly in the NMJ. This globulin was reported to occur in the serum of some 18-68% of patients with the disease (Strauss et al., 1960; Namba and Grob, 1966; Shulman et al., 1966). Binding activities of the globulin appeared to be greater in patients with more severe myasthenia gravis and in those patients with a thymoma. Others have shown that the muscle binding antibody which occurs in some patients with myasthenia gravis does not bind to NMJs or block neuromuscular transmission. Furthermore, there was no correlation between the activity of the myasthenic blood and the severity of the muscle weakness and fatigue. The activity of the blood samples on the rat preparation following thymectomy were also variable.

Later it was found that myasthenic serum globulins with anti-muscle activity also reacted with thymic epithelial cells indicating common antigenic components (Van der Geld et al., 1964). However, additional studies revealed that not all patients with anit-muscle antibodies had myasthenia gravis, that patients with thymoma and antibodies to muscle and thymus also had no evidence of myasthenia gravis (McFarlin et al., 1966) so that the conclusion was inescapable that the anti-muscle and anti-thymic antibodies probably were not the cause of the disease. They may however represent a consequence of abnormal NMJ function and possibly indicate focal muscle destruction. Rule et al, (1973) found that the antigenic sites related to humoral antibody formation in myasthenic patients are in the myosin fraction.

Namba et al. (1969) injected lymphocytes from patients with myasthenia gravis into rats and found that the foreign lymphocytes produced local neutrophilic and lymphocytic infiltration in the injected rat muscle. Lymphorrhages, eosinophilic infiltrates and fibroblasts were also found. The reactions in the rat muscle appeared more intense when lymphocytes from myasthenic patients were injected than from normal humans, normal rabbits, sensitized rabbits or sera from normal patients or myasthenic patients. Increase in the mean diameter of soleplates and changes in the ultrastructure of the NMJs occurred. These changes in the ultrastructure of the NMJs occurred. These changes consisted of an increase in the mean diameter 2 hours after injection followed by a second phase of increased soleplate diameter on the 9th day which became maximal on the 22nd day after injection. There was also an increased proportion of tortuous preterminal fibers and multiple terminals. There were unusual innervation patterns including preterminal branching at the final node of Ranvier and double NMJs innervated by either a nerve terminal in series or by branches from another terminal. Goldstein and Whittingham (1966) claimed that they could produce a myasthenic syndrome in guinea pigs by innoculation of thymic tissue or skeletal muscle in Freund's adjuvant.

Goldstein (1971) has suggested that the thymus secretes a hormone called "thymin" that can depress neuromuscular transmission and that autoimmune inflammation causes hypersecretion of this hormone. However, "thymin" has not been isolated. If this hypothesis is correct, the existence of thymin would provide the rationalization of thymectomy as therapy for myasthenia gravis. The concept of myasthenia gravis as an autoimmune disease had led to therapy with immunosuppressive drugs, particularly in Europe. Szobor and Petranyi (1970) treated 25 myasthenic patients with the cytostatic drug mesoerythrite and claimed definite improvement in 15. All had severe disease that had shown poor response to standard therapy. Similar encouraging results were reported by Mertens et al. (1969) who used 6 MP, azathioprine, actinomycin C and methotrexate to treat 38 patients. They claimed significant improvement in 22 patients. The response of myasthenic patients to immunosuppressive treatment appears to be unrelated to the results of available immunoserological tests. Treatment of large numbers of patients will be required before this therapy can be evaluated because of the well known variability and incidence of spontaneous remissions that occur in myasthenic patients. However Vetters et al. (1969) were unable to confirm the work of Goldstein and Whittingham (1966). Thus this contribution offered by Dr. Simpson's group concludes with the statement in the summary that "these findings constitute a failure to confirm an immunological hypothesis for myasthenia gravis put forward by other workers in 1966". Although considerable information of interest concerning muscle antibodies in patients with myasthenia gravis was derived from the concept of a possible autoimmune etiology of myasthenia gravis, most investigators have now concluded that circulating antimuscle antibodies play no direct etiologic role. With respect to possible autoimmune etiology of myasthenia gravis possibly mediated by cell-bound antibodies, it is notable that there has been only one report of actual lymphocytic infiltration of NMJs in myasthenic muscle (Wiesendanger and D'Alessandri, 1963). This should be common if sensitized lymphocytes are responsible for NMJ injury. Kawanami and Mori (1972) reported myasthenic EMG responses in mice immunized with thymus extract and the passive transfer of this effect by Lymph node cells. Recently, Patrick and Lindstrom (1973) have produced neuromuscular blockade that is abolished by neostigmine in rabbits injected with highly purified AchR from the electric eel.

Blocking Agents in Myasthenia Gravis

Numerous attempts have been made to demonstrate a circulating blocking agent, possibly of thymic origin, in the blood of patients with myasthenia gravis. The occurrence of neonatal myasthenia gravis with subsequent improvement with time and the experiment of increasing myasthenic weakness by exercising a limb with obstructed venous outflow has prompted several searches for such an agent (Bergh, 1953). Since the studies of Wilson and Wilson (1955) this kind of investigation has been redirected toward isolation of abnormal antibodies.

Parks and McKinna (1966) tested whole blood, plasma, red cells and a "globulin fraction" from myasthenic patients on the rat nerve-muscle preparation. They reported that plasma samples from 7 of 18 myasthenic patients produced 30% or greater depression of rat muscle contraction amplitude on stimulation at frequencies of 30 c.p.m. and 15 c.p.m. They ascribed the failure of neuromuscular transmission to elements of competition and depolarization. The induced block was reversed by cholinesterase inhibitors. Parks and McKinna (1966) found no evidence that the material contained in their crude globulin preparation had antibody activity.

Morphology of Myasthenic Neuromuscular Junctions

Early pathologic study of the central and peripheral nervous systems in patients dying of myasthenia gravis yielded surprisingly few lesions. Oppenheim (1887), who performed the first post-mortem examination on such a patient, called myasthenia gravis a progressive paralysis without anatomic findings. Mott and Barrada (1923) noted minor changes in the central nervous system (focal increase in neuroglia, occasional cells with vacuoles and chromatolysis, "lipoid changes"), which they were inclined to correlate with the clinical syndrome. The NMJs stained by methylene blue, appeared to be normal. Their conclusions were generally attacked in the discussion that followed their paper. McAlpine (1929) reported finding inflammatory changes in the spinal cord consisting of slight gliosis of the anterior horns, and "mucocytic degeneration." Adams et al. (1962) reported difficulty in staining the telodendria of NMJs (by a silver method) in two cases of myasthenia gravis.

Histochemical staining for AchE activity has revealed no decrease in the apparent enzyme activity in human extraocular muscles in myasthenic patients (Cohen and Zacks, 1959).

Woolf et al. (1956) reported various abnormalities in the terminal arborizations of NMJs obtained from a single case of myasthenia gravis. The methylene blue-stained NMJs were composed of terminal nerve fibers resembling those seen in myopathic disease. Beaded sprouts similar to those observed in cases of Werdnig-Hoffmann disease (Woolf and Till, 1955) were also present. Woolf and his co-workers were unable to reach a conclusion as to the specificity of these NMJ abnormalities.

Coërs and Desmedt (1958, 1959) reported on six cases of myasthenia gravis in which biopsy specimens were stained with methylene blue and the Koelle method for AchE activity. Two kinds of abnormal NMJs were found. The first consisted of "dystrophic endings" (Fig. 112B, 114),

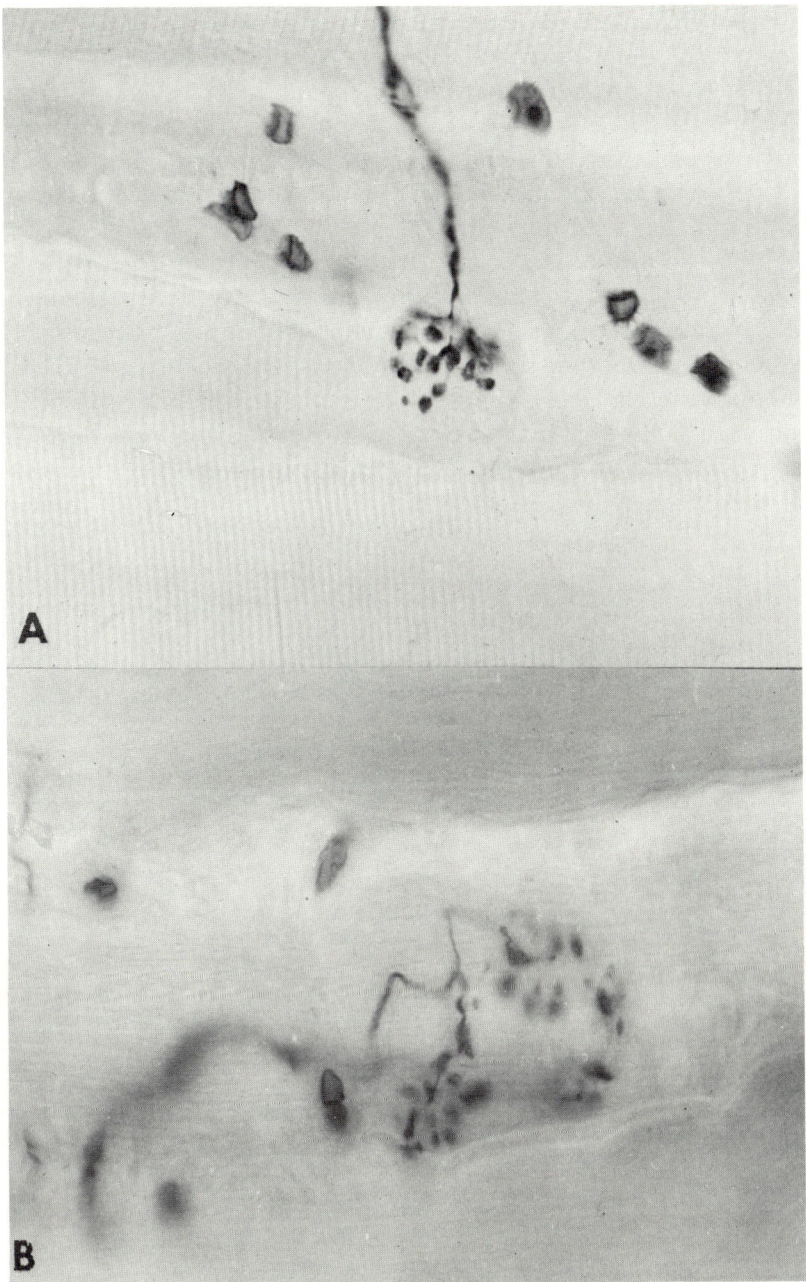

Figure 112. A, photomicrograph of a normal human neuromuscular junction stained by the methylene blue method. *B* illustrates "dystrophic" changes in a NMJ from a patient with polymyositis. (approximately X 1,000.) (From Coërs and Desmedt, 1959.)

that were characterized by abnormally profuse ramifications of the terminal arborization. In several cases the NMJs were greatly expanded, with several arborizations on a single nerve fiber. However, this change was not regarded as specific since it occurred in dystrophia myotonica and nonspecific myositis. These changes were present in three of the six myasthenic cases examined, all of which showed considerable variability. In only one of the muscle biopsy specimens studied were "dystrophic" endings clearly related to degenerating muscle fibers. The second kind, the "dysplastic" abnormality (Fig. 113), consisted of elongation of motor endings in one direction without side branching. This was found in four of the six myasthenic cases. The incidence of this kind of abnormality was 5 to 45 per cent of the total number of NMJs in each biopsy specimen. That these changes were not due to muscle degeneration is indicated by the essentially normal muscle fibers present in the

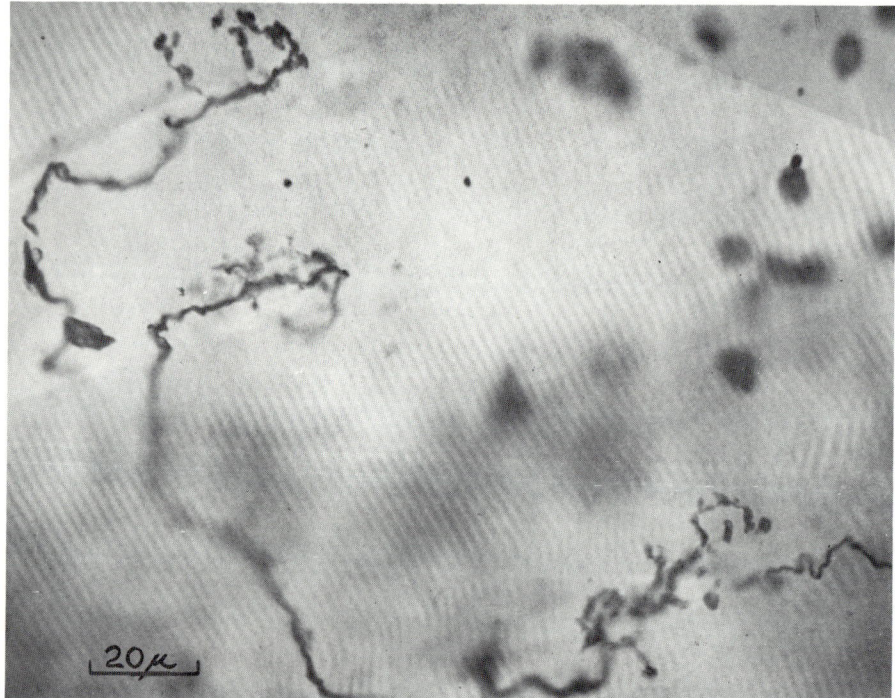

Figure 113. Photomicrograph of a neuromuscular junction stained with methylene blue from a patient with myasthenia gravis. These NMJs illustrate the "dysplastic" abnormality thought by Woolf to be characteristic of this disease. Note the extreme elongation of the terminal axons without significant evidence of axonal sprouting. The terminal expansions may also be shrunken in such NMJs. (After Woolf, 1963.)

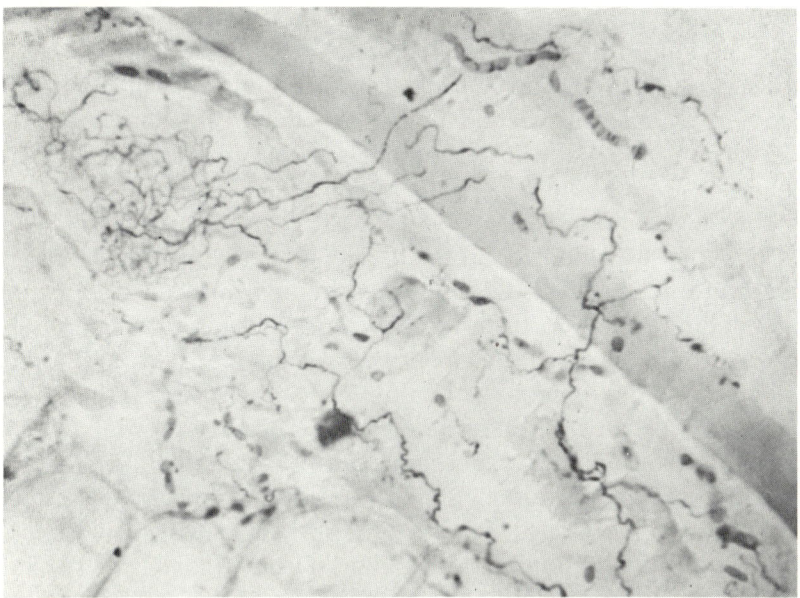

Figure 114. Photomicrograph of NMJs from a case of myasthenia gravis illustrating the "dystrophic" or "myositic" type of abnormality. In this methylene blue stained preparation, there is a remarkable degree of proliferation of subterminal nerve fibers and many beaded sprouts have small and abnormal terminal expansions. (X 220.) (From Woolf et al., 1956.)

biopsy preparations. Coërs and Desmedt concluded that the occurrence of "dysplastic" NMJs represents the specific abnormality in myasthenia gravis, since it was not observed in other disease entities.

In a later report Bickerstaff and Woolf (1960) described muscle biopsy specimens from seven cases of myasthenia gravis studied by methylene blue and AchE staining. They separated their cases into two groups: (I) slightly affected muscles without evidence of inflammation or degenerative change; and (II) muscles with lymphorrhages, variation in muscle fiber size, and degeneration. In two cases of the three in group I, NMJs were remarkably elongated and were frequently multiple. These changes, which were never observed in normal NMJs, resembled the appearance of NMJs in the congenital case of myasthenia gravis reported by Coërs and Woolf (1954). Double or quadruple NMJs arising from a single axon on single muscle fibers were found, and the terminal arborization was often in the form of a peculiar semicircular disc. NMJs joined together, forming single, much enlarged, and elaborate terminal arborization, were also present. Other NMJs were unusually long, with terminal arborizations arising on either side of a single filament originating from a terminal axon in a T-shaped fashion. In the second case in group I, terminal arborizations were elaborate and composed of coarsely beaded fibers. The third case had occasional NMJs with shrunken and fused terminal arborizations similar to those seen in cases of myositis (Coërs and Woolf, 1959). Figure 114 illustrates the "myositic" kind of NMJ.

The cases classified in group II had elongated NMJs similar to those in group I but were distinguished by their marked disorganization of the innervation pattern resulting from collateral axon sprouting (Bickerstaff and Woolf, 1960). In a typical example of this condition (case 4), marked proliferation of terminal nerve fibers with beaded sprouts and small or bizarre terminal expansions were present. Cholinesterase staining demonstrated some normal subneural apparatuses, whereas others were unusually small and widely dispersed. In this particular case lymphorrhages, hypertrophy, and atrophy were present, as well as focal degeneration of muscle fibers. Degenerative axon swelling was also noted in the vicinity of lymphorrhages. Similar changes were also observed in dermatomyositis and various neuropathies (e.g. carcinomatous, thyrotoxic). Such NMJs are regarded as resulting from degeneration of muscle fibers and the presence of inflammatory exudates (Bickerstaff and Woolf, 1960). These influences are thought to encourage multiple innervation patterns. A biopsy specimen from a second case in group II (case 5), a 19 year old girl, showed atrophic muscle fibers and small lymphorrhages. NMJ AchE was difficult to demonstrate histochemically even when the incubation time was prolonged and the pH of the incubation medium was increased from 4.4 to 5. The AchE activity was frequently spread over areas as great as 300μ. Methylene blue staining revealed many minute terminal arborizations with fine ultraterminal collateral sprouts arising from NMJs or terminal branches. This produced unduly elaborate and elongated NMJs. The final result in these cases is an excess of nerve fibers over muscle fibers with concomitant reduction of the functional terminal innervation ratio. However, these NMJ changes are not as functionally useful as the kind of sprouting that occurs before the emergence of the subterminal nerve fibers from the terminal nerve bundles, as in cases of primary degeneration of the lower motor neuron. This latter kind of sprouting results in collateral reinnervation, which tends to raise the functional terminal innervation ratio. Bickerstaff and Woolf (1960) suggested that even the "myopathic" type of sprouting seen in group II cases of myasthenia gravis may have some functional value by tending to increase the area of the synapses. These investigators interpret the evidence of increased dispersion of AchE activity in these NMJs as support for this hypothesis. However, the observed abnormalities in AchE staining might be due to loss of structural integrity of AchE molecules within the subsynaptic clefts, or possibly the presence of newly formed AchE molecules in abnormal sites unrelated to the synaptic clefts. A suggestion by Bickerstaff and Woolf (1960), that each AchE focus demonstrated histochemically at the site of contact of an axonal tip with a muscle fiber corresponds to a miniature synapse, is unlikely and requires confirmation. Certainly we cannot conclude that each of these foci corresponds to the structure of the normal subneural apparatus without electron microscopic confirmation. That abnormal and "immature" subsynaptic clefts may be observed in NMJs from cases of myasthenia gravis (Zacks et al., 1961, 1962) does not necessarily support the histochemical findings of Bickerstaff and Woolf (1960). It is possible that only portions of degenerating or regenerating myasthenic NMJs contain AchE activity and therefore produce the appearance of discontinuous AchE staining.

On the basis of methylene blue staining and localization of AchE activity, Bickerstaff and Woolf (1960) concluded that there is a primary NMJ abnormality in longstanding cases of myasthenia gravis consisting of elongated and multiple "dysplastic" NMJs, that tend to increase the synaptic area. In cases with a short history of myasthenia, elongation of NMJs tends to be absent, although some NMJs are shrunken. The occurrence of bizarre hemispherical terminal arborizations arising from a central filament, that was also observed in a congenital case of myasthenia gravis (Coërs and Woolf, 1954), was regarded as quite different from the usual appearance of NMJs in acquired myasthenia gravis (Bickerstaff and Woolf, 1960). The "myopathic" changes characterized by severe sprouting were regarded as a nonspecific abnormality, because similar multiple NMJs also occur in dystrophia myotonica and myotonia congenita, in which muscle hypertrophy is a common feature.

MacDermot (1960) used the methylene blue-staining method to study NMJ structure in muscle biopsy specimens from eight myasthenic patients, ranging in age from 30 to 60 years, with symptoms of myasthenia gravis ranging from two months to 15 years. All these patients had abnormal NMJs, although the biopsy specimens were taken from muscles that were electromyographically and clinically normal. Focal muscle atrophy was found in two cases, and all but two cases had increased numbers of subsarcolemmal nuclei. The NMJs were characterized by irregular axon swellings and finely beaded nonmyelinated nerve fibers. Abnormal branching and complex terminal arborizations were present in all the cases. All the NMJs were abnormally elongated and some were very small. Nerve branches arising from NMJs were present, and there was a tendency for the telodendria to degenerate and disappear in many of the NMJs. MacDermot concluded that the distal nerve abnormalities were unrelated to clinical fatigability and weakness. Similarly, the distal nerve changes failed to correlate with muscle fiber abnormalities, age of the patient, or duration of symptoms. Furthermore, no change in NMJ morphology could be observed in patients following thymectomy. However, all the patients had a common feature: namely, abnormal responses of the myasthenic subjects to decamethonium (C_{10}) and Tensilon tests. MacDermot suggested that the abnormal structure of the myasthenic NMJs might be related to their abnormal responses to decamethonium. She also stated that the presence of numerous ultraterminal fibers indicated evidence of previous degeneration and regeneration. Reske-Nielsen et al. (1964) described elongated, bizarre shaped NMJs stained by methylene blue or cholinesterase histochemical methods and Iwayama and Ohta (1969) employed silver and cholinesterase staining techniques as well as electron microscopy to study biopsies from 2 cases of myasthenia gravis. After staining with silver, NMJs had decreased terminal branching and abnormally simple subneural apparatuses were observed following cholinesterase staining.

Electron Microscope Studies of Myasthenic Neuromuscular Junctions

Because Bickerstaff et al. (1959) were reluctant to accept the pronounced and apparently irreversible changes revealed in myasthenic NMJs by methylene blue staining as the primary abnormality in this disease, they extended their investigations of myasthenic NMJs to include electron microscopic observations. It was clear that the methylene blue-staining method, which chiefly stains terminal nerve branches, and the histochemical method, which demonstrates AchE activity in the subneural apparatus, yielded little information concerning the structure of the subneural apparatus. This first electron microscopic study revealed the existence of a compound synaptic membrane in the subneural apparatus of human NMJs that is similar in structure to that seen in other animals. Bickerstaff et al. (1959) were unable to find significant differences when myasthenic NMJs were compared with normal NMJs. The electron micrographs in this report reveal extensive preparation artefacts that would obscure all but gross structural differences between normal and myasthenic junctions. In a more extensive investigation Bickerstaff et al. (1960) reported the results of their electron microscopic study of the NMJs in two myasthenic patients. The NMJs were located by electrical stimulation and recording and blocks of muscle containing the junctions were prepared for electron microscopic examination.

Of the two cases examined, the first had normal-appearing nerve fibers, with the exception perhaps of increased amounts of collagen within the nerve bundles. The axoplasm, mitochondria, and synaptic vesicles were normal. Similarly, no abnormalities were found in the terminal arborization. The synaptic clefts contained the five layers described by Robertson (1956). In their second case, the terminal arborizations appeared less "turgid" and the synaptic vesicles seemed abnormally large (640 to 800 A).

Bickerstaff and his co-worders also noted few intact mitochondria in the axoplasm and soleplate, a result more likely due to preparation artefact than to significant anatomic differences from previously described human NMJs (deHarven and Coërs, 1959). The electron micrographs provided show artefacts consisting of apparent leaching out of axoplasm and empty mitochondria. "Explosion" damage is also visible. Bickerstaff et al. (1959) concluded that the fine structure of NMJs in patients with myasthenia gravis is essentially normal.

This conclusion was challenged by Zacks et al. (1961, 1962), who studied the fine structure of NMJs in five myasthenic patients, including one child and four adults. Biopsy specimens were obtained at operation and were fixed immediately without use of electrical stimulation and recording or methylene blue staining. We hoped to avoid artefacts by taking the biopsy specimens with a minimum of manipulation. For example, Del Castillo (1960) observed that recording from methylene blue-stained NMJs with microelectrodes reveals a high rate of miniature endplate potential discharge, which he believed was due to depolarization of the synaptic membrane. This phenomenon may be due to inhibition of AchE by methylene blue, a potent anticholinesterase (Massart and Dufait, 1941; Zacks and Welsh, 1951).

Patients with myasthenia gravis of short duration appeared to have a subtle abnormality consisting of patchy decrease in density of the post junctional membrane a change which is now regarded as a fixation or embedding artefact. The NMJs were more severely disorganized in patients with longer duration of the disease. The subneural apparatus appeared to be particularly affected (Zacks et al., 1962). Additional morphologic evidence suggesting trophic or degenerative changes in myasthenic NMJs was reported by Johnson and Woolf (1965) who found shrunken axoplasmic expansions with partial replacement by Schwann cell cytoplasm in a case of severe myasthenia gravis that was resistant to anticholinesterase medication. In this case, the terminal axons measured less than 1μ in diameter and the axonal mitochondria were extremely electron dense. Synaptic vesicles were present and in some cases appeared increased. More recent ultrastructure studies by Iwayama and Ohta (1969) revealed absence of synaptic vesicles in the terminal axon and increased width of the primary synaptic cleft and reduction in the number of secondary synaptic clefts. Dense granular material was also described within the external lamina of the subneural apparatus. Similar findings have been reported by Fardeau and Godet-Gaillain (1970), Edwards (1970), Engel and Santa (1971), Santa et al, (1972). Sakimoto and Cheng-Minoda (1970) found widened subneural clefts in myasthenic extraocular muscle NMJs and surprisingly, increased junctional folding.

Re-examination of the fine structure of NMJs in muscle biopsy specimens from myasthenic patients after improved fixation has revealed convincing ultrastructure evidence of denervation and reinnervation. Earlier descriptions of the fine structure of myasthenic NMJs included widening and shortening of secondary synaptic clefts (Zacks et al., 1966) that resembled the changes in NMJs in a dog with a myasthenic syndrome. Study of the muscle biopsy specimens from myasthenic patients has yielded several examples where the subneural apparatus consists of an abnormal primary synaptic cleft and greatly distorted, shortened and widened secondary synaptic clefts (Fig. 115). The changes in these soleplates resemble the abnormal structure of denervated soleplates in experimental animals (Saito and Zacks, 1969a, b). Furthermore, deep primary clefts associated with local myofiber membrane thickening and minute surface invaginations (Fig. 115) closely resemble areas of *de novo* formation of NMJs in experimental animals. (Fig. 105). Similar findings were reported by Engel and Santa (1971). This data corresponds to the previously observed occurrence of myofiber atrophy in myasthenic patients and the histochemical evidence of denervation and reinnervation in muscle biopsy specimens. There have

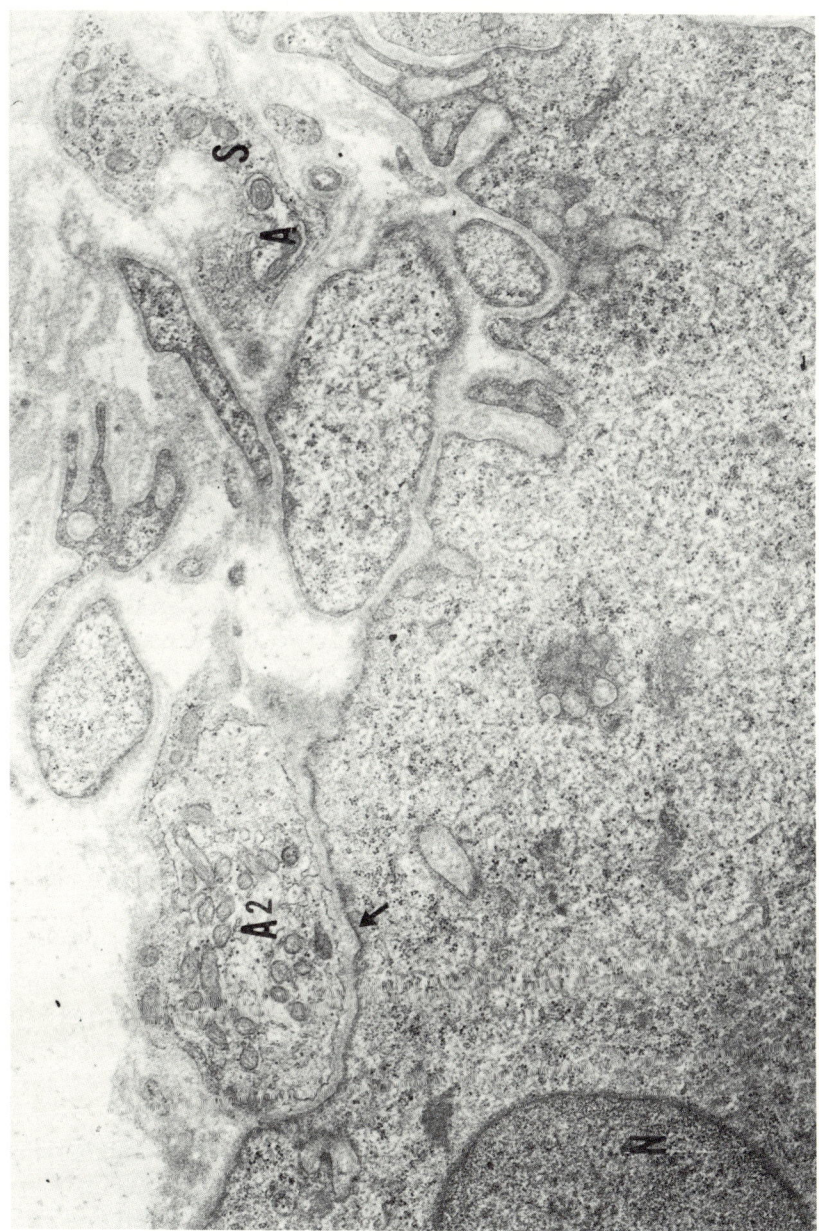

Figure 115. Electron micrograph of a neuromuscular junction from a patient with severe myasthenia gravis. The junctional region in the top of the illustration shows disorganization, shortening and widening of the subneural apparatus. Possible early reinnervation is shown at A_2. (X 20,000.)

been several reports of scattered atrophic myofibers in biopsy specimens from myasthenic patients (Russell, 1953) and of groups of atrophic fibers (Russell, 1953; Lowenberg-Scharenberg, 1962; Steidel et al., 1962; Fenichel and Shy, 1963; Brody and Engel, 1964; Brownell et al., 1972). These groups of atrophic myofibers suggest that denervation and reinnervation, probably by collateral sprouting (Bickerstaff and Woolf, 1960; McDermot, 1960) are important aspects of myasthenia gravis. Also, the peculiar "dysplastic" terminal axons described by Woolf et al. (1956) and Coërs and Desmedt (1959) may reflect abnormal axon growth during NMJ regeneration.

Recently, data has been obtained by McComas et al. (1971) indicating that the entire motor unit is affected in myasthenic patients. The size and numbers of motor units were investigated in ten myasthenic patients and 50 normal individuals, as was the isometric twitch tension and motor nerve impulse conduction. Five of the 10 myasthenic patients had reduced numbers of functioning motor units in the extensor digitorum brevis muscle indicating previous denervation. Amplitude of muscle potentials were consistent with collateral reinnervation of previously denervated myofibers. Also, there was slowing of isometric twitches in some of the myasthenic muscles. The authors concluded that the defect in myasthenia gravis may affect the motor unit more centrally with respect to the axon or cell body than had previously been considered.

The chief objective of anatomic study of myasthenic NMJs is to attempt to correlate structural abnormalities with the known abnormalities of function. This has been an exceedingly difficult task. We believe that morphologic and other evidence indicates that degeneration and replacement of NMJs occur in myasthenia gravis. This appears to be a secondary effect rather than the cause of the disease. These changes may result from abnormal secretion of Ach or another substance from the terminal axons. This process may proceed to total destruction of NMJs and, to a varying degree, formation of new NMJs. The axonal sprouting, elongated NMJs, and other abnormalities demonstrated by methylene blue staining may reflect various stages in the degeneration and regeneration of the NMJs. For the sake of speculation, such an hypothesis of ebbing and waning of NMJ destruction and regeneration could account for several of the commonly observed clinical features of myasthenia gravis. The exacerbations and remissions so typical of myasthenia gravis may reflect the relative proportion of injured NMJs. Thus at any given time the degree of weakness may be due to the relative proportion of structurally intact and functional junctions. Muscles that reflect relatively slight weakness in the form of detectable clinical signs and symptoms, such as the extraocular muscles, serve as the first indicators of the disease, whereas the effects on muscles with greater reserves are less easily detected until a relatively large proportion of the NMJs are affected. Myasthenic crisis and periodic failure to respond to anticholinesterase medication may also be due to destruction of a sufficient number of NMJs. Furthermore, single myofiber and group atrophy occurs late in the course of myasthenia gravis, especially in cases of long duration. This may result from long-standing denervation resulting from many irreversibly injured NMJs.

AN ANIMAL MODEL OF MYASTHENIA GRAVIS

Myasthenic Syndrome in a Dog

An electron microscopic study of an unusual case of a myasthenic syndrome in a dog (Zacks et al., 1966) was the first ultrastructure study of this rare syndrome. The only other case had been published as a clinical report (Omrod, 1961). Because of its rarity, this dog's syndrome is described in some detail.

An eight month old mixed breed male dog was examined at the University Veterinary Clinic because of vomiting. This dog was the largest and only survivor of a litter of 7. The others had died between 3 and 4 weeks of age of unknown causes. The mother did poorly after delivery and was destroyed three weeks later. There were no post mortem examinations of either the puppies or the mother. The first indication that the surviving dog was abnormal was noted at 5 weeks of age when he vomited repeatedly approximately an hour after feeding. By three months, his bark was abnormally high pitched and there was a tendency for the animal to limp, loose balance and fall on his hind legs. On some occasions, the dog had great difficulty arising from the prone position. At the age of 7 months, the dog was examined by a veterinarian who discovered megaesophagus by x-ray examination. When examined at the University, the dog was thin, apprehensive and had a fluctuant swelling of the left side of the neck thought to be the esophagus. The dog stood with difficulty due to weakness of all 4 legs (Fig. 116). His gait became progressively unsteady until he was

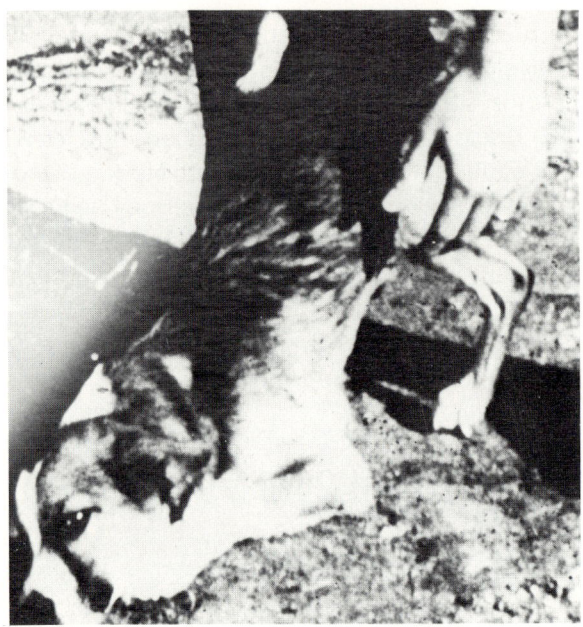

Figure 116. Photograph of dog with myasthenic syndrome illustrating severe weakness. The dog is unable to support his weight on his forelegs.

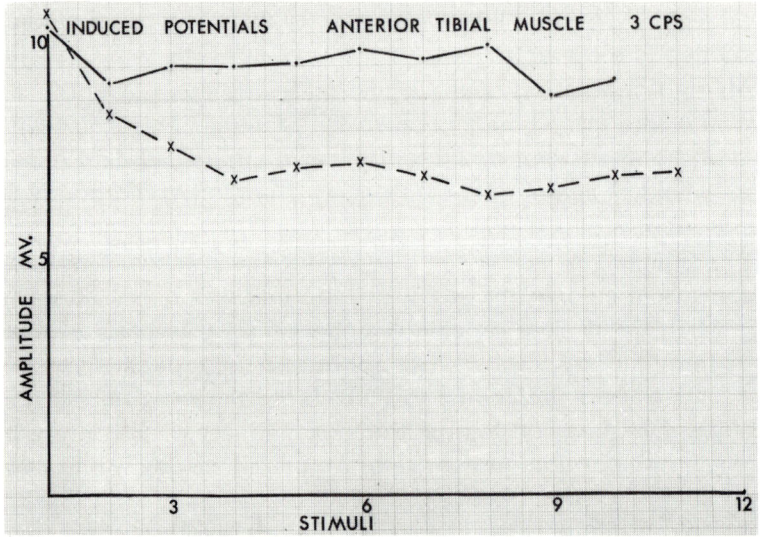

Figure 117. Chart of induced potentials from the anterior tibial muscle of a dog with a myasthenic syndrome. The dashed line indicates amplitude *(MV)* without medication and the solid line shows the response following prostigmine medication.

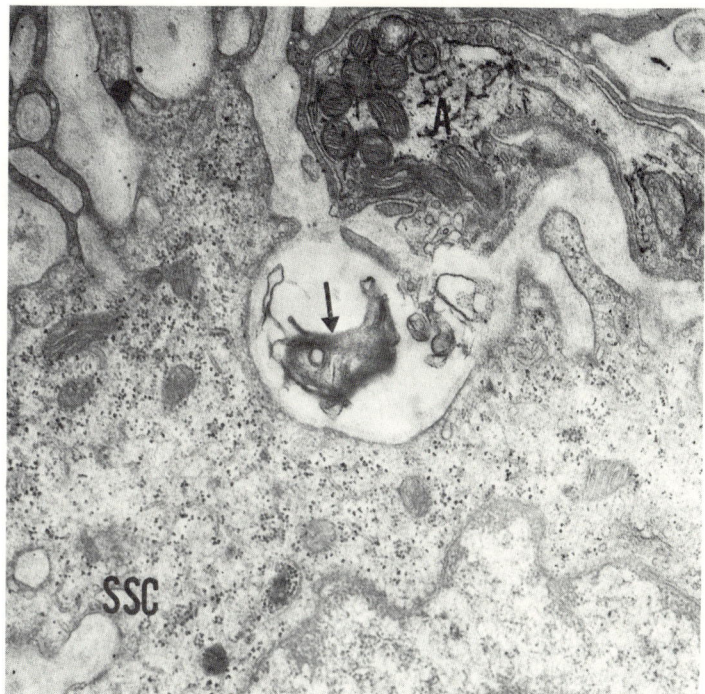

Figure 118. Electron micrograph from a NMJ from the dog with the myasthenic syndrome. Note the retraction of the terminal axon *(A)* and the membranous debris (arrow) in the widened primary synaptic cleft. There is also widening of the secondary synaptic clefts *(SSC).* (X 18,000.)

unable to stand. After rest in his cage he was able to take a few steps before repetition of the cycle. In the following 2 weeks, weakness increased significantly and he would stand only during defecation and urination and his dysphagia continued. One mg. of edrophonium was given intravenously over a 15 second period following which there was immediate salivation and bradycardia, constriction of the pupils and a marked increase in muscle strength. The dog was able to stand and walk normally after a minute. However, 12 minutes later he was again unable to stand. Three days later, he was too weak to lift his head and he had respiratory difficulty, with slight cyanosis. One mg. of neostigmine was given intramuscularly and again, after 4 minutes, the dog was able to walk and bark. A dosage regimen of pyridostigmine 45 mg. every 12-24 hours was begun. Electromyograms made at this time demonstrated a typical myasthenic reaction (Fig. 117). Gradually, the dog's requirement for medication was reduced and he was admitted for a Heller-Ramstedt operation to relieve the megaesophagus. At this time, biopsy specimens were obtained from intercostal, esophageal and leg muscles for conventional optical and electron microscopy. Following operation, the dog's recovery was uneventful and he was able to eat solid foods without vomiting. There was no further requirement for anticholinesterase medication and as of January 1965 the dog was still in remission. We have not been able to obtain additional follow-up.

Paraffin sections from the muscle biopsy specimens stained with routine stains revealed no abnormalities. There was no muscle destruction nor were lymphorrhages found. The fine structure of the dog's intercostal NMJs consisted of $1\text{-}2\mu$ terminal axons containing moderate numbers of typical synaptic vesicles and mitochondria. Some of the axons contained abnormal aggregates of electron dense granular material that in some areas seemed to be related to neurofilaments. The most striking abnormality was marked widening of primary and secondary synaptic clefts and disorganization of the normally radiating structure of the secondary synaptic clefts of the subneural apparatus. One NMJ had a greatly dilated primary synaptic cleft containing masses of electron dense laminated membrane profiles resembling myelin bodies (Fig. 118). For comparison, this report also included electron micrographs from a case of severe myasthenia gravis in a young woman. NMJs from this patient's intercostal muscles also had widened primary synaptic clefts and markedly abnormal secondary synaptic clefts which were widely dilated and lined by amorphous external lamina. Also there were decreased numbers of mitochondrial profiles in the soleplate sarcoplasm.

Although it is not fair to state that the disease described in the dog is identical to the disease in man, the close parallelism to myasthenia gravis with regard to the pattern of weakness, response to anticholinesterase medication and electromyographic findings, suggests that valuable information might be obtained from study of this syndrome in such an animal model. However, efforts to arrange mating of the dog reported by Ormond and the present dog came to no avail. Unfortunately the spontaneous occurrence of this myastenic syndrome in dogs is too infrequent to serve as a useful model for research.

The changes in the subneural apparatus that occurred in the NMJs of the "myasthenic" dog may be interpreted as a kind of atrophy or degeneration that resembles the changes that occur in denervated NMJs.

Primary Diseases of Muscle

Continuing in our plan of arbitrarily distinguishing various levels of disease of the motor neuron, we encounter a group of diseases that appear chiefly to involve the structure and function of the muscle fiber itself.

Myotonia

A phenomenon associated with two diseases, which appears chiefly to involve the muscle itself rather than the NMJ, is myotonia. In patients with myotonia, the motor nerve impulse evokes tetanic instead of a twitch contraction. That this is not due to an abnormal Ach mechanism is demonstrated by the persistence of the myotonic reaction after curare block and even after section of the motor nerve (Lanari, 1947; Floyd et al., 1955; Brown and Harvey, 1939). There appears to be an abnormal delay in relaxation after cessation of either voluntary, mechanical, or electrical stimulation. The two diseases characterized by this phenomenon are myotonia congenita (Thomsen, 1876) and myotonic dystrophy (Steinert, 1909).

Myotonia Congenita

This relatively benign disease is not accompanied by muscular dystrophy. It is inherited as a mendelian dominant in approximately 25 per cent of the cases and is manifested as generalized myotonia early in life. Histologically the muscles are hypertrophic without striking histologic changes. Two cases studied by Coërs and Woolf (1959) showed marked distal branching of subterminal nerve fibers and frequent multiple innervation, which they believed was a result of muscle hypertrophy. Unlike NMJs in myotonic dystrophy, there was no neurocladism — reflecting muscle degeneration — in cases of Thomsen's disease.

Myotonic Dystrophy

Of greater importance is myotonic dystrophy, a slowly progressive myopathy of late onset with moderate myotonic features. It tends to be genetically dominant and does not occur in the pedigrees of patients with Thomsen's disease. Distal muscles are usually involved, with ultimate progression to facial, extraocular, and bulbar muscles. Other dystrophic features, including cataracts, bone changes and testicular atrophy, also occur in these patients. Electromyographic studies reveal bursts of high frequency potentials during attempted relaxation that are thought to arise from changes in the muscle fiber rather than in the NMJs (Adams et al., 1962).

Study of the NMJs by the methylene blue method (Coërs, 1952b) revealed that the proximal parts of the intramuscular nerve fibers were normal but there was an excessive degree of sprouting from subterminal fibers. Some of the sprouts were very fine and beaded, whereas others were normal and ended in normal NMJs. Occasionally there were more than one NMJ on a muscle fiber. The NMJs were large and, in some areas, neurocladism was observed. Occasional subterminal nerve fibers were seen that formed anastomoses with other nerve fibers, producing NMJs at the junction of two nerve fibers. In other cases large terminal arborizations were derived from single subterminal nerve fibers. Occasional beaded nerve fibers ran parallel to muscle fibers and gave off collateral sprouts ending in elongated, darkly stained terminal arborizations. Staining for AchE activity demonstrated expanded subneural apparatuses.

Coërs and Woolf (1959) concluded that the absolute terminal innervation ratio was increased in these cases but that the functional terminal innervation ratio was decreased. Though sprouting was seen in other forms of muscular dystrophy and myositis, it was most pronounced in myotonic dystrophy and was especially associated with large, well formed soleplates as demonstrated by AchE staining. These investigators suggested that there is probably some substance arising from degenerating muscle that stimulates axon sprouting.

Kamieniecka and Ojak (1964) found no abnormalities in AchE staining in NMJs in primary muscular dystrophy but Allen (1969) detected abnormal NMJs by means of methylene blue staining and electron microscopy. Schroder (1970) described peculiar sarcolemmal indentations resembling junctional folds in muscles from a patient with myotonic dystrophy that he interpreted as probable sites of denervation. We have observed similar structures in a case of muscular atrophy caused by porphyria (Fig. 119). Unmistakable denervation changes were also observed in a case of myotonic dystrophy studied in our laboratory (Fig. 120).

Progressive Muscular Dystrophy

This group of diseases is characterized by slow, progressive weakness and wasting of skeletal muscle due to primary muscle degeneration (Adams et al., 1962). They are usually heredofamilial, although some sporadic cases occur. The proximal muscles are usually affected first, but all muscles may ultimately be involved. Their etiology is unknown.

These muscle diseases may be grouped according to their clinical pattern. The histologic appearance of muscle biopsy specimens is similar in all of them.

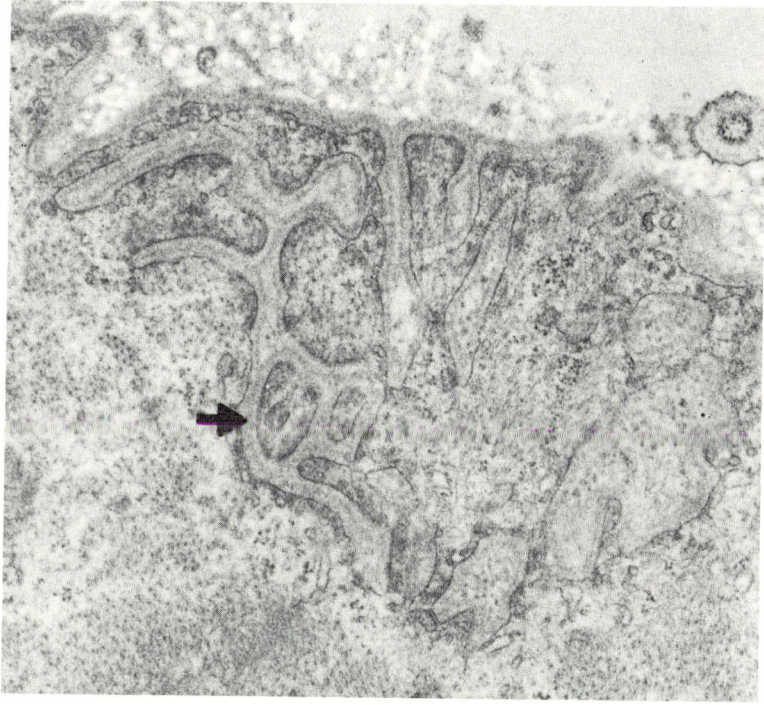

Figure 119. Electron micrograph of an area resembling the subneural apparatus of a denervated NMJ from a patient with porphyria. The primary synaptic cleft is flattened and covered by collagen filaments and the secondary synaptic cleft is widened and irregular (arrow). (X 24,600.)

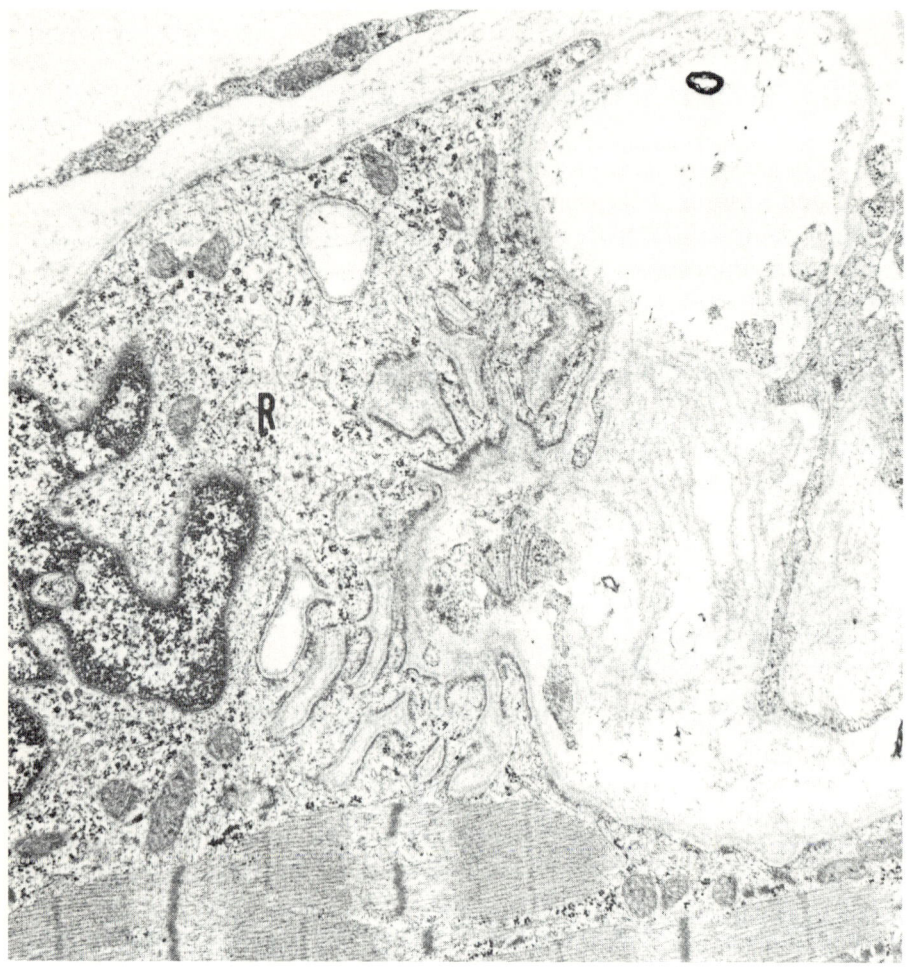

Figure 120. Electron micrograph of a NMJ from a patient with myotonic dystrophy. Note the disorganization of the primary synaptic and secondary synaptic clefts and the absence of a normal terminal axon. Myofibers present in this illustration show minimal dystrophic changes. Numerous clusters of ribosomes are present in the junctional sarcplasm *(R)*. (X 25,000.)

Pseudohypertrophic Muscular Dystrophy (Duchenne)

This is a disease of childhood, usually affecting the pelvic girdle muscles and later the shoulder muscles but not the face. It is a severe, progressive disorder apparently associated with a sex-linked recessive gene.

Fascioscapulohumeral Dystrophy (Landouzy-Dejerine)

This occurs in either males or females, usually in the second decade, is slowly progressive and involves the shoulder girdle and facial muscles. Other disease patterns demonstrating similar muscular changes are juvenile scapulohumeral type (Erb) and ocular myopathy. Histologic features of these diseases are muscle atrophy, hypertrophy, and degeneration with little evidence of regeneration. Eventually the increased perimysial connective tissue and fat replaces the degenerating muscle fibers. Usually there is no inflammation. Cardiac but not smooth muscle may also be involved. Biochemical abnormalities in these diseases seem to be nonspecific and are related to muscle wasting.

Falin and Kanarejkin (1941) employed silver staining (Gros-Bielschowsky) to study NMJs from cases of pseudohypertrophic and juvenile scapulohumeral muscular dystrophy. They observed fine collateral sprouts in NMJs from patients with scapulohumeral muscular dystrophy, and small NMJs with poor terminal arborizations in patients with the Landouzy-Dejerine form of the disease. All the changes in NMJs were interpreted as secondary reactions to primary muscle disease.

Other studies, employing methylene blue staining, by Coërs and Woolf (1959) have demonstrated similar abnormalities in the terminal innervation pattern regardless of the clinical pattern of the dystrophic process. The intermuscular nerve bundles were essentially normal, although the small branches appeared tortuous. This appearance was due to the loss of muscle fibers and the increase of perimysial connective tissue. Nerve fibers that had lost contact with their muscles tended to have fusiform swellings and finely beaded nerve fibers wandered between and parallel to surviving muscle fibers. In some areas, a plexiform pattern of globules was formed from these wandering nerve branches. In some biopsy specimens the terminal arborization and subneural apparatus appeared to be shrunken. However, in the pseudohypertrophic form of muscular dystrophy, very large and complex NMJs were seen lying on hypertrophied muscle fibers. In a few specimens, especially from patients with muscle weakness, axonic sprouting and multiple NMJs similar to the type seen in myositis were observed. That these changes are not specific is indicated by the presence of similar changes in thyrotoxic myopathy and the neuromyopathy associated with solitary myeloma. Falin and Kanarejkin (1941) also concluded that NMJ abnormalities in muscular dystrophy are reactive in nature and are due to primary changes in the innervated muscle. In muscular degeneration occurring in guinea pigs deficient in vitamin E, Rogers et al. (1931) were unable to demonstrate abnormal NMJs (using a silver-staining method) despite the severe changes present in the muscle fibers. Adams et al. (1962), however, do not accept this experimental disease as being equivalent to spontaneous muscular dystrophy.

Muscular Dystrophy: Abnormalities in Neuromuscular Junctions

Although it is generally accepted that the primary abnormality in muscular dystrophy is primary in the myofibers, both morphologic and physiologic evidence has accumulated to indicate that abnormalities are also present in NMJs in both human and murine muscular dystrophy. Coërs and Woolf (1959) found swelling of subterminal nerve fibers and shrinkage of terminal arborizations (methylene blue stain) that were similar to changes that they had observed in primary peripheral nerve disease. In an early electron microscope study, Wechsler and Hager (1961b) described abnormal NMJ ultrastructure in muscle biopsy specimens from patients with myotonic dystrophy. Jedrzejowska et al. (1965) used both supravital staining with methylene blue and ultrastructure methods to study NMJs in pseudohypertrophic muscular dystrophy. They described pale staining of the NMJs and abnormal terminal axon expansions that were swollen, fused and simplified. Dark staining of the axon terminal expansions was observed in NMJs on atrophic myofibers. In the electron microscope, the synaptic vesicles appeared normal in terminal axons, but the subneural apparatus contained widened and irregular secondary synaptic clefts, or no clefts in some NMJs. The authors suggested that since the abnormal NMJs occurred only on myofibers undergoing degeneration, the changes in the subneural apparatus were probably secondary to myofiber degeneration. Nara (1965) described large vacuoles in the subneural sarcoplasm in the biopsy specimens from two patients with progressive muscular dystrophy. These morphologic changes are all consistent with the appearance of denervated (Fig. 86) or in some cases, reinnervated NMJs (Fig. 106). Widening and shortening of the secondary synaptic clefts occurs in denervation and simplified subneural clefts are an early stage of *de novo* NMJ formation. Furthermore, this hypothesis is supported by physiologic data indicating that denervation is a component of some forms of muscular dystrophy. McComas et al. (1971) studied 17 patients with myotonic dystrophy and found prolonged contraction and half relaxation times in the isometric twitches from the extensor digitorum brevis muscle. With increase in age, the patients' muscles became weaker, due to progressive loss of motor units, a result supported by the histologic demonstration of axon degeneration (MacDermot, 1961). Two patients had a myasthenic response to repetitive nerve stimulation indicating the probability of malfunction of the NMJs. Prolongation of the twitch contraction and relaxation phases in dystrophic muscle has also been reported in the limb girdle and Duchenne types of muscular dystrophy (Sica and McComas, 1971; McComas et al., 1971). These data have raised doubts that muscular dystrophy is a primary disease of myofibers. Although McComas et al. (1971) has suggested that muscular dystrophy may be a primary neuronal disease, a concept that could be explained by some abnormal trophic influences from the nerve, it is also possible that severe myofiber changes may sufficiently alter the postsynaptic membrane in NMJs to be equivalent to denervation.

Mouse Muscular Dystrophy

Abnormal neuromuscular transmission has been found in an hereditary animal model of muscular dystrophy that occurs in (dy) mice (Michelson et al., 1955). These mice are extremely sensitive to cholinesterase inhibition by low doses of neostigmine which causes intense spontaneous twitching of the muscles (Baker, 1960). Other anticholinesterase drugs are also effective in producing this result and several drugs were effective in inhibiting spontaneous twitching without blocking neuromuscular transmission (Baker, 1963). Similar spontaneous activity occurs in the human disease (McComas and Mossawy, 1965). Studies using intracellular electrodes by McComas and Mossawy (1966) revealed that the level of membrane depolarization necessary to elicit the action potential was lower in the dystrophic mice. There was also indirect evidence for reduced membrane conductance since the dystrophic myofibers had a longer membrane time constant. Ach quanta secretion also appeared to be reduced (Conrad and Glaser, 1964). In a later study, McComas and Mrozek (1967) suggested that denervation may be an important aspect of mouse dystrophy, a suggestion supported by the morphologic studies of Coërs and Woolf (1959) who found reactive branching of terminal axons in patients with muscular dystrophy and Curtis et al. (1961) found elongation and fragmentation of NMJs in mouse dystrophy.

I am unaware of an ultrastructure investigation of early changes in dystrophic muscle that might help in the decision as to whether severe myofiber changes must be present before the NMJs are affected. More recently, Harris and Wilson (1971) have suggested that denervation is a major factor in mouse dystrophy as well as in the human diseases, dystrophia myotonica (Campbell et al., 1970) and progressive muscular dystrophy (McComas et al., 1970; McComas and Sica, 1970).

Hereditary muscular dystrophy in the chicken (Asmundson and Julian, 1956) is characterized by hypertrophied pectoral myofibers (McMurty et al., 1972) but this report does not include description of the motor innervation. Information concerning NMJ fine structure would be of interest because Albuquerque and Warnick (1971) observed increase in membrane resistance and capacitance and increased duration of MEPPs.

RARE FORMS OF MYOPATHY

Nemaline Myopathy

With the increasing use of the electron microscope to study muscle biopsy specimens, a group of new myopathies with varying ultrastructure features have been described. In 1963, a myopathy characterized by the presence of threadlike or rod bodies in the myofibers was described by Conen et al. (1963) and Shy (1963). This disease occurred in flaccid infants with delayed motor development, who had proximal limb weakness and reduced muscle bulk. It was usually discovered when the child made initial attempts to walk although some cases were recognized because of their severe hypotonia during the neonatal period. Other abnormalities in these children included kyphosis and scoliosis as well as high arched palate. Although originally thought to be congenital and determined by a dominant (autosomal) gene, rod-like bodies have also been described in non-inherited, late onset and relatively progressive myopathies. Rod structures may also occur in some cases of myositis. Although there has been extensive investigation of the rods, consideration of neuromuscular innervation has been secondary. Heffernan et al. (1968) illustrated a single electron micrograph of a NMJ from such a biopsy. This micrograph (Fig. 121) demonstrates striking widening of some of the secondary synaptic clefts similar to the changes that have been reported in some cases of myasthenia gravis. An electron micrograph illustrating a contribution by Karpati et al. (1971) shows NMJs with normal or slight abnormalities in the subneural apparatus. An unidentified structure (Fig. 122) adjacent to the axon was filled with elongated vesicles, some of which contained electron dense material. A portion of identifiable Schwann cell cytoplasm covering the axon is also separate from this structure and it does not appear to be part of the terminal axon.

Vacuolar Myopathy

As with the other kinds of changes that occur in abnormal skeletal muscle, vacuolization of myofibers is also nonspecific. It tends to occur in various forms of muscular injury including acute necrosis from

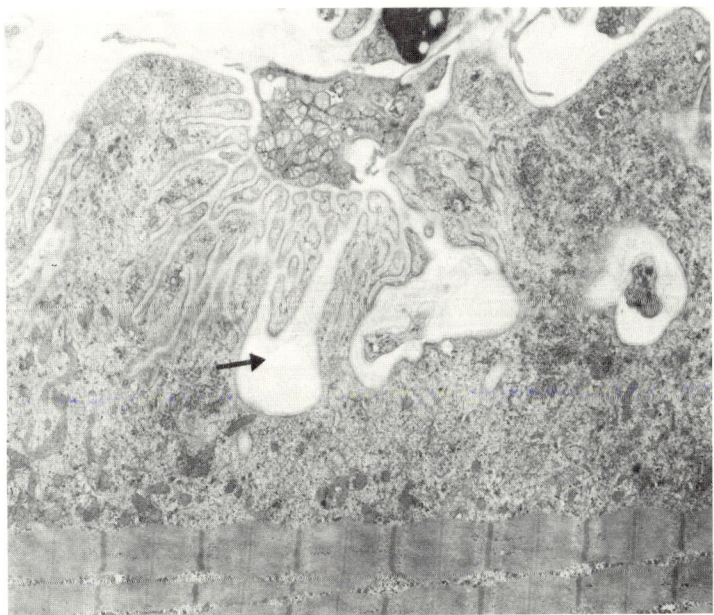

Figure 121. Electron micrograph illustrating a NMJ from a patient with nemaline myopathy. The terminal axon contains numerous mitochondria and the underlying subneural apparatus is distorted with prominently widened secondary clefts (arrow). (From Heffernan et al., *Arch. Neurol. 18,* 1968.) (X 10,800.)

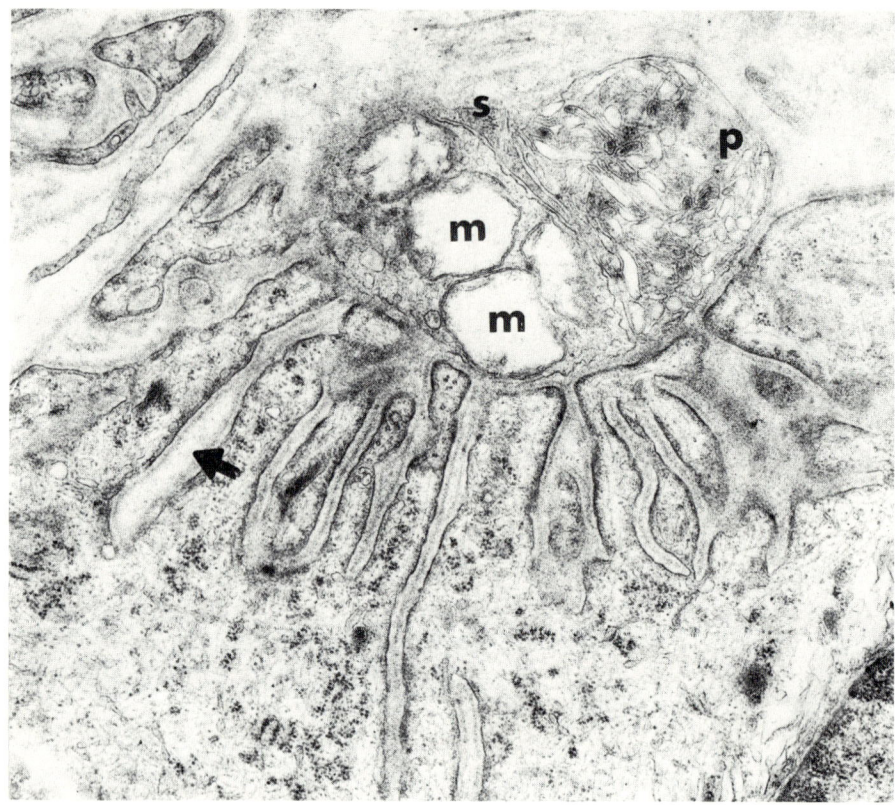

Figure 122. Electron micrograph of a neuromuscular junction from a child with nemaline myopathy. The axon contains artefactually swollen mitochondria *(M)* and adjacent to it is an unidentified structure *(P)* filled with elongated vesicles that is tentatively identified as a Schwann cell process. Some widening and distortion of secondary synaptic clefts is also present (arrows). (X 15,000.) (After Karpati et al., *Arch Neurol.* 24:291, 1971.)

trauma or anoxia or in some forms of myositis and polymyositis. Vacuolar myopathy also occurs in systemic lupus erythematosus, as a complication of choloroquine therapy and in various kinds of familial periodic paralysis. Coërs et al. (1971) reported on the clinical and histologic features of a patient with vacuolar myopathy and steatorrhea with low plasma potassium. The patient developed quadriparesis that was reversed by electrolyte therapy. Muscle biopsy specimens stained by the methylene blue technique and a thiocholine method for cholinesterase activity revealed normal appearance of intramuscular nerve fibers and occasional small and widened terminal arborizations in some NMJs. Other junctions were extremely large and abnormally expanded and there was slight increase in collateral sprouting of subterminal axons. Deficiency of neuromuscular transmission was indicated by decreased amplitude and duration of evoked muscle potentials on repetitive stimulation. Both clinical and EMG evidence of muscle hyperexcitability was evident in the muscle spasms that occurred and the high frequency discharges of short duration resembling fibrillation potentials and increased insertion activity. Apparent enlargement of the observed NMJs was of the nonspecific kind that had previously been reported in various myopathies. Several investigators have atrributed increase of soleplate area as a reactive or compensatory response to prolonged or reduced refractoriness of the muscle membrane to stimulation. In adult celiac disease with peripheral neu-

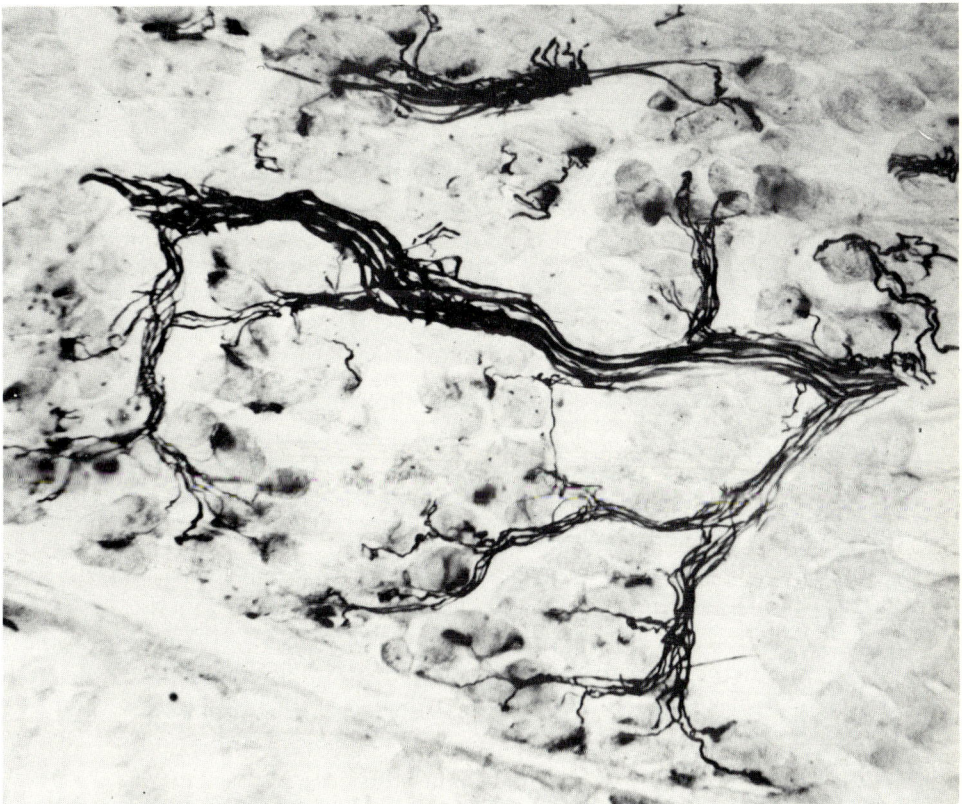

Figure 123. Photomicrograph of intercostal muscle from a mouse with MED myopathy illustrating nerve trunks, branches and NMJs innervating the myofibers. Stained by the combined silver and cholinesterase method. Note the normal innervation pattern. (X 150.)

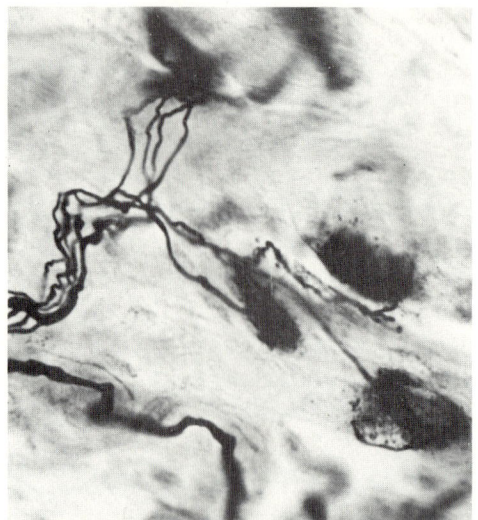

Figure 124. Photomicrograph of neuromuscular junctions in a MED mouse illustrating the arrangement of normal appearing terminal axons and cholinesterase activity in the subneural apparatus. (X 440.)

ropathy, Cooke et al. (1966) described swelling and fusion of terminal axonal expansions within NMJs. One of the biopsy specimens studied in the cases reported by Coërs et al. (1971), revealed diffuse irregular swellings of small intramuscular nerve fibers. Since no ultrastructure studies were performed on these muscles, the finer details of axonal organelles and membranes of the NMJ were not evaluated.

An Animal Model of Hereditary Myopathy: MED Myopathy

Duchen et al. (1967) reported a fatal hereditary disease of mice characterized by progressive weakness of the skeletal muscle beginning approximately 8 days after birth. Because of claimed abnormalities in the terminal nerve fibers and NMJs, this autosomal recessive gene was named NED for "Motor Endplate Disease". Duchen et al. (1967) reported muscle atrophy and increased complexity and marked sprouting of the terminal axons and elongation of terminal arborizations in silver-stained sections. The structure of the subneural apparatus was not demonstrated.

Using mice contributed by that laboratory, Zacks et al. (1969) studied the morphology, histochemistry, and ultrastructure of MED muscles as well as some physiologic properties of the NMJs. The general clinical pattern of the disease was confirmed in this study but combined staining with silver and for AchE activity demonstrated minimal changes in the terminal axons (Figs. 123, 124). Early in the course of the disease (8-9 days), the fine structure of NMJs was normal. Even at 20 days, when the animals were nearly paralyzed, there were no changes in the fine structure of the NMJs (Fig. 125).

The MED mice are smaller than their heterozygous litter mates and the size of individual myofibers in intercostal, diaphragm and leg muscles of MED mice are also smaller than the corresponding muscles in their heterozygous litter mates of the same age. However, there was no evidence of individual myofiber or group atrophy such as occurs in denervation atrophy and there was no evidence of active degeneration of

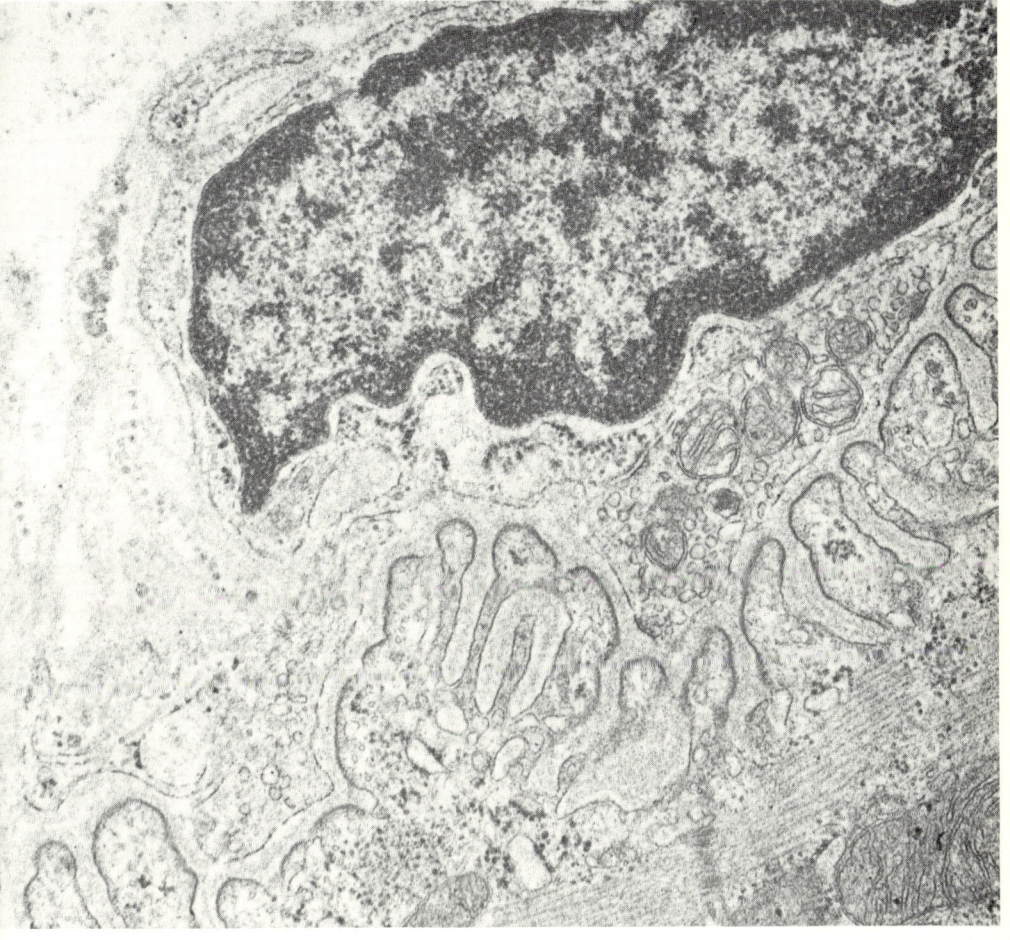

Figure 125. Electron micrograph illustrating the normal appearing structure of a neuromuscular junction from a MED mouse with severe muscular weakness. (X 24,000.)

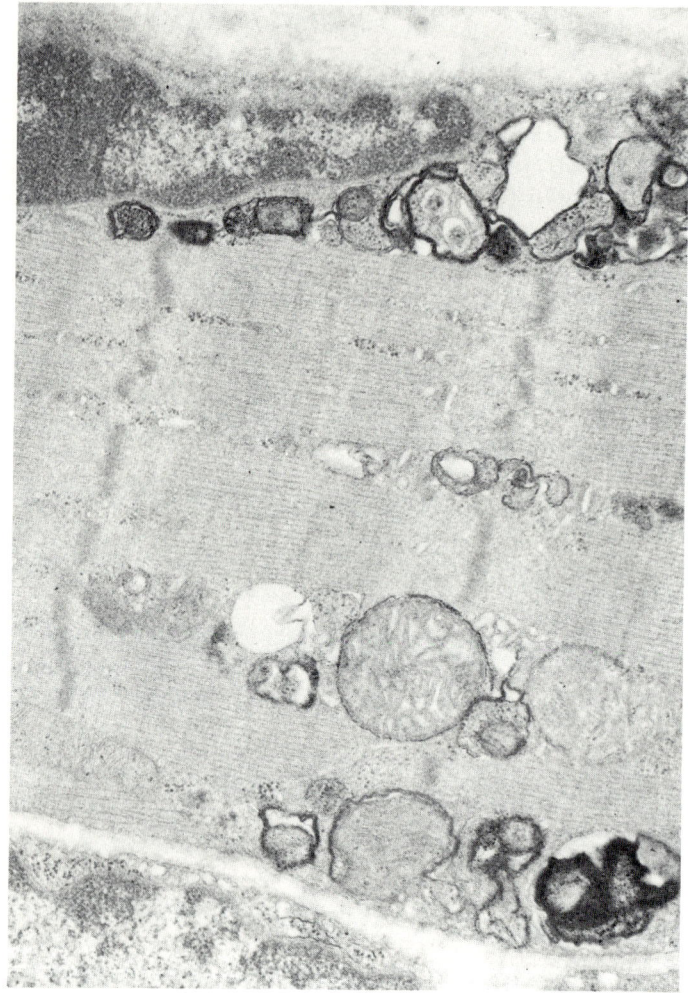

Figure 126. Electron micrograph illustrating "spheromembranous" degeneration of skeletal muscle from a MED mouse. Note the proliferation of membranes, incorporation of sarcoplasm and mitochondria by the membranes and abnormalities in the interfibrillar mitochondria. (X 22,000.)

myofibers evidenced by fraying myofilaments as occurs in some forms of myopathic atrophy in the early course of the disease. Later (12-20 days) there is focal myofibrillar degeneration and a striking increase in the number of autophagic vacuoles containing acid phosphatase activity in the homozygous MED animals (Fig. 126). Biochemical assay for this enzyme in animals from 8 to 20 days of age revealed progressive increase of the enzyme that correlated with an ultrastructure pattern resembling "spheromembranous degeneration" that occurs in vincristine myopathy. In a second contribution, Duchen (1970) provided additional details concerning the histological, histochemical and electron microscopic examination of homozygous MED mice, 10-29 days of age. Optical microscopy revealed "atrophy" of skeletal myofibers with most severe changes in the short head of the biceps brachii whereas the long head of the same muscle, triceps, tibialis anterior and gastrocnemius muscle were said to be less involved. Clinically, the earliest signs of weakness occurred in the hind limbs indicating general involvement of skeletal musculature. Although not described as lysosomes, a micrograph from a 23 day animal illustrated in this report shows myofibrillar destruction and organelles resembling lysosomes. Unlike Zacks et al. (1969), Duchen found marked sprouting of motor nerve fibers after silver impregnation and reported markedly abnormal size and shape of soleplates stained for cholinesterase activity by a modified thiocholine method. An illustration provided by the authors show little detail of the subneural apparatus in apparent areas of innervation but instead, general spread of esterase activity along the axons. The ultrastructure of the NMJ in 11-13 day old mice was normal. Beyond 18 days, the reported abnormalities in NMJs consisted of an increased number of normal terminals and some NMJs with increased numbers of subneural folds. Although the author suggested that these were newformed terminals, the illustrations offered show mature terminals with no early evidence of *de novo* formation.

The discrepancy between the essential normal fine structure of the NMJs and their interpretation of the small fibers as "atrophic" suggested that the abnormality in the MED NMJs resembled the abnormality in local botulinum poisoned muscles where transmission failure and muscle atrophy occur without NMJ degeneration (Duchen and Stritch, 1968; Duchen, 1970). The absence of changes indicating denervation led the authors to conclude that MED disease is due to a progressive functional denervation of skeletal muscle resulting from transmitter deficiency. This report (Duchen, 1970) cites unpublished electrophysiologic supporting data. However, in the work reported by Zacks et al. (1969), repetitive supermaximal stimulation of whole muscles *in vivo* for considerable periods of time revealed no gross failure of neuromuscular transmission or increased fatigability as measured by both recordings of the mechanical and electrical responses of indirectly stimulated muscles (Fig. 127). The method used, however, would not

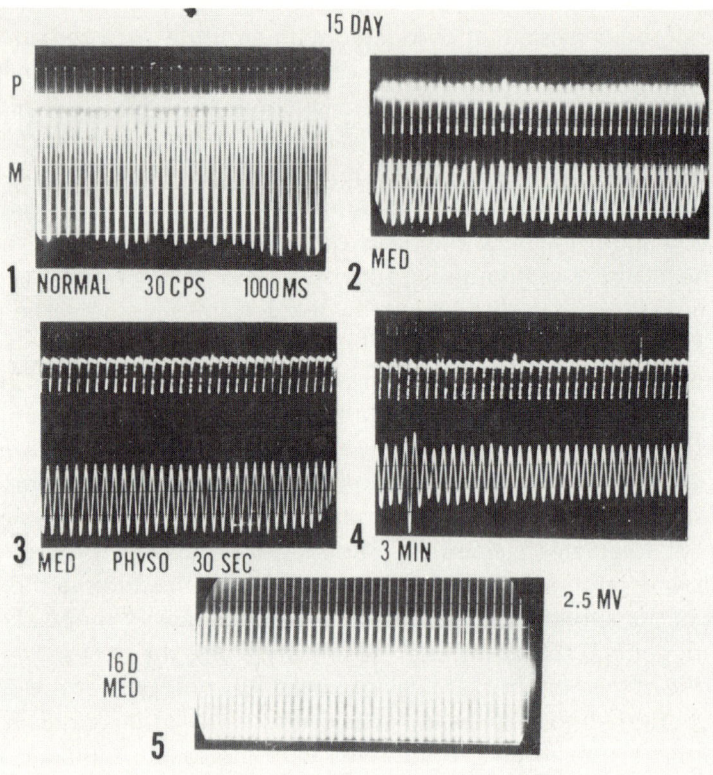

Figure 127. Electromyographic recordings from affected MED and normal litter mates. Membrane potentials *(P)* and mechanogram *(M)* are shown in *(1)* for a normal mouse stimulated at 30hZ. *2* illustrates corresponding recordings from a severely affected MED mouse. Note the approximately similar amplitude of the evoked potentials *(P)* and the marked amplitude reduction in the mechanogram *(M)*. Treatment of both the control *(3)* and the MED mouse *(4)* with physostigmine produces no differences in either the control or the experimental animals. At *5*, repetitive stimulation of a weak 16 day old MED mouse reveals no evidence of neuromuscular fatigue.

detect subtle changes in transmission. Zacks et al. (1969) concluded that the membrane and probable Ach release mechanism were normal but that there was deficient myofiber contractility probably due to a primary myopathy.

Because of the multiple genes carried by the original MED mice, Zacks et al. (1969) bred the MED gene into a black C57BL6J Bar Harbor strain and have maintained the strain through 17 generations. This strain of MED mice does not have the numerous other genes producing neurologic disease that were carried by the original colony of MED mice. However, the typical lesions in the myofibers were found in the C57BL6J strain. Zacks and Sheff (1970) have performed biochemical studies on oxidative metabolism, ion fluxes and uptake of amino acids by MED myofibers. No abnormalities were found in overall oxidative or glycolytic metabolism in MED mice in the 8-10 day period when symptoms first occur in homozygous animals and electrolyte and water content were within the range of normal with no evidence of changes characteristic of denervation.

Recent results of microphysiological studies on isolated MED nerve-muscle preparations (Duchen and Stefani, 1971) has provided more detailed data on neuromuscular transmission in this disease. Microelectrode recordings revealed the presence of MEPPs in nearly every myofiber studied and there was increased frequency of MEPPs in many. Also the postsynaptic membrane was hypersensitive to Ach, indicating that Ach is secreted by the terminals and combines with the postsynaptic receptors. Evidence for a presynaptic defect was the failure of single or repetitive stimuli to increase MEPP frequency. Increased external potassium concentrations did increase MEPP frequency, indicating that the presynaptic membrane could be depolarized. These data suggest that the terminal axons in MED mice are capable of secreting Ach when stimulated since MEPPs can be recorded and that these molecules perform their usual function when bound to the postsynaptic membrane. That increased stimuli fail to produce increased MEPP frequency was interpreted by Duchen and Stefani (1971) as evidence that the nerve action potential did not invade the terminal axons normally. Since the receptors in the postsynaptic membrane play an essential role in generation of MEPPs, other explanations of the MED abnormality might be sought in this area. Additional studies of myofiber protein metabolism in our laboratory employing radio-labelled histidine reveal that there is no defect in transport of this amino acid through the myofiber cell membrane but once inside, incorporation of histidine into contractile as well as non-contractile protein is greatly reduced. Our observation that this defect occurs only *in vivo* and our demonstration that histidine incorporation in normal muscle is inhibited by extracts of MED nervous system suggest that a factor in the MED nervous system, possibly transported in peripheral nerves, is responsible for abnormal protein synthesis.

The data obtained by the different approaches of the two laboratories may be reconciled by some common factor, possibly a genetically determined trophic substance from the nerve, that affects both protein synthesis and both pre- and postsynaptic junctional membrane characteristics in the NMJ.

Myositis and Polymyositis

In this group of loosely defined disease entities, the outstanding clinical features are muscle tenderness and weakness. These symptoms are sometimes associated with skin changes, as in the acute form of dermatomyositis. Subacute and chronic forms of polymyositis that lack skin changes are now recognized. The principal disease entities in this group are dermatomyositis, polymyositis, scleroderma, and sarcoid (Walton and Adams, 1958).

Electromyograph recordings from affected muscles demonstrate a myopathic pattern. Microscopic examination of affected muscles reveals variable degrees of degeneration, regeneration, and inflammation. It is sometimes difficult to distinguish polymyositis from muscular dystrophy solely on the basis of histopathology. The principal difference between these two disease groups is the presence of inflammation in muscle affected by polymyositis and its usual absence in muscular dystrophy.

NMJ Pathology in Myositis

Coërs and Woolf (1959) observed several types of abnormalities in the methylene blue-stained terminal nerve fibers of muscles affected with myositis. In areas free of inflammation or muscle degeneration, degenerative changes were observed that consisted of transformation of the normal delicate structure of the terminal arborization into swollen subterminal nerve fibers and coarse globules that stained intensely with methylene blue. In the most severely affected areas, the subterminal nerve fibers were thickened, angulated, and tortuous. In fibrotic areas, the NMJs were small and the terminal nerve branches were shrunken (Fig. 128).

In addition to these degenerative changes, reactive changes were observed in NMJs in myositic muscle biopsy specimens. These changes were less specific than the degenerative changes and consisted of sprouting of the distal nerve fiber, producing multiple enlarged NMJs which increased the absolute terminal innervation ratio.

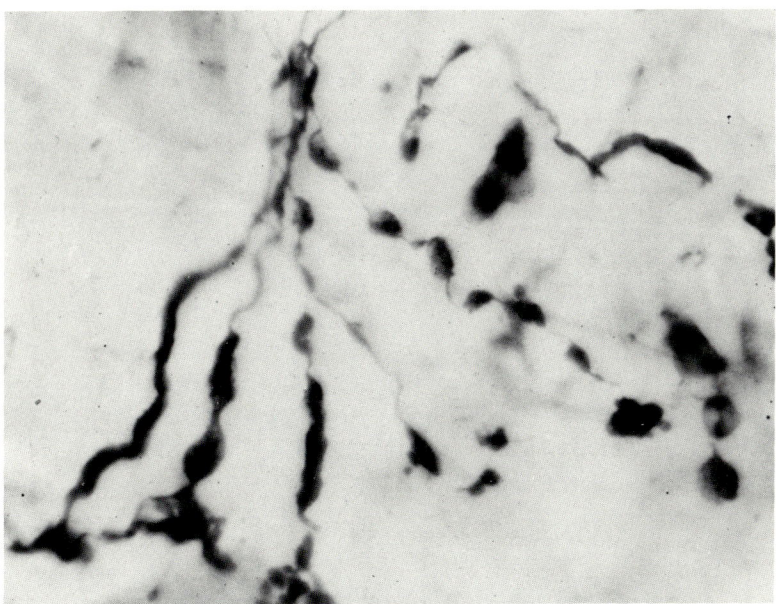

Figure 128. Photomicrograph of an NMJ from a patient with dermatomyositis illustrating the characteristic distortion of the NMJ structures and the varicose swelling of the subterminal nerve fibers. (From Coërs and Woolf, 1959.) (approximately X 1,000.)

Some of the fine nerve sprouts were found to wander for considerable distances. These NMJ abnormalities resembled those seen in muscular dystrophy. NMJs stained for AchE activity demonstrated apparent expansion of the soleplates. Another abnormality found in myositic muscle biopsy specimens resembled the changes observed in cases of neural atrophy. This consisted of collateral reinnervation with increase of both functional and absolute terminal innervation ratios. As we have discussed previously, collateral reinnervation is indicative of more proximal involvement of the motor nerve fibers. Thus several changes can be observed in NMJs in myositic muscle: degeneration of terminal axons, apparently due to a local process (inflammation), changes related to degeneration of terminal axons, changes related to myofiber degeneration, and apparent restorative efforts consisting of collateral reinnervation. Secondary degeneration of NMJs also occurs in experimental myositis produced by drugs such as paraphenylene diamine, plasmocid and calvacin (Anderson and Song, 1966).

Appendix

GOLD-STAINING METHODS

RANVIER (GRAY, 1954)

Reagents

1. fresh filtered lemon juice
2. 1% gold chloride
3. 0.2% acetic acid
4. 20% formic acid
5. triple distilled water
6. glycerin

Method

Hang muscle by nerve in lemon juice until it becomes transparent (2 to 12 hours). Rinse in triple distilled water, drain, and place in 60 ml. of 1% gold chloride with gentle agitation for 20 minutes. The muscle will become light brown. Rinse and transfer preparation with glass hook into 0.2% acetic acid. The amount of incident light is critical at this stage. Reflected light, diffuse but not bright, is recommended. After 1 to 2 days, the muscle should become dull purple. If mauve-colored or dark purple, the intensity of light has been too small or too great. Then place the muscle into 20% formic acid in the dark for 2 days. Glycerol is then placed in the bottom of a tube and 20% formic acid is layered over it. The muscle is then transferred to the upper layer of the tube. After 24 hours, the muscle, which first floated at the formic acid-glycerol interface, should sink to the bottom of the tube. The formic acid is pipetted out when no more formic acid is seen rising from the submerged muscle. Glycerol is added to the tube after removal of the formic acid. When the muscle sinks to the bottom, it is transferred to fresh glycerol, teased, and mounted in glycerol jelly. Such preparations are impermanent.

Result

NMJs are stained red-violet. Nerve fibers, terminal axons, granules of Kühne, and soleplate structures should be visible.

SIMPLIFIED GOLD METHOD

COLE, 1955

Reagents

1. 10% citric acid
2. 1% gold chloride
3. 20% formic acid

Method

Four-millimeter blocks of fresh muscle are fixed for 10 minutes in 10% citric acid and then placed without rinsing in 1% gold chloride for 60 minutes. The muscle is then placed in 20% aqueous formic acid for 48 hours. Storage in a mixture of equal parts of glycerin and 95% methyl alcohol preserves the preparations. Mounts are made by teasing the muscle fibers in glycerin and mounting in glycerin or glycerin jelly.

Result

NMJs stain red-violet and appear very similar to those stained by the more complex Ranvier method. We have found it simple and reliable.

CAREY METHOD (1942)

Reagents

1. lemon juice (fresh)
2. 1% gold chloride (aged 1 to 2 days)
3. 1 part concentrated formic acid to 3 parts aq. dist.
4. 50% glycerin in 95% ethanol

Method

Place strips of muscle 3 to 5 mm. thick in fresh filtered lemon juice for 10 to 15 minutes. Decant the lemon juice and pour on 1% gold chloride without rinsing. Keep preparation in dark until golden (10 to 60 minutes). Then transfer to formic acid solution in dark for 8 to 12 hours. Wash, soak in mixture of 50% glycerin and 50% alcohol, tease, and mount.

Result

Similar to previous methods. Nerve fibers and soleplate are stained.

SILVER STAINING OF NEUROMUSCULAR JUNCTIONS

CAJAL (GRAY, 1954)

Reagents

1. 1.5% silver nitrate
2. Balbuena developer
    alcoholic extract of amber

hydroquinone	2.5 gm.
in aq. dist.	250 ml.
3. Balbuena toning solution	
sodium borate	2.5 gm.
in aq. dist.	250 ml.
gold chloride (dark bottle)	0.25 gm.

Method

Fresh muscle with or without prior exposure to 95% alcohol (24 hours) is blotted and placed in 1.5% silver nitrate for 4 or 5 days at 35°C. Rinse the muscle in aq. dist. and place in Balbuena developer for 24 hours. Paraffin sections are then prepared in the usual way and brought to water. The sections may be optionally toned with the Balbuena toning solution. Dehydrate and mount in balsam or other comparable medium.

Result

NMJs are indicated by brown-black staining of the terminal arborizations.

Comment

This method is included chiefly for historical interest because it is somewhat capricious and utilizes an unusual reagent (Balbuena developer). Particular attention must be given to the purity of the reagents and chemically clean glassware is required.

GROS-BIELSCHOWSKY STAIN

Reagents

1. 10% silver nitrate
2. 20% formalin
3. ammoniacal silver solution
    To 30 ml. 20% silver nitrate, add concentrated ammonium

hydroxide until the brown precipitate first formed disappears. Add 15 additional drops of ammonium hydroxide.
4. 20% aq. ammonia
5. 1% acetic acid
6. 0.02% gold chloride (yellow)
7. 5% sodium thiosulfate
8. alum carmine (counterstain)

Method

Frozen sections are cut from blocks fixed for 24 hours in 10% formol-saline and washed for 1 hour in aq. dist. Then place the sections in 10% silver nitrate for 45 minutes. Without washing, the sections are transferred to 20% formalin that has previously been neutralized with magnesium carbonate. If the solution becomes cloudy, fresh formalin is substituted. After 15 minutes, wash a few sections in aq. dist. and place in ammoniacal silver solution for 1 to 3 hours. If no staining can be observed in the microscope after 2 hours, drop 20% formalin into the staining dish and agitate gently.

When staining is suitable, place sections in 20% aq. ammonia, wash in aq. dist., and place briefly in 1% acetic acid. Rinse, place in 0.02% gold chloride for 30 to 60 minutes, rinse in aq. dist., and fix in sodium thiosulfate for a few seconds. The sections are then washed, dried on albumenized slides, dehydrated in the usual way, and mounted. An alum carmine counterstain may be used if desired.

Result

Nerve fibers and terminal arborizations of NMJs are stained black. Adjacent muscle, nuclei, and other structures are gray.

ADDISON (1939)

Reagents

1. fixative
   chloral hydrate   5 gm.

absolute alcohol	25 ml.
aq. dist.	75 ml.
2. ammoniated alcohol	
absolute ethanol	50 ml.
ammonium hydroxide	4 drops
3. 1.5% silver nitrate	
4. reducer	
hydroquinone	1-2 gm.
40% neutral formalin	5-10 ml.
aq. dist.	100 ml.
5. gold chloride toning solution	
gold chloride	1 gm.
in aq. dist.	500 ml.
6. sodium thiosulfate 5-10% aq. solution	

Method

Fix muscle in chloral hydrate alcohol for 24 hours. Wash rapidly in aq. dist. and place in ammoniated alcohol. Wash and silver in 100 ml. of 1.5% silver nitrate (in the dark) at 37°C. for 3 to 5 days. Rinse in aq. dist. and place in reducer. Then tone in toning solution, wash, and place in sodium thiosulfate for 30 seconds. After washing, dehydrate, embed in paraffin, cut sections, and mount.

Result

Similar to other silver-staining methods.

METHYLENE BLUE-STAINING METHODS

DENZ (1951)

Reagents

1. staining solution
    0.8% sodium chloride
    0.2% glucose

0.02% magnesium bromide
0.02% methylene blue (2BS-I.C.I.)
in phosphate buffer pH 6
2. fixative
ammonium molybdate, saturated in aq. dist.

Method

Muscles are infiltrated with the staining solution at 37°C. for 20 minutes. The degree of bluing is controlled with the microscope. After staining, fixation with ammonium molybdate or ammonium picrate for 24 hours is used. Frozen sections are cut, dehydrated in n-butanol, cleared in xylene, and mounted in balsam.

COËRS (1952)

Reagents

1. 0.02-0.03% methylene blue in physiologic saline (sterile)
2. ammonium molybdate saturated in aq. dist.
3. 10% neutral formalin

Method

At operation, a muscle bundle is infiltrated with methylene blue-staining solution, allowed to remain in situ for 10 minutes, and then the biopsy sample is excised. The muscle biopsy specimen is kept moist with saline and exposed to air or pure oxygen for 30 to 60 minutes. The muscle is then fixed in saturated ammonium molybdate solution for 24 hours at 0°C. Wash in three changes of aq. dist. and fix in 10% neutral formalin for 3 to 5 days. Frozen sections are cut and mounted on albumenized slides. Counterstaining with 1% carmalum may be done at this stage. Then dehydrate in 90% alcohol, absolute alcohol, and clear in toluene. Mount in a neutral synthetic resin medium.

Result

The muscle fibers are pale green or light blue, the sarcolemma is often somewhat darker, and the nerve fibers are the most deeply stained. The nuclei do not stain. NMJs have blue-stained terminal arborizations. Experince indicates *in vivo* infiltration is unnecessary. See below.

METHYLENE BLUE STAINING *(in vitro)*

EVANS et al. (1970)

Reagents

1. saline solution

NaCl	8.900 gm.
KCl	0.429 gm.
NaHCO$_3$	1.000 gm.
CaCl$_2$	0.222
MgCl$_2$·5H0	0.203
glucose	2.000
aq. dist.	1000.00 ml.

2. methylene blue
   0.015% in 0.89% NaCl
3. ammonium molybdate $(NH_4)_2MoO_4$ saturated in aq. dist. Filter before use.

Method

Freshly excised biopsy specimen transferred in saline solution that is oxygenated with 96% O_2/4% CO_2 mixture. Within an hour, the muscle is pinned to cork board and methylene blue solution is injected via 26 gauge needle into one of the cut ends of the specimen using 10-20 ml. for a 3 × 5 cm. specimen. After 5 minutes, divide the muscle into longitudinal strips 2-3 mm. wide and expose to air at room temperature for 30-60 minutes. When staining is complete, place in ammonium molybdate overnight, wash in tap H_2O, flatten, dehydrate, clear and mount.

Result

Axons including terminal branches are stained blue.

Comment

The original method required injection of methylene blue at the time of operation. The present method eliminates this necessity.

JANUS GREEN B STAINING

COUTEAUX (1947)

Reagents

1. Janus green B 1:1000, 1:10,000
2. 10% ammonium molybdate
3. Ringer's solution

Method

Blocks of muscle are stained with Janus green B dissolved in Ringer's or Tyrode's solution. Removal of external connective tissue facilitates staining. High temperatures must be avoided. Fixation with 10% ammonium molybdate is followed by sectioning at 3μ.

Result

The nerve fibers and subneural apparatus of NMJs are stained blue-green. Some pale staining of muscle fibers occurs.

PARAPHENYLENE DIAMINE METHOD FOR OSMIUM FIXED, PLASTIC-EMBEDDED, SECTIONS

ESTABLE-PUIG, et al., J. Neuropath. Exp. Neurol. 24:531-535, 1965)

Reagent

1. paraphenylene diamine 1% in aq. dist.

Method

0.5-2μ sections embedded in Epon are dried on glass slides and are stained in freshly filtered solution 1 for 15 minutes to 1 hour. Then, rinse in aq. dist. for 2 minutes, dehydrate in graded ethanol, dry and mount in permount.

Result

Muscle fibers are brown, nerve fibers and nuclei are dark brown.

ALDEHYDE FUCHSIN-ALCIAN BLUE METHOD

SPICER AND MEYER (Am. J. Clin. Path. 33:453-460, 1960)

Reagents

1. sulfation solution
    H_2SO_4 concentrated   10 ml.
    acetic acid   30 ml.
        made fresh before each use

2. aldehyde fuchsin solution
basic fuchsin	2.0 gm.
paraldehyde	4.0 gm.
HCl concentrated	6.0 ml.
ethanol 6%	400 ml.

    ripen 24 hours — store at 4°C.
3. alcian blue solution
alcian blue	0.3 gm.
acetic acid 3%	100 ml.

Method

The 10% neutral formalin-fixed tissue is embedded in paraffin and cut 3-7μ. Then remove paraffin with xylol 2 times 5 minutes. Hydrate through graded ethanol to distilled H 0. Sulfate 8 minutes in solution 1, rinse in acetic acid, and aq. dist. Stain in solution 2 for 60 minutes 25°C., rinse in distilled H_2O, 70% ethanol and stain in solution 3 for 40 minutes. Rinse in aq. dist., dehydrate in graded ethanol, clear in xylol and mount in permount.

Result

Myofibers are outlined by red-stained external lamina which extends into subneural apparatus of NMJs and interdigitations of the MTJs. Connective tissue stains blue.

METHOD FOR LEAD-REACTIVE SUBSTANCE IN NEUROMUSCULAR JUNCTIONS

SAVÁY AND CSILLIK (1958)

Reagents

1. lead nitrate	5 gm.
in 8% formalin	100 ml.

2. sodium sulfide	2 gm.
in aq. dist.	100 ml.

Method

Fresh muscle is fixed for 15 minutes in the lead nitrate-formalin solution. Frozen sections (30 to 40μ) are cut, washed rapidly in aq. dist., and placed in 2% sodium sulfide solution.

Result

The NMJs are stained brown-black against a nearly colorless background.

POLARIZATION OPTICAL METHOD FOR NEUROMUSCULAR JUNCTIONS

CSILLIK (1963)

Reagents

1. lead nitrate	3.3 gm.
2. aq. dist.	100 ml.
3. 0.1 M glycerol-acetic acid	

Method

Small blocks of skeletal muscle are fixed in 3.3% lead nitrate solution for 30 minutes at room temperature. The blocks are then washed for 2 hours in distilled water. Frozen sections (7 to 20μ) are cut, mounted in glycerol-acetic acid solution or other media of varying refractive indices. The sections are examined in a polarizing microscope equipped with a variable compensator of the Barek type. To determine imbibition curves, sections containing endplates are selected by use of the phase microscope and an area no greater than 2 by 2 mm. is cut out by means of a small knife and glass needles. The pattern of the subneural apparatuses within the square is diagrammed, and the square is successively examined in various media of different refractive index. Refractive indices used range from water (n=1.33) to glue (n=1.52). A minimum of 2 hours is required in each medium for complete imbibition. The optical retardation of several junctional folds is determined in each medium and plotted against the refractive index.

This procedure is repeated for each specimen after treating the section with warm acetone at 56°C. for 6 hours to extract lipids.

Result

Lead-stained NMJs appear as bright birefringent objects against the pale birefringence of the striated muscle fibers. The birefringence of the latter is greatly reduced by use of acetic acid in the mounting medium.

RUTHENIUM RED METHOD

LUFT (1971)

Fixation

1. glutaraldehyde 3.6% aq.	0.5 ml.
2. 0.2 M cacodylate buffer, pH 7.3	0.5 ml.
3. ruthenium red stock solution 1500 ppm in H_2O	0.5 ml.

Post Fixation

1. 5% OSO₄ in aq. dist.   0.5 ml.
2. 0.2 M cacodylate buffer, pH 7.3   0.5 ml.
3. ruthenium red stock solution   0.5 ml.
    1500 ppm made up immediately before use

Method

Fix for 1 hour in solution 1, 25°C. Rinse three times 4 minutes in 0.15 M cacodylate buffer. Post fix 3 hours in solution 2. Rinse with buffer, dehydrate with ethanol and embed in Epon. Fresh tissue blocks may be placed directly into solution 2. Other buffers except phosphate may be substituted.

Result

Optical microscopy: brown-black deposits at sites of reaction. Electron microscopy: electron dense granules corresponding to sites visible in optical microscope.

DEMONSTRATION OF CONNECTIONS BETWEEN THE T SYSTEM AND THE SUBNEURAL APPARATUS BY MEANS OF LANTHANUM

modified from REVEL AND KARNOVSKY (J. Cell. Biol. 33:67, 1967)

Reagents

1. lanthanum nitrate: $(La(NO_3) \cdot 6H_2O$
    1 gm. in 100 ml. of 0.85% NaCl

2. fixative for perfusion: 3% glutaraldehyde in 0.1 M phosphate buffer (pH 7.4) containing O.5% NaCl and 1% sucrose
3. post fixative: 1% OSO_4 in phosphate buffer (pH 7.4)

Method

Inject mouse muscle *in vivo* with 0.2 ml. of solution 1 using small (27 gauge) needle. After 5 minutes, perfuse with solution 2 via the left ventricle. Excise blocks of NMJ-containing muscle and fix for an additional 20 minutes in solution 1. Wash with buffered 0.85% saline 3 times 5 minutes, post fix with solution 3 for 15 minutes, rinse in 50% ethanol and dehydrate through graded ethanol, propylene oxide and embed in Epon.

ZINC-IODIDE—OSMIUM METHOD FOR SYNAPTIC VESICLES

KAWANA et al. (*Brain Res. 16:*325-331, 1969)

Reagents

Fixation: Tissue may be place fresh into the incubation solutions but better preservation of fine structure results if aldehyde fixation is used.
1. paraformaldehyde fixative
   perfusion with 4% paraformaldehyde in 0.05 M phosphate buffer, pH 7.4
2. stock buffer (Martin et al., *Brain Res. 15:*1-16, 1969)
    a. NaCl   3.3 gm.
    b. $CaCl_2$ 0.06 gm.
    c. $MgCl_2 \cdot 6H_2O$ 0.31 g.
    d. Tris-HCl buffer   100 ml. (pH 7.4)
3. ZIO mixture
    a. zinc powder   6 gm.

b. iodine resublimate 2 gm.
c. water 40 ml.
Take 4 ml. of this filtered solution and add to 4 ml. of Tris-Hcl buffer (pH 7.4) containing
   3.3 gm. NaCl
   0.06 g. $CaCl_2$
   0.31 g. $MgCl_2 \cdot 6H_2O$
   0.605 gm. Tris in 50 ml. H_2O
4. osmium tetroxide
   2% solution in stock buffer (2)

Method

Small blocks of tissue are post fixed in 6.25% glutaraldehyde, 0.1 M phosphate buffer pH 7.4 for 2 hours. Wash 3 times 5 minutes in stock buffer (2) and impregnate 16 hours at 4°C. in ZIO mixture prepared by mixing solution 3 with 2 ml. of solution 4 shortly before use (pH 6.25). Dehydrate and embed in Epon.

HISTOCHEMICAL METHODS FOR ESTERASES

THIOCHLINE METHOD (KOELLE, 1951, Modified)

Reagents

1. copper glycine solution
   glycine 3.75 gm.
   copper sulfate ($CuSO_4 \cdot 5H_2O$) 2.50 gm.
   aq. dist. 100 ml.
2. maleate buffer
   monosodium maleate 9.60 gm.
   N sodium hydroxide 52.20 ml.
   aq. dist. 100 ml.

3. sodium sulfate 40% in buffer pH 6
   (stored at 38°C.)
4. magnesium chloride   9.52 gm.
   in aq. dist.   100 ml.
5. acetylthiocholine solution
   - acetylthiocholine iodide   23 mg.
   - aq. dist.   1.2 ml.
   - 0.1 M copper sulfate   0.4 ml.
   - centrifuge; save supernatant
6. butyrylthiocholine solution
   - butyrylthiocholine iodide
   - aq. dist.   1.8 ml.
   - 0.1 M copper sulfate   0.6 ml.
   - centrifuge; save supernatant
7. copper thiocholine solution
   Incubation solutions are filtered immediately after removal of slides, stored at 38°C. for 2 to 4 days, and centrifuged. The precipitate is collected and washed with aq. dist.
8. rinse solution 1
   20% sodium sulfate saturated with copper thiocholine
9. rinse solution 2
   10% sodium sulfate saturated with copper thiocholine
10. rinse solution 3
    water saturated with copper thiocholine
11. copper sulfide-ammonium sulfide solution
    Half strength ammonium hydroxide solution saturated with hydrogen sulfide is stored at 4°C. until used. Immediately before use, dilute 1:25 and saturate with copper sulfide.
12. fixative: 10% formalin saturated with sulfide

Method

Frozen sections are cut at 20 to 35μ and stored in the following solutions prior to incubation. All are kept at 30 to 35°C.

    a. storage solution, di-isopropyl fluorophosphate (DFP)
        aq. dist.   4.5 ml.
        40% sodium sulfate solution   9.0 ml.
        10^{-6} M DFP   1.5 ml.

b. storage solution
 aq. dist. 6.0 ml.
 40% sodium sulfate solution 9.0 ml.
c. storage solution
 aq. dist. 4.5 ml.
 40% sodium sulfate solution 10.5 ml.

Demonstration of Acetylcholinesterase Activity. Sections to be stained for AchE activity and controls are placed in storage solution DFP (storage solution a) for 30 minutes and transferred to storage solution b until placed in the incubation solution. To demonstrate AchE activity, sections are then incubated in the following mixture for 5 to 60 minutes at 38°C.

1. copper glycine solution 0.6 ml.
2. aq. dist. 2.1 ml.
3. maleate buffer 1.5 ml.
4. sodium sulfate 9.0 ml.
5. magnesium chloride 0.6 ml.
6. copper thiocholine trace
7. acetylthiocholine 1.2 ml.

After completion of the reaction, the sections are rinsed in the sodium sulfate-copper thiocholine solution for 5 minutes and in 10% sodium sulfate saturated with copper thiocholine for an additional minute. The final rinse is in water saturated with copper thiocholine. The sections are then placed in copper sulfide-saturated ammonium sulfide solution for 20 seconds, rinsed rapidly in water, and fixed in 10% formalin saturated with copper sulfide. The blocks are dehydrated through copper sulfide-saturated alcohol and xylol and mounted in permount. The preparations may be counterstained with hematoxylin and eosin or brilliant cresyl violet.

Controls are incubated in the following mixture:
1. copper glycine 0.4 ml.
2. aq. dist. 1.4 ml.
3. maleate buffer 1.0 ml.
4. sodium sulfate solution 6.0 ml.
5. magnesium chloride solution 0.4 ml.
6. copper thiocholine trace
7. acetylthiocholine none
8. butyrylthiocholine 0.8 ml.

Demonstration of Cholinesterase. For nonspecific ChE, sections are stored in storage solution c (40% sodium sulfate) and then incubated in the following solution for 5 to 60 minutes at 38°C.:

1. copper glycine solution	0.6 ml.
2. aq. dist.	0.6 ml.
3. maleate buffer	1.5 ml.
4. sodium sulfate solution	10.5 ml.
5. magnesium chloride	0.6 ml.
6. copper thiocholine	trace
7. butyrylthiocholine	1.2 ml.

The subsequent steps are the same as in the AchE technique. All solutions are allowed to incubate 15 minutes after addition of copper thiocholine. The substrates acetylthiocholine and butyrylcholine are added immediately before filtering of the final reaction mixture.

Result

Sites of AchE and ChE activity are indicated by a granular dark brown precipitate.

ACETYLTHIOCHOLINE METHOD
(KOELLE — MODIFIED BY COUTEAUX, 1951)

Reagents

1. amino-acetic acid solution		
amino-acetic acid	3.75	gm.
aq. dist.	100	ml.
2. copper sulfate (0.1 M)		
copper sulfate	24.9	gm.
aq. dist.	1000	ml.
3. acetate buffer (pH 5) solution		
0.1 N acetic acid	3	ml.
0.1 N sodium acetate	6	ml.

4. acetylthiocholine solution
    acetylthiocholine iodide   15   mg.
    aq. dist.   0.75 ml.
    solution 2 (copper sulfate)   0.3 ml.

Method

Muscle blocks are fixed in 10% formol-saline for 6 hours and frozen sections are cut at 50μ. Sections are incubated for 45 minutes at 37°C. in the following mixture:

1. amino-acetic acid solution (reagent 1)   0.2 ml.
2. 0.1 M copper sulfate (reagent 2)   0.2 ml.
3. acetate buffer (reagent 3)   5.0 ml.
4. aq. dist.   3.8 ml.
5. acetylthiocholine solution (reagent 4)   0.8 ml.

At the end of the staining period the sections are removed from the staining solution, washed in aq. dist., and placed in 5% ammonium sulfide. Wash, dehydrate, clear and mount in neutral media.

Result

Sites of esterase activity are indicated by a brown granular precipitate.

THIOCHOLINE FERRICYANIDE METHOD
(KARNOVSKY AND ROOTS, 1964)

Reagents

1. 5 mg. substrate (acetyl or butyrylthiocholine iodide) dissolved in 6.5 ml. 0.1 M sodium hydrogen maleate buffer pH 5.0 (other buffers acceptable: phosphate, acetate phthalate)
2. add with stirring in order:
    a. 0.5 ml. 0.3 M sodium citrate
    b. 1.0 ml. 30mM copper sulphate

c. 1.0 ml. water
   d. 1.0 ml. 5mM potassium ferricyanide
3. eserine inhibitor may be added 1 ml. freshly prepared 1 M solution instead of water following copper sulfate

Method

Blocks of tissue are fixed overnight in cold 10% formalin containing 1% CaCl and stored in 0.88 M sucrose — 1% gum arabic solution. Wash tissue for 5 minutes in aq. dist., blot and quick frozen in isopentane — acetone — dry ice. The cryostat sections are mounted on gelatinized slides and incubated 15 minutes in reaction mixture.

Result

Brown deposits (Hatchett's Brown) of insoluble copper ferrocyanide at sites of enzyme activity.

GOLD THIOCHOLINE METHOD
(KOELLE AND GROMADZKI, 1966)

Fixation

4% formaldehyde in maleate buffer (0.028 M, pH 7.4) containing 7.5% sucrose:

Reagents

1. $AuNa_3(S_2O_3)$ H_2O 0.1 M
2. acetylthiocholine 0.05 M
   46 mg. acetylthiocholine iodide dissolved in 2.00 ml. H_2O
   add 1.15 ml. 0.1 M $AgNO_3$, shake and allow AgCl ppt to settle
   50 mg. butyrylthiocholine iodide may be substituted for acetylthiocholine

3. inhibitors:
   eserine salicylate 10^{-3} M
   BW 284 10^{-3} M
   Nu 683 10^{-3} M
4. $NaH_2PO_4 \cdot H_2O$ and K_2HPO_4 6 M
5. DFP 0.10-0.3 M in anhydrous propylene glycol for inhibitor ChE (10^{-8}, 10^{-7}M) for AchE (10^{-5}M)
6. gold thiocholine phosphate — allow incubation solutions to undergo complete spontaneous hydrolysis 2-3 days at 37°C. and collect ppt.
7. acid-alcoholic $(NH_4)_2S$
   3.6 ml.   yellow $(NH_4)_2S$
   20.0 ml.   absolute ethanol
   6.0 ml.   acetic a
   q.s. 30 ml. with alcohol
   1 drop $AuNa_3(S_2O_3)_2$
   mix. adjust pH 5.4-5.6 — filter #3 Whatman
8. alcohol — formalin solution
   2.0 ml.   40% formaldehyde
   4.0 ml.   dist. H_2O
   to 20 ml.   absolute ethanol
9. preincubation solution:
   0.4 ml.   solution 1
   2.9 (2.8) ml. H_2O
   4.6 ml. NaH_2PO_4
   2.1 ml. K_2HPO_4
   pH adjusted to 5.6 ± 0.05
10. incubation solution:
    0.4 ml.   solution 1
    2.1 (2.0) ml. H_2O
    0.8 ml.   thiocholine (.004)
    (0.1 ml.   inhibitor (10^{-5}M)
    4.6 ml. NaH_2PO
    2.1 ml. K_2PO_4
    stand 20-40 minutes until colloidal
    filter immediately before use
    pH adjusted to 5.6 ± 0.05
11. rinse solution:
    3.3 ml. H_2O
    4.6 ml. NaH_2PO_4

2.1 ml. K_2HPO_4
saturate with filtered gold thiocholine phosphate
with inhibitor (eserine or BW 284)

Method

Fresh tissue is fixed 2 hours in cold (4°C.) 4% formaldehyde maleate (0.028 M) fixative at pH 7.4 containing 7.5% sucrose. Rinse in same solution without formaldehyde 30 minutes to 40 hours. Frozen sections (10-20μ) are cut in cryostat and dried on slides. Preincubate for 15 minutes in preincubation solution (9). Incubate for 15 to 60 minutes in incubation solution (10). Then rinse for 10 minutes in rinse solution (11), and place in acid-alcoholic ammonium sulphide solution (7) for 10 minutes. Then rinse in alcoholic formalin (8) for 10 minutes, dehydrate in graded ethanol and mount in permount.

Result

Brown reaction product granules at sites of enzyme activity.

GOLD ACETYLTHIOCHOLINE METHOD FOR ELECTRON MICROSCOPY

DAVIS AND KOELLE (1965, 1967)

Fixation

4% formol-sucrose (7.5%) maleate buffer (0.028 M, pH 7.4)

Reagents

1. preincubation solution:
    solution 2 with substrate Au thiocholine omitted
2. incubation solution
    0.004 M $AuNa_3(S_2O_3)_2$
    0.004 M   AThCh (or BuThCh)
    4.0 M NaH_2PO_4-K_2HPO_4 (pH 5.6)
3. postincubation solution:
    as in 2 but omit substrate and gold salt
    solutions 1 and 3 are saturated with the primary reaction product

4. acid-alcoholic $(NH_4)_2S$

5. acidic 4% formaldehyde solution

6. 1% osmium tetroxide solution

Method

Fixed muscle is washed in cold sucrose — maleate buffer 30 minutes to 18 hours. Then cut frozen sections (50-100μ) in cryostat and incubate in solution 1 for 15 minutes (room temperature 22-24°C.) and solution 2 for 10 seconds to 15 minutes. Then place in solution 3 for 15 minutes. Immerse sections in acid-alcoholic $(NH_4)_2S$ solution, rinse in acidic 4% formaldehyde solution and post fix 30-60 minutes cold buffered 1% OSO_4. Dehydrate and embed in Epon.

Result

Electron dense precipitate at sites of AchE activity in pre- and postsynaptic membranes.

AZO DYE METHOD

RAVIN et al. (1953)

Reagents

staining solution
β-naphthyl acetate	10 mg.
tetrazotized diorthoanisidine (Diazo blue B)	40 mg.
barbital buffer pH 7.8	50 ml.
calcium chloride 3%	5 ml.
acetone	1 ml.

Method

Fresh frozen sections are cut at 6 to 20 μ and dried onto glass slides. The sections are incubated for 10 to 20 minutes in the staining solution, washed, and mounted in glycerogel. Incubation with eserine (10^{-5}M), sodium arsenilate (10^{-3}M), and sodium taurocholate (10^{-3}M) may be used prior to staining to identify the activities of various esterases since the substrate β-naphthyl acetate is not specific for AchE.

Result

Blue granules of azo dye are precipitated in the region of NMJs.

Comment

This method will demonstrate low levels of AchE activity in frozen sections but is not specific for AchE, and the final dye product tends to diffuse where large amounts of lipid are present. It stains NMJs well but does not have sufficient resolution to demonstrate the rodlets of the subneural apparatus. Now chiefly of historic interest, this method is still useful for rapid survey work.

INDOXYL ACETATE METHOD

HOLT AND WITHERS (1952)

Reagents

    staining solution
o-acetyl-5-bromoindoxyl	1.3 mg.
ethanol	0.1 ml.

    dissolve and add

0.1 M tris (hydroxymethyl) amino-methane-hydrochloric acid buffer	2.0 ml.
0.05 M potassium ferricyanide	1.0 ml.
0.05 M potassium ferrocyanide	1.0 ml.
0.1 M calcium chloride	1.0 ml.

    add aq. dist. or 1.0 M sodium chloride to 10 ml.

Method

Fix small blocks of muscle in 5% neutral formalin in 1% saline at 4°C. for 24 hours. Cut frozen sections at 10 to 15μ and incubate in staining solution at 37°C. for 10 seconds to several hours. Use the microscope to follow the progress of the reaction. Counterstain with carmalum if desired. Rinse in water, mount on slides in glycerogel or dehydrate in graded ethanol, clear in carbolxylene, and mount in neutral mounting medium.

Result

A blue indigo precipitate forms at the site of esterase activity.

Comment

This method is capable of demonstrating the subneural apparatus. It is nonspecific, however, and inhibitors must be used where mixtures of esterases are present. This method has been supplanted by the more specific methods.

OSMIOPHILIC POLYMER METHODS

BERGMAN et al. (1967)

Reagents

    2.5% 2-naphthylthiolacetate (NTA) in acetone
    2.5% 2-thiolacetoxybenzanilide (TAB) in acetone
    2.5% 2-thiolpropionoxybenzanilide (TPB)

Fixation

1. 10% formalin buffered with 0.1 M phosphate buffer (pH 7.4) containing 0.22 M sucrose 4°C.
2. freeze in isopentane (-70°C.)
3. cut 25μ frozen sections floated on 0.44 M sucrose solution 30 minutes
4. incubation: 0°C.
    a. phosphate buffer (0.1 M pH 7.4)   10.0 ml.
    b. substrate   0.1 ml.
    c. fast blue BBN   5 mg.
    d. sucrose   0.75 gm.
    incubate 5-20 minutes with NTA, 5-30 minutes with TAB and 5-40 minutes with TPB

Method

    Freshly prepared incubation solution is made by dissolving 0.75 gm. sucrose in 10 ml. phosphate buffer (pH 7.4) and add 0.1 ml. of 2.5% substrate solution prepared in acetone. Add 5 mg. fast blue BBN, shake and filter. After incubation, sections washed in chilled 0.22 M sucrose solution (1-2 minutes), place on cover slips and post fix with OSO_4 vapor 10-20 minutes (osmium crystals and a small amount of distilled water heated to 50°C. on a sand bath). Transfer to 70% ethanol, dehydrate in graded ethanol and embed in Epon.

Result

Osmium black outlines the subneural apparatus. In the electron microscope, there are droplets of electron dense reaction product at sites of esterase activity.

MEDNICK et al. (1971)

I. p-Acetylthiolbenzenediazonium (ATBD) method:

Reagents

1. p-Acetylthiolanilinium chloride   102 mg. in 1.0 ml.
2. add 1.0 ml. of 1.0 M HCl diluted with 2 ml. H_2O with 1.0 ml. water rinse at 0-4°C.
3. add 34.4 mg. $NaNO_2$ in 3.0 ml. H_2O followed by 1 min. rinse
4. swirl for 5 minutes and add urea 2.1 mg. in 0.5 ml. and swirl for 2 minutes
5. dilute with 190 ml. 0.1 M sodium phosphate buffer (pH 7.2 at 25°C.) and use immediately.

ATBD Method

Frozen or fixed sections (cold 1% glutaraldehyde for 60 minutes) are incubated in ATBD medium at 4°C. for 2 hours. Rinse in 20% $(Na)_2SO_4$ for 1-3 minutes, post fix in OSO_4 vapor for 40-45 minutes at 50°C. and dehydrate in ethanol. Mount in permount or embed in Epon for electron microscopy.

II. α-Acetylthiol-m-toluenediazonium ion (ATTD) method:

Reagents

1. 25 mg. of α-acetylthiol-m-toluidinium chloride diazotized at 0-4°C. in ice bath by dissolving amine hydrochloride in 0.5 ml. 4% HCl (0.05 M) and add 0.5 ml. 1.7% $NaNO_2$. After 5 minutes, add 1ml. 1.0 M NaAc and bring to 10 ml. with distilled water
2. the pH is 5.0-5.5
3. add 2.5 ml. of the freshly prepared diazonium mixture to an incubation solution containing 5 ml. 0.1 M phosphate buffer (pH 7.2) and 2.5 ml. H_2O

ATTD Method

Incubate tissue sections in ATTD medium for 20 minutes at 37°C. Then rinse in water for 1-3 minutes and post fix in OSO_4 vapor at 50°C. Dehydrate in graded ethanol, clear in xylol and mount in permount.

Result

The sites of enzyme activity are indicated by electron dense amorphous deposits. (See also Davis et al J. Histochem. Cytochem 1972.)

THIOLACETIC ACID METHOD

BARRNETT AND PALADE (1959)

Reagents

1. 0.12 M thiolacetic acid (practical, not purified) (Eastman Kodak)   0.23 ml.
2. 1 N sodium hydroxide

3. cacodylate buffer
    a. stock sodium cacodylate 42.899 gm.
       in aq. dist. 1000 ml.
    b. 0.2 M hydrochloric acid
    Take 50 ml. of a and 39.2 ml. of b and dilute to 200 ml. with aq. dist. Final pH is 5.6
4. lead nitrate 830 mg.
   aq. dist. 100ml.
5. 0.2 M manganese chloride
6. 0.2 M calcium chloride
7. 0.2 M magnesium chloride

Method

Take 0.23 ml. of thiolacetic acid in fume hood and add about 4 ml. of 1 N sodium hydroxide drop by drop until the pH is 5.6. Bring to 25 ml. with cacodylate buffer (pH 5.6). Then add 1 ml. lead nitrate and 0.5 ml. each of manganese, magnesium and calcium chloride solutions. Blocks of fresh muscle or whole muscles from small animals are placed in the staining solution. For light microscopy 5 to 10 minutes' incubation at room temperature is sufficient. For electron microscopy 30 seconds' to 2 minutes' incubation suffices. The blocks may be sectioned and examined in the light microscope or fixed in osmium tetroxide and embedded for electron microscopy.

Result

NMJs are sharply outlined by black lead sulfide precipitate when viewed in the light microscope. In electron micrographs, a minutely granular (approximately 30 to 100 Å) precipitate is deposited at or near the sites of esterase activity. The method is extremely sensitive in fresh tissue and the precipitate is very dense and very fine in electron micrographs. Glutaraldehyde fixation prior to incubation with thiolacetic acid gives somewhat different results (Sabatini et al., 1963). As with many of the other methods that do not employ specific substrates, this method lacks specificity.

GOLD THIOLACETIC ACID METHOD

KOELLE AND GROMADZKI (1966)

Reagents

1. $AuNa_3(S_2O_3) \cdot 2H_2O$ 0.1 M
2. $MgCl_2 \cdot 6H_2O$ 1 M
3. maleate buffer   0.703 M
   4.80 gm. NaH maleate in 26.1 ml. NaOH q.s. 50 ml.
4. thiolacetic acid   0.2 M
   0.288 ml. thiolacetic acid (E.K. practical) in 3.6 ml. N NaOH q.s. with cold, freshly boiled distilled H_2O
5. HCl   1 N
6. inhibitors: DFP 0.10–0.30 M in 0.85% NaCl
   BW 284 + eserine 10^{-3}M stock solutions
7. $(NH_4)_2S$ yellow   0.3/100

1. Preincubation Solution:

   a. $AuNa_3(S_2O_3)_2$ 0.3 ml.
   b. H_2O 8.2 ml. (8.1)*
   c. $MgCl_2$ 0.32 ml.
   d. maleate   0.8 ml.
   e. thiolacetic acid   0.3 ml.
   f. HCl   0.12 ml.
   g. (inhibitor)   0.1 ml.
      pH 6.2 ± 0.05

2. Incubation Solution:

   a. $AuNa_3(S_2O_3)_2$ 0.3 ml.
   b. H_2O 6.5 ml. (6.4)*
   c. $MgCl_2$ 0.32 ml.
   d. maleate   0.8 ml.
   e. thiolacetic acid   2.0 ml.
   f. HCl   0.12 ml.
   g. (inhibitor)   0.1 ml.
   h. $(NH_4)_2S$ 1 drop

3. Post-incubation Solution:
As in incubation solution with omission of gold salt and thiolacetic acid and addition of 4% formaldehyde.

Method

Whole strips of muscle are fixed 2 hours in cold 4% formol (7.5%) maleate buffer (0.028 M pH 7.4). Preincubate in solution 1 for 30 minutes, incubate in solution 2 for 1-4 hours (2-4°C.) and solution 3 for 15 minutes. Cut blocks with NMJs in solution 3 and post fix 1-2% buffered OSO_4 4-6°C. 2-4 hours. Dehydrate and embed in Epon.

Inhibitors

1. DFP 10^{-7} to 3×10^{-7} in sucrose maleate buffer.
   Incubate 30 minutes prior to solution 1 used to inhibit nsChE
2. ambenomium chloride $10^{-6}M$ prior to solution 1 inhibits AchE. BW 284 can not be used.

Result

Fine electron dense particles at sites of enzyme activity.

COMBINED STAINING FOR AXONS AND CHOLINESTERASE ACTIVITY

CHOLINESTERASE — BIELSCHOWSKY STAINING METHOD

GWYN AND HEARDMAN (1965)

1. **Fixative:** 10% formol-saline
2. **Incubation Solution:**
   a. $CuSO_4$ 0.1 M   0.2 ml.
   b. aminoacetic acid 0.5 M   0.1 ml.

c. acetate buffer 0.1 M pH 4.7   5 ml.
d. supernatant 0.8 ml. from 3 volumes 2% acetylthiocholine iodide solution and 1 volume 0.1 M $CuSO_4$

3. **Ammoniacal $AgNO_3$ Solution:**
add NH_4OH until precipitate forms, then add 3 drops in excess after solution clears.

Method

Fix pieces less than 5 mm. thick for 6 hours in formol-saline 20-25°C. (1) and wash in aq. dist. 16 hours. Cut 50μ frozen sections in 10% sucrose, wash 1 hour in distilled H_2O and incubate 15 minutes at 37°C. in incubation solution (2). Then wash 5 minutes in aq. dist. and place in 5% $(NH_4)_2S$ solution for 2 minutes. Wash in aq. dist. for 1 hour and place in 10% neutral formalin containing 2% pyridine for at least 15 days. Then wash in tap water 1 hour and stain in 10% $AgNO_3$ 1.5 hours at 37°C. in the dark. Wash in 10% formalin in tap H_2O until white precipitate removed. Warm sections in 10 ml. ammoniacal $AgNO_3$ solution (3) for 1 minute, rinse in 1% ammoniated H_2O for 2 minutes, 3% $Na_2S_2O_3$ for 5 minutes and aq. dist. for 30 minutes. Dehydrate and mount.

Result

Black Ag_2S deposits in NMJs and black-stained axons.

CHOLINESTERASE — SILVER STAINING METHOD

NAMBA et al. (1967)

1. frozen sections 30-50μ from blocks frozen in dry ice-isopentane
2. place on coverslip and thaw in formalin vapor at 25°C.

Reagents

1. fixative for sections
   a. 10 ml. formalin
   b. 1 gm. $CaCl_2$
   c. 0.5 gm. $MgCl_2 6H_2O$
   d. 0.1 gm. $CdCl_2 \cdot 2½H_2O$
   in 100.0 ml. 0.07 M Veronal-acetate buffer (pH 6.45)
2. **Thiocholine solution:**
   a. 0.15 gm. acetylthiocholine iodide in 7.8 ml. H_2O
   b. 0.06 gm. $CuSO_4 \cdot 5H_2O$ in 2.6 ml. H_2O
   c. 0.05 M Veronal-acetate buffer (pH 6.1)
      containing 0.075 gm. glycine and 0.05 gm. $CuSO_4 \cdot 5H_2O$ in 92 ml.
3. **Potassium ferricyanide solution:**
   0.25 gm. in 100 ml. distilled H_2O
4. **Silver nitrate solution:**
   1. $AgNO_3$ — 10 gm.
   2. $CuSO_4 \cdot 5H_2O$ — 0.05 gm.
   3. $CaCO_3$ — 0.1 gm.
   4. distilled H_2O — 100 ml.
5. **Reducing solution:**
   1. hydroquinone — 1.0 gm.
   2. Na_2SO_3 — 10 gm.
   3. distilled H_2O — 100 ml.

Method

Fix sections 60 minutes in solution 1. Rinse in aq. dist. for 60 minutes at 4°C. (may be stored for days). Then incubate 60 minutes at 37°C. in 8 ml. of supernatant from thiocholine solution 2 followed by rinse in aq. dist. for 30 seconds. Place in potassium ferricyanide solution (3) for 10 minutes at 25°C. and rinse twice for 5 minutes in aq. dist. Then place in silver nitrate solution (4) for 90 minutes at 37°C. Rinse with aq. dist. for 5 seconds and place in reducing solution (5) for 10 minutes with gentle shaking during the first minute. Wash twice 5 minutes in aq. dist., dehydrate in 90% ethanol, absolute ethanol, clear in xylol and mount.

Bibliography

Aagenaes, O. and Moe, H.: Light and electron microscopic study of skin capillaries of diabetics. Diabetes *10:* 253-259, 1961.

Aarseth, P., Barstad, J.A.B., Rogne, O. and Oksne, S.: A quaternary carbon analogue of acetylthiocholine as substrate for cholinesterases. Histochemie *15:* 229-233, 1968.

Abel, J.J., Firor, W.M. and Chalian, W.: Researches on tetanus. IX. Further evidence to show that tetanus toxin is not carried to central neurones by way of the axis cylinders of motor nerves. Bull. Johns Hopkins Hosp. *63:* 373-403, 1938.

Abrams, H.K., Hamblin, D.O. and Marchand, J.F.: Pharmacology and toxicology of certain organic phosphorus insecticides. 4. Clinical experience. J.A.M.A. *144:* 107-108, 1950.

Acheson, G.H.: Physiology of neuro-muscular junctions: chemical aspects. Fed. Proc. *7:* 447-457, 1948.

Adams, D.H. and Whittaker, V.P.: The cholinesterases of human blood. I. The specificity of the plasma enzyme and its relation to the erythrocyte cholinesterase. Biochim. et Biophys. Acta *3:* 358-366, 1949.

Adams, R.D., Denny-Brown, D. and Pearson, C.M.: Diseases of Muscle: A Study in Pathology. Paul B. Hoeber, Inc., New York, 1962, p. 492.

Addison, W.H.F.: Neurological technique, *in* Microscopic Technique (McClung, C.V., ed.). 2nd edition, Paul B. Hoeber, New York, 1939.

Agostini, B. and Noetzel, H.: Morphological study of muscle fibres and motor endplates in tetanus. *in* Muscle Diseases Proc. Int. Congress Milan 1969 Excerpta Med. Int. Congress Ser. *199:* 123-127, 1970.

Aitken, J.T.: Growth of nerve implants into voluntary muscle. J. Anat. (Lond.) *84:* 38-49, 1950.

Akert, K. and Sandri, C.: An electron-microscopic study of zinc iodide osmium impregnation of neurons. I. Staining of synaptic vesicles at cholinergic junctions. Brain Res. *7:* 286-295, 1968.

Albuquerque, E.X.: The mode of action of batrachotoxin Fed. Proc. *31:*1133-1138, 1972.
Albuquerque, E.X., Barnard, E.A., Chiu, T.H., Lapa, A.J. et al: Acetylcholine receptor and ion conductance modulator sites at the murine neuromuscular junction: evidence for specific toxin reactions. Proc. Nat. Acad. Sci. (U.S.) *70:*949-953, 1973a.
Albuquerque, E.X. and McIsaac, R.J.: Early development of acetylcholine receptors in fast and slow mammalian skeletal muscle. Life Sci. *8:*409-416, 1969.
Albuquerque, E.X. and McIsaac, R.J.: Fast and slow mammalian muscles after denervation. Exp. Neurol. *26:*183-202, 1970.
Albuquerque, E.X., Sasa, M. and Avner, B.P.: Possible site of action of batrachotoxin. Nature New Biology *234:*93-94, 1971.
Albuquerque, E.X., Schuh, F.T. and Kauffman, F.C.: Early membrane depolarization of the fast mammalian muscle after denervation. Pflüger's Arch. *328:*36-50, 1971.
Albuquerque, E.X. and Warnick, J.E.: Electrophysiological observations in normal and dystrophic chicken muscles. Science *172:*1260-1263, 1971a.
Albuquerque, E.X., Warnick, J.E. and Sansone, F.M.: The pharmacology of batrachotoxin. II. Effect on electrical properties of the mammalian nerve and skeletal muscle membranes. J. Pharm. Exp. Therap. *176:*511-528, 1971c.
Albuquerque, E.X., Warnick, J.E., Sansone, and Daly, J.: The pharmacology of batrachotoxin v. A comparative study of membrane properties and the effect of batrachotoxin on sartorius muscles of the frogs *Phyllobates aurotaenia* and *Rana pipiens.* J. Pharm. Exp. Therap. *184:*315-329, 1973b.
Alexandrowicz, J.S.: Receptor organs in thoracic and abdominal muscles of crustacea. Biol. Rev. *42:*288-326, 1967.
Allen, D.E., Johnson, A.G. and Woolf, A.L.: The intramuscular nerve endings in dystrophia myotonica — a biopsy study by vital staining and electron microscopy. J. Anat. *105:*1-26, 1969.
Alles, G.A. and Hawes, R.C.: Cholinesterase in the blood of man. J. Biol. Chem. *133:*375-390, 1942.
Altamirano, M., Schleyer, W.L. and Nachmansohn, D.: Electrical activity in electric tissue. I. The difference between tertiary and quaternary nitrogen compounds in relation to their chemical and electrical activities. Biochim. et Biophys. Acta *16:*268-282, 1955.
Ambache, N., Morgan, R.S. and Wright, G.P.: The action of tetanus toxin on the rabbit's iris. J. Physiol. (Lond.) *107:*45-53, 1948.
Ammon, R.: Die Hemmungskörper der Cholinesterase. Ergebn. Enzfor., *9:*35-69, 1943.
Anderson, P.J. and Song, S.K.. Experimental myositis: a cytochemical and electron microscopic study of drug-induced degeneration. *in* Proc. V Internat. Congr. Neuropath., (Luthy, F. and Bischoff, A., eds.). Internat. Congr. Series No. 100, Excerpta Med. Found. Amsterdam, pp. 687-693, 1966.
Anderson, P.J., Song, S.K. and Slotwiner, P.: The fine structure of spheromembranous degeneration of skeletal muscle induced by vincristine. J. Neuropath. & Exper. Neurol. *26:*15-24, 1967.
Andersson-Cedergren, E.: Ultrastructure of motor endplate and sarcoplasmic components of mouse skeletal muscle fiber. J. Ultrastr. Res., suppl. *1:*5-181, 1959.
Andres, K.H.: Mikropinozytose im Zentralnerven system. Z. Zellforsch. *64:*63-73, 1964.
Andrews, J.M. and Maxwell, D.S.: Ultrastructure features of anterior horn cell degeneration in the Wobbler (wr) mouse. Anat. Rec. *157:*206, 1967.

Aran, F.A.: Recherches sur une maladie non encore décrite du système musculaire (atrophie musculaire progressive). Arch. Gén. Méd. 24:5-35, 1850.
Aranow, H., Hoefer, P.F.A. and Rowland, L.P.: The long-acting anticholinesterase drugs in the management of myasthenia gravis. J. Chron. Dis. 6:457-474, 1957.
Ariëns, R.J., Van Rossum, J.M. and Simonis, A.M.: Affinity, intrinsic activity and drug interactions. Pharmacol. Rev. 9:218-236, 1957.
Askanas, V., Shafiq, S.A. and Milhorat, A.T.: Histochemistry of cultured aneural chick muscle morphological maturation without differentiation of fiber types. Exper. Neurology 37:218-230, 1972.
Asmundson, V.S. and Julian, L.M.: Inherited muscular abnormality in the domestic fowl. J. Hered. 47:248-252, 1956.
Atsumi, S.: The histogenesis of motor neurons with special reference to the correlation of their endplate formation. I. The development of endplates in the intercostal muscle of the chick embryo. Acta Anat. 80:161-182, 1971.
Atwood, H.L. and Johnson, H.S.: Neuromuscular synapses of a crab motor axon. J. Exp. Zool. 167:457-470, 1968.
Atwood, H.L., Luff, A.R., Morin, W.A. and Sherman, R.G.: Dense-cored vesicles at neuromuscular synapses of anthropods and vertebrates. Experientia 27:816-817, 1971.
Auerbach, A. and Betz, W.: Does Curare Affect transmitter release? J. Physiol. (Lond.) 213:691-705, 1971.
Augustinsson, K.B.: Cholinesterase — a study in comparative enzymology. Acta Physiol. Scand. 15 (suppl. 52):1-181, 1948.
Averell, P.R. and Norris, M.V.: Estimation of small amounts of 0,0-diethyl 0,p-nitrophenyl thiophosphate. Analyt. Chem. 20:753-756, 1948.
Awad, E.A.: Motor-point biopsies in carcinomatous neuropathy. Arch Phys. Med. 49:643-649, 1968.
Axelsson, J. and Thesleff, S.: A study of supersensitivity in denervated mammalian skeletal muscle. J. Physiol. (Lond.) 147:178-193, 1959.

Baker, N.: Supersensitivity to neostigmine and resistance to d-tubocurarine in mice with hereditary myopathy. Am. J. Physiol. 198:926-930, 1960.
Baker, N.: Supersensitivity to acetylcholinesterases of an isolated nerve-muscle preparation from hereditarily dystrophic mice. J. Pharm. & Exp. Therap. 141:223-229, 1963.
Bárány, M. and Close, R.I.: The transformation of myosin in cross innervated rat muscles. J. Physiol. (Lond.) 213:455-474, 1971.
Barets, A.: Différences dans le mode d'innervation des diverses portions du muscle latéral et leurs rapports avec la structure musculaire chez le poisson-chat. (Ameiurus nebulosus Les). Arch. Anat. Micros. et de Morph. Exptl. 41:305-331, 1952.
Barets, A.: Caractéristiques morphologiques des deux types d'innervation motrice du muscle latéral des Téléosteens. C.R. Soc. Biol. 149:1420-1422, 1955.
Barker, D.: L'innervation motrice du muscle strie des vertebres. Actualities Neurophysiol. 8:23-71, 1968.
Barker, D. and Ip, M.C.: The probable existence of a process of motor endplate replacement. J. Physiol. (Lond.) 176:11-12P, 1965.
Barker, D. and Ip, M.C.: Sprouting and degeneration of mammalian motor axons in normal and de-afferented skeletal muscle. Proc. Roy. Soc. B. 163:538-554, 1966.

Barnard, E.A. and Rogers, A.W.: Determination of the number, distribution and some in situ properties of cholinesterase molecules in the motor endplate, using labeled inhibitor methods. Ann. N.Y. Acad. Sci. 144:584-612, 1967.

Barondes, S.H.: Delayed appearance of labelled protein in isolated nerve endings and axoplasmic flow. Science 146:779-781, 1964.

Barrantes, F.J.: The neuromuscular junctions of a pulmonate mollusc. I. Ultrastructure study. Z. Zellforsch. 104:205-212, 1970.

Barrnett, R.J.: The fine structural localization of acetylcholinesterase at the myoneural junction. J. Cell Biol. 12:247-262, 1962.

Barrnett, R.J. and Palade, G.E.: Enzymatic activity in the M-bands. J. Biophys. & Biochem. Cytol. 6:163-169, 1959.

Barrnett, R.J. and Seligman, A.M.: Histochemical demonstration of esterases by production of indigo. Science 114:579-582, 1951.

Barron, K.D., Ordinario, A.T., Bernsohn, J., Hess, A.R. and Hedrick, M.T.: Cholinesterases and nonspecific esterases of developing and adult (normal and atrophic) rat gastrocnemius. I. Chemical assay and electrophoresis. J. Histochem. Cytochem. 16:346-361, 1968.

Bartels, E., Deal, W., Karlin, A. and Mautner, H.G.: Affinity oxidation of the reduced acetylcholine receptor. Biochem. Biophys. Acta 203:568-571, 1970.

Bartels, E., Wassermann, N.H. and Erlanger, B.F.: Photochromic activators of the acetylcholine receptor. Proc. U.S. Nat. Acad. Sci. 68:1820-1823, 1971.

Bass, L. and Moore, W.J.: Electrokinetic mechanism of miniature postsynaptic potentials. Proc. U.S. Nat. Acad. Sci. 55:1214-1217, 1966.

Bauer, W.C., Blumberg, J.M. and Zacks, S.I.: Short and Long Term Ultrastructure Changes in Denervated Mouse Motor Endplates. Proc. IV Int. Congress of Neuropathology, Munich, 1962. Georg Thieme Verlag, Stuttgart, 1962, pp. 16-18.

Bauwens, P.: Electrodiagnosis in motor unit dysfunction. Proc. Roy. Soc. Med. 48:194-197, 1955.

Bauwens, P.: Electrodiagnostic features of distal pathology in the motor unit. Symposium on Innervation of Muscle. Utrecht, 1957.

Beams, H.W. and Evans, T.C.: Electron micrographs of motor endplates. Proc. Soc. Biol. & Med. 82:344-346, 1952.

Beckett, E.B. and Bourne, G.H.: Some histochemical observations on enzyme reactions in goat foetal cardiac and skeletal muscle and some human foetal muscle. Acta Anat. 35:224-253, 1958.

Begliomini, A. and Moriconi, A.: Sull' epoca della comparsa e della localizzazione della colinesterasi nel musculo striato dell' embrione di pollo. Riv. Biol. 51:517-530, 1959.

Bellamy, D.: The distribution of bound acetylcholine and choline acetylase in rat and pigeon brain. Biochem. J. 72:165-168, 1959.

Belleau, B.: A molecular theory of drug action based on induced conformational perturbations of receptors. J. Med. Chem. 7:776-784, 1964.

Benda, P., Tsuji, S., Daussant, J. and Changeux, J.P.: Localization of acetylcholinesterase by immunofluorescence in eel electroplax. Nature 225:1149-1150, 1970.

Bennett, H.S. and Porter, K.P.: An electron microscopic study of sectioned breast muscle of the domestic fowl. Am. J. Anat. 93:61-105, 1955.

Berg, D.K., Kelly, R.B., Sargent, P.B., Williamson, P. and Hall, Z.W.: Binding of α-bungarotoxin to acetylcholine receptors in mammalian muscle. Proc. U.S. Nat. Acad. Sci. 69:147-151, 1972.

Bergh, N.P.: Studies on reaction of isolated phrenic nerve diaphragm preparation of various species to certain agents causing neuromuscular block. Scand. J. Clin. Lab. Invest. 5 (1 suppl.):5, 1953.

Bergman, R.A.: Motor nerve endings of twitch muscle fibers in Hippocampus hudsonius. J. Cell Biol. 32:751-757, 1967.

Bergman, R.A., Ueno, H., Morizono, Y., Hanker, J.S. and Seligman, A.M.: Ultrastructural demonstration of acetylcholinesterase activity of motor endplates via osmiophilic diazothioethers. Histochemie 11:1-12, 1967.

Bergner, A.D.: Histochemical demonstration of the effect of nerve section on cholinesterase activity at motor endplates in the gastrocnemius muscle of the guinea pig. Br. J. Exp. Path. 38:160-163, 1957.

Bergner, A.D.: Histochemical detection of fatal anticholinesterase poisoning the reactivation of cholinesterase in cadavers of rats. Am. J. Path. 35:807-817, 1959.

Bergner, A.D. and Durlacher, S.H.: Histochemical detection of fatal anticholinesterase poisoning. Am. J. Path. 27:1011-1021, 1951.

Bergstrand, A. and Bucht, H.: Electron microscopic investigations on the glomerular lesions in diabetes mellitus (diabetic glomerulosclerosis). Lab. Invest. 6:293-299, 1957.

Bernard, C.: Leçons sur les effets des substances toxiques et medicamenteuses. Paris, 1857.

Bernstein, J.J. and Guth, L.: Nonselectivity in establishment of neuromuscular connections following nerve regeneration in the rat. Exp. Neurol. 4:262-275, 1961.

Bernstein, S.: Über den zietliche Verlauf der negativen Schwankung des Nervenstroms. Arch. Ges. Physiol. 1:173-207, 1868.

Bessis, M. and Breton-Gorius, J.: Différents aspects du fer dan l'organisme. I. Ferritine et micelles ferrugineuses. J. Biophys. & Biochem. Cytol. 6:231-236, 1959.

Betz, W. and Sakmann, B.: "Dysjunction" of frog neuromuscular synapses by treatment with proteolytic enzymes. Nature New Biology 232:94-95, 1971.

Beuhler, H.J., Schantz, E.J. and Lamanna, C.: The elemental and amino acid composition of crystalline Clostridium botulinum type A toxin. J. Biol. Chem. 169:295-302, 1947.

Bickerstaff, E.R., Evans, J.V. and Woolf, A.L.: Ultrastructure of the myoneural junction in myasthenia gravis. Nature 184:1500, 1959.

Bickerstaff, E.R., Evans, J.V. and Woolf, A.L.: The ultrastructure of human myasthenic and non-myasthenic motor endplates. Brain 83:638-647, 1960.

Bickerstaff, E.R. and Woolf, A.L.: Carcinomatous sensory neuropathy associated with a pin-head-sized anaplastic carcinoma and plasma cell "encephalitis". Bgham. Med. Rev. 20:355-360, 1958.

Bickerstaff, E.R. and Woolf, A.L.: The intramuscular nerve endings in myasthenia gravis. Brain 83:10-23, 1960.

Bidstrup, P.L., Bonnell, J.A. and Beckett, A.G.: Paralysis following poisoning by a new organic phosphorus insecticide (mipafox). Report of two cases. Brit. Med. J. 1:1068-1072, 1953.

Birks, R.J.: The role of sodium ions in the metabolism of acetylcholine. Canad. J. Biochem. Physiol. 41:2573-2579, 1963.

Birks, R.I.: The fine structure of motor nerve endings at frog myoneural junctions. Ann. N.Y. Acad. Sci. 135:8-26, 1966.

Birks, R.I. and Brown, L.M.: A method for locating the cholinesterase of a mammalian neuromuscular junction by electron microscopy. J. Physiol. (Lond.) *152*:5-7, 1960.

Birks, R., Huxley, H.E. and Katz, B.: The fine structure of the neuromuscular junction of the frog. J. Physiol. (Lond.) *150*:134-144, 1960.

Birks, R., Katz, B. and Miledi, R.: Physiological and structural changes at the amphibian myoneural junction in the course of nerve degeneration. J. Physiol. (Lond.) *150*:145-168, 1960.

Birks, R. and MacIntosh, F.C.: Acetylcholine metabolism of a sympathetic ganglion. Canad. J. Biochem. Physiol. *39*:787-827, 1961.

Bishop, G.H. and Bronfenbrenner, J.J.: The site of action of botulinus toxin. Am. J. Physiol. *117*:393-404, 1936.

Bittner, G.D. and Kennedy, D.: Quantitative aspects of transmitter release. J. Cell Biol. *47*:585-592, 1970.

Blaustein, M.P. and Goldman, D.E.: The action of certain polyvalent cations on the voltage-clamped lobster axon. J. Gen. Physiol. *51*:279-291, 1968.

Blechschmidt, E. and Daikoku, S.H.: Die Entstehung der motorischen innervation in der menschlichen Zugenmuskulatur. Electronen mikroskopie der embryonalen Endplatte. Acta Anat. (Basel) *63*:179-198, 1966.

Blioch, Z.L., Glagoleva, I.M., Liberman, E.A. and Nemashev, V.A.: A study of the mechanism of quantal transmitter release at a chemical synapse. J. Physiol. (Lond.) *199*: 11-35, 1968.

Bloodworth, J.M.B. and Epstein, N.: Diabetic amyotrophy: light and electron microscopic investigation. Diabetes *16*:181-190, 1967.

Bloom, F.E.: Ultrastructural identification of catecholamine containing central synaptic terminals. J. Histochem. and Cytochem. *21*:333-348, 1973.

Blumcke, S. and Niedorf, H.R.: Elektronenoptische untersuchungen an Wachstumsendkolben regenerierender peripherer nervenfasern. Virchow's Archiv Path. Anat. *340*: 93-104, 1965.

Blumenthal, H.T.: A histo- and immunologic analysis of the small vessel lesion of diabetes in the human and in the rabbit, *in* Conference on Small Blood Vessel Involvement in Diabetes Mellitus, Airlie House Conference, Warrenton, Virginia, 1963. American Institute of Biological Sciences Monograph.

Bodansky, O.: Cholinesterase. Ann. N.Y. Acad. Sci. *47*:521-547, 1946.

Boeke, J.: Die motorischen Endplatte bei den höheren Vertebraten, ihre Entwickelung, Form und Zusammenhang mit der Muskelfaser. Anat. Anz. *35*:193-226, 1909.

Boeke, J.: Beiträge zur Kenntniss der motorischen Nervenendigungen. I. Die Form und Struktur der motorischen Endplatte der quergestreiften Muskelfasern bei den höheren Vertebraten. II. Die akzessorischen Fasern und Endplättchen. Int. Monatschr. Anat. u. Physiol. *28*:377-443, 1911.

Boeke, J.: Studien zur Nervenregeneration. I. Die Regeneration der motorischen Nervenelementen und die Regeneration der Nerven der Muskelspindeln. Verhand. Kon. Akad. Wetensch Amsterdam, Tweede Sectic, Deel *18*:#6, 1916, pp. 1-120.

Boeke, J.: Die morphologische Grundlage der sympathischen Innervation der quergestreiften Muskelfasern. Z. Mikr. Anat. Forsch. *8*:561-639, 1927.

Boeke, J.: Nerve endings, motor and sensory, *in* Cytology and Cellular Pathology of the Nervous System (Penfield, W., ed.). Paul B. Hoeber, Inc., New York, 1932, vol. 1, pp. 243-315.

Boeke, J.: The sympathetic endformation, its synaptology, the interstitial cells, the periterminal network, and its bearing on the neurone theory. Discussion and critique. Acta Anat. 8:18-61, 1949.

Boeke, J. and Noël, R.: Sur la cytologie des plaques motrices dans les muscles de la lange, chez le chat. C.R. Soc. Biol. (Paris) 92:263-265, 1925.

Boell, E.J. and Nachmansohn, D.: Localization of choline esterase in nerve fibers. Science 92:513-514, 1940.

Bonichon, A.: Localisation de l'acétylcholinestérase dans les muscles stries au cours du developpement chez e' embryon du poulet. Ann. Histochim. 2:301-309, 1957.

Bornstein, M.B. and Breitbart, L.B.: Anatomical studies of mouse embryo spinal cord-skeletal muscle in long term tissue culture. Anat. Rec. 148:362, 1964.

Bornstein, M.B., Iwanami, H., Lehrer, G.M. and Breitbart, L.: Observations on the appearance of neuromuscular relationships in cultured mouse tissues. Z. Zellforsch. 92:197-206, 1968.

Bowden, R.E.M.: Factors influencing functional recovery in peripheral nerve injuries. M.R.C. Special Reports Series 282:298-353, 1954.

Bowden, R.E.M. and Gutmann, E.: Denervation and reinnervation of human voluntary muscle. Brain 67:273-313, 1944.

Bowman, W.C. and Zaimis, E.: The effects of adrenalin, noradrenaline and isoprenaline on skeletal muscle. J. Physiol. (Lond.) 144:92-107, 1958.

Boyd, I.A. and Martin, A.R.: Spontaneous subthreshold activity at mammalian neuromuscular junctions. J. Physiol. (Lond.) 132:61-73, 1956.

Braganca, B.: Neurochemical effects of snake venoms, in Neurochemistry: The Chemical Dynamics of Brain and Nerve (Elliot, K.A.C., Page, I.H. and Quastel, J.H., eds.). Charles C. Thomas, Springfield, Ill., 1955, pp. 612-663.

Braganca, B.M. and Quastel, J.H.: Action of snake venom on acetylcholine synthesis in brain. Nature 169:695-697, 1952.

Brain, W.R. and Henson, R.A.: Neurological syndromes associated with carcinoma. The carcinomatous neuromyopathies. Lancet 2:971-974, 1958.

Brandt, S.: Werdnig-Hoffmann's Infantile Progressive Muscular Atrophy. Manksgaard, Copenhagen, 1950.

Brazil, O.V. and Corrado, A.P.: The curariform action of streptomycin. J. Pharmacol. 120:452-459, 1957.

Brazil, O.V. and Prado-Francheschi, J.: The nature of neuromuscular block produced by neomycin and gentamicin. Arch. int. Pharmacodyn. 179:78-85, 1969.

Bremer, L.: Über die Endigungen der markhaltigen und marklosen Nerven im quergestreiften Muskel. Arch. Mikr. Anat. 21:165-201, 1882.

Brody, I.A.: Effect of denervation on the lactate dehydrogenase isozymes of skeletal muscle. Nature 205:196, 1965.

Brody, I.A. and Engel, W.K.: Denervation of muscles in myasthenia gravis. Arch. Neurol. 11:350-354, 1964.

Brooke, M.H. and Kaiser, K.K.: Muscle fiber types: How many and what kind? Arch. Neurol. 23:369-379, 1970.

Brooks, V.B.: An intracellular study of the action of repetitive nerve volleys and of botulinum toxin on miniature endplate potentials. J. Physiol. (Lond.) 134:264-277, 1956.

Brooks, V.B., Curtis, D.R. and Eccles, J.C.: The action of tetanus toxin on the inhibition of motor neurones. J. Physiol. (Lond.) 135:655-672, 1957.

Brown, G.L. and Harvey, A.M.: Congenital myotonia in the goat. Brain 62:341-363, 1939.
Brown, L.M.: A thiocholine method for locating cholinesterase activity by electron microscopy. Histochemistry of cholinesterase symposium. Bibliotheca Anat. (Basel) 2:21-33, 1961.
Brown, M.C. and Matthews, P.B.C.: An investigation into the possible existence of polyneural innervation of individual skeletal muscle fibers in certain hind-limb muscles of the cat. J. Physiol. (Lond.) 151:436-457, 1960.
Brownell, B., Oppenheimer, D.R. and Spalding, J.M.K.: Neurogenic muscle atrophy in myasthenia gravis. J. Neurol. Neurosurg. & Psychiat. 35:311-322, 1972.
Bruchhausen, F.V. and Merker, H.J.: Morphologischer und Chemischer aufbau Isolierter Basalmembranen aus der Nierenrinde der Ratte. Histochemie 8:90-108, 1967.
Brunton, T.L. and Fayrer, J.: On the nature and physiological action of the poison of *Naja tripudians* and other Indian venomous snakes. I. Proc. Roy. Soc. Med. 21:358-375, 1873.
Bryant, S.V., Fyfe, D. and Singer, M.: The effects of denervation on the ultrastructure of young limb regenerates in the newt, *Triturus*. Develop. Biol. 24:577-595, 1971.
Brzin, M. and Majcen-Tkačev, Ž.: Cholinesterase in denervated endplates and muscle fibers. J. Cell Biol. 19:349-358, 1963.
Brzin, M., Tennyson, V.M. and Duffy, P.E.: Acetylcholinesterase in frog sympathetic and dorsal root ganglia. A study by electron microscope cytochemistry and microgasometric analysis with the magnetic diver. J. Cell Biol. 31:215, 1966.
Brzin, M. and Zajicek, J.: Quantitative determination of cholinesterase activity in individual endplates of normal and denervated gastrocnemius. Nature 181:226-242, 1958.
Brzin, M. and Župančič, A.O.: On the mode of action of tubocurarine. Brit. J. Pharmacol. 11:428-430, 1956.
Buchthal, F., Guld, C. and Rosenfalck, P.: Multielectrode study of the territory of a motor unit. Acta Physiol. Scand. 39:83-104, 1957.
Buchthal, F. and Lindhard, J.: Transmission of impulses from nerve to muscle fiber. Acta Physiol. Scand. 4:136-148, 1942.
Buckley, G.A. and Heaton, J.: A quantitative study of cholinesterase in myoneural junctions from rat and guinea-pig extraocular muscles. J. Physiol. (Lond.) 199:743-749, 1968.
Buckley, G.A. and Heaton, J.: Cholinesterase in motor endplate during postnatal development. J. Physiol. (Lond.) 207.55P-56P, 1970.
Buckley, G.A. and Heaton, J.: Cholinesterase activity of myoneural junctions from twitch and tonic muscles of the domestic fowl. Nature 231:154-155, 1971.
Buller, A.J., Eccles, J.C. and Eccles, R.M.: Interactions between motorneurones and muscles in respect of the characteristic speeds of their responses. J. Physiol. (Lond.) 150:417-439, 1960.
Buller, A.J., Mommaerts, W.F.H.M. and Seraydarian, K.: Enzymic properties of myosin in fast and slow twitch muscles of the cat following cross-innervation. J. Physiol. (Lond.) 205:581-597, 1969.
Buller, A.J., Ranatunga, K.W. and Smith, J.: Influence of temperature on the isometric myograms of cross innervated mammalian fast twitch and slow twitch skeletal muscles. Nature 218:877-878, 1968.
Bunch, W., Kallsen, G., Berry, J. and Edwards, C.: The effect of denervation on incorporation of ^{32}P and [^3H] glycerol by the muscle membrane. J. Neurochem. 17:613-620, 1970.

Burgen, A.S.V., Dickens, F. and Zatman, L.J.: The action of botulinum toxin on the neuromuscular junction. J. Physiol. (Lond.) *109:*10-24, 1949.
Burke, R.E., Levine, D.N. and Zajac, F.E.: Mammalian motor units: physiological-histochemical correlation in three types in cat gastrocnemius. Science *174:*709-712, 1971.
Burt, A.M.: A histochemical procedure for the localization of choline acetyltransferase activity. J. Histochem. Cytochem. *18:*408-415, 1970.
Burton, R.M.: Gangliosides and acetylcholine of the central nervous system. III. The binding of radioactive acetylcholine by subcellular particles of the brain. Internat. J. Neuropharmacol. *3:*13-21, 1964.
Buzzard, E.F. and Greenfield, J.G.: Pathology of the Nervous System. London, 1921.

Cajal, R.S.: Variaciónes morfológicas, normales y patológicas del retículo neurofibrilar. Trab. Inst. Cajal Invest. Biol. (Madrid) *3:*(fasc. 1), 9-15, 1904.
Cajal, R.S.: Studien über Nervenregeneration. J.A. Barth, Leipzig, 1908.
Cajal, R.S.: Histologie du Système Nerveux de l'Homme et des Vertébrés. Maloine, Paris, 1909.
Cajal, R.S.: Quelques remarques sur les plaques motrices de la langue des mammiferes. Trab. Inst. Cajal Invest. Biol. (Madrid) *23:*245-254, 1925.
Cajal, R.S.: Degeneration and Regeneration of the Nervous System. Oxford University Press, London, 1928.
Camougis, G., Takman, B.H. and Tasse, J.R.: Potency difference between the Zwitterion form and the cation forms of tetrodotoxin. Science *156:*1625-1627, 1967.
Canal, N. and Frattola, L.: Changes in muscular glycogen synthetase activity following denervation. Nature *211:*416-417, 1966.
Carafoli, E., Margreth, A. and Buffa, P.: Biochemical changes in pigeon breast muscle mitochondria following nerve section. Nature *196:*1101-1102, 1962.
Carafoli, E., Margreth, A. and Buffa, P.: Early biochemical changes in mitochondria from denervated muscle and their relation to the onset of atrophy. Exp. Mol. Path. *3:*171-181, 1964.
Carey, E.J.: Experimental pleomorphism of motor nerve plates as a mode of functional protoplasmic movement. Anat. Rec. *81:*393-413, 1941a.
Carey, E.J.: Effect of CO_2 on amoeboid changes in motor nerve plates in intercostal muscle. Proc. Soc. Exp. Biol. & Med. *47:*67-72, 1941b.
Carey, E.J.: Pleomorphism of the myoneural junction. Biodynamica *3:*379-393, 1942.
Carey, E.J.: Morphologic effects of poliomyelitis virus upon motor endplates in the monkey, Proc. Soc. Exp. Biol. & Med. *53:*3-5, 1943a.
Carey, E.J.: Studies on amoeboid motion of motor endplates. Am. J. Path. *18:*327-390, 1943b.
Carey, E.J.: Studies on amoeboid motion and secretion of motor endplates. III. Experimental histopathology of motor endplates produced by quinine, curare, prostigmine, acetylcholine, strychnine, tetraethyl lead, and heat. Am. J. Path. *20:*341-393, 1944a.
Carey, E.J.: Studies on amoeboid motion and secretion of motor endplates. IV. Anatomic effects of poliomyelitis on the neuromuscular mechanism in the monkey. Am. J. Path. *20:*961-995, 1944b.
Carey, E.J.: Studies on amoeboid motion and secretion of motor endplates. X. Effects of

slow nervous action and disuse on the structure of nerve endings, neurosomes, and muscle fibers. Am. J. Path. *24:*135-175, 1948.

Carey, E.J., Downer, E.M., Toomey, F.B. and Haushalter, E.: Morphologic effects of DDT on nerve endings, neurosomes, and fiber types in voluntary muscles. Proc. Soc. Exp. Biol. & Med. *62:*76-83, 1946.

Carey, E.J. and Massopust, L.C.: Sudden destruction of motor endplates by lactic acid. Proc. Soc. Exp. Biol. & Med. *55:*194-197, 1944.

Carey, E.J., Massopust, L.C., Haushalter, E., Sweeney, J., Saribalis, C. and Raggio, J.: Studies on amoeboid motion and secretion of motor endplates. VIII. Experimental morphologic pathology of the chemical transmitter of nerve impulses in the course of Wallerian degeneration. Am. J. Path. *22:*1205-1285, 1946.

Carey, E.J., Massopust, L.C., Zeit, W. and Haushalter, E.: Studies on amoeboid motion and secretion of motor endplates. VII. Experimental pathology of the secretion mechanism of motor endplates in thermal shock. Am. J. Path. *22:*175-233, 1946.

Carey, E.J., Massopust, L.C., Zeit, W., Haushalter, E., Hamel, J. and Jeub, R.: Studies on amoeboid motion and secretion of motor endplates. VI. Pathologic effects of traumatic shock on motor and sensory nerve endings in skeletal muscle of unanesthetized rats in the Noble-Collip drum. Am. J. Path. *21:*935-1005, 1945.

Causey, E. and Hoffman, H.: Axon sprouting in partially deneurotized nerves. Brain *78:*661-668, 1955.

Cavallito, C.J.: Some speculations on the chemical nature of postjunctional membrane receptors. Fed. Proc. *26:*1647-1654, 1967.

Cavanagh, J.B.: The toxic effects of tri-ortho-cresyl phosphate on the nervous system. An experimental study in hens. J. Neurol. Neurosurg. & Psychiat. *17:*163-172, 1954.

Cavanagh, J.B., Thompson, R.H.S. and Webster, G.R.: The localization of pseudocholinesterase activity in nervous tissue. Q. J. Exp. Physiol. *39:*185-197, 1954.

Ceccarelli, B., Hurlbut, W.P. and Mauro, A.: Depletion of vesicles from frog neuromuscular junctions by prolonged tetanic stimulation. J. Cell Biol. *54:*30-38, 1972.

Ceccarelli, B., Hurlbut, W.P. and Mauro, A.: Turnover of transmitter and synaptic vesicles at the frog neuromuscular junction. J. Cell BioL. *57:*499-524, 1973.

Chagas, C.: Studies on the mechanism of curarization. Ann. N.Y. Acad. Sci. *81:*345-357, 1959.

Chagas, C.: Studies on nervous transmission in the electric organ of *Electrophorus electricus* (L.), *in* Bioelectrogenesis: A Comparative Survey of its Mechanisms with Particular Emphasis on Electric Fishes (Chagas, C., and de Carvalho, A.P., eds.). Elsevier, Amsterdam and New York, 1961, pp. 341-352.

Chagas, C., Penna-Franca, E., Nishie, K., Crocker, C. and Miranda, M.: Sur la fixation du triiodoethylate de gallamine radio actif au niveau des electroplaques de l'Electrophorus electricus. C.R. Acad. Sci. *242:*2671-2674, 1956.

Chain, E.: Inhibition of dehydrogenases by snake venom. Biochem. J. *33:*407-411, 1939.

Chakrin, L.W. and Whittaker, V.P.: The subcellular distribution of (N-Me-^{3}H) acetylcholine synthesized by brain *in vivo.* Biochem. J. *113:*97-107, 1969.

Chambers, R. and MacDermot, V.: Polyneuritis as a cause of "amyotonia congenita". Lancet *1:*397-401, 1957.

Chang, C.C. and Lee, C.Y.: Isolation of neurotoxins from the venom of *Bungarus multicinctus* and their modes of neuromuscular blocking action. Arch. Internat. Pharmacodyn. *144:*241-257, 1963.

Chang, C.C. and Lee, C.Y.: Electrophysiological study of neuromuscular blocking action of cobra neurotoxin. Br. J. Pharm. and Chemotherap. 28:172-181, 1966.
Changeux, J.P., Podleski, T.R. and Wofsy, L.: Affinity labeling of the acetylcholine receptor. Proc. U.S. Nat. Acad. Sci. 58:2063-2070, 1967.
Changeux, J.P. and Podleski, T.R.: On the excitability and cooperativity of the electroplax membrane. Proc. U.S. Nat. Acad. Sci. 59:944-950, 1968.
Changeux, J.P., Ryter, A. and Leuzinger, W.: On the association of tyrocidine with acetylcholinesterase. Proc. U.S. Nat. Acad. Sci. 62:986-993, 1969.
Charcot, J.M. and Joffroy, A.: Deuz cas d'atrophie musculaire progressive avec lésions de la substance grise es des faisceaux antérolatéraux de la moëlle épinière. Arch. Physiol. Norm. and Path. 2:354, 629-744, 1869.
Charcot, J.M. and Marie, P.: Sur une forme particulière d'atrophie musculaire progressive souvent familiale débutante par les pieds et les jambes et atteignant plus tard les mains. Rev. Méd. (Paris) 6:97-138, 1886.
Chatterjee, A.K.: Studies on snake venoms. I. The isolation of an inhibitor of the cytochrome-cytochrome oxidase system from cobra venom and study of the effects of pH, temperature and ultra-violet rays on its stability. Indian J. M. Res. 37:241-248, 1949.
Chen, I.-Li and Lee, C.Y.: Ultrastructural changes in the motor nerve terminals caused by β bungarotoxin. Virchow's Archiv. B. 6:318-325, 1970.
Cheng, K., Ozawa, T. and Liebowitz, A.: Ultrastructural changes in the extraocular muscles of rabbit after denervation. Invest. Opthalmol. 6:210, 1967.
Cheng-Minoda, K., Davidowitz, J., Liebowitz, A. and Breinin, G.M.: Fine structure of extraocular muscle in rabbit. J. Cell Biol. 39:193-196, 1968.
Cheng-Minoda, K., Ozawa, T. and Breinin, G.M.: Ultrastructural changes in rabbit extraocular muscles after oculomotor nerve section. Invest. Opthalmol. 7:599-616, 1968.
Chessick, R.D.: Histochemical study of the distribution of cholinesterases. J. Histochem. & Cytochem. 1:471-485, 1953.
Chessick, R.D.: The histochemical specificity of cholinesterases. J. Histochem. & Cytochem. 2:258-273, 1954.
Cheymol, J., Barme, M., Bourillet, F. and Roch-Arveiller, M.: Action neuromusculaire de trois venins d'hydrophiides. Toxicon 5:111-119, 1967.
Chicheportiche, R., Rochat, C., Sampieri, F. and Lazdunski, M.: Structure-function relationships of neurotoxins isolated from Naja haje venom. Physicochemical properties and identification of the active site. Biochemistry 11:1681-1690, 1972.
Chokroverty, S., Parameswar, K.S. and Co, C.: Nonspecific esterases in the myoneural junction of human striated muscle. J. Histochem. Cytochem. 19:798-800, 1971.
Chor, H.: Nerve degeneration in poliomyelitis. VI. Changes in the motor nerve endings. Arch. Neurol. & Psychiat. 29:344-358, 1933.
Chor, H., Dolkart, R.E. and Davenport, H.E.: Chemical and histological changes in denervated skeletal muscle of the monkey and cat. Am. J. Physiol. 118:580-587, 1937.
Chu, C.H.U.: A histochemical study of staining the axis cylinder with fuchsin-sulfurous acid (Schiff's reagent). Anat. Rec. 108:723-745, 1950.
Churchill-Davidson, H.C. and Wise, R.P.: Neuromuscular transmission in the newborn infant. Anesthesiology 24:271-278, 1963.
Clark, A.W., Hurlbut, W.P. and Mauro, A.: Changes in the fine structure of the neuromuscular junction of the frog caused by black widow spider venom. J. Cell Biol. 52: 1-14, 1972.

Clark, A.W., Mauro, A., Longenecker, H.E., Jr. and Hurlbut, W.P.: Effects of black widow spider venom on the frog neuromuscular junction. Nature 225:703-705, 1970.
Clark, D.G., Macmurchie, D.D., Elliott, E., Wolcott, R.G., Landel, A.M. and Raftery, M.A.: Elapid neurotoxins. Purification, characterization and immunochemical studies of α-bungarotoxin. Biochemistry 11:1663-1668, 1972.
Clark, D.G., Wolcott, R.G. and Raftery, M.A.: Partial characterization of an α-bungarotoxin-binding component of electroplax membranes. Biochem. & Biophys. Res. Comm. 48:1061-1067, 1972.
Claude, A.: A fraction from normal chick embryo similar to the tumor-producing fraction of chicken tumor. I. Proc. Soc. Exp. Biol. & Med. 39:398-403, 1938.
Close, R.: Dynamic properties of fast and slow skeletal muscles of the rat during development. J. Physiol. (Lond.) 173:74-95, 1964.
Close, R.: Dynamic properties of fast and slow skeletal muscles of the rat after nerve cross-union. J. Physiol. (Lond.) 204:331-346, 1969.
Coërs, C.: The vital staining of muscle biopsies with methylene blue. J. Neurol., Neurosurg. and Psychiat. 15:211-215, 1952a.
Coërs, C.: La dystrophie myotonique. Étude clinique, électromyographique et histologique de quatre cas. Acta Clin. Belg. 7:407-444, 1952b.
Coërs, C.: Contribution à l'étude de la jonction neuromusculaire. Données nouvelles concernant la structure de l'arborisation terminale et de l'appareil sousneural chez l'homme. Arch. Biol. (Paris) 64:133-147, 1953a.
Coërs, C.: Note sur une technique de prelevement des biopsies musculaires. Acta Neurol. Belg. 53:759-765, 1953b.
Coërs, C.: La detéction histochimique de la cholinesterase au niveau de la jonction neuromusculaire. Rev. Belge. Path. Méd. Exp. 22:306-315, 1953c.
Coërs, C.: L'exploration fonctionelle et l'étude histologique quantitative des muscles atrophiés. Acta Clin. Belg. 10:244-265, 1955a.
Coërs, C.: Les variations structurelles normales et pathologiques de la jonction neuromusculaire. Acta Neurol. Belg. 55:741-866, 1955b.
Coërs, C.: Personal communication, 1962.
Coërs, C.: Structure and organization of the myoneural junction in Internat. Rev. Cytol. 22:239-264, 1967.
Coërs, C. and Desmedt, J.E.: Abnormal endplates in myasthenic muscle. Lancet 2:1124, 1958.
Coërs, C. and Desmedt, J.E.: Mise en évidence d'une malformation caractéristique de la jonction neuromusculaire dans la myasthénie. Acta Neurol. Belg. 59:539-561, 1959.
Coërs, C. and Durand, J.: La repartition des appareils cholinestérasiques en cupule dans divers muscles striés. Arch. Biol. (Paris) 68:209-215, 1957.
Coërs, C. and Hildebrand, J.: Latent neuropathy in diabetes and alcoholism. Electrophysiological and histological study. Neurology 15:17-38, 1965.
Coërs, C., Joffroy, A., Capon, A., Hildebrand, J. and Carbone, F.: Indentification electromyographique et morphologique des neuropathies sub-clinques in Proc. VII Internat. Congr. Neurol. Vienna II 443, 1965, Wiener Medizinische Adakemie, Vienna.
Coërs, C. and Pelc, S.: Un cas d'amyotonie congénitale caractérisé par une anomalie histologique et histochimique de la jonction neuromusculaire. Acta Neurol. Belg. 54:166-173, 1954.

Coërs, C., Teberman-Toppet, N. and Cremer, M.: Regressive vacuolar myopathy in steatorrhea. Arch. Neurol. *24*:217-227, 1971.

Coërs, C. and Woolf, A.L.: Étude histologique et histochimique de la jonction neuromusculaire dans deux cas de myasthénie. Comptes-rendus du Congres des Médecins Aliénistes et Neurologistes, Liège, July 19-26, 1954.

Coërs, C. and Woolf, A.L.: The Innervation of Muscle: A Biopsy Study. Blackwell Scientific Publications, Oxford, 1959.

Cohen, E.N., Rubinstein, L.J., Corbascio, A.N. and Hood, N.: Localization of d-tubocurarine-H^3 at the motor endplate. J. Pharmacol. & Expermtl. Therap. *157*:170-174, 1967.

Cohen, L.B., Hille, B. and Keynes, R.D.: Changes in axon birefringence during the action potential. J. Physiol. (Lond.) *211*:495-515, 1970.

Cohen, M.J. and Hess, A.: Fine structural differences in "fast" and "slow" muscle fibers of the crab. Am. J. Anat. *121*:285-304, 1967.

Cohen, R.B. and Zacks, S.I.: Myasthenia gravis. II. Histochemical demonstration of acetylcholinesterase activity in motor endplates of extraocular muscle in patients with myasthenia gravis. A post-mortem study. Am. J. Path. *35*:399-405, 1959.

Cole, W.V.: Motor endings in the striated muscle of vertebrates. J. Comp. Neurol. *102*: 671-716, 1955.

Cole, W.V.: Structural variations of nerve endings in the striated muscles of the rat. J. Comp. Neurol. *108*:445-464, 1957.

Collier, B.: The preferential release of newly synthesized transmitter by a sympathetic ganglion. J. Physiol. (Lond.) *205*:341-352, 1969.

Conen, P.E., Murphy, E.G. and Donohue, W.L.: Light and electron microscopic studies of myogranules in a child with hypotonia and muscle weakness. Canad. Med. Assn. J. *89*:983-986, 1963.

Conrad, J.T. and Glaser, G.H.: Spontaneous activity at myoneural junction in dystrophic muscle. Arch. Neurol. *11*:310-316, 1964.

Cooke, W.T., Johnson, A.G. and Woolf, A.L.: Vital staining and electron microscopy of the intramuscular nerve endings in the neuropathy of adult coeliac disease. Brain *89*:663-682, 1966.

Coombs, J.S., Ecc.es, J.C. and Fatt, P.: Excitatory synaptic action in motorneurones. J. Physiol. (Lond.) *130*:374-395, 1955.

Coupland, R.E. and Holmes, R.L.: The use of cholinesterase techniques for the demonstration of peripheral nervous structures. Quart. J. Micr. Sci. *98*:327-330, 1957.

Couteaux, R.: Sur l'origine de la sole des plaques motrices. C.R. Soc. Biol. (Paris) *127*: 218-221, 1938.

Couteaux, R.: Recherches sur l'histogénèse des muscles striés des mammifères et la formation des plaque motrices. Bull. Biol. *75*:103-239, 1941.

Couteaux, R.: La cholinestérase des plaques motrices après section du nerf moteur. Bull. Biol. *76*:1-44, 1942.

Couteaux, R.: Contribution à l'étude de la synapse myoneurale. Rev. Canad. Biol. *6*: 563-711, 1947.

Couteaux, R.: Remarques sur les méthodes actuelles de détection histochimique des activités cholinestérasiques. Arch. Int. Physiol. *59*:526-537, 1951.

Couteaux, R.: Particularités histochimiques des zones d'insertion du muscle strié. C.R. Soc. Biol. (Paris) *147*:1974-1976, 1953.

Couteaux, R.: Morphological and cytochemical observations on the postsynaptic membrane at motor endplates and ganglionic synapses. Exp. Cell Res., suppl. 5:294-322, 1958.

Couteaux, R.: Motor endplate structure, in Muscle (Bourne, G.H. ed.). Academic Press, New York, 1960, I, pp. 337-378.

Couteaux, R.: The differentiation of synaptic areas. Proc. Roy. Soc. B. 158:457-480, 1963.

Couteaux, R. and Katz, B.: Discussion in Symposium sur la microphysiologie comparee des elements excitables. Colloq. Int. Nat. Rech. Sci. (Paris), 67:255-258, 1957.

Couteaux, R. and Nachmansohn, D.: Changes of cholinesterase at endplate of voluntary muscle following section of sciatic nerve. Proc. Soc. Exp. Biol. & Med. 43:177-181, 1940.

Couteaux, R. and Pecot-Dechavassine, M.: Vesicules synaptiques et poches au niveau des zones actives de la jonction neuromusculaire. C.R.H. Acad. Sci. Ser. D 271:2346-2349, 1970.

Couteaux, R. and Taxi, J.: Recherches histochimiques sur la distribution des activités cholinestérasiques au niveau de la synapse myoneurale. Arch. Anat. Micr. 41:352-392, 1952.

Crain, S.M.: Development of functional neuromuscular connections between separate explants of fetal mammalian tissues after maturation in culture. Anat. Rec. 160:466, 1968.

Crain, S.M.: Bioelectric interactions between cultured fetal rodent spinal cord and skeletal muscle after innervation in vitro. J. Exp. Zool. 173:353-370, 1970.

Crain, S.M., Alfei, L. and Peterson, E.R.: Neuromuscular transmission in cultures of adult human and rodent skeletal muscle after innervation in vitro by fetal rodent spinal cord. J. Neurobiol. 1:471-489, 1970.

Crevier, M. and Bélanger, L.F.: Simple method for histochemical detection of esterase activity. Science 122:556, 1955.

Csillik, B.: Submikroskopische Organisation der post-synaptischen Membranen. Acta Physiol. Acad. Sci. Hung. 16:(suppl.)27, 1959.

Csillik, B.: Contributions to the development of the myoneural synapses. Ontogenic aspects of the subneural apparatus. Z. Zellforsch. 52:150-162, 1960.

Csillik, B.: Submicroscopic organization of the post-synaptic membrane in the myoneural junction A polarization optical study. J. Cell Biol. 17:571-586, 1963.

Csillik, B.: Functional structure of the post synaptic membrane in the myoneural junction. Budapest Akademiai Kiadó, 1965.

Csillik, B. and Davis, R.: Electron microscopic localization of the "lead reactive substance" in the myoneural junction. Acta Biol. Hung. 15:203-211, 1964.

Csillik, B., Haarstad, V.B. and Knyihar, E.: Autoradiographic localization of ^{14}C hemicholinium: an approach to locate sites of acetylcholine synthesis. J. Histochem. Cytochem. 18:58-60, 1970.

Csillik, B., Joó, F., Juhász, K., Kálmán, Gy., Kása, P. and Savay, Gy.: Über die Wirkung der denervation auf den submikroskopischen bau der postsynaptischen membran in der Myoneuralen Junktion. Acta Morph. 12:212-226, 1963.

Csillik, B. and Knyihár, E.: On the effect of motor nerve degeneration on the fine structural localization of esterases in the mammalian motor endplate. J. Cell Sci. 3:529-538, 1968.

Csillik, B. and Savay, B.: Die Regeneration des subneuralen apparates der motorischen endplatten. Acta Neuroveg. 19:41-52, 1958.

Csillik, B. and Savày, G.: Release of calcium in the myoneural junction. Nature 198:399, 1963.
Cuajunco, F.: Development of the human motor endplate. Contrib. Embryol., #195, 30: 129-151, 1942.
Curtis, R.L., Abrams, M.T. and Harman, P.J.: The myoneural junction in dystrophic and atrophic mouse muscle. Anat. Rec. 139:219, 1961.
Cushney, A.R. and Yagi, S.: On the action of cobra venom. I. The cause of death (Cushney), 1-19. II. Action on individual organs (Yagi), 19-36. Phil. Trans. Roy. Soc. (Lond.) B, 208:1-36, 1918.

Dahlbäck, O., Elmqvist, D., Johns, T.R., Rader, S. and Thesleff, S.: An electrophysiologic study of the junction in myasthenia gravis. J. Physiol. (Lond.) 156:336-343, 1961.
Dale, H.H.: The action of certain esters and ether of choline and their relation to muscarine. J. Pharmacol. 6:147-190, 1914.
Dale, H.H. and Dudley, H.W.: The presence of histamine and acetylcholine in the spleen of the ox and the horse. J. Physiol. (Lond.) 68:97-123, 1929.
Davenport, H.K., Ranson, S.W. and Stevens, E.: Microscopic changes of muscle in myostatic contracture caused by tetanus toxin. Arch. Path. 7:978-992, 1929.
Davenport, H.K. and Ranson, S.W.: Contracture resulting from tenotomy. Arch. Surg. 21:995-1014, 1930.
Davis, D.A., Wasserkrug, H.L., Heyman, I.A., Padmanabhan, K.C., Seligman, G.A., Plapinger, R.E. and Seligman, A.M.: Comparison of ultrastructural cholinesterase demonstration in the motor endplate with α-acetylthiol-m-toluenediazonium ion (ATTD) and 3-acetoxy-5-indolediazonium ion (AID). J. Histochem. Cytochem. 20: 161-172, 1972.
Davis, L.E., Burnett, A.L. and Haynes, J.F.: Histological and ultrastructural study of the muscular and nervous systems in Hydra. II. Nervous system. J. Exp. Zool. 167:295-332, 1968.
Davis, R. and Koelle, G.E.: Electron microscopic localization of acetylcholinesterase (AchE) at the motor endplate by the gold-thiolacetic acid (ThAc) and gold-thiocholine (ThCh) method. J. Histochem. Cytochem. 13:703-704, 1965.
Davis, R. and Koelle, G.E.: Electron microscopic localization of acetylcholinesterase and nonspecific cholinesterase at the neuromuscular junction by the gold thiocholine and gold-thiolacetic acid methods. J. Cell Biol. 34:157-171, 1967.
Dawson, D.M., Goodfriend, T.L. and Kaplan, N.O.: Lactic dehydrogenases: functions of the two types. Science 143:929-933, 1964.
Dawson, D.M. and Kaplan, N.O.: Factors influencing the concentration of enzymes in various muscles. J. Biol. Chem. 240:3215-3221, 1965.
De Anda, G., Rebollo, M.A. and Achaval, M.: Differentiation of the skeletal muscle in the chicken. II. Development of the myoneural synapse. Acta Neurol. Latinoamer. 9:93-101, 1963.
Debré, R. and Thieffry, S.: Remarques sur le syndrome de Guillain-Barré chez l'enfant. (À propos de 32 observations personnelles.) Arch. Franc. Pédiatr. 8:357-364, 1951.
De Duve, C., Wattiaux, R. and Baudhuin, P.: Distribution of enzymes between subcellular fractions in animal tissues. in Adv. Enzymol. (Nord, R.F., ed.). 291-358 Interscience, New York, 1962.

De Harven, E. and Coërs, C.: Electron microscope study of the human neuromuscular junction. J. Biophys. & Biochem. Cytol. 6:7-10, 1959.

De Iraldi, P. and Guedet, R.: Action of reserpine on the osmium tetroxide zinc iodide reactive site of synaptic vesicles in the pineal nerves of the rat. Z. Zellforsch. 91:178-185, 1968.

del Castillo, J.: The transmission of excitation from nerve to muscle in neuromuscular disorders (the motor unit and its disorders). A Res. Nerv. & Ment. Dis. Proc. 38:90-143, 1960.

del Castillo, J. and Engbaek, L.: The nature of the neuromuscular block produced by magnesium. J. Physiol. (Lond.) 124:370-384, 1954.

del Castillo, J. and Katz, B.: Facilitation at the nerve-muscle junction due to anodic polarization of nerve endings. J. Physiol. (Lond.) 123:8P, 1954a.

del Castillo, J. and Katz, B.: The effect of magnesium on the activity of motor nerve endings. J. Physiol. (Lond.) 124:553-559, 1954b.

del Castillo, J. and Katz, B.: Statistical factors involved in neuromuscular facilitation and depression. J. Physiol. (Lond.) 124:574-585, 1954c.

del Castillo, J. and Katz, B.: Changes in endplate activity produced by presynaptic polarization. J. Physiol. (Lond.) 124:586-604, 1954d.

del Castillo, J. and Katz, B.: Local activity at a depolarized nerve-muscle junction. J. Physiol. (Lond.) 128:396-411, 1955.

del Castillo, J. and Katz, B.: Localization of active spots within the neuromuscular junction of the frog. J. Physiol. (Lond.) 132:630-649, 1956a.

del Castillo, J. and Katz, B.: Biophysical aspects of neuromuscular transmission. Progr. Biophys. 6:121-170, 1956b. (Pergamon Press, London).

del Castillo, J. and Stark, L.: The effect of calcium ions on the motor endplate potentials. J. Physiol. (Lond.) 116:507-515, 1952.

del Rio Hortega, P.: Phénomènes de régénération nerveuse dans le ramollissement cérébral. C.R. Soc. Biol. (Paris) 93:1018-1020, 1925.

Denny-Brown, D.: Primary sensory neuropathy with muscular changes associated with carcinoma. J. Neurol. Neurosurg. Psychiat. 11:73-87, 1948.

Denny-Brown, D. and Brenner, C.: Lesion in peripheral nerve resulting from compression by spring clip. Arch. Neurol. & Psychiat. 52:1-19, 1944.

Denz, F.A.: Myoneural junction and toxic agents. J. Path. & Bact. 63:235-247, 1951.

Denz, F.A.: On the histochemistry of the myoneural junction. Brit. J. Exp. Path. 34:329-339, 1953.

Denz, F.A.: Cholinesterase inhibition at the myoneural junction. Brit. J. Exp. Path. 35:459-471, 1954.

de Quatrefages, A.: Mémoire sur l'Elodine paradoxale. Ann. Sci. Nat., 2nd series, 19:274-312, 1843.

De Robertis, E.: Submicroscopic changes in synapses after nerve section in the acoustic ganglion of the guinea pig. J. Biophys. & Biochem. Cytol. 2:503-512, 1956.

De Robertis, E.: Submicroscopic morphology and function of the synapse. Exp. Cell Res. suppl. 5:347-369, 1958.

De Robertis, E.: Ultrastructure and cytochemistry of the synaptic region. Science 156:907-914, 1967.

De Robertis, E.: Molecular biology of synaptic receptors. Science 171:963-971, 1971.

De Robertis, E. and Bennett, H.S.: Submicroscopic vesicular component in the synapse. Fed. Proc. 13:35, 1954.

De Robertis, E. and Bennett, H.S.: Some features of the submicroscopic morphology of synapses in frog and earthworm. J. Biophys. & Biochem. Cytol. *1*:47-58, 1955.

De Robertis, E., Fiszer de Plazas, S. and Soto, E.F.: Cholinergic binding capacity of proteolipids from isolated nerve ending membranes. Science *158*:928-929, 1967.

De Robertis, E. and Fiszer de Plazas, S.: Acetylcholinesterase and acetylcholine proteolipid receptor: Two different components of electroplax membranes. Biomembranes *219*:388, 1970.

De Robertis, E. and Franchi, C.M.: Electron microscope observations on synaptic vesicles in synapses of the retinal rods and cones. J. Biophys. & Biochem. Cytol. *2*:307-318, 1956.

De Robertis, E., Pellegrino de Iraldi, A., Rodriguez de Lores Arnaiz, G. and Salganicoff, L.: Cholinergic and non-cholinergic nerve endings in rat brain. I. Isolation and subcellular distribution of acetylcholine and acetylcholinesterase. J. Neurochem. *9*:23-35, 1962.

De Robertis, E., Salganicoff, L., Zieher, M. and Rodriguez de Lores Arnaiz, G.: Acetylcholine and cholinacetylase content of synaptic vesicles. Science *140*:300-301, 1963.

Desmedt, J.E.: Sur le type de l'anomalie neuromusculaire observe's dans la myasthénie. J. Physiol. (Paris) *48*:511-512, 1956.

Desmedt, J.E.: The physiopathology of neuromuscular transmission and the trophic influences of motor innervation. Am. J. Phys. Med. *38*:248-261, 1959.

Desmedt, J.E.: Neuromuscular defect in myasthenia gravis: electrophysiological and histopathological evidence, *in* Myasthenia Gravis. The Second International Symposium Proceedings, (H.R. Viets, ed.). Charles C. Thomas, Springfield, Ill., 1961, pp. 150-178.

Desmedt, J.E.: Données récentes sur la pathogénie de la myasthénie grave. Bull. Acad. Roy. Med. Belg. *2*:213-267, 1962a.

Desmedt, J.E.: Identification and titration of myasthenic defect by nerve stimulation. Electroenceph. Clin. Neurophysiol., suppl. *22*:63-64, 1962b.

Desmedt, J.E.: Presynaptic mechanisms in myasthenia gravis. Ann. N.Y. Acad. Sci. *135*:209-246, 1966.

Desmedt, J.E., Borenstein, S. and Lambert, C.: L'action du calcium sur la transmission neuromusculaire dans la myasthénie. Rev. Neurol. *112*:331-335, 1965.

Dettbarn, W.: Mechanism of action of tetrodotoxin (TTX) and saxitoxin (STX) *in* Neuropoisons their pathophysiological action *1*:169-186, 1971 (L.L. Simpson, ed.). Plenum Press, New York and London.

de Villaverdes, J.M.: Les lésions des plaques motrices dans l'intoxication par le plomb. Trab. Inst. Cajal Invest. Biol. (Madrid) *24*:267-287, 1926.

Diamond, J. and Mellanby, J.: The effect of tetanus toxin in the goldfish. J. Physiol. (Lond.) *215*:727-741, 1971.

Diamond, J. and Miledi, R.: Sensitivity of foetal and new-born rat muscle to acetylcholine. J. Physiol. (Lond.) *149*:50, 1959.

Diamond, J. and Miledi, R.: A study of foetal and new-born rat muscle fibres. J. Physiol. (Lond.) *162*:393-408, 1962.

Di Carlo, V.: Ultrastructure of the membrane of synaptic vesicles. Nature *213*:833-835, 1967.

Dickson, E.C. and Shevky, R.: Botulism. Studies on the manner in which the toxin of *Clostridium botulinum* acts upon the body. I. The effect upon the autonomic nervous system. J. Exp. Med. *37*:711-731, 1923a.

Dickson, L.M.: The development of nerve endings in the respiratory muscles of the sheep. J. Anat. 74:268-276, 1940.

Diehl, J.F. and Jones, R.R.: Effects of denervation and muscular dystrophy on amino acid transport in skeletal muscle. Am. J. Physiol. 210:1080-1085, 1966.

Dixon, W.E.: Vagus inhibition. Brit. Med. J. 2:1807, 1906.

Dixon, W.E.: On the mode of action of drugs. Med. Magazine 16:454-457, 1907.

Dodge, F.A., Jr., Miledi, R. and Rahamimoff, R.: Strontium and quantal release of transmitter at the neuromuscular junction. J. Physiol. (Lond.) 200:267-283, 1969.

Dodge, F.A., Jr. and Rahamimoff, R.: Cooperative action of calcium ions in transmitter release at the neuromuscular junction. J. Physiol. (Lond.) 193:419-433, 1967.

Dogiel, A.S.: Methylenblautinktion der motorischen Nervendigungen in den Muskeln der Amphibien und Reptilien. Arch. Mikrosk. Anat. 35:305-320, 1890.

Domonkos, J. and Heiner, L.: Effect of denervation and immobilization on carbohydrate metabolism in tonic and tetanic muscles. I. Glycolytic mechanism. Acta Physiol. Hung. 28:227-236, 1965.

Dorsett, D.A.: The sensory and motor innervation of Nereis. Proc. Roy. Soc. B. 159:652-667, 1964.

Douglas, L.T.: Thiocholine techniques: I. Modification for demonstration of acetylcholinesterase in Schistosoma mansoni (Trematoda) and in Hymenolysis diminuta (Cestoda). Acta Histochem. (Jena) 24:301-306, 1966.

Doyère, M.: Mémoire sur les Tardigrades. Ann. Sci. Nat., ii, 14:269-361, 1840.

Drachman, D.B.: The developing motor endplate: pharmacological studies in the chick embryo. J. Physiol. (Lond.) 169:707-712, 1963.

Drachman, D.B.: Atrophy of skeletal muscle in chick embryos treated with botulinum toxin. Science 145:719-721, 1964.

Drachman, D.B.: Is acetylcholine the trophic neuromuscular transmitter? Arch. Neurol. 17:206-218, 1967.

Drachman, D.B. and Romanul, F.C.A.: Effects of neuromuscular blockade on enzymatic activities of muscles. Arch. Neurol. 23:85-89, 1970.

Drachman, D.B. and Witzke, F.: Trophic regulation of acetylcholine sensitivity of muscle. Effect of electrical stimulation. Science 176:514-516, 1972.

Drahota, Z. and Gutmann, E.: The effects of use and disuse on neuromuscular functions. p. 143 Prague, Czech. Acad. Sci., 1963.

Droz, B. and Barondes, S.H.: Nerve endings: rapid appearance of labelled protein shown by electron microscopic radioautography. Science 165:1131-1133, 1969.

Dryden, W.F.: Development of acetylcholine sensitivity in cultured skeletal muscle. Experientia 26:984-986, 1970.

Dublin, W.B., Bede, B.A. and Brown, B.A.: Pathologic findings in nerve and muscle in poliomyelitis. Am. J. Clin. Path. 14:266-272, 1944.

DuBois-Reymond, E.: Vorläufiger Abriss einer Untersuchung über den sogenannten Froschstrom und über die elektromotorischen Fische. Ann. Physik. u. Chem. 58:1-30, 1843.

DuBois-Reymond, E.: Untersuchungen über theirische Elektricitat. Georg Reimer, Berlin, 1843-1849.

Dubowitz, V.: Enzymic maturation of skeletal muscle. Nature 197:1215, 1963.

Dubowitz, V. and Newman, D.L.: Change in enzyme pattern after cross innervation of fast and slow skeletal muscle. Nature 214:840-841, 1967.

Dubowitz, V. and Pearse, A.G.E.: Reciprocal relationship of phosphorylase and oxidative enzymes in skeletal muscle. Nature 185:701-702, 1960.
Duchen, L.W.: The effects of botulinum toxin on the pattern of innervation of skeletal muscle in the mouse. Q.J. Exp. Physiol. 53:84-89, 1968.
Duchen, L.W.: Hereditary motor endplate disease in the mouse: light and electron microscope studies. J. Neurol. Neurosurg. Psychiat. 33:238-250, 1970a.
Duchen, L.W.: Changes in motor innervation and cholinesterase localization induced by botulinum toxin in skeletal muscle of the mouse: differences between fast and slow muscles. J. Neurol. Neurosurg. Psychiat. 33:40-54, 1970b.
Duchen, L.W.: The effect in the mouse of nerve crush and regeneration on the innervation of skeletal muscles paralysed by Clostridium botulinum toxin. J. Path. 102:9-14, 1970c.
Duchen, L.W.: An electron microscopic study of the changes induced by botulinum toxin in the motor endplates of slow and fast skeletal muscle fibres of the mouse. J. Neurol. Sci. 14:47-60, 1971a.
Duchen, L.W.: Changes in the electron microscopic structure of slow and fast skeletal muscle fibres of the mouse after local injection of botulinum toxin. J. Neurol. Sci. 14: 61-74, 1971b.
Duchen, L.W., Searle, A.G. and Strich, S.: An hereditary motor endplate disease in the mouse. J. Physiol. (Lond.) 189:4-6P, 1967.
Duchen, L.W. and Stefani, E.: Electrophysiological studies of neuromuscular transmission in hereditary "motor endplate disease" of the mouse. J. Physiol. (Lond.) 212: 535-548, 1971.
Duchen, L.W., Stolkin, C. and Tonge, D.A.: Light and electron microscopic changes in slow and fast skeletal muscle fibres and their motor endplates in the mouse after local injection of tetanus toxin. J. Physiol. (Lond.) 222:136-137P, 1972a.
Duchen, L.W., Stolkin, C. and Tonge, D.A.: Changes in neuromuscular transmission in slow and fast skeletal muscles of the mouse after local injection of tetanus toxin. J. Physiol. (Lond.) 222:147-148P, 1972b.
Duchen, L.W. and Strich, S.: Changes in the pattern of motor innervation of skeletal muscle in the mouse after local injection of Clostridium botulinum toxin. J. Physiol. (Lond.) 189:2P, 1967.
Dutchen, L.W. and Strich, S.: The effect of botulinum toxin on the pattern of innervation of skeletal muscle in the mouse. Qt. J. Exp. Physiol. 53:84-89, 1968a.
Duchen, L.W. and Strich, S.J.: An hereditary motor neurone disease with progressive denervation of muscle in the mouse: the mutant "Wobbler". J. Neurol. Neurosurg. Psychiat. 31:535-542, 1968b.
Duchenne, G.B.: Étude comparée des lésions anatomiques dans l'atrophie musculaire progressive et dans la paralysie-générale. Union Méd. 7:202-203, 1853.
Duff, J.T., Klerer, J., Bibler, R.H., Moore, D.E., Gottfried, C. and Wright, G.G.: Studies on immunity to toxins of Clostridium botulinum. II. Production and purification of type B toxin for toxoid. J. Bact. 73:597-601, 1957.
Dulhunty, A. and Gage, P.W.: Selective effects of an octopus toxin on action potentials. J. Physiol. (Lond.) 218:433-445, 1971.
Durell, J., Garland, J.T. and Friedel, R.O.: Acetylcholine action: Biochemical aspects. Science 165:862-866, 1969.
Düring, M.: Über die Feinstruktur der motorischen Endplatte von höheren Wirbeltieren. Z. Zellforsch. 81:74-90, 1967.

Dustin, A.P.: Le Rôle des tropismes et de l'odogenèse dans la régénération du système nerveux. Arch. Biol. (Paris) *25:*269-288, 1910.

East, E.W.: An anatomical study of the initiation of movement in rat embryos. Anat. Rec. *50:*201-219, 1931.
Eaton, L.M. and Lambert, E.H.: Electromyography and electric stimulation of nerves in diseases of motor unit: observations on the myasthenic syndrome associated with malignant tumours. J.A.M.A. *163:*1117-1124, 1957.
Eccles, J.C.: Investigations on muscle atrophies arising from disuse and tenotomy. J. Physiol. (Lond.) *103:*253-266, 1944.
Eccles, J.C.: An electrical hypothesis of synaptic and neuromuscular transmission. Nature *156:*680-683, 1945.
Eccles, J.C.: Specificity of Neural influence on speed of muscle contraction. in The Effect of Use and Disuse on Neuromuscular Functions. (E. Gutmann and P. Hńik, eds.). Czech. Acad. Sci. *111-128*, 1963, Prague.
Eccles, J.C., Eccles, R.M. and Kozak, W.: Further investigations on the influence of motor neurones on the speed of muscle contraction. J. Physiol. (Lond.) *163:*324-339, 1962.
Eccles, J.C., Eccles, R.M. and Magni, F.: Monosynaptic excitatory action on motoneurones regenerated to antagonistic muscles. J. Physiol. (Lond.) *154:*68-88, 1960.
Eccles, J.C. and Jaeger, J.C.: The relationship between the mode of operation and the dimensions of the junctional regions at synapses and motor end organs. Proc. Roy. Soc. B. *148:*38-56, 1958.
Edds, M.V., Jr.: Collateral regeneration of residual motor axons in partially denervated muscles. J. Exp. Zool. *113:*517-551, 1950.
Edelstein, S.J.: An allosteric mechanism for the acetylcholine receptor. Biochem. & Biophys. Res. Comm. *48:*1160-1165, 1972.
Edmunds, C.W. and Long, P.H.: Contribution to the pathologic physiology of botulism. J.A.M.A. *81:*542-547, 1923.
Edstrom, L. and Kugelberg, E.: Histochemical composition, distribution of fibres and fatiguability of single motor units. J. Neurol., Neurosurg. & Psychiat. *31:*424-433, 1968.
Edwards, C., Bunch, W., Marfey, P., Marois, R. and Meter, D. van: Studies on the chemical properties of the acetylcholine receptor site of frog neuromuscular junctions. J. Membrane Biol. *2:*119-126, 1970.
Edwards, G.A.: The fine structure of a multiterminal innervation of an insect muscle. J. Biophys. & Biochem. Cytol. *2:*241-244, 1959.
Edwards, W.: Ultrastructural changes in the human motor endplate in myasthenia gravis. in Proc. VI Internat. Congr. Neuropath. Masson and Cie, Paris, pp. 751-752, 1970.
Ehrenpreis, S.: Isolation and identification of the acetylcholine receptor protein from electric tissue. Biochem. et Biophys. Acta *44:*561-577, 1960a.
Ehrenpries, S.: Isolation and identification of the acetylcholine receptor protein from electric organ of electric eel, in Bioelectrogenesis, a Comparative Survey of its Mechanism with Particular Emphasis on Electric Fishes (Chagas, C. and deCarvalho, A.P., eds.). Elsevier, Amsterdam and New York, 1961, pp. 379-396.
Ehrenpreis, S.: Immunohistochemical localization of drug binding protein in the tissues of the electric eel. Nature *194:*586-587, 1962.

Ehrenpreis, S.: Isolation and properties of a drug binding protein from electric tissue of electric eel. Proc. First Int. Pharmacol. Meeting 7:119-133, 1963. Pergamon Press, Oxford.
Ehrenpreis, S.: Possible nature of the cholinergic receptor. Ann. N.Y. Acad. Sci. 144:720-736, 1967.
Ehrenpreis, S.: Molecular aspects of cholinergic mechanisms. in Drugs Affecting the peripheral nervous system. 1:1-78, 1967, (Burger, A., ed.). Marcel Dekker, Inc., New York.
Ehrenpreis, S. and Fishman, M.M.: The interaction of quaternary ammonium compounds with chondroitin sulfate. Biochim. et Biophys. Acta 44:577-585, 1960b.
El-Badawi, A. and Schenk, E.A.: Histochemical methods for separate, consecutive and simultaneous demonstration of acetylcholinesterase and norepinephrine in cryostat sections. J. Histochem. Cytochem. 15:580-588, 1967.
Eldefrawi, M.E., Britten, A.G. and Eldefrawi, A.T.: Acetylcholine binding to Torpedo electroplax: relationship to acetylcholine receptors. Science 173:338-340, 1971.
Elliott, T.R.: On the action of adrenalin. J. Physiol. (Lond.) 31:20P, 1904.
Elmqvist, D. and Feldman, D.S.: Calcium dependence of spontaneous acetylcholine release at mammalian motor nerve terminals. J. Physiol. (Lond.) 181:487-497, 1965.
Elmqvist, D., Hofmann, W.W., Kugelberg, J. and Quastel, D.M.J.: An electrophysiological investigation of neuromuscular transmission in myasthenia gravis. J. Physiol. (Lond.) 174:417-434, 1964.
Elmqvist, D. and Josefsson, J.O.: The nature of the neuromuscular block produced by neomycin. Acta Physiol. Scand. 54:105-110, 1962.
Elmqvist, D. and Lambert, E.H.: Detailed analysis of neuromuscular transmission in a patient with the myasthenic syndrome sometimes associated with bronchogenic carcinoma. Mayo Clin. Proc. 43:689-713, 1968.
Elsberg, C.A.: Experiments on motor nerve regeneration and the direct neurotization of paralysed muscles by their own and foreign nerves. Science 45:318-320, 1917.
Elul, R., Miledi, R. and Stefani, E.: Neurotrophic control of contracture in slow muscle fibers. Nature 217:1274-1275, 1968.
Emmelin, N. and Malm, L.: Development of supersensitivity as dependent on the length of degenerating nerve fibers. Q. J. Exp. Physiol. 50:142-145, 1965.
Emmelin, N., Nordenfelt, I. and Perec, C.: Rate of fall in choline acetyltransferase activity in denervated diaphragms as dependent on the length of the degenerating nerve. Experientia 22:725-726, 1966.
Emmert, F.C.: Über die Endigungsweise der Nerven in den Muskeln, Nach Eigenen Untersúchen. C.A. Jenni, Bern, 1836, pp. 1-35.
Emmons, P. and McLennan, H.: Failure of acetylcholine release in tick paralysis. Nature 183:474-475, 1959.
Engel, A.G. and Santa, T.: Histometric analysis of the ultrastructure of the neuromuscular junction in myasthenia gravis and the myasthenic syndrome. Ann. N.Y. Acad. Sci. 183:46-63, 1971.
Engel, W.K.: The essentiality of histo- and cytochemical studies of skeletal muscle in the investigation of neuromuscular disease. Neurology 12:778-794, 1962.
England, J.M.: The localization of endplates in unstained muscle. J. Anat. 106:311-321, 1970.
Englehart, E. and Loewi, O.: Fermentative Azetylcholinspaltung in Blut und ihre Hemmung durch Physostigmin. Arch. Exp. Path. u. Pharmakol. 150:1-13, 1930.

Eränkö, O.: Specific demonstration of acetylcholinesterase and non-specific cholinesterase in the adrenal gland of the rat. Histochemie 1:257-266, 1959.
Eränkö, O.: Histochemistry of nervous tissues: catecholamines and cholinesterases. Ann. Rev. Pharm. 7:203-222, 1967.
Eränkö, O., Härkönen, M., Kokko, A. and Räisänen, L.: Histochemical and starch gel electrophoretic characterization of desmo- and lyoesterases in the sympathetic and spinal ganglia. J. Histochem. & Cytochem. 12:570-581, 1964.
Eränkö, O., Koelle, G.B. and Räisänen, L.: A thiocholine-lead ferrocyanide method for acetylcholinesterase. J. Histochem. Cytochem. 15:674-679, 1967.
Eränkö, O. and Teräväinen, H.: Distribution of esterases in the myoneural junction of the striated muscles of the rat. J. Histochem. Cytochem. 15:399-403, 1967a.
Eränkö, O. and Teräväinen, H.: Cholinesterases and eserine-resistant carboxylic esterases in degenerating and regenerating motor endplates of the rat. J. Neurochem. 14:947-954, 1967b.
Erb, W.: Zur Pathologie und pathologischen Anatomie peripherischen Paralysin. Arch. Clin. Med. 4:535-578, 1868.
Erminio, F., Buchthal, F. and Rosenfalck, P.: Motor unit territory and muscle fiber concentration in paresis due to peripheral nerve injury and anterior horn cell involvement. Neurology 9:657-671, 1959.
Esplin, D.W., Phillip, C.B. and Hughes, L.E.: Impairment of muscle stretch reflexes in tick paralysis. Science 132:958-959, 1960.
Estable-Puig, J.F., Bauer, W.C. and Blumberg, J.M.: Technical note. Paraphenylenediamine staining of osmium fixed plastic-embedded tissue for light and phase microscopy. J. Neuropath. & Exp. Neurol. 24:531-535, 1965.
Evans, R.H., Haynes, J., Morris, C.J. and Woolf, A.L.: In vitro staining of intramuscular nerve endings. J. Neurol. Neurosurg. Psychiat. 33:783-785, 1970.
Exner, S.: Notiz zu der Fage von der Faserverthelung mehreren nerven in einem Muskeln. Pflüg. Arch. ges. Physiol. 36:572-576, 1855.
Eyzaquirre, C., Espildora, J. and Luco, J.V.: Alterations of neuromuscular synapses during Wallerian degeneration. Acta Physiol. latinoam. 2:213-227, 1952.
Ezerman, E.B. and Ishikawa, H.: Differentiation of the sarcoplasmic reticulum and T system in developing chick skeletal muscle in vitro. J. Cell Biol. 35:405-420, 1967.

Faeder, I.A., O'Brien, R.D. and Salpeter, M.M.: A reinvestigation of evidence for cholinergic neuromuscular transmission in insects. J. Exp. Zool. 173:187-202, 1970.
Falconer, D.S.: Mouse News Letter 15:23, 1956.
Falin, L. and Kanarejkin, L.: Histopathologie der motorischen nervenendigungen bei Myopathie und einegen Verwandten Erkrankungen. Virchow's Arch. Path. Anat. 307:523, 1940.
Falk, G. and Fatt, P.: Linear electrical properties of striated muscle fibres observed with intercellular electrodes. Proc. Roy. Soc. B. 160:69-123, 1960.
Fambrough, D.M.: Acetylcholine sensitivity of muscle fiber membranes: mechanisms of regulation by motor neurons. Science 168:372-373, 1970.
Fambrough, D.M. and Hartzell, H.C.: Acetylcholine receptors: Number and distribution at neuromuscular junctions in rat diaphragm. Science 176:189-191, 1972.
Fambrough, D. and Rash, J.E.: Development of acetylcholine sensitivity during myogenesis. Developmental Biol. 26:55-68, 1971.

Fardeau, M. and Godet-Guillain, J.: Etude ultrastructurale des plaques motrices du muscle squelettique et de leurs modifications pathologiques. *in* Proc. Sixth Internat. Congr. Neuropathol. Paris 746:1970 (abstr.).
Farrant, J.L.: An electron microscopic study of ferritin. Biochim. et Biophys. Acta 13: 569-576, 1954.
Fatt, P.: Electromotive action of acetylcholine at the motor endplates. J. Physiol. (Lond.) 111:408-422, 1950.
Fatt, P. and Katz, B.: Some observations on biological noise. Nature 166:597-598, 1950.
Fatt, P. and Katz, B.: An analysis of the endplate potential recorded with an intracellular electrode. J. Physiol. (Lond.) 115:320-370, 1951.
Fatt, P. and Katz, B.: Spontaneous subthreshold activity at motor nerve endings. J. Physiol. (Lond.) 117:109-128, 1952.
Fawcett, D.W.: The identification of particulate glycogen and ribonucleoprotein granules in electron micrographs. J. Histochem. & Cytochem. 6:95-96, 1958.
Feigin, G.A., Peterson, N.S., Hoffman, W.W., Genther, G.H. and Van Heyningen, W.E.: The effect of impure tetanus toxin on the frequency of miniature endplate potentials. J. Gen. Microbiol. 33:489-495, 1963.
Feist, B.: Beiträge zur Kenntniss der vitalen Methylenblaufärburg des Nervengewebes. Arch. Anat. u. Physiol. 116:184, 1890.
Feldberg, W.: Present views on the mode of action of acetylcholine in the central nervous system. Physiol. Rev. 25:596-642, 1945.
Feldberg, W. and Fessard, A.: The cholinergic nature of the nerves to the electric organ of the Torpedo (*Torpedo marmorata*). J. Physiol. (Lond.) 101:200-215, 1942.
Feldman, D.S.: Calcium dependence of spontaneous acetylcholine release at mammalian motor nerve terminals. J. Physiol. (Lond.) 179:33-34P, 1965.
Feng, T.P. and Ting, Y.C.: Studies on the neuromuscular junctions. A note on the local concentration of cholinesterase at the motor nerve endings. Chin. J. Physiol. 13:141-144, 1938.
Fenichel, G.M. and Shy, G.M.: Muscle biopsy experience in myasthenia gravis. Arch. Neurol. 9:237-243, 1963.
Fernand, V.S.V. and Hess, A.: The occurrence, structure and innervation of slow and twitch muscle fibers in the tensor tympani and stapedius of the cat. J. Physiol. (Lond.) 200:547-554, 1969.
Fex, S., Sonesson, B., Thesleff, S. and Zelená, J.: Nerve implants in botulinum poisoned mammalian muscle. J. Physiol. (Lond.) 184:872-882, 1966.
Fex, S. and Thesleff, S.: The time required for innervation of denervated muscles by nerve implants. Life Sciences 6:635-639, 1967.
Fidziańska, A.: Electron microscopic study of the development of human foetal muscle, motor endplate and nerve. Acta Neuropath. 17:234-247, 1971.
Fields, H.L. and Kennedy, D.: Functional role of muscle receptor organs in the crayfish. Nature 206:1235-1237, 1965.
Fields, W.S.: Myasthenia Gravis. Ann. N.Y. Acad. Sci. 183:1-385, 1971.
Filogamo, G. and Gabella, G.: Cholinesterase behavior in the denervated and reinnervated muscles. Acta Anat. 63:199-214, 1966.
Filogamo, G. and Gabella, G.: The development of neuromuscular correlations in vertebrates. Arch. Biol. (Liège) 78:9-60, 1967.

Fischer, E. and Ramsey, V.W.: Changes in muscle proteins during muscular atrophy. Arch. Phys. Therap. 25:709-716, 1944.

Fischer, E. and Ramsey, V.W.: Changes in protein content and in some physicochemical properties of the protein during muscular atrophies of various types. Am. J. Physiol. 145:571-582, 1946.

Fischer, G.: Inhibierung und Restitution der Azetylcholinesterase an der motorischen Endplatte im Zwerchfell der Ratte Nach Intoxikation mit Soman. Histochemie 16: 144-149, 1968.

Fleckenstein, A., Tippelt, H. and Kroner, H.: Über die Dehydrasen-hemmende Wirkung von Bienengift. Arch. Exp. Path. u. Pharmacol. 210:380-388, 1950.

Flood, P.R.: A peculiar mode of muscular innervation in amphioxus. Light and electron microscopic studies of the so called ventral roots. J. Comp. Neurol. 126:181-218, 1966.

Floyd, K.: Muscular innervation junction between muscle fibres in cat extraocular muscle. Nature 227:185-186, 1970.

Floyd, W.F., Kent, P. and Page, F.: An electromyographic study of myotonia. Electroenceph. Clin. Neurophysiol. 7:621-630, 1955.

Foldes, F.: Production of the myasthenic state in man and its possible significance in the pathogenesis of myasthenia gravis. in Myasthenia Gravis (Viets, H.R., ed.). Springfield, Ill., 1961, pp. 119-126.

Fonnum, F.: Choline acetyltransferase binding to and release from membranes. Biochem. J. 109:389-398, 1968.

Fonnum, F.: Surface charge of choline acetyltransferase from different species. J. Neurochem. 17:1095-1100, 1970.

Forssman, J.: Über die Ursachen, welche die Wachsthumsrichtung der peripheren Nervenfasern bei der Regeneration bestimmen. Bietr. Path. Anat. 24:56-100, 1898.

Francois, C.: Tetanus toxin and muscle relaxation. Toxicon 8:247-248, 1970.

Frank, G.B. and Inoue, F.: Large miniature endplate potentials in partial denervated skeletal muscle. Nature 212:596-598, 1966.

Friede, R.: Electrophoretic production of "reactive" axon swellings in vitro and their histochemical properties. Acta Neuropath. 3:217-228, 1964.

Fukuhara, N., Takamori, M., Gutmann, L. and Chou, S.M.: Eaton-Lambert syndrome. Ultrastructural study of the motor endplates. Arch. Neurol. 27:67-78, 1972.

Fulpius, B. and Klett, R.P.: Acetylcholine receptor of the electric eel: biochemical and pharmacological properties. Fed Proc. (in press) 1973.

Furshpan, E.J. and Potter, D.D.: Transmission at the giant motor synapses of the crayfish. J. Physiol. (Lond.) 145:289-325, 1959.

Furukawa, T., Takagi, T. and Sugihara, T.: Depolarization of endplates by Ach externally applied. Jap. J. Physiol. 6:98-107, 1956.

Gage, P.W. and Quastel, D.M.J.: Influence of sodium ions on transmitter release. Nature 206:1047-1048, 1965.

Gage, P.W.: The effect of methyl, ethyl, and n-propyl alcohols on neuromuscular transmission in the rat. J. Pharmacol. & Exp. Therap. 150:236-243, 1965.

Gage, P.W. and Hubbard, J.I.: Evidence for a poisson distribution of miniature endplate potentials and some implications. Nature 208:395-396, 1965.

Galindo, A.: Curare and pancuronium compared: Effects on previously undepressed mammalian myoneural junctions. Science *178:*753-755, 1972.

Gautrelet, J. and Corteggiani, E.: Libération de l'acétylcholine du complexe acétylcholinique du cerveau des mammifères par le venin de cobra. C.R. Séance Acad. Sci. *207:*465-466, 1938.

Geld, H. Van der, Feltkamp, I.E.W. and Oosterhuis, H.J.G.H.: Reactivity of myasthenia gravis serum and globulin with skeletal muscles and thymus demonstrated by immunofluorescence. Proc. Soc. Exp. Biol. and Med. *115:*782-785, 1964.

Gentner, D.R. and Rosenberg, R.N.: Choline acetyltransferase and acetylcholinesterase. Their role in the causes of myasthenia gravis Arch. Neurol. *27:*521-525, 1972.

Genuit, H. and Labenz, K.: Über die Wirksamkeit der cholinesterase im intakten Herzmuskel des Warmbluters und ihre Beeinfluszbarkeit durch verschiedene. Pharmaka, besonders die Narkotica. Arch. Exp. Path. u. Pharmakol. *198:*369-384, 1941.

Gerard, R.W.: The acetylcholine system in neural function. Recent Progr. Hormone Res. *5:*37-61, 1950.

Gerebtzoff, M.A.: Recherches histochimiques sur les acétylcholines et cholinestérases. I. Introduction et technique. Acta Anat. *19:*366-379, 1953.

Gerebtzoff, M.A.: Development of cholinesterase activity in the nervous system *in* Waelsch, H. Biochemistry of the Developing Nervous System. Academic Press, New York, pp. 315-320, 1955.

Gerebtzoff, M.A.: Cholinesterase. A histochemical contribution to the solution of some functional problems. Pergamon Press, London, 1959.

Gerebtzoff, M.A., Philippot, E. and Dallemagne, M.J.: Recherches histochimiques sur les acétylcholine et choline estérases. 2. Activité enzymatique dans les muscles lents et rapides des mammifères et des oiseaux. Acta Anat. *20:*234-257, 1954.

Gerebtzoff, M.A. and Ueten, L.: Présence d'appareils cholinestérasiques musculotendineux chez divers mammifères, notamment chez l'homme, et leur persistances apres dénervation. C.R. Soc. Biol. (Paris) *148:*1896-1898, 1954.

Gerebtzoff, M.A. and Vandermissen, L.: Étude de la relation spatiale entre acétylcholinesterase et récepteur de l'acétylcholine. Ann. Histochim. *1:*221-229, 1956.

Gersh, I. and Catchpole, G.W.: The organization of ground substance and basement membranes and its significance in tissue injury, disease and growth. Am. J. Anat. *85:*457-478, 1949.

Ghiretti, F.: Toxicity of octopus saliva against crustacea. Ann. N.Y. Acad. Sci. *90:*726-741, 1960.

Ghosh, B.N. and Chatterjee, A.K.: Effect of snake venom on the oxidation of glucose and its metabolites in cell suspensions. J. Indian Chem. Soc. *25:*359-364, 1948.

Ghosh, B.N., De, S.S. and Chowdhury, D.K.: Enzymes in snake venom. Ann. Biochem. & Exp. Med. *1:*31-42, 1941.

Giacobini, G.: Embryonic and postnatal development of choline acetyltransferase activity in muscles and sciatic nerve of the chick. J. Neurochem. *19:*1401-1403, 1972.

Ginsborg, B.L.: Some properties of avian skeletal muscle fibres with multiple neuromuscular junctions. J. Physiol. (Lond.) *154:*581-598, 1960.

Ginsborg, B.L. and Mackay, B.: A histochemical demonstration of two types of motor innervation in avian skeletal muscle. Bibl. Anat. (Basel) *2:*174-181, 1961.

Goldberg, A.L. and Singer, J.J.: Evidence for a role of cyclic AMP in neuromuscular transmission. Proc. U.S. Nat. Acad. Sci. *64:*134-141, 1969.

Goldman, D.E.: A molecular structural basis for the excitation properties of axons. Biophys. J. *4*:167-188, 1964.

Goldspink, D.F., Harris, J.B., Park, D.C., Parsons, M.E. and Pennington, R.J.: Quantitative enzyme studies in denervated extensor digitorum longus and soleus muscles of rats. Internat. J. Biochem. *2*:427-433, 1971.

Goldstein, D.J.: Some histochemical observations of human striated muscle. Anat. Rec. *134*:217-232, 1959.

Goldstein, G.: Myasthenia gravis and the thymus. Ann. Rev. Med. *22*:119-124, 1971.

Goldstein, G. and Whittingham, S.: Experimental autoimmune thymitis. An animal model of human myasthenia gravis. Lancet *2*:315-318, 1966.

Gomori, G.: Microtechnical demonstration of sites of lipase activity. Proc. Soc. Exp. Biol. & Med. *58*:362-364, 1945.

Gomori, G.: Histochemical demonstration of sites of cholinesterase activity. Proc. Soc. Exp. Biol. & Med. *68*:354-358, 1948.

Gomori, G.: The histochemistry of esterases. Int. Rev. Cytol. *1*:323-335, 1952a.

Gomori, G.: Microscopic Histochemistry. University of Chicago Press, Chicago, Ill., 1952b.

Gonzalez, A.W.A.: The prenatal development of behavior in the albino rat. J. Comp. Neurol. *55*:395-442, 1932.

Göpfert, H. and Schaefer, H.: Über den direkt und indirekt erregten Aktionsstrom und die Funktion der motorischen Endplatten. Pflüg. Arch. Ges. Physiol. *239*:597-619, 1938.

Govier, W.C. and Holland, W.C.: Effects of ouabain on tissue calcium and calcium exchange in pacemaker in turtle heart. Am. J. Physiol. *207*:195-198, 1964.

Graff, G.L.A., Hudson, A.J. and Strickland, K.P.: Biochemical changes in denervated skeletal muscle. I. the effect of denervation atrophy on the main phosphate fractions of the rat gastrocnemius muscle. Biochim. Biophys. Acta *104*:524-531, 1965.

Grampp, W., Harris, J.B. and Thesleff, S.: Inhibition of denervation changes in mammalian skeletal muscle by actinomycin D. J. Physiol. (Lond.) *221*:743-754, 1972.

Granbacher, N.: Relation between the size of muscle fibers, motor endplates and nerve fibers during hypertrophy and atrophy. Zts. f. Anat. u. Entwicklungsges. *135*:76-87, 1971.

Gray, E.G.: The spindle and extrafusal innervation of a frog muscle. Proc. Roy. Soc. B. *146*:416-430, 1957.

Gray, E.G. and Guillery, R.W.: The basis for silver staining of synapses of the mammalian spinal cord: A light and electron microscope study. J. Physiol. (Lond.) *157*:581-588, 1961.

Gray, E.P. and Whittaker, V.P.: The isolation of synaptic vesicles from the central nervous system. J. Physiol. (Lond.) *153*:35-37, 1960.

Gray, P.: The Microtomist's Formulary and Guide. Blakiston Co., Inc., New York, 1954.

Graziadei, P.: Endplates in cephalopod muscles. J. Physiol. (Lond.) *179*:9P, 1965.

Graziadei, P.: The ultrastructure of the motor nerve ending in the muscles of a cephalopod. J. Ultrastr. Res. *15*:1-13, 1966.

Graziadei, P. and de Rubeis, S.R.: Sur l'innervation des muscles adducteurs et des du man trau chez *Ostrea edulis*. Acta Anat. *53*:60-80, 1963.

Greef, K. and Westermann, E.: Untersuchungen über die muskellahmenden Wirkung des Strophanthins. Arch. Exp. Pharm. Pharmakol. *226*:103-113, 1955.

Greenfield, J.G.: The Spino-cerebellar Degenerations. Blackwell Scientific Publications, Oxford, 1954.
Greenfield, J.G., Blackwood, W., McMenemey, W.H., Meyer, A. and Norman, R.M.: Neuropathology. Edward Arnold Publishers, Ltd., London, 1960.
Greenfield, J.G. and Carmichael, E.A.: The peripheral nerves in cases of subacute combined degeneration of the cord. Brain 58:483-491, 1935.
Grob, D., Garlick, W.L. and Harvey, A.M.: The toxic effects in man of the anticholinesterase insecticide parathion (p-nitrophenyl diethyl thionophosphate). Bull. Johns Hopkins Hosp. 87:106-229, 1950.
Grob, D. and Harvey, A.M.: Effect of adrenocorticotrophic hormone (ACTH) and cortisone administration in patients with myasthenia gravis and report of onset of myasthenia gravis during prolonged cortisone administration. Bull. Johns Hopkins Hosp. 91:124-136, 1952.
Grob, D. and Johns, R.: Further studies on the mechanism of the defect in neuromuscular transmission in myasthenia gravis, with particular reference to the acetylcholine insensitive block, in Myasthenia Gravis, The Second International Symposium Proceedings (Viets, H.R., ed.). Charles C. Thomas, Springfield, Ill., 1961, pp. 127-149.
Grob, D., Johns, R.J. and Harvey, A.M.: Studies in neuromuscular function. IV. Stimulating and depressant effects of acetylcholine and choline in patients with myasthenia gravis, and their relationship to the defect in neuromuscular transmission. Bull. Johns Hopkins Hosp. 99:153-181, 1956.
Grob, D., Namba, T. and Feldman, D.S.: Alterations in reactivity to acetylcholine in myasthenia gravis and carcinomatous myopathy. Ann. N.Y. Acad. Sci. 135:247-275, 1966.
Gruber, H.: Structure and innervation of the striated muscle fibres of the esophagus of the rat. Z. Zellforsch. 91:236-247, 1968.
Grundfest, H.: The mechanisms of discharge of the electric organs in relation to general and comparative electrophysiology. Progr. Biophys. 7:1-85, 1957.
Günther, P.G.: Die Innervation der tetanischen und tonischen Fasern der quergestreiften Skeletmuskulatur der Wirbeltiere. I. Die Innervation des M. sartorius und des M. ileofibularis des Frosches. Anat. Anz. 97:175-191, 1949.
Guth, L.: "Trophic" influences of nerve on muscle. Physiol. Rev. 48:645-680, 1968.
Guth, L.: Effect of immobilization on soleplate and background cholinesterase of rat skeletal muscle. Exper. Neurol. 24:508-513, 1969.
Guth, L., Albers, R.W. and Brown, W.C.: Quantitative changes in cholinesterase activity of denervated muscle fibers and soleplates. Exper. Neurol. 10:236-250, 1964.
Guth, L. and Brown, W.C.: The sequence of changes in cholinesterase activity during reinnervation of muscle. Exper. Neurol. 12:329-336, 1965a.
Guth, L. and Brown, W.C.: Changes in cholinesterase activity following partial denervation and hyperneurotization of muscle. Exper. Neurol. 13:198-205, 1965b.
Guth, L., Dempsey, J. and Cooper, T.: Maintenance of neurotrophically regulated proteins in denervated skeletal and cardiac muscle. Exper. Neurol. 32:478-488, 1971.
Guth, L., Samaha, F.J. and Albers, R.W.: The neural regulation of some phenotypic differences between fiber types of mammalian skeletal muscle. Exper. Neurol. 26:126-135, 1970.
Guth, L. and Watson, P.K.: The influence of innervation on the soluble proteins of slow and fast muscles of the rat. Exper. Neurol. 17:107-117, 1967.

Guth, L., Watson, P.K. and Brown, W.C.: Effects of cross-innervation on some chemical properties of red and white muscles of rat and cat. Exper. Neurol. 20:52-69, 1968.
Guth, L. and Wells, J.B.: Physiological and histochemical properties of the soleus muscle after denervation of its antagonists. Exper. Neurol. 36:463-471, 1972.
Guth, L. and Zalewski, A.A.: Disposition of cholinesterase following implantation of a nerve into innervated and denervated muscle. Exper. Neurol. 2:316-326, 1963.
Guth, L., Zalewski, A.A. and Brown, W.C.: Quantitative changes in cholinesterase activity of denervated soleplates following implantation of nerve into muscle. Exper. Neurol. 16:136-147, 1966.
Guth, P.S.: Acetylcholine binding by isolated synaptic vesicles in vitro. Nature 224: 384-385, 1969.
Gutmann, E.: The Denervated Muscle. Prague, Czech. Acad. Sci., 1962.
Gutmann, E., Gutmann, L., Medawar, P.B. and Young, J.Z.: The rate of regeneration of nerve. J. Exper. Biol. 19:14-44, 1942.
Gutmann, E. and Hanzlíková, V.: Age changes of motor endplates in muscle fibers of the rat. Gerontologia 11:12-24, 1965.
Gutmann, E. and Hanzlíková, V.: Effects of accessory nerve supply to muscle achieved by implantation into muscle during regeneration of its nerve. Physiol. bohemoslov. 16:244-250, 1967.
Gutmann, E., Hanzlíková, V. and Vyskocil, F.: Age changes in cross striated muscle of the rat. J. Physiol. (Lond.) 219:331-343, 1971.
Gutmann, E., Vodická, Z. and Zelená, J.: Changes in striated muscle after section of nerve, as a function of the length of the peripheral segment. Czech. Fiziol. 4:200-204, 1955.
Gutmann, E. and Vrbová, G.: Die Physiologie des tenotomierten muskels. Physiol. bohemoslov. 1:205-219, 1952.
Gutmann, E. and Young, J.Z.: The reinnervation of muscle after various periods of atrophy. J. Anat. 78:15-41, 1944.
Guy, E., Lefebvre, J., Lerique, J. and Scherrer, J.: Les signes électromyographiques des dermatomyosites. Rev. Neurol. 83:278-279, 1950.
Guyton, A.C. and MacDonald, M.A.: Physiology of botulinus toxin. Arch. Neurol. & Psychiat. 57:578-592, 1947.
Gwyn, D.G. and Aitken, J.T.: The formation of new motor endplates in mammalian skeletal muscle. J. Anat. (Lond.) 100:111-126, 1966.
Gwyn, D.G. and Heardman, V.: A cholinesterase-bielschowsky staining method for mammalian motor endplates. Stain Technol. 40:15-18, 1965.

Haggqvist, G.: On cholinesterase in skeletal muscles. Anat. Anz. 111:250-257, 1962.
Hagstrom, J.W.C., Roseman, D.M. and Ellis, J.T.: Debilitating muscular weakness and steroid therapy. Arch. Neurol. 5:60-67, 1961.
Hajek, I., Gutmann, E. and Syrovy, I.: Changes of proteolytic activity of proteins following denervation in the anterior and posterior latissimus dorsi of the chicken. Physiol. behemoslov. 15:1-6, 1966.
Hall, Z.: Acetylcholine receptors of normal and denervated muscle. Fed. Proc. 1973 (in press).

Hall, Z.W. and Kelly, R.B.: Enzymatic detachment of endplate acetylcholinesterase from muscle, Nature New Biology 232:62, 1971.

Hall-Graggs, E.C.B.: Observations on the fate of muscle fibers temporarily isolated by transection of a muscle belly. Z. Zellforsch. 119:68-76, 1971.

Hanker, J.S., Katzoff, L., Rosen, H.R., Seligman, M.L., Ueno, H. and Seligman, A.M.: Osmiophilic reagents: New cytochemical principle for light and electron microscopy. Science 146:1039-1043, 1964.

Hanker, J.S., Katzoff, L., Rosen, H.R., Seligman, M.L., Ueno, H. and Seligman, A.M.: Design and synthesis of thiolesters for histochemical demonstration of esterase and lipase via formation of osmiophilic diazothioethers. J. Med. Chem. 9:288-291, 1966.

Harkin, J.C.: Localization of the cellular site of collagen synthesis in peripheral nerves by electron microscopic autoradiography using H^3 proline. Proc. Fifth Internat. Congr. Neuropath. Zurich 1965 (Luthy, F. and Bischoff, A., eds.). Excerpta Medica Found. Amsterdam and New York, pp. 861-863, 1966.

Härkönen, M.: Carboxylic esterases, oxidative enzymes and catecholamines in the superior cervical ganglion of the rat and the effect of pre- and post ganglionic nerve division. Acta Physiol. Scand. 63: suppl. 237:9-94, 1964.

Harris, A.J. and Miledi, R.: Prolonged survival of isolated frog muscle and its sensitivity to acetylcholine. Nature 209:716-717, 1966.

Harris, A.J. and Miledi, R.: The effect of type D botulinum toxin on frog neuromuscular junctions. J. Physiol. (Lond.) 217:497-515, 1971.

Harris, C.: The morphology of the myoneural junction as influenced by neurotoxic drugs. Am. J. Path. 30:501-519, 1954.

Harris, E.J. and Nicholls, J.G.: The effect of denervation on the rate of entry of potassium into frog muscle. J. Physiol. (Lond.) 131:473-476, 1956.

Harris, J.B. and Thesleff, S.: Denervation — Relation of nerve stump length to membrane changes in skeletal muscle. Nature New Biology 236:60-61, 1972.

Harrison, R.G.: The outgrowth of the nerve fiber as a mode of protoplasmic movement. J. Exp. Zool. 9:787-848, 1910.

Hartzell, H.C. and Fambrough, D.M.: Acetylcholine receptors. Distribution and extrajunctional density in rat diaphragm after denervation correlated with acetylcholine sinsitivity. J. Gen. Physiol. 60:248-262, 1972.

Hartzell, H.C. and Fambrough, D.M. Acetylcholine receptor production and incorporation into membranes of developing muscle fibers. Develop. Biol. 31:153-165, 1973.

Harvey,, A.M.: The peripheral action of tetanus toxin. J. Physiol. (Lond.) 96:348-365, 1939.

Hassón, A.: Interaction of quaternary ammonium bases with a purified acid polysaccharide and other macromolecules from the electric organ of electric eel. Biochim. Biophys. Acta 56:275-292, 1962.

Hassón-Voloch, A.: Curare and acetylcholine receptor substance. Nature 218:330-333, 1968.

Hatsuyama, Y.: Histological studies on the reinnervation of denervated muscle with special reference to the collateral branching. J. Jap. Orth. Assn. 38:375-394, 1964.

Hearn, G.R.: Succinate-cytochrome c reductase, cytochrome oxidase, and aldolase activities of denervated rat skeletal muscle. Am. J. Physiol. 196:465-466, 1959.

Heaton, J., Buckley, G.A., and Evans, R.H.: The cholinesterase activity of myoneural junctions from frog twitch and tonic muscles Experientia 28:503-504, 1972.

Hebb, C.O., Krnjević, K. and Silver, A.: Acetylcholine and choline acetyltransferase in the diaphragm of the rat. J. Physiol. (Lond.) *171*:504-513, 1964.
Hebb, C.O. and Silver, A.: The effect of transection on the level of choline acetylase in the goat's sciatic nerve. J. Physiol. (Lond.) *169*:41-42P, 1963.
Hebb, C.O. and Smallman, B.N.: Intracellular distribution of choline acetylase. J. Physiol. (Lond.) *134*:385-392, 1956.
Hebb, C.O. and Waites, G.M.H.: Choline acetylase in antero- and retrograde degeneration of a cholinergic nerve. J. Physiol. (Lond.) *132*:667-671, 1956.
Hebb, C.O. and Whittaker, V.P.: Intracellular distribution of acetylcholine and choline acetylase. J. Physiol. (Lond.) *142*:187-196, 1958.
Heffernan, L.P., Rewcastle, N.B. and Humphrey, J.G.: The spectrum of rod myopathies. Arch. Neurol. *18*:529-542, 1968.
Heines, H.M., Wehrmacher, W.H. and Thomson, J.D.: Functional changes in nerve and muscle after partial denervation. Am. J. Physiol. *145*:48-53, 1945.
Heller, I.H. and Hesse, S.: The activating substances in peripheral nerve. Exp. Neurol. *10*:133-139, 1964.
Henneman, E. and Olson, C.B.: Relations between structure and function in the design of skeletal muscles. J. Neurophysiol. *28*:558-598, 1965.
Herzen, A. and Odier, R.: Altérations fibres et filaments nerveux par le curare. Arch. Int. Physiol. *1*:364-372, 1904.
Hess, A.: The structure of extrafusal muscle fibers in the frog and their innervation studied by the cholinesterase technique. Am. J. Anat. *107*:129-152, 1960.
Hess, A.: The structure of slow and fast extrafusal muscle fibers in the extraocular muscles and their nerve endings in guinea pigs. J. Cell. & Comp. Physiol. *58*:63-80, 1961.
Hess, A.: Further morphological observations of "en plaque" and "en grappe" nerve endings on mammalian extrafusal muscle fibers with the cholinesterase technique. Rev. Canad. Biol. *21*:241-248, 1962.
Hess, A.: Two kinds of extrafusal muscle fibers and their nerve endings in the garter snake. Am. J. Anat. *113*:347-364, 1963.
Hess, A.: The sarcoplasmic reticulum, the T system, and the motor terminal of slow and twitch muscle fibers in the garter snake. J. Cell Biol. *26*:467-476, 1965.
Hess, A.: The fine structure of the striated muscle fibers and their nerve terminals in the avian iris morphological "twitch-slow fibers". Anat. Rec. *154*:357, 1966.
Hess, A. and Pillar, G.: Slow fibers in the extraocular muscles of the cat. J. Physiol. (Lond.) *169*:780-798, 1963.
Heuser, J.E.: Structural changes with stimulation of frog neuromuscular junctions. Am. Soc. Cell Biol. abstr. #240, 1971.
Heuser, J.E., Katz, B. and Miledi, R.: Structural and functional changes of frog neuromuscular junctions in high calcium solutions. Proc. Roy. Soc. B. (Lond.) *178*:407-415, 1971.
Heuser, J.E. and Miledi, R.: Effects of lanthanum on the frog neuromuscular junction. J. Cell Biol. *47*:87a (abstr.), 1970.
Heuser, J.E. and Miledi, R.: Effect of lanthanum ions on function and structure of frog neuromuscular junctions. Proc. Roy. Soc. B. (Lond.) *179*:247-260, 1971.
Heuser, J.E. and Reese, T.S.: Evidence for recycling of synaptic vesicle membrane during transmitter release at the frog neuromuscular junction. J. Cell Biol. *57*:315-344, 1973.

Hikida, R.S. and Bock, W.S.: Effect of denervation on pigeon slow skeletal muscle. Z. Zellforsch. *128:*1-18, 1972.

Hildebrand, J. and Coërs, C.: The neuromuscular function in patients with malignant tumors: Electromyographic and histological study. Brain *90:*67-82, 1967.

Hildebrand, J., Joffroy, A. and Coërs, C.: Myoneural changes in experimental isoniazid neuropathy. Arch. Neurol. *19:*60-70, 1968.

Hildebrand, J., Joffroy, A., Graff, G. and Coërs, C.: Neuromuscular changes with alloxan hyperglycemia. Arch. Neurol. *18:*633-641, 1968.

Hill, R.B. and Usherwood, P.N.R.: The action of 5-hydroxytryptamine and related compounds on neuromuscular transmission in the locust *Schistocera gregaria*. J. Physiol. *157:*393-401, 1961.

Hines, H.M. and Knowlton, G.C.: Changes in the skeletal muscle of the rat following denervation. Am. J. Physiol. *104:*379-391, 1933.

Hines, H.M., Thompson, J.D. and Lazere, B.: A comparative study of muscle atrophies caused by denervation and acute inanition. Am. J. Physiol. *140:*115-118, 1943.

Hines, M.: A histochemical study of the localization of cholinesterase in skeletal muscle during its regeneration. Anat. Rec. *138:*283, 1960.

Hinsey, J.C.: The innervation of skeletal muscle. Physiol. Rev. *14:*514-585, 1934.

Hirano, H.: Fine structures of the neuromuscular junction in the skeletal muscle of the chick. *in* Proc. VI Int. Congress for Electron Microscopy, Kyoto, Japan, 1966.

Hirano, H.: A histochemical study of the cholinesterase activity in the neuromuscular junction in developing chick skeletal muscles. Arch. Histol. Jap. *28:*89-101, 1976a.

Hirano, H.: Ultrastructural study on the morphogenesis of the neuromuscular junction in the skeletal muscle of the chick. Z. Zellforsch. *79:*198-208, 1967b.

Hńik, P.: The effect of deafferentiation upon muscle atrophy due to tenotomy in rats. Physiol. bohemoslov. *13:*209-215, 1964.

Hńik, P. Beranek, R., Vyklický, L. and Zelená, J.: Sensory outflow from chronically tenotomized muscles. Physiol. bohemoslov. *12:*23, 1963.

Hńik, P., Jirmanová, I., Vyklický, L. and Zelená, J.: Fast and slow muscles of the chick after nerve cross union. J. Physiol. (Lond.) *193:*309-325, 1967.

Hodgkin, A.L. and Huxley, A.F.: Resting and action potentials in single nerve fibers. J. Physiol. (Lond.) *104:*176-195, 1945.

Hodgkin, A.L. and Huxley, A.F.: A quantitative description of membrane current and its application to conduction and excitation in nerve. J. Physiol. (Lond.) *117:*500-544, 1952.

Hodgkin, A.L., Huxley, A.F. and Katz, B.: Ionic currents underlying activity in the giant axon of the squid. Arch. Sci. Physiol. *3:*129-150, 1949.

Hoffman, H.: Local reinnervation in partially denervated muscle: A histophysiological study. Austral. J. Exp. Biol. & Med. Sci. *28:*393-397, 1950.

Hoffman, H.: Fate of interrupted nerve fibers regenerating into partially denervated muscles. Austral. J. Exp. Biol. & Med. Sci. *29:*211-219, 1951a.

Hoffman, H.: A study of the factors influencing innervation of muscles by implanted nerves. Austral. J. Exp. Biol. & Med. Sci. *29:*289-308, 1951b.

Hoffman, H. and Springell, P.H.: An attempt at the chemical identification of "neurocletin" (the substance evoking axon sprouting). Austral. J. Exp. Biol. & Med. Sci. *29:*417-423, 1951.

Hoffmann, J.: Über chronische spinale Muskelatrophie im Kindsalter, auf familiärer Basis. Deutsche Z. Nervenh. *3:*427-470, 1893.

Hofmann, W.W., Thesleff, S. and Zelená, J.: Innervation of botulinum poisoned skeletal muscles by accessory nerves. J. Physiol. (Lond.) *171:*27-28P, 1964.
Hogan, E.L., Dawson, D.M. and Romanul, F.C.A.: Enzymatic changes in denervated muscle. II. Biochemical studies. Arch. Neurol. *13:*274-282, 1965.
Hogenhuis, L.A.H. and Engel, W.K.: Histochemistry and cytochemistry of experimentally denervated guinea pig muscle. Acta Anat. *60:*39-65, 1965.
Hoh, J.F.Y.: Selective reinnervation of fast-twitch and slow-graded muscle fibers in the toad. Exper. Neurol. *30:*263-276, 1971.
Hoh, J.F.Y. and Salafsky, B.: Effects of nerve cross-union on rat intracellular potassium in fast-twitch and slow-twitch rat muscles. J. Physiol. (Lond.) *216:*171-179, 1971.
Hokin, L.E. and Hokin, M.R.: Enzymatic secretion and the incorporation of P^{32} into phospholipids of pancreas slices. J. Biol. Chem. *203:*967-977, 1953.
Hokin, L.E. and Hokin, M.R.: Studies on the carrier function of phosphatidic acid in sodium transport. I. The turnover of phosphatidic acid and phosphoinositide in the avian salt gland on stimulation of secretion. J. Gen. Physiol. *44:*61, 1960.
Hokin, M.R. and Hokin, L.E.: Phosphatidic acid metabolism and active transport of sodium. Fed. Proc. *22:*8-18, 1963.
Holmes, W.: Silver staining of nerve axons in paraffin sections. Anat. Rec. *86:*157-187, 1943.
Holmstedt, B.: A modification of the thiocholine method for the determination of cholinesterase. Acta Physiol. Scand. *40:*322-337, 1957.
Holmstedt, B. and Sjöqvist, F.: Some principles about histochemistry of cholinesterases with special references to the thiocholine method. Bibl. Anat. *2:*1, 1961.
Holt, S.J.: A new principle for the histochemical localization of hydrolytic enzymes. Nature *169:*271-273, 1952.
Holt, S.J.: A new approach to the cytochemical localization of enzymes. Proc. Roy. Soc. B. (Lond.) *142:*160-169, 1954.
Holt, S.J. and Hicks, R.M.: The importance of osmiophilia in the production of stable azoindoxyl complexes of high contrast for combined enzyme cytochemistry and electron microscopy. J. Cell Biol. *29:*361-366, 1966.
Holt, S.J. and Withers, R.F.J.: Cytochemical localization of esterases using indoxyl derivatives. Nature *170:*1012-1014, 1952.
Holtzman, E., Freeman, A.R. and Kashner, L.A.: Stimulation dependent alterations in peroxidase uptake at lobster neuromuscular junctions. Science *173:*733-735, 1971.
Houssay, B.A., Negrete, J. and Mazzocco, P.: Action des venins de serpents sur le nerf et le muscle isolés. C.R. Soc. Biol. (Paris) *87:*823-824, 1922.
Houssay, B.A. and Pavé, S.: Action curatisante des venins de serpents chez la grenouille. C.R. Soc. Biol. (Paris) *87:*821-823, 1922.
Howell, J.N., Fairhurst, A.S. and Jenden, D.J.: Alterations of the calcium accumulating ability of striated muscle following denervation. Life Sci. *5:*439-446, 1966.
Hoyle, G. and McNeill, P.A.: Correlated physiological and ultrastructural studies on specialized muscles. I. Neuromuscular junctions in the eye stalk levator muscles of *Podophthalmus vigil* (Weber). J. Exp. Zool. *167:*523-550, 1968.
Hubbard, J.I.: The effect of calcium and magnesium on the spontaneous release of transmitter from mammalian motor nerve endings. J. Physiol. (Lond.) *159:*507-517, 1961.
Hubbard, J.I.: Mechanism of transmitter release. Prog. Biophys. Mol. Biol. *21:*33-124, 1970.

Hubbard, J.I. and Gage, P.W.: The abolition of post-tetanic potentiation. Nature *202:* 299-300, 1964.

Hubbard, J.I., Jones, S.F. and Landau, E.M.: The relationship between the state of nerve-terminal polarization and liberation of acetylcholine. Ann. N.Y. Acad. Sci. *144:* 459-469, 1967.

Hubbard, J.I., Jones, S.F. and Landau, E.M.: On the mechanism by which calcium and magnesium affect the spontaneous release of transmitter from mammalian motor nerve terminals. J. Physiol. (Lond.) *194:*381-407, 1968a.

Hubbard, J.I., Jones, S.F. and Landau, E.M.: On the mechanism by which calcium and magnesium affect the release of transmitter by nerve impulses. J. Physiol. (Lond.) *196:*75-87, 1968b.

Hubbard, J.I., Jones, S.F. and Landau, E.M.: The effect of temperature change upon transmitter release, facilitation and post-tetanic potentiation. J. Physiol. (Lond.) *216:*591-609, 1971.

Hubbard, J.I. and Kwanbunbumpen, S.: Evidence for the vesicle hypothesis. J. Physiol. (Lond.) *194:*407-420, 1968.

Hubbard, J.I., Llinas, R. and Quastel, C.M.J.: Electrophysiological analysis of synaptic transmission. Williams and Wilkins, Co., 1969, Baltimore.

Hubbard, J.I. and Schmidt, R.F.: An electrophysiological investigation of mammalian motor nerve terminals. J. Physiol. (Lond.) *166:*145-167, 1963.

Hubbard, J.I. and Willis, W.D.: The effects of depolarization of motor nerve terminals upon the release of transmitter by nerve impulses. J. Physiol. (Lond.) *194:*381-405, 1968.

Hubbard, J.I. and Wilson, D.F.: Reduction of the quantum content of endplate potentials by atropine. Experientia *26:*1234-1235, 1970.

Hughes, A.: The growth of embryonic neurites. A study of cultures of chick neural tissues. J. Anat. *87:*150-162, 1953.

Hunt, R.: Further observations on the blood pressure-lowering bodies in extracts of the suprarenal gland. Am. J. Physiol. *5:*6-7, 1901.

Hunt, R. and Taveau, R. de M.: On the physiological action of certain choline derivatives and new methods for detecting choline. Brit. Med. J. *2:*1788-1791, 1906.

Hurlbut, W.P., Longenecker, H.B., Jr. and Mauro, A.: Effect of calcium and magnesium on the frequency of miniature endplate potentials during prolonged tentanization. J. Physiol. (Lond.) *219:*17-38, 1971.

Ing, H.R. and Wright, W.M.: Further studies on the pharmacological properties of onium salts. Proc. Roy. Soc. B. *114:*48-63, 1933.

Ip, M.C.: A combined method for demonstrating the cholinesterase activity and the nervous structure of mammalian peripheral motor endings in teased preparations. J. Physiol. (Lond.) *192:*801-803, 1967.

Israël, M.: Localisation de l'acetylcholine des synapses myoneurales et nerf electroplaque. Arch. d'Anat. Micros. Morp. Exper. *59:*67-98, 1970.

Israël, M. and Gautron, J.: Cellular and subcellular localization of acetylcholine in electric organs. Symp. Int. Soc. Cell Biol. *8:*137-152, 1969 Academic Press, New York.

Iwanaga, I.: Studien über die motorischen Nervendigungen. I. Ihre Histogenese. Mitt. Allg. Path. u. Path. Anat. (Sendai) *2:*257-342, 1925.

Iwasaki, S.: Effect of DNP on neuro-muscular junction of frog. Tohoku J. Exp. Med. *83:*309-324, 1964.

Iwayama, T.: Electron microscopic study on cholinesterase at the neuromuscular junction. Okajima Folia Anat. Japon. *42*:329-353, 1966.

Iwayama, T. and Ohta, M.: Morphology in neuromuscular junction in myasthenia gravis. Proc. Myasthenia Gravis Symposium (Kyoto) *1*:41-46, 1969.

Iyengar, N.K., Sehra, K.B., Mukerji, B. and Chopra, R.N.: Choline esterase in cobra venom. Current Sci. (India Inst. Sci.) *7*:51-53, 1938.

James, D.W. and Tresman, R.L.: *De novo* formation of neuromuscular junctions in tissue culture. Nature *220*:384-385, 1968.

James, D.W. and Tresman, R.L.: An electron microscopic study of the *de novo* formation of neuromuscular junctions in tissue culture. Z. Zellforsch. *100*:126-140, 1969.

Järlfors, U. and Smith, D.S.: Association between synaptic vesicles and neurotubules. Nature *224*:710-711, 1969.

Jarman, M.: Electrical activity in the muscle cells of *Ascaris lumbricoides*. Nature *184*: 1244, 1959.

Jedrzejowska, H., Johnson, A.G. and Woolf, A.L.: The intramuscular nerve endings in muscular dystrophy. Acta. Neuropath. *5*:225-242, 1965.

Jenkinson, D.H.: The nature of the antagonism between calcium and magnesium ions at the neuromuscular junction. J. Physiol. (Lond.) *138*:434-444, 1957.

Jirmanová, I., Sobotkova, M., Thesleff, S. and Zelená, J.: Atrophy in skeletal muscles poisoned with botulinum toxin. Physiol. bohemoslov. *13*:467-472, 1964.

Jirmanová, I. and Zelená, J.: Effect of denervation and tenotomy on slow and fast muscles of the chicken. Z. Zellforsch. *106*:333-347, 1970.

Johns. T.R. and Thesleff, S.: Effects of motor inactivation on the chemical sensitivity of skeletal muscle. Acta Physiol. Scand. *51*:136-141, 1961.

Johnson, A.G. and Woolf, A.L.: Replacement at the neuromuscular synapse of the terminal axonic expansion by the Schwann cell. Acta. Neuropath. *4*:436-441, 1965.

Jolly, F.: Über Myasthenia gravis pseudoparalytica. Berl. Klin. Wochschr. *32*:1-7, 1895.

Jonecko, A.: Über die Hemmung der histochemischen Azetylcholinesterase — reaktion an den motorischen Endplatten durch Einspritzungen von Neostigmin und physostigmin. Acta histochem. *16*:375-381, 1963.

Jonecko, A.: Die histochemische Darstellung der Endplatten-Esterase im mutterlichen und fotalen skeletmuskel nach akuten Vergiftungen mit Cholinestease-Inhibitoren. Acta Histochem. *20*:149-160, 1965a.

Jonecko, A.: Histochemische Untersuchungen mit Hilfe der Thioessigsaure-Methode über die Hemmung der Endplattenesterase durch Injektionen von irreversibel wirkenden Anticholinesterasen. Acta Histochem. *20*:39-44, 1965b.

Jonecko, A.: Über die PAS-Substanz an der motorischen Endplatte und myotendinosen Junktion. Acta Histochem. *36*:113-118, 1970.

Jones, S.F. and Kwanbunbumpen, S.: Some effects of nerve stimulation and hemicholinium on quantal transmitter release at the neuromuscular junction. J. Physiol. (Lond.) *207*:31-50, 1970a.

Jones, S.F. and Kwanbunbumpen, S.: The effects of nerve stimulation and hemicholinium on synaptic vesicles at the mammalian neuromuscular junction. J. Physiol. (Lond.) *207*:51-62, 1970b.

Joó, F., Gajo, M., Kalman, G. and Csillik, B.: Lipoprotein substances in the postsynaptic membrane of the myoneural junction. Acta Histochem. *20*:280-285, 1965.

Joó, F., Sávay, G. and Csillik, B.: A new modification of the Koelle-Friedenwald method for the histochemical demonstration of cholinesterase activity. Acta Histochem. Jena 22:40-45, 1965.

Josefsson, J.O. and Thesleff, S.: Electromyographic findings in experimental botulinum intoxication. Acta Physiol. Scand. 51:163-168, 1961.

Juntunen, J. and Teräväinen, H.: Structural development of myoneural junctions in the human embryo. Histochemie 32:107-112, 1972.

Kaeser, H.E., Muller, H.R. and Friedrich, B.: The nature of tetraplegia in infectious tetanus. Europ. Neurol. 1:17-27, 1968.

Kai, M., Salway, J.G., Mitchell, R.H. and Hawthorne, J.N.: The biosynthesis of triosphosphoinositide by rat brain in vitro. Biochem. Biophys. Res. Comm. 22:370-375, 1966.

Kaire, G.H.: Isolation of tick paralysis toxin from Ixodes hyolcyclus. Toxin 4:91-97, 1966.

Kamieniecka, Z.: The stages of development of human foetal muscle with reference to some muscular diseases. J. Neurol. Sci. 7:319-329, 1968.

Kamieniecka, Z. and Ojak, M.: Acetylcholinesterase (AchE) in the motor plates in diseases of the muscles. Patol. Polska 15:121-129, 1964.

Kano, M. and Shimada, Y.: Innervation of skeletal muscle cells differentiated in vitro from chick embryo. Brain Res. 27:402-405, 1971.

Kano, M. and Shimada, Y.: Innervation and acetylcholine sensitivity of skeletal cells differentiated in vitro. J. Cell Physiol. 78:233-242, 1971.

Kao, C.Y. and Nishiyama, A.: Actions of saxitoxin on peripheral neuromuscular systems. J. Physiol. (Lond.) 180:50-66, 1965.

Karlin, A.: Chemical distinctions between acetylcholinesterase and the acetylcholine receptor. Biochim. Biophys. Acta 139:358-362, 1967.

Karlin, A. and Bartels, E.: Effects of blocking sulfhydryl groups and of reducing disulfide bonds on the acetylcholine activated permeability system of the electroplax. Biochim. Biophys. Acta 126:525-535, 1966.

Karlin, A., Prives, J., Deal, W. a nd Winnik, M.: Affinity labeling of the acetylcholine receptor in the electroplax. J. Mol. Biol. 61:175-188, 1971.

Karlsson, U.L. and Anderson-Cedergren, E.: Motor myoneural junctions in frog intrafusal muscle fibre. J. Ultrastr. Res. 14:191-211, 1966.

Karnovsky, M.J. and Roots, L.: A "direct-coloring" thiocholine method for cholinesterases. J. Histochem. Cytochem. 12:219-221, 1964.

Karpati, G., Carpenter, S. and Andermann, F.: A new concept of childhood nemaline myopathy. Arch. Neurol. 24:291-304, 1971.

Karpati, G. and Engel, W.K.: Transformation of the histochemical profile of skeletal muscle by "foreign" innervation. Nature 215:1509-1510, 1967.

Karpati, G. and Engel, W.K.: Correlative histochemical study of skeletal muscle after suprasegmental denervation, peripheral nerve section, and skeletal fixation. Neurology 18:681-692, 1968.

Kása, P., Mann, S.P. and Hebb, C.: Localization of choline acetyltransferase. Nature 226:812-814, 1970a.

Kása, P., Mann, S.P. and Hebb, C.: Ultrastructural localization in spinal neurones. Nature 226:814-816, 1970b.

Kato, G., Yung, J. and Ihnat, M.: Nuclear magnetic resonance studies on acetylcholinesterase. Molec. Pharmacol. 6:588-596, 1970.

Katz, B.: Microphysiology of the neuromuscular junction. Bull. Johns Hopkins Hosp. 102:275-312, 1958.

Katz, B.: Nerve, muscle and synapse. McGraw Hill Book Co., New York, 1966.
Katz, B. and Miledi, R.: Spontaneous subthreshold activity at denervated amphibian endplates. J. Physiol. (Lond.) *146*:44-45P, 1959.
Katz, B. and Miledi, R.: The development of acetylcholine sensitivity in nerve-free segments of skeletal muscle. J. Physiol. (Lond.) *170*:389-396, 1964.
Katz, B. and Miledi, R.: Release of acetylcholine from a nerve terminal by electric pulses of variable strength and duration. Nature *207*:1097-1098, 1965a.
Katz, B. and Miledi, R.: The effect of temperature on the synaptic delay at the neuromuscular junction. J. Physiol. (Lond.) *181*:656-670, 1965b.
Katz, B. and Miledi, R.: Tetrodotoxin-resistant electrical activity in presynaptic terminals. J. Physiol. (Lond.) *203*:459-487, 1969.
Katz, B. and Thesleff, S.: A study of the desensitization produced by acetylcholine at the motor endplates. J. Physiol. (Lond.) *138*:63-80, 1;957.
Katz, N.L. and Edwards, C.: The effect of scorpion venom on the neuromuscular junction of the frog. Toxicon *10*:133-137, 1972.
Kawana, E., Akert, K. and Sandri, C.: Zinc iodide-osmium tetroxide impregnation of nerve terminals in the spinal cord. Brain Res. *16*:325-331, 1969.
Kalwanami, S. and Mori, R.: Experimental myasthenia in mice. The role of the thymus and lymphoid cells. Clin. and Exp. Immunol. *12*:447-454, 1972.
Kaye, G.I., Donahue, S. and Pappas, G.D.: Electron microscopical evidence for the uptake of colloidal particles by Schwann cells in situ. J. de Micros. *2*:605-612, 1963.
Kellaway, C.H.: The peripheral action of the Australian snake venoms. 3. The reversibility of the curari-like action. Austral. J. Exp. Biol. & Med. Sci. *10*:195-202, 1932.
Kellaway, C.H.: Snake venoms. II. Their peripheral action. Bull. Johns Hopkins Hosp. *60*:20-39, 1937.
Kellaway, C.H., Cherry, R.O. and Williams, F.E.: The peripheral action of the Australian snake venoms. 2. The curari-like action in mammals. Austral. J. Exp. Biol. & Med. Sci. *10*:181-194, 1932.
Kellaway, C.H. and Holden, F.: The peripheral action of the Australian snake venoms. 1. The curari-like action of frogs. Austral. J. Exp. Biol. & Med. Sci. *10*:167-179, 1932.
Kelly, A.M.: The development of the motor endplate in the rat. J.Cell Biol. *31*:58a, 1966.
Kelly, A.M. and Zacks, S.I.: Motor endplate lead binding in immature and adult rats. J. Histochem. Cytochem. *13*:704, 1965.
Kelly, A.M. and Zacks, S.I.: Neuromuscular development in intercostal muscle of the foetal and newborn rat. J. Neuropath. Exp. Neurol. *27*:109, 1968.
Kerkut, G.A. and Cottrell, G.A.: Acetylcholine and 5-hydroxytryptamine in the snail brain. Comp. Biochem. Physiol. *8*:53-63. 1963.
Kerkut, G.A., Shapira, A. and Walker, R.J.: The transport of ^{14}C labelled material from CNS ⇌ muscle along a nerve trunk. Comp. Biochem. Physiol. *23*:729-748, 1967.
Kernan, R.P.: Active transport in innervated and denervated mammalian skeletal muscle. J. Physiol. (Lond.) *179*:63P, 1965.
Kerr, D.M.S. and Muir, A.R.: A demonstration of the structure and disposition of ferritin in the human liver cell. J. Ultrastr. Res. *3*:313-319, 1960.
Key, A. and Retzius, G.: Studien in der Anatomie des Nervensystems. Arch. Mikr. Anat. *9*:308-386, 1873.
Keynes, R.D. and Lewis, P.R.: The intracellular calcium contents of some invertebrate nerves. J. Physiol. (Lond.) *134*:399-407, 1956.

Khera, K.S. and Laham, Q.N.: Cholinesterases and motor endplates in developing duck skeletal muscle. J. Histochem. Cytochem. *13*:559-565, 1965.

King, R.: The effects of fatigue and curare on the morphology of the motor endplates. Anat. Rec. *91*:286, 1945.

Kita, H. and Van der Kloot, W.: The quantitative relation between extracellular calcium and acetylcholine release at the frog neuromuscular junction. Brain Research *49*: 205-207, 1973.

Knowlton, G.C. and Hines, H.M.: The respiratory metabolism of atrophic muscle. Am. J. Physiol. *109*:200-208, 1934.

Knowlton, G.C. and Hines, H.M.: Kinetics of muscle atrophy in different species. Proc. Soc. Exp. Biol. & Med. *35*:394-398, 1936.

Knyazeva, G.D.: Morphological and histochemical features of the neuromuscular synapsis in guinea pigs suffering from diptheritic polyneuritis. Biull. Eksp. Biol. Med. (Eng.) *52*:1080-1084, 1962.

Koblinger, W., Kraupp, O., Stormann, H. and Clodi, P.H.: Einflusz des lokalen Wundstarrkramp-fes auf die Kalium-freisetzung aus der Skeletmuskulatur durch Acetylcholin. Arch. Exp. Path. Pharmakol. *228*:425-433, 1956.

Koelle, G.B.: The histochemical differentiation of types of cholinesterases and their localizations in tissues of the cat. J. Pharm. & Exp. Therap. *100*:158-179, 1950.

Key, A. and Retzius, G.: Studien in der Anatomie des Nervensystems. Arch. Mikr. Anat. *9*:308-386, 1873.

Keynes, R.D. and Lewis, P.R.: The intracellular calcium contents of some invertebrate nerves. J. Physiol. (Lond.) *134*:399-407, 1956.

Khera, K.S. and Laham, Q.N.: Cholinesterases and motor end plates in developing duck skeletal muscle. J. Histochem. Cytochem. *13*:559-565, 1965.

King, R.: The effects of fatigue and curare on the morphology of the motor endplates. Anat. Rec. *91*:286, 1945.

Kita, H. and Van der Kloot, W.: The quantitative relation between extracellular calcium and acetylcholine release at the frog neuromuscular junction. Brain Research *49*: 205-207, 1973.

Knowlton, G.C. and Hines, H.M.: The respiratory metabolism of atrophic muscle. Am. J. Physiol. *109*:200-208, 1934.

Knowlton, G.C. and Hines, H.M.: Kinetics of muscle atrophy in different species. Proc. Soc. Exp. Biol. & Med. *35*:394-398, 1936.

Knyazeva, G.D.: Morphological and histochemical features of the neuromuscular synapsis in guinea pigs suffering from diptheritic polyneuritis. Biull. Eksp. Biol. Med. (Eng.) *52*:1080-1084, 1962.

Koblinger, W., Kraupp, O., Stormann, H. and Clodi, P.H.: Einflusz des lokalen Wundstarrkrampfes auf die Kalium-freisetzung aus der Skeletmuskulatur durch Acetylcholin. Arch. Exp. Path. Pharmakol. *228*:425-433, 1956.

Koelle, G.B.: The histochemical differentiation of types of cholinesterases and their localizations in tissues of the cat. J. Pharm. & Exp. Therap. *100*:158-179, 1950.

Koelle, G.B.: The elimination of enzymatic diffusion artefacts in the histochemical localization of cholinesterases and a survey of their cellular distributions. J. Pharm. & Exp. Therap. *103*:153-171, 1951.

Koelle, G.B.: The histochemical identification of acetylcholinesterase in cholinergic, adrenergic and sensory neurons. J. Pharmacol. Exp. Therap. *114*:167-184, 1955.

Koelle, G.B.: Histochemical and pharmacological evidence of the physiological role of acetylcholinesterase, in Bioelectrogenesis: A Comparative Survey of its Mechanisms with Particular Emphasis on Electric Fishes. (Chagas, C. and de Carvalho, A.P., eds.). Elsevier, Amsterdam and New York, 1961, pp. 310-319.

Koelle, G.B.: Functional anatomy of synaptic transmission. Anesthesiology 29:643-653, 1968.

Koelle, G.B., Davis, R. and Devlin, M.: Acetyl disulfide, $(CH_3 COS)_2$, and Bis — (thioacetoxy) aurate (I) complex, Au $(CH_3 COS)_2$, histochemical substrates of unusual properties with acetylcholinesterase. J. Histochem. and Cytochem. 16:754-764, 1968.

Koelle, G.B. and Friedenwald, J.S.: A histochemical method for localizing cholinesterase activity. Proc. Soc. Exp. Biol. and Med. 70:617-622, 1949.

Koelle, G.B. and Gromadzki, C.G.: Comparison of the gold-thiocholine and gold-thiolacetic acid methods for the histochemical localization of acetylcholinesterase and cholinesterases. J. Histochem. Cytochem. 14:443-454, 1966.

Koelle, G.B. and Horn, R.S.: Acetyl disulfide $(CH_3COS)_2$, a major active component in the thiolacetic acid histochemical method for acetylcholinesterase. J. Histochem. Cytochem. 16:743-753, 1968.

Koelle, W.A., Hossaini, K.S., Akbarzadeh, P. and Koelle, G.B.: Histochemical evidence and consequences of the occurrence of isoenzymes of acetylcholinesterase. J. Histochem. Cytochem. 18:812-819, 1970.

Koenig, E.: Synthetic mechanisms in the axon. I. Local axonal synthesis of acetylcholinesterase. J. Neurochem. 12:343-356, 1965.

Koenig, J.: Innervation motrice expérimentale d'une portion de muscle strie normalement dé pourvu de plaques motrices chez le rat. C.R. Acad. Sci. (Paris) 256:2918, 1963.

Koenig, J.: Ultrastructure des plaques motrices en voie de neoformation et de reinnervation chez le rat. C.R. Acad. Sci. (Paris) 271:997-999, 1970a.

Koenig, J.: Morphological study of the endplates in chicken's latissimus dorsi anterior and posterior after cross innervation. Arch. d'Anat. Micros. et Morph. Exp. 59:403-426, 1970b.

Koenig, J.: Contribution a l'étude de la neoformation experimentale des plaques motrices de rat. Arch. d'Anat. Micros. et Morph. Exp. 60:1-26, 1971.

Koenig, J. and Pecot-Dechavassine, M.: Relations entre l'apparition des potentiels miniatures spontanés et l'ultrastructure des plaques motrices en voie de reinnervation et de neoformation chez le rat. Brain Res. 27:43-57, 1971.

Koike, H., Eisenstadt, M. and Schwartz, J.H.: Axonal transport of newly synthesized acetylcholine in an identified neuron of Aplysia. Brain Research 37:152-159, 1972.

Kokko, A.: Histochemical and cytophotometric observations on esterases in the spinal ganglion of the rat. Acta Physiol. Scand. 66: suppl. 261:7-76, 1965.

Kokko, A., Mautner, H.G. and Barrnett, R.J.: Fine structural localization of acetylcholinesterase using acetyl β-methyl thiocholine and acetylselenocholine as substrates. J. Histochem. Cytochem. 17:625-640, 1969.

Kono, T. and Collowick, S.P.: Isolation of skeletal muscle cell membrane and some of its properties. Arch. Biochem. and Biophys. 93:520-533, 1961.

Kono, T., Kakuma, F., Homa, M. and Fukuda, S.: The electron microscopic structure and chemical composition of the isolated sarcolemma of the rat skeletal muscle cell. Biochim. et Biophys. Acta 88:155-176, 1964.

Korneliussen, H.: ultrastructure of normal and stimulated motor endplates, with comments on the origen and fate of synaptic vesicles. Z. Zellforsch. 130:28, 1972.

Korneliussen, H., Barstad, J.A.B. and Lilleheil, G.: Vesicle hypothesis: Effect of nerve stimulation on the synaptic vesicles of motor endplates. Experientia 28:1055-1057, 1972.
Kornfield, P., Somlyo, A. and Osserman, K.E.: Role of calcium in myasthenia gravis. Arch. Neurol. 21:466-470, 1969.
Korr, I.M., Wilkinson, P.N. and Chornock, F.W.: Axonal delivery of neuroplasmic components to muscle cells. Science 155:342-345, 1967.
Kosower, E.M. and Werman, R.: New step in transmitter release at the myoneural junction. Nature New Biology 233:121-122, 1971.
Kovács, T., Kővér, A. and Balogh, G.: Studies on the localization of cholinesterase in various types of muscle. J. Cell Comp. Physiol. 57:63-71, 1961.
Krause, W.: Über die Endigung der Muskelnerven. Z. rat. Med. 18:136-160, 1863.
Kreutzberg, G.: Lokalisierter Oxydereduktasenanstieg bei der Wallerschen Degeneration das peripheren Nerven. Naturwissenschaften 50:96, 1963.
Kristensson, K.: Transport of fluorescent protein tracer in peripheral nerves. Acta Neuropath. 16:293-300, 1970.
Kruckenberg, P. Pontzen, W., Sandweg, R. and Bauer, H.: Zur Storung der Erregungsubertragung bei Myasthenia Gravis. Z. Neurol. 200:158-173, 1971.
Krüger, P.: Die Innervation der tetanischen und tonischen Fasern der quergestreifen Skeletmuskulatur der Wirbeltiere. Anat. Anz. 97:169-175, 1949.
Krüger, P.: Untersuchungen am Vogelflügel. Zool. Anz. 145:445-460, 1950.
Krüger, P. and Gunther, P.G.: Fasern mit "Fibrillenstruktur" und Fasern mit "Felderstruktur" in der quergestreiften Skeletmuskulatur der Säuger und des Menschen. Z. Anat. Entw.-Gesch. 118:313-323, 1955.
Krüger, P. and Gunther, P.G.: Innervation und pharmakologisches Verhalten des M. gastrocnemius und M. pectoralis major der Vögel. Acta Anat. 33:325-338, 1958.
Kryzhanovsky, G.N.: The mechanism of action of tetanus toxin: Effect on synaptic processes and some particular features of toxin binding by the nervous tissue. Nauyn-Schmiedeberg's Arch. Pharmacol. 276:247-270, 1973.
Kuba, K.: Effects of catecholamines on the neuromuscular junctions in the rat diaphragm. J. Physiol. (Lond.) 211:551-570, 1970.
Kuffler, S.W.: Physiology of neuromuscular junctions: electrical aspects. Fed. Proc. 7:437-446, 1948.
Kuffler, S.W. and Vaughan Williams, E.M.: Small-nerve junctional potentials. The distribution of small motor nerves to frog skeletal muscle, and the membrane characteristics of the fibers they innervate. J. Physiol. (Lond.) 121:289-317, 1953.
Kugelberg, E. and Welander, L.: Heredofamilial-juvenile muscular atrophy simulating muscular dystrophy. A.M.A. Arch. Neurol. Psychiat. 75:500-509, 1956.
Kühne, W.: Über die chemische Reizung der Muskeln und Nerven und ihre Bedeutung für die Irritabilitätsfrage. Arch. Anat. Physiol. (Leipzig) 315-354, 1860.
Kühne, W.: Über die peripherischen Endorgane der motorischen Nerven. Engelmann, Leipzig, 1862.
Kühne, W.: Über den feineren Bau der peripherischen Endorgane der motorischen Nerven. Virchow's Arch. Path. Anat. 29:433-449, 1864.
Kühne, W.: Die Verbindung der Nervenscheiden mit dem Sarkolemm. Z. Biol. 19:501-534, 1883.
Kühne, W.: Die motorische Nervendigung. Verh. Nat.-Med. Vereins (Heidelberg) 3:223-231, 1886a.

Kühne, W.: Über Form, Structur und Entwicklung der motorischen Nervenendigungen. Verh. Nat.-Med. Vereins (Heidelberg) 3:276-285, 1886b.

Kühne, W.: Neue Untersuchungen uber motorische Nervendigungen. Z. Biol. 23:1-148, 1887.

Kulchitsky, N.: Nerve endings in muscles. J. Anat. (Lond.) 58:152-159, 1924.

Kuno, M., Turkanis, S.A. and Weakly, J.N.: Correlation between nerve terminal size and transmitter release at the neuromuscular junction of the frog. J. Physiol. (Lond.) 213:545-556, 1971.

Kupfer, C. and Koelle, G.B.: A histochemical study of choline esterase during formation of the motor endplate of the albino rat. J. Exp. Zool. 116:397-414, 1951.

Kura, N. and Kamesawa, S.: Über die Veränderung der peripheren Nervenfasern und ihrer Endigungen durch das Tetanustoxin. Trans. Jap. Path. Soc. 18:330-331, 1928.

Kuriyama, K., Roberts, E. and Vos, J.: Some characteristics of binding of γ-aminobutyric acid and acetylcholine to a synaptic vesicle fraction from mouse brain. Brain Res. 9:231-252, 1968.

Lagos, J.C. and Thies, R.E.: Tick paralysis without muscle weakness. Arch. Neurol. 21: 471-474, 1969.

Lamanna, C. and Carr, C.J.: The botulinal, tetanal, and enterostaphylococcal toxins: A review. J. Clin. Pharmacol. Therap. 8:286-332, 1967.

Lambert, D.H. and Parsons, R.L.: Influence of polyvalent cations on the activation of muscle endplate receptors. J. Gen. Physiol. 56:309-321, 1970.

Lanari, A.: La contracción miotónica en el hombre después de curarización completa. Medicina (Buenos Aires) 7:21-26, 1947.

Landau, E.M. and Kwanbunbumpen, S.: Morphology of motor nerve terminals subjected to polarizing currents. Nature 221:171-272, 1969.

Landmesser, L.: Pharmacological properties, cholinesterase activity and anatomy of nerve-muscle junctions in vagus-innervated frog sartorius. J. Physiol. (Lond.) 220: 243-256, 1972.

Landsteiner, K. and Botteri, A.: Über Verbindungen von Tetanustoxin mit lipoiden. IV. Mitteilung über Adsorptionsverbindungen. Zentralbl. Bakt. I. Abt. Orig. 42:562-566, 1906.

Lane, C.E. and Dodge, E.: The toxicity of Physalia nematocysts. Biol. Bull. 115:219-226, 1958.

Lang, F.: Ultrastructure of neuromuscular junctions in Limulus heart. Z. Zellforsch. 130:481-488, 1972.

Langley, J.N.: Observations on the physiological action of extracts of the supra-renal bodies. J. Physiol. (Lond.) 27:237-256, 1901.

Langley, J.N.: On the reaction of cells and of nerve endings to certain poisons chiefly as regards the reaction of striated muscle to nicotine and to curari. J. Physiol. (Lond.) 33:374-413, 1905.

Langley, J.N.: On the contraction of muscle, chiefly in relation to the presence of "receptive" substances. IV. The effect of curari and of some other substances on the nicotine response of the sartorius and gastrocnemius muscles of the frog. J. Physiol. (Lond.) 39:235-295, 1909.

Lapicque, L.: L'Excitabilité en Fonction du Temps. Paris, 1926.

Lapicque, L.: Has the muscular substance a longer chronaxie than the nervous substance? J. Physiol. (Lond.) 73:189-214, 1931.
Laskowski, M.B. and Thies, R.: Interactions between calcium and barium on the spontaneous release of transmitter from mammalian motor nerve terminals. Internat. J. Neuroscience 4:11-16, 1972.
Lawrentjew, B.J.: Studien über den feineren Bau der Nervenendigungen in der quergestreiften Muskulatur des Frosches. I. Bau der Normalen motorischen Nervenendigungen in der Skeletmuskulatur. Z. Mikr. Anat. Forsch. 13:388-409, 1928.
Lazarow, A. and Speidel, E.: The chemical composition of the glomerular basement membrane and its relationship to the production of diabetic complications. p. 127-150, in Conference on Small Blood Vessel Involvement in Diabetes Mellitus, Airlie House Conference, Warrenton, Virginia, 1963 (Siperstein, M.D., ed.). American Institute of Biological Sciences Monograph.
Lee, C.Y.: Mode of action of cobra venom and its purified toxins. in Neuropoisons their Pathophysiological actions. 1:21-70, 1971 (Simpson, L.L., ed.). Plenum Press, New York.
Leffvin, J.Y., Pickard, W.F., McCullough, W.S. and Pitts, W.: The theory of passive ion flux through axon membranes. Nature 202:1338-1339, 1964.
Lehrer, G.M. and Ornstein, L.: A diazo coupling method for the electron microscopic localization of cholinesterase. J. Biophys. & Biochem. Cytol. 6:399-406, 1959.
Lentz, T.L.: Cytological studies of muscle dedifferentiation and differentiation during limb regeneration of the newt Triturus. Am. J. Anat. 124:447-480, 1969a.
Lentz, T.L.: Development of the neuromuscular junction. I. Cytological and cytochemical studies of the neuromuscular junction of differentiating muscle in the regenerating limb of the newt, Triturus. J. Cell Biol. 42:431-443, 1969b.
Lentz, T.L.: Development of the neuromuscular junction. II. Cytological and cytochemical studies on the neuromuscular junction of dedifferentiating muscle in the regenerating limb of the newt Triturus. J. Cell Biol. 47:423-436, 1970.
Lentz, T.L.: Development of the neuromuscular junction. III. Degeneration of motor endplates after denervation and maintenance in vitro by nerve explants. J. Cell Biol. 55:93-103, 1972.
Lester, H.A.: Post synaptic action of cobra venom at the myoneural junction. Nature 227:727-728, 1970.
Lester, H.A.: Blockade of acetylcholine receptors by cobra toxin: Electrophysiological Studies. Molec. Pharmacol. 6:623-631, 1972.
Levi-Montalcini, R. and Angeletti, P.U.: Growth control of the sympathetic system by a specific protein factor. Quant. Rev. Biol. 36:99-108, 1961.
Lewandowsky, M.: Über die Wirkung des Nebennierenextractes auf die glatten Muskeln, im Besonderen des Auges. Arch. Anat. u. Physiol. (Leipzig) 2:360-366, 1899.
Lewis, P.R. and Hughes, A.F.W.: Patterns of myoneural junctions and cholinesterase activity in the muscles of tadpoles of Xenopus laevis. Quart. J. Micr. Sci. 101:55-67, 1960.
Lewis, P.R. and Shute, C.D.: Demonstration of cholinesterase activity with the electron microscope. J. Physiol. (Lond.) 175:5P, 1964.
Lewis, P.R. and Shute, C.D.: The distribution of cholinesterase in cholinergic neurons demonstrated with the electron microscope. J. Cell Sci. 1:381-390, 1966.
Liesegang, R.E.: Die Kolloidchemie der histologischen Silberfärbungen. Kolloid, Beih. 3:1-46, 1911.

Liévremont, M., Czajka, M. and Tazieff-Depierre, F.: Étude in situ d'unes fixation de calcium et de sa liberation á la jonction neuromusculaire. C.R. Acad. Sci. (Paris) D. 267:1988-1991, 1968.
Liley, A.W.: An investigation of spontaneous activity at the neuromuscular junction of the rat. J. Physiol. (Lond.) 132:65-666, 1956a.
Liley, A.W.: The effects of presynaptic polarization on the spontaneous activity at the mammalian neuromuscular junction. J. Physiol. (Lond.) 134:427-443, 1956b.
Lindstrom, J.M., Singer, S.J. and Lennox, E.S.: Study of frog sartorius muscle acetylcholine receptor using the irreversible inhibitor TDF. J. Membrane Biol. 9:155-176, 1972.
Lissák, K., Dempsey, E.W. and Rosenblueth, A.: The failure of transmission of motor nerve impulses in the course of Wallerian degeneration. Am. J. Physiol. 128:45-56, 1939.
Liu, H.C. and Maneely, R.B.: Some cutaneous nerve endings in the soft-shelled turtle of South China. J. Comp. Neurol. 119:381-390, 1962.
Liu, H.C. and Maneely, R.B.: The development of motor endplates in the embryonic and regenerative tail of Hemidactylus bouringi (Gray). Acta Anat. 71:249-267, 1968.
Liu, J.H. and Nastuk, W.L.: The effects of UO^{2+} ions on neuromuscular transmission and membrane conduction. Fed. Proc. 25:570, 1966.
Loe, P.R. and Florey, E.: The distribution of acetylcholine and cholinesterase in the nervous system and in innervation organs of Octopus dofleini. Comp. Biochem. & Physiol. 17:509-522, 1966.
Loewi, O.: Über humorale Übertragbarkeit der Herznervenwirkung. I. Mitteilung. Pflüg. Arch. Ges. Physiol. 189:239-242, 1921.
Loewi, O.: Uber humoral Ubertragbarkeit der Herznervenwirkung. II. Mitteilung. Pflüg. Arch. Ges. Physiol. 193:201-213, 1922.
Loewi, O. and Navratil, E.: Über humorale Übertragbarkeit der Herznervenwirkung. X. Mitteilung. Über das Schicksal des Vagusstoffs. Pflüg. Arch. Ges. Physiol. 214:678-688, 1926a.
Loewi, O. and Navratil, E.: Über humorale Übertragbarkeit der Herznervenwirkung. XI. Mitteilung. Über den Mechanismus der Vaguswirkung von Physostigmin und Ergotamin. Pflüg. Arch. Ges. Physiol. 214:689-696, 1926b.
Lomo, T. and Rosenthal, J.: Control of Ach sensitivity by muscle activity in the rat. J. Physiol. (Lond.) 221:493-513, 1972.
London, E.S. and Pesker, D.J.: Über die Entwicklung des peripheren Nervensystems bei Saugetieren (weissen Mausen). Arch. Mikr. Anat. 67:303-318, 1906.
Longenecker, H.E., Hurlbut, W.P., Mauro, A. and Clark, A.W.: Effects of the black widow spider venom on the frog neuromuscular junction. Nature 225:701-705, 1970.
Lowenberg-Scharenberg, K.: Degeneration of peripheral nerves and muscles in myasthenia gravis. Trans. Amer. Neurol. Assn. 87:235-237, 1962.
Lowenstein, J.M.: in Oxygen in the Animal Organism. (Duchens, F. and Neil, E., eds.). p. 163, Pergamon Press, Oxford, England, 1964.
Lubińska, L.: Mechanisms of Neural regeneration. in Progress in Brain Res. 13:1-71, (Singer, M. and Shade, J.P., eds.). Elsevier, 1964.
Lubińska, L. and Zelená, J.: Formation of new sites of acetylcholinesterase activity in denervated muscles of young rats. Nature 210:39-41, 1966.
Lubińska, L. and Zelená, J.: Acetylcholinesterase at muscle-tendon junctions during post-natal development in rats. J. Anat. (Lond.) 101:295-308, 1967.

Luco, J.V. and Eyzaquirre, C.: Fibrillation and hypersensitivity to acetylcholine in denervated muscle: effect of degenerating nerve fibers. J. Neurophysiol. *18:*65-73, 1955.
Luft, J.H.: The fine structure of electric tissue. Exp. Cell Res. suppl. *5:*168-182, 1958.
Luft, J.H.: Ruthenium red staining of the striated muscle cell membrane and the myotendinal junction. *in* Electron Microscopy, Proc. 6th Internat. Congress, Kyoto, vol. 2 Biology (Uyeda, R., Ed.). Maruzen Co. Ltd., Tokyo, pp. 60-65, 1966.
Luft, J.H.: Ruthenium red and violet. II. Fine structural localization in animal tissues. Anat. Rec. *71:*369-416, 1971.
Luse, S.: Electron Microscopic observations of the central nervous system. J. Biophys. O Biochem. Cytol. *2:*531-542, 1956.

McAlpine, D.: A form of myasthenia gravis with changes in the central nervous system. Brain *52:*6-22, 1929.
McArdle, J.J. and Albuquerque, E.X.: A study of reinnervation of fast and slow mammalian muscles. J. Gen. Physiol. *61:*1-23, 1973.
McCollester, D.L.: A method for isolating skeletal muscle cell membrane components. Biochim. Biophys. Acta *57:*427-437, 1962.
McComas, A.J. and Mrozek, K.: Denervated muscle fibres in hereditary mouse dystrophy. J. Neurol. Neurosurg. & Psychiat. *30:*526-530, 1967.
McComas, A.J., Campbell, M.J. and Sica, R.E.P.: Electrophysiological study of dystrophia myotonica. J. Neurol. Neurosurg. & Psychiat. *34:*132-139, 1971.
McComas, A.J., Fawcett, P.R.W., Campbell, M.J. and Sica, R.E.P.: Electrophysiological estimation of the number of motor units within a human muscle. J. Neurol. Neurosurg. & Psychiat. *34:*121-131, 1971.
McComas, A.J. and Mossawy, S.J.: Electrophysiological investigation of normal and dystrophic muscles in mice. *in* Research in muscular dystrophy, Proc. Third Symposium of the Muscular Dystrophy Group. pp. 317-341, Pitman Med. Publ. Co., London, 1965.
McComas, A.J. and Mossawy, S.J.: Excitability of muscle fibre membranes in dystrophic mice. J. Neurol. Neurosurg. & Psychiat. *29:*440-445, 1966.
McComas, A.J., Sica, R.E.P. and Brown, J.C.: Myasthenia gravis: Evidence for a "central" defect. J. Neurol. Sci. *13:*107-113, 1971.
McComas, A.J., Sica, R.E.P. and Currie, S.: Muscular dystrophy: Evidence for a neural factor? Nature *226:*1263-1264, 1970.
MacDermot, V.: The changes in the motor endplates in myasthenia gravis. Brain *83:*24-36, 1960.
MacDermot, V.: The histology of the neuromuscular junction in dystrophia myotonica. Brain *84:*75-84, 1961.
McFarlin, D.E., Barlow, M. and Strauss, A.J.L.: Antibodies to muscle and thymus in nonmyasthenic patients with thymoma. N.E.J.M. *275:*1322-1326, 1966.
MacIntosh, F.C.: Effect of HC-3 on acetylcholine turnover. Fed. Proc. *20:*562-568, 1961.
MacKay, B., Muir, A.R. and Peters, A.: Observations on the terminal innervation of segmental muscle fibres in Amphibia. Acta Anat. *40:*1-12, 1960.
MacKay, B. and Peters, A.: Terminal innervation of segmental muscle fibres. Histochemistry of cholinesterase. Bibl. Anat. (Basel) *2:*182-193, 1961.
MacKay, B., Harrop, T.J. and Muir, A.R.: The fine structure of the muscle tendon junction in the rat. Acta Anat. *73:*588-604, 1969.

McLennan, H.: Synaptic Transmission. 2nd Edn. W.B. Saunders, Phila., 1970.
McMahan, U.J., Spitzer, N.C. and Peper, K.: Visual identification of nerve terminals in living isolated skeletal muscle. Proc. Roy. Soc. B. *181:*421-430, 1972.
McManus, J.F.A.: Histological and histochemical uses of periodic acid. Stain Tech. *23:* 99-108, 1948.
McManus, J.F.A., Saunders, J.C., Penton, G.B. and Cason, J.E.: A hitherto undescribed coloring reaction of certain human nerve fibers. Science *111:*155, 1950.
McMinn, R.M.H. and Vrbová, G.: Morphological changes in red and pale muscles following tenotomy. Nature *195:*509, 1962.
McMurtry, S.L., Julina, L.M. and Asmundson, V.S.: Hereditary muscular dystrophy of the chicken. Arch. Path. *94:*217-224, 1972.
McPherson, A. and Tokunaga, J.: The effects of cross-innervation on the myoglobin concentration of tonic and phasic muscles. J. Physiol. (Lond.) *188:*121-129, 1967.
Mackereth, M.B. and Scott, D.J.: Local tetanus in the rat diaphragm. Dunedin. N.Z. U. Otago Med. Sch. Proc. *32:*13-14, 1954.
Madsen, T.: Über Tetanolysin. Z. f. Hygiene *32:*214-238, 1899.
Maillet, M.: La technique de Champy a l'osmium ioduré de potassium et la modification de Maillet a l'osmium-ioduré de zinc. Trab. Inst. Cajal Invest. Biol. *54:*1-36, 1962.
Mair, W.G.P. and Tomé, F.M.S.: The ultrastructure of the adult and developing human musculotendinous junction. Acta Neuropath. *21:*239-252, 1972.
Mallart, A. and Martin, A.R.: An analysis of facilitation of transmitter release at the neuromuscular junction of the frog. J. Physiol. (Lond.) *193:*679-694, 1967.
Malmgren, H. and Sylvén, B.: On the chemistry of the thiocholine method of Koelle. J. Histochem. & Cytochem. *3:*441-445, 1955.
Malvey, J.E., Schottelius, D.D. and Schottelius, B.A.: Energy reserves and chemical changes in denervated anterior and posterior latissimus dorsi muscles of the chicken. Exp. Neurol. *33:*171-180, 1971.
Manchester, K.L. and Harris, E.J.: Effect of denervation on the synthesis of ribonucleic acid and deoxyribonucleic acid in rat diaphragm muscle. Biochem. J. *108:*177-183, 1968.
Mann, P.J.G., Tennenbaum, M. and Quastel, J.H.: On the mechanism of acetylcholine formation in brain, *in vitro.* Biochem. J. *32:*243-261, 1938.
Manolov, S.: Topography and cholinesterase activity of the nerve endings in striated muscles. Acta Neuroveg. *25:*427-434, 1963.
Manolov, S., Ivanov, D.P. and Itchev, K.: Recherches histochimiques et morphologiques sur les terminaisons nerveuses motrices du muscle vocal du chat. Acta Anat. *60:*406-421, 1965.
Marchbanks, R.M.: Exchangeability of radioactive acetylcholine with the bound acetylcholine of synaptosomes and synaptic vesicles. Biochem. J. *106:*87-95, 1968.
Marchesi, V.T. and Andrews, E.P.: Glycoproteins: isolation from cell membranes with lithium diiodosalicylate. Science *174:*1247-1248, 1971.
Marchisio, P.C.: Configuration of the blood capillaries and their relation to the motor endplates (Rouget) of the tongue musculature in some mammalian species. Anat. Anz. *114:*79-85, 1964.
Margreth, A., Salviati, G., DiMauro, S. and Turati, G.: Early biochemical consequences of denervation in fast and slow skeletal muscles and their relationship to neural control over muscle differentiation. Biochem. J. *126:*1099-1110, 1972.

Marinskaya, L.F.: Evolutionary and morphological changes in vertebrate junctions. Arkh. Anat. Gistol. i Embriol. 43:3-15, 1962, trans. in Fed. Proc. 22:994-1008, 1963.

Mark, R.F.: Matching muscles and motoneurones. A review of some experiments on motor nerve regeneration. Brain Res. 14:245-254, 1969.

Marnay, A. and Nachmansohn, D.: Choline esterase in voluntary muscle. J. Physiol. (Lond.) 92:37-47, 1938.

Marotte, L.R. and Mark, R.F.: The mechanism of selective reinnervation of fish eye muscle. I. Evidence from muscle function during recovery. Brain Res. 19:41-51, 1970.

Martin, K.: Effects of quaternary ammonium compounds on choline transport in red cells. Br. J. Pharmacol. 36:458-469, 1969.

Martini, E. and Torda, K.: Die Cholinesterase des denervierten Muskels. Klin. Wochenschr. 16:824-825, 1937.

Massart, L. and Dufait, R.P.: Hemmung der Acetylcholin Esterase durch Farbstoffe und durch Eserin. Enzymologia 9:364-368, 1941.

Matthes, K.: The action of blood on acetylcholine. J. Physiol. (Lond.) 70:338-348, 1930.

Maurel, P. and Galzigna, L.: Dipole moment of acetylcholine and its relevance to the chemical synaptic transmission. Biophys. J. 11:550-557, 1971.

Mautner, H.G., Bartels, E. and Webb, G.D.: Sulfur and selenium isologs related to acetylcholine and choline to activity in the electroplax preparation. Biochem. Pharmacol. 15:187-193, 1966.

Max, S.R., Nelson, P.G. and Brady, R.O.: The effect of denervation on the composition of muscle gangliosides. J. Neurochem. 17:1517-1520, 1970.

Maynard, E.A.: Electrophoretic studies of cholinesterases in brain and muscle of the developing chicken. J. Exp. Zool. 161:319-335, 1966.

Mayr, R.: Structure and distribution of fibre types in the external eye muscles of the rat. Tissue and Cell 3:433-462, 1971.

Mayr, R., Stockinger, L. and Zenker, W.: Elektronen mikroskopische untersuchungen an unterschiedlich innervierten muskelfasern der Ausseren Augenmuskulatur des Rhesus affen. Z. Zellforsch. 75:434-452, 1966.

Mednick, M.L., Petrali, J.P., Thomas, N.C., Sternberger, L.A., Plapinger, R.E., Davis, D.A., Wasserkrug, H.L. and Seligman, A.M.: Localization of acetylcholinesterase via production of osmiophilic polymers: new benzenediazonium salts with thiolacetate functions. J. Histochem. Cytochem. 19:155-160, 1971.

Meiri, U. and Rahamimoff, R.: Neuromuscular transmission: inhibition by manganese ions. Science 176:308-309, 1972.

Mellanby, J. and Thompson, P.A.: The effect of tetanus toxin at the neuromuscular junction in the goldfish. J. Physiol. (Lond.) 224:407-420, 1972.

Mendel, B., Mundell, D.B. and Rudney, H.: Studies on cholinesterase. 3. Specific tests for true cholinesterase and pseudocholinesterase. Biochem. J. 37:473-476, 1943.

Mendel, B. and Rudney, H.: Studies on cholinesterase. 1. Cholinesterase and pseudocholinesterase. Biochem. J. 37:59-63, 1943.

Mertens, H.G., Balzereit, F. and Leipert, M.: The treatment of severe myasthenia gravis with immunosuppressive agents. European Neurol. 2:321-339, 1969.

Meyer, H. and Ransom, F.: Untersuchungen über den Tetanus. Arch. Exper. Path. u. Pharmakol. 49:369-416, 1903.

Meyer, K.H.: La perméabilité des membranes. V. Sur l'origine des courants bioélectriques. Helv. Chim. Acta 20:634-647, 1937.

Miani, N., diGirolamo, A. and diGirolamo, M.: Sedimentation characteristics of axonal RNA in rabbits. J. Physiol. (Lond.) *207*:507-528, 1970.

Michel, H.O.: An electrometric method for the determination of red blood cell and plasma cholinesterase activity. J. Lab. & Clin. Med. *34*:1564-1568, 1949.

Michelazzi, L., Mor, M.A. and Dianzani, M.U.: Adenosine triphosphate concentration in guinea pig muscle after denervation. Experientia *13*:117-118, 1957.

Michelson, A.M., Russell, E.S. and Harman, P.J.: Dystrophia muscularis: Hereditary primary myopathy in house mouse. Proc. U.S. Nat. Acad. Sci. *41*:1079-1084, 1955.

Miledi, R.: Junctional and extrajunctional acetylcholine receptors in skeletal muscle fibers. J. Physiol. (Lond.) *151*:24-30, 1960a.

Miledi, R.: The acetylcholine sensitivity of frog muscle fibres after complete or partial denervation. J. Physiol. (Lond.) *151*:1-23, 1960b.

Miledi, R.: Induced innervation of endplate free muscle segments. Nature *193*:281-282, 1962.

Miledi, R.: Formation of extra nerve-muscle junctions in innervated muscle. Nature *199*: 1191-1192, 1963.

Miledi, R.: Electron microscopical localization of products from histochemical reactions used to detect cholinesterase in muscle. Nature *204*:293-295, 1964.

Miledi, R.: Lanthanum ions abolish the "calcium response" of nerve terminals. Nature *229*:410-411, 1971.

Miledi, R., Molinoff, P. and Potter, L.T.: Isolation of the cholinergic receptor protein of Torpedo electric tissue. Nature *229*:554-557, 1971.

Miledi, R. and Orkand, P.: Effect of a fast nerve in slow muscle fibres in the frog. Nature *209*:717-718, 1966.

Miledi, R. and Potter, L.T.: Acetylcholine receptors in muscle fibres. Nature *233*:599-603, 1971.

Miledi, R. and Slater, C.R.: A study of rat nerve-muscle junctions after degeneration of the nerve. J. Physiol. (Lond.) *167*:23-24P, 1963.

Miledi, R. and Slater, C.R.: Electrophysiology and electron microscopy of rat neuromuscular junctions after nerve degeneration. Proc. Roy. Soc. B. *169*:289-306, 1968.

Miledi, R. and Slater, C.R.: On the degeneration of rat neuromuscular junctions after nerve section. J. Physiol. (Lond.) *207*:507-528, 1970.

Miledi, R., Stefani, E. and Zelená, J.: Neural control of acetylcholine sensitivity in rat muscle fibres. Nature *220*:497-498, 1968.

Miledi, R. and Stefani, E.: Miniature potentials in denervated slow muscle fibres of the frog. J. Physiol. (Lond.) *209*:179-186, 1970.

Miledi, R. and Zelená, J.: Sensitivity to acetylcholine in rat slow muscle. Nature *210*: 855-856, 1966.

Milhaud, G., Chagas, C., Jacob, J. and Esquibel, M.A.: Étude de la fixation de curares a fonction ammonium quaternaire sur le mucopolysaccharide acide extrait de l'organe electrique d'*Electrophorus Electricus* et comparaison, avec leur action inhibitrice sur la décharge reflexe. Biochem. Biophys. Acta *58*:19-26, 1962.

Misra, R.P. and Berman, L.B.: Studies on glomerular basement membrane. II. Isolation and chemical analysis of diseases glomerular basement membrane. Lab. Invest. *18*: 131-138, 1968.

Mitchell, J.F. and Silver, A.: The spontaneous release of acetylcholine from the denervated hemidiaphragm of the rat. J. Physiol. (Lond.) *165*:117-129, 1963.

Miura, N.: Untersuchungen über die motorischen Nervenendigungen der quergestreiften Muskelfasern. Virchow's Arch. Path. Anat. *105:*129-135, 1886.
Moldaver, J.: Tourniquet paralysis syndrome. A.M.A. Arch. Surg. *68:*136-144, 1954.
Monod, J., Changeux, J.P. and Jacob, F.: Allosteric proteins and cellular control systems. J. Mol. Biol. *6:*306-329, 1963.
Monod, J., Wyman, J. and Changeux, J.P.: On the nature of allosteric transitions: a plausible model. J. Mol. Biol. *12:*88-118, 1965.
Morax, V. and Marie, A.: Recherches sur l'absorption de la toxine tétanique. Ann. de l'Inst. Pasteur *17:*335-342, 1903.
Morbidity and Mortality. U.S. Dept. Health, Education & Welfare Weekly Report, September 18, 1965.
Morris, C.J.: The significance of intermediate fibres in reinnervated human skeletal muscle. J. Neurol. Sci. *11:*129-136, 1970.
Morris, D.D.B.: Recovery in partially paralysed muscles. J. Bone and Jt. Surg. *35B:*650-660, 1953.
Mott, F.W.: In Peripheral neuritis (Sharkey, S.J.), Brit. Med. J. *1:*456-458, 1896.
Mott, F.W. and Barrada, Y.A.: Pathological findings in the central nervous system of a case of myasthenia gravis. Brain *46:*237-244, 1923.
Mountford, S.: Effects of light and dark adaptation on the vesicle populations of receptor-bipolar synapses. J. Ultrastr. Res. *9:*403-418, 1963.
Muchnick, S. and Rubinstein, E.H.: Mechanism of the local tetanus induced by intramuscular tetanus toxin. Acta Physiol. latino Amer. *17:*166-174, 1967.
Mukino, K.: The fine structure of the human extraocular muscles. I. A "laminated structure" in the muscle fibers. J. of Electron Micros. (Japan) *15:*227-236, 1966.
Mumenthatler, M. and Engel, W.K.: Cytological localization of cholinesterase in developing chick embryo skeletal muscle. Acta Anat. *47:*274-299, 1961.
Murata, F. and Ogata, T.: The ultrastructure of neuromuscular junctions of human red, white and intermediate striated muscle fibers. Tohoku J. exp. Med. *99:*289-301, 1969.
Murnaghan, M.F.: Neuroanatomical site in tick paralysis. Nature *181:*131, 1958.
Murnaghan, M.F.: Site and mechanism of tick paralysis. Science *131:*418-419, 1960.
Musick, J. and Hubbard, J.I.: Release of protein from mouse motor nerve terminals. Nature *237:*279-281, 1972.
Myers, D.K. and Mendel, B.: Investigations on the use of eserine for the differentiation of mammalian esterases. Proc. Soc. Exp. Biol. & Med. *71:*357-360, 1949.

Nachlas, M.M. and Seligman, A.M.: The histochemical demonstration of esterase. J. Nat. Cancer Inst. *9:*415-425, 1949.
Nachmansohn, D.: Choline esterase in voluntary muscle. J. Physiol. (Lond.) *95:*29-35, 1939.
Nachmansohn, D.: Studies on permeability in relation to nerve function. I. Axonal conduction and synaptic transmission. Biochem. et Biophys. Acta *4:*78-95, 1950.
Nachmansohn, D.: Mechanisms of impulse transmission across neuromuscular junctions. Am. J. Phys. Med. *34:*33-45, 1955.
Nachmansohn, D.: Chemical and molecular basis of nerve activity. Academic Press, New York and London, p. 37, 1959.
Nachmansohn, D.: Proteins in excitable membranes. Science *168:*1059-1066, 1970.

Nachmansohn, D. and Machado, A.L.: The formation of acetylcholine. A new enzyme: "Cholineacetylase". J. Neurophysiol. 6:397-403, 1943.

Nachmias, V. and Padykula, H.: A histochemical study of normal and denervated red and white muscle of the rat. J. Biophys. Biochem. Cytol. 4:47-54, 1958.

Nadol, J.B., Jr. and deLorenzo, A.J.D.: Observations on the abdominal stretch receptor and the fine structure of association axo-dendrite synapses and neuromuscular junctions in Homarus. J. Comp. Neurol. 132:419-444, 1968.

Nagy, I.Z. and Salanki, J.: Histochemical investigations of cholinesterase in different molluscs with reference to functional conditions. Nature 206:842-843, 1965.

Naik, N.T.: Technical variations in Koelle's histochemical method for demonstrating cholinesterase activity. Q. J. Micr. Sci. 104:89-100, 1963.

Nakai, J.: The development of neuromuscular junctions in cultures of chick embryo tissues. J. Exp. Zool. 170:85-106, 1969.

Nakai, J., Takata, C. and Kawasaki, Y.: Neuromuscular junction formed in vitro. Acta Anat. Nippon. 36:356-357, 1961.

Nakajima, Y.: Fine structure of red and white muscle fibers and their neuromuscular junctions in the snake fish (Ophiocephalus argus). Tissue and Cell 1:229-246, 1969.

Nakamura, T., Namba, T. and Grob, D.: Motor endplate reactivity to divalent metal ions. Histochemical studies. J. Histochem. Cytochem. 15:276-284, 1967.

Nakata, T. and Nishijima, S.: Combined staining by thiolacetic and Bielschowsky methods. Stain Tech. 46:151-153, 1971.

Namba, T.: Cholinesterase activity of muscle fibers and motor endplates: comparative studies. Exper. Neurol. 33:322-328, 1971.

Namba, T., Arimoi, S. and Grob, D.: Lymphocytes of patients with myasthenia gravis. Arch. Neurol. 21:285-295, 1969.

Namba, T. and Grob, D.: Autoantibodies and myasthenia gravis with special reference to muscle ribonucleoprotein. Ann. N.Y. Acad. Sci. 135:606-630, 1966.

Namba, T. and Grob, D.: Ribonucleoprotein in human skeletal muscle with affinity for d-tubocurarine and acetylcholine. Biochem. Pharmacol. 16:1135-1138, 1967.

Namba, T. and Grob, D.: Cholinesterase activity of the motor endplate in isolated muscle membrane. J. Neurochem. 15:1445-1454, 1968.

Namba, T., Nakamura, T. and Grob, D.: Staining for nerve fiber cholinesterase activity in fresh frozen sections. Am. J. Clin. Path. 47:74-77, 1967.

Namba, T., Nolte, C.T., Jackrel, J. and Grob, D.: Poisoning due to organophosphate insecticides. Am. J. Med. 50:475-492, 1971.

Nara, T.: Electron microscopical study on the fine structure and cholinesterase activity of the neuromuscular junction in progressive muscular dystrophy. Arch. Jap. Chir. 34:1213-1220, 1965.

Narahashi, T., Albuquerque, E.X. and Deguchi, T.: Effects of batrachotoxin on membrane potential and conductance of squid giant axons. J. Gen. Physiol. 58:54-70, 1971.

Nastuk, W.L.: Activation and inactivation of muscle postjunctional receptors. Fed. Proc. 26:1639-1646, 1967.

Nastuk, W.L. and Liu, J.H.: Muscle postjunctional membrane: changes in chemosensitivity produced by calcium. Science 154:266-267, 1966.

Nastuk, W.L., Plescin, O.J. and Osserman, K.E.: Changes in serum complement activity in patients with myasthenia gravis. Proc. Soc. Exp. Biol. Med. 105:177-184, 1960.

Nathaniel, E.J.H.: Fibrillogenesis by reactive Schwann cells in regenerating dorsal roots. Proc. Fifth Int. Congr. Electron Microscopy, Philadelphia, 2:N7, 1962. Academic Press, N.Y.

Nathaniel, E.J.H. and Pease, D.C.: Collagen and basement membrane formation by Schwann cells during nerve regeneration. J. Ultrastr. Res. 9:550-560, 1963.

Needham, A.E.: Regeneration and Wound-healing. Methuen Monograph, London, 1952.

Neet, K.E. and Friess, S.L.: Curare-binding macromolecules from medullated nerve tissue. Arch. Biochem. Biophys. 99:484-493, 1962.

Negrete, J., del Castillo, J., Escobar, I. and Yankelevich, G.: Spreading activation of endplate receptors by single transmitter quanta. Nature New Biology 235:158-159, 1972.

Nickel, E. and Potter, L.T.: Synaptic vesicles in freeze-etched electric tissue of *Torpedo*. Brain Res. 23:95-100, 1970.

Nickel, E., Vogel, A. and Waser, P.G.: Coated vesicles in der umgebung der neuromuskularen synapsen. Z. Zellforsch. 78:261-266, 1967.

Nickel, E. and Waser, P.G.: Elektronenmikroskopische Untersuchungen am Diaphragma der Maus nach einsteitiger phrenikotomie. I. Die degenerierende motorische Endplatte. Z. Zellforsch. 88:278-296, 1968.

Nickel, E. and Waser, P.G.: An electron microscopic study of denervated motor endplates after zinc-iodide-osmium impregnation. Brain Res. 13:168-176, 1969.

Noël, R.: La structure de la substances protoplasmiques dans les plaques motrices des vertébrés. Bull. Histol. Appl. et Tech. Microscop. 2:124-133, 1925.

Noël, R.: La zone de jonction myoneurale; contribution a l'étude morphologique des synapses. Biol. Méd. (Paris) 39:273-317, 1950.

Noël, R.: Telosomes et manchon péritéloneuritique. Acta Anat. 30:530-541, 1957.

Norris, F.H.: Neuromuscular transmission in thyroid disease. Ann. Int. Med. 64:81-86, 1964.

Novak, J. and Salafsky, B.: Early electrophysiological changes after denervation of slow skeletal muscle. Exper. Neurol. 19:388-400, 1967.

Nyberg-Hansen, R., Rinvik, E., Aarseth, P. and Barstad, J.A.B.: Electron microscopic localization of cholinesterase at the neuromuscular junction by a quaternary carbon analogue of acetylthiocholine as substrate. Histochemie 20:40-45, 1969.

Nyström, Bo.: Histochemical studies of endplate bound esterases in "slow-red" and "fast-white" cat muscles during post natal development. Acta Neurol. Scand. 44: 295-318, 1968.

O'Brien, R.D., Eldefrawi, M.E. and Eldefrawi, A.T.: Isolation of acetylcholine receptors. Ann. Rev. Pham. 12:19-34, 1972.

Ogata, T.: A histochemical study on the structural differences of motor endplate in the red, white and intermediate muscle fibers of mouse limb muscle. Acta Med. Okayama 19:149-153, 1965.

Ogata, T., Hondo, T. and Seito, T.: An electron microscopic study on differences in the fine structures of motor endplate in red, white and intermediate muscle fibers of rat intercostal muscle. Acta Med. Okayama 21:327-338, 1967.

Ogata, T. and Mori, M.: Histochemical study of oxidative enzymes in vertebrate muscle. J. Histochem. & Cytochem. 12:171-182, 1964.

Ogata, T. and Murata, F.: Fine structure of motor endplate in red, white and intermediate fibers of mammalian fast muscle. Tohoku J. Exp. Med. *98:*107-115, 1969.

Ogata, T., Seito, T. and Hino, H.: A cytological study of the effect of reinnervation and cross-innervation on rat striated muscle. Acta Med. Okayama *22:*219-226, 1968.

Okada, K.: Effects of divalent cations on the spontaneous transmitter release at the amphibian neuromuscular junction in the presence of ethanol. Jap. J. Physiol. *20:*97-111, 1970.

Okamoto, M., Longenecker, H.E., Riker, W.F., Jr. and Song, S.K.: Destruction of mammalian motor nerve terminals by black widow spider venom. Science *172:*733-736, 1971.

Oppenheim, H.: Über einen Fall von chronischer progressiver Bulbarparalyse ohne anatomischen Befund. Virchow's Arch. Path. Anat. *108:*522-530, 1887.

Oppenheim, H.: Über allgemeine und localisierte Atonie der Muskulatur (myatonie) im frühen Kindesalter. Mschr. Psychiat. Neurol. *8:*232-233, 1900.

Orfanos, C.: On the micromorphology of the neuromuscular junction of the afibrillar-tonic skeletal muscle fiber in the frog (*Rana temporaria* L.). Z. Zellforsch. *56:*387-, 403, 1962.

Ormrod, A.N.: Myasthenia gravis in a cocker spaniel. Vet. Rec. *73:*489-490, 1961.

Osserman, K.E.: Myasthenia Gravis. Grune & Stratton, New York, 1958.

Ostrowski, K., Barnard, E.A., Stocka, Z. and Darzynkiewicz, Z.: Autoradiographic methods in enzyme cytochemistry. I. Localization of acetylcholinesterase activity using a ^{3}H-labeled irreversible inhibitor. Exp. Cell Res. *31:*89-99, 1963.

Overton, E.: Über die osmotischen Eigenschaften der lebenden Pflanzen und Tierzelle. Vierteljahrschr. Naturforsch. Gesell. (Zurich) *40:*159-201, 1895.

Padykula, H. and Gauthier, G.: The ultrastructure of the neuromuscular junction of mammalian red, white and intermediate skeletal muscle fibers. J. Cell Biol. *46:*27-41, 1970.

Page, S.G. and Slater, C.R.: Observations on fine structure and rate of contraction of some muscles from the chicken. J. Physiol. (Lond.) *179:*58-59P, 1965.

Palade, G.E.: Electron microscope observations of interneural and neuromuscular synapses. Anat. Rec. *118:*335-336, 1954.

Palay, S.L.: Synapses in the central nervous system. J. Biophys. & Biochem. Cytol. suppl. *2:*193-202, 1956.

Palay, S.L.: The morphology of synapses in the central nervous system. Exp. Cell Res. suppl. *5:*275-293, 1958.

Pappas, G.D., Peterson, E.R., Masurovsky, E.B. and Crain, S.M.: Electron microscopy of the *in vitro* development of mammalian motor endplates. Ann. N.Y. Acad. Sci. *183:* 33-45, 1971.

Parkes, J.D. and McKinna, J.A.: Neuromuscular blocking activity in the blood of patients with myasthenia gravis. Lancet *1:*388-391, 1966.

Parsons, R.L., Hofmann, W.W. and Feigin, G.A.: Mode of action of tetanus toxin on the neuromuscular junction. Am. J. Physiol. *210:*84-90, 1966.

Paton, W.D.M. and Zaimis, E.J.: The methonium compounds. Pharm. Rev. *4:*219-253, 1952.

Patrick, J. and Lindstorm, J.: Autoimmune response to acetylcholine receptor. Science *180:*871-872, 1973.

Peachey, L.D.: Muscle. Ann. Rev. Physiol. *30:*401-440, 1968.
Pearce, J. and Harriman, O.G.F.: Chronic spinal muscular atrophy. J. Neurol. Neurosurg. & Psychiat. *29:*509-520, 1966.
Pearse, A.G.E.: Histochemistry — Theoretical and Applied. Little, Brown & Co., Boston, 1960.
Pelligrino, C. and Franzini, C.: An electron microscope study of denervation atrophy in red and white skeletal muscle fibers. J. Cell Biol. *17:*327-349, 1963.
Perdrup, A.: Electromyographic investigations of the mode of action of tetanus toxin. Acta Pharmacol. et Toxicol. *2:*121-137, 1946.
Perroncito, A.: Sur la terminaison des nerfs dans les fibres musculaires striées. Arch. Ital. Biol. *36:*245-254, 1901.
Péterfi, T.: Untersuchungen über die Beziehungen der Myofibrillen zu den Sehnenfibrillen. Arch. Mikr. Anat. *83:*1-42, 1913.
Péterfi, T. and Kapel, O.: Die Wirkung des Anslechens auf das Protoplasma der in vitro gezüchteten Gewebezellen. III. Anstichversuche and den Nervenzellen. Arch. Exp. Zellforsch. *5:*341-348, 1928.
Peters, A. Experiments on the mechanism of silver staining. I. Impregnation. Q. J. Micr. Sci. *96:*84-102, 1955.
Peterson, E.R. and Crain, S.M.: Innervation in cultures of fetal rodent skeletal muscle by organotypic explants of spinal cord from different animals. Z.Zellforsch. *106:*1-21, 1970.
Peterson, R.P. and Pepe, F.A.: The fine structure of inhibitory synapses in the crayfish. J. Biophys. & Biochem. Cytol. *11:*157-169, 1961.
Petty, C.S.: Histochemical proof of organic phosphate poisoning. A.M.A. Arch. Path. *66:* 458-463, 1958a.
Petty, C.S.: Organic phosphate insecticide poisoning. Residual effects in two cases. Am. J. Med. *24:*467-470, 1958b.
Pezard, A. and May, R.M.: Les terminaisons nerveuses du muscle couturier de la grenouille et la question de sa partie aneurale. Ann. Physiol. Physiochem. Biol. *13:*460-473, 1937.
Pillar, G. and Hess, A.: Differences in internal structure and nerve terminals of the slow and twitch muscle fibers in the cat superior oblique. Anat. Rec. *154:*243-252, 1966.
Pommé, B. and Noël, R.: La zone de jonction myoneurale dans quelques cas pathologiques. Rev. Neurol. *2:*1-30, 1934.
Potapova, T.V.: The effect of neostigmine and atropine on the equilibrium potentials of the endplate current on the frog muscle. Biofizika *14:*757-759, 1969.
Potter, L.T.: Synthesis storage and release of [^{14}C] acetylcholine in isolated rat diaphragm muscles. J. Physiol. (Lond.) *206:*145-166, 1970.
Prabhu, V.G. and Oester, Y.T.: Electromyographic changes in skeletal muscle due to tetanus toxin. J. Pharm. & Exp. Therap. *138:*241-248, 1962.
Preusser, H.J.: Die Ultrastruktur der motorischen Endplatte im Zwerchfell der Ratte und Veränderungen nach Inhibierung der acetylsholinesterase. Z. Zellforsch. *80:*436-457, 1967.
Price, Z. and Nishi, Y.: Effect of tetanus toxin on mitochondria of the proximal convoluted tubule of the mouse. Traveling Exhibit of the Electron Microscope Society of America, 1961.
Prineas, J.: Triorthocresyl phosphate myopathy. Arch. Neurol. *21:*150-156, 1969a.

Prineas, J.: The pathogenesis of dying back polyneuropathies: I. An ultrastructural study of tri-ortho-cresyl phosphate intoxication in the cat. J. Neuropath. Exp. Neurol. *28:* 571-597, 1969a.

Prineas, J.: The pathogenesis of dying back polyneuropathies: II. An ultrastructural study of experimental acrylamide intoxication in the cat. J. Neuropath. Exp. Neurol. *28:*598-621, 1969b.

Prineas, J.: Peripheral nerve changes in thiamine deficient rats. Arch. Neurol. *23:*541-548, 1970.

Quastel, D.M.J., Hackett, J.T. and Cooke, J.D.: Calcium: Is it required for transmitter secretion? Science *172:*1034-1036, 1971.

Quastel, J.H., Tennenbaum, M. and Wheatley, A.H.M.: Choline ester formation in, and choline esterase activities of, tissues *in vitro.* Biochem. J. *30:*1668-1681, 1936.

Raftery, M.A.: Isolation of acetylcholine receptor α-bungarotoxin complexes from *Torpedo Californica* electroplax. Arch. Biochem. Biophys. *154:*270-276, 1973.

Rambourg, A.: Morphological and histochemical aspects of glycoproteins at the surface of animal cells Internat. Rev. Cytol. *31:*57-114, 1971.

Rambourg, A., Hernandez, W. and Leblond, C.P.: Detection of complex carbohydrates in the Golgi apparatus of rat cells. J. Cell Biol. *40:*395-414, 1969.

Rambourg, A. and Leblond, C.P.: Electron microscope observations on the carbohydrate-rich cell coat present at the surface of cells in the rat. J. Cell Biol. *32:*27-54, 1967.

Rand, M.J. and Whaler, B.C.: Impairment of sympathetic transmission by botulinum toxin. Nature *206:*588-591, 1965.

Rang, H.R. and Ritter, J.M.: The effect of disulfide bond reduction on the properties of cholinergic receptors in chick muscle. Molec. Pharmacol. *7:*620-631, 1971.

Ranvier, L.: Leçons sur l'histologie du système nerveux. Savy, Paris, 1878.

Rash, J.E. and Fambrough, D.: Ultrastructural and electrophysiological correlates of cell coupling and cytoplasmic fusion during myogenesis *in vitro.* Developmental Biol. *30:*166-186, 1973.

Ravin, H.A., Zacks, S.I. and Seligman, A.M.: The histochemical localization of acetylcholinesterase in nervous tissue. J. Pharm. & Exp. Therap. *107:*37-53, 1953.

Redfern, P.A.: Neuromuscular transmission in newborn rats. J. Physiol. *209:*701-709, 1970.

Redfern, P. and Thesleff, S.: Action potential generation in denervated rat skeletal muscle. I. Quantitative aspects. Acta physiol. Scand. *81:*557-564, 1971.

Reger, J.F.: Electron microscopy of the motor endplate in intercostal muscle of the rat. Anat. Rec. *118:*344, 1954.

Reger, J.F.: Electron microscopy of the motor endplate in rat intercostal muscle. Anat. Rec. *122:*1-16, 1955.

Reger, J.F.: The fine structure of neuromuscular synapses of gastrocnemii from mouse and frog. Anat. Rec. *130:*7-14, 1958.

Reger, J.F.: Studies on the fine structure of normal and denervated neuromuscular junction from mouse gastrocnemius. J. Ultrastr. Res. *2:*269-282, 1959.

Reger, J.F.: The fine structure of neuromuscular junctions and the sarcoplasmic reticulum of extrinsic eye muscles of *Fundulus heterocletus.* J. Biophys. Biochem. Cytol. *10:*4 suppl. 111-121, 1961.

Reger, J.F.: The fine structure of neuromuscular junctions and contact zones between body wall muscle cells of *Ascaris lumbricoides* (Var. Suum). Z. Zellforsch. *67:*196-210, 1965.

Reiter, M.J., Cowburn, D.A., Prives, J.M. and Karlin, A.: Affinity labeling of the acetylcholine receptor in the electroplax: electrophoretic separation in sodium dodecyl sulfate. Proc. US Nat. Acad. Sci. *69:*1168-1172, 1972.

Renaut, J.: Traite d'Histologie Pratique. *2:*972, 1899, Rueff, Paris.

Reske-Nielsen, E., Coërs, C. and Harmsen, A.: Qualitative and quantitative histological study of neuromuscular biopsies from healthy young men. J. Neurol. Sci. *10:*369-384, 1970.

Reske-Nielsen, E., Dalby, A. and Dalby, M.: Studies on the innervation of muscles in muscular and neuromuscular diseases. An attempt of diagnosis by comparing biopsy and endplate studies with clinical and electromyographic findings. Acta Neurol. Scand. *41:* suppl. *13:*289-296, 1965.

Revel, J.P. and Karnovsky, M.J.: Hexagonal array of subunits in intercellular junctions of the mouse heart and liver. J. Cell Biol. *33:*C7, 1967.

Richardson, A.T.: Clinical and electromyographic aspects of polymyositis. Proc. Roy. Soc. Med. *49:*111-114, 1956.

Ricther, D. and Croft, P.G.: Blood esterases. Biochem. J. *36:*746-757, 1942.

Ricker, G. and Ellenbeck, J.: Beiträge zur Kenntniss der Veränderungen des Muskels nach der Durchscheidung seiner Nerven. Arch. Path. Anat. u. Physiol. *158:*199-253, 1899.

Ridge, R.M.A.P.: The differentiation of conduction velocities of slow twitch and fast twitch muscle motor innervations in kittens and cats. Q. J. Exper. Physiol. *52:*293-304, 1967.

Ritchie, A.K. and Goldberg, A.M.: Vesicular and synaptoplasmic synthesis of acetylcholine. Science *169:*489-490, 1970.

Robbins, N. and Yonezawa, T.: Developing neuromuscular junctions: First signs of chemical transmission during formation in tissue culture. Science *172:*395-398, 1971a.

Robbins, N. and Yonezawa, T.: Physiological studies during formation and development of rat neuromuscular junctions in tissue culture. J. Gen. Physiol. *58:*467-481, 1971b.

Robert, E.D. and Oester, Y.T.: Nerve impulses and trophic effect. Arch. Neurol. *22:*57-63, 1970.

Robertson, J.D.: The ultrastructure of a reptilian myoneural junction. J. Appl. Phys. *25:*1466-1467, 1954.

Robertson, J.D.: Recent electron microscope observations on the ultrastructure of the crayfish median-to-motor giant synapse. Exp. Cell Res. *8:*226-229, 1955a.

Robertson, J.D.: Some features of the ultrastructure of reptilian skeletal muscle. J. Biophys. & Biochem. Cytol. *2:*369-379, 1955b.

Robertson, J.D.: The ultrastructure of a reptilian myoneural junction J. Biophys. & Biochem. Cytol. *2:*381-394, 1956.

Robertson, J.D.: New observations on the ultrastructure of the membranes of frog peripheral nerve fibers. J. Biophys. & Biochem. Cytol. *3:*1043-1047, 1957.

Robertson, J.D.: Ultrastructure of cell membranes and their derivatives *in* The Structure and Function of Subcellular Components. Biochemical Society Symposium (Crook, E.M., ed.). Cambridge University Press, New York, 1959, vol. 16, pp. 3-43.

Robertson, J.D.: Electron microscopy of the motor endplate and the neuromuscular spindle. Am. J. Phys. Med. *39:*1-43, 1960.

Roepke, M.H.: A study of choline esterase. J. Pharmacol. Exp. Therap. 59:264-276, 1937.
Rogers, A.W., Darzynkiewicz, Z., Barnard, E.A. and Salpeter, M.M.: Number and location of acetylcholinesterase molecules at motor endplates of the mouse. Nature 210: 1003, 1966.
Rogers, A.W., Darzynkiewicz, M., Salpeter, M.M., Ostrowski, K. and Barnard, E.A.: Quantitative studies on enzymes in structures in striated muscles by labelled inhibitor methods. I. The number of acetylcholinesterase molecules and other DFP-reactive sites at motor endplates, measured by radioautography. J. Cell Biol. 41:665-685, 1969.
Rogers, P.C.: Fine structure of smooth muscle and neuromuscular junction in the optic tentacles of Helix aspersa and Limax flanus. Z. Zellforsch. 89:80-94, 1968.
Rogers, W.M., Pappenheimer, A.M. and Goettsch, M.: Nerve endings in nutritional muscular dystrophy. J. Exp. Med. 54:167-169, 1931.
Rogers, W.M. and Parrack, H.O.: Influence of age on functional survival of severed mammalian nerves. Am. J. Physiol. 126:195-196, 1939.
Rohr-Hadorn, I.: Beziehungen zwischen cholinergischen receptor und acetylcholinesterase der Endplatte, untersucht während der Degeneration und Regeneration des Mäusezwerchfells. Hev. Physiol. Acta 19:119-134, 1961.
Rojas, P., Szepsenwol, J. and Resta, L.S.: Influence du curare et de l'excitation sur ls structure de la plaque motrice. C.R. Soc. Biol. (Paris) 131:295-296, 1939.
Romanes, G.J.: The staining of nerve fibers in paraffin sections with silver. J. Anat. (Lond.) 84:104-115, 1950.
Romanul, F.C.A. and Meulen, J.P. van der: Slow and fast muscles after cross innervation. Enzymatic and physiological changes. Arch. Neurol. 17:387-402, 1967.
Romhányi, Gy. and Jobst, K.: Polarisationsmikroskopische Untersuchungen über saurebedingte intramolekulare Strukturänderung der Desoxyribonukleinsäure. Acta Histochem. 3:308-317, 1956.
Rose, S. and Glow, P.H.: Denervation effects on the presumed de novo synthesis of muscle cholinesterase and the effects of acetylcholine availability on retinal cholinesterase. Exper. Neurol. 18:267-275, 1967.
Rosenberg, R.N., Dalosso, D.J., Tromblay, J. and Woodman, D.: Kinetics of acetylcholine synthesis and hydrolysis in myasthenia gravis. Science 173:644-645, 1971.
Rosenblueth, A.: The Transmission of Nerve Impulses. Technology Press and J. Wiley & Sons, Inc., Cambridge and New York, 1950.
Rosenblueth, A., Lissak, K. and Lanari, A.: An explanation of the five stages of neuromuscular and ganglionic synaptic transmission. Am. J. Physiol. 128:31-44, 1939.
Rosenbluth, J.: Myoneural junctions of two ultrastructurally distinct types in earthworm body wall muscle. J. Cell Biol. 54:566-579, 1972.
Ross, I.C.: An experimental study of tick paralysis in Australia. Parisitology 18:410-429, 1926.
Rossi, P.G. and Cortesina, G.: Multi-motor endplate muscle fibres in the human vocalis muscle. Nature 206:629-630, 1965.
Roth, Th. F. and Porter, K.R.: Specialized sites on the cell surface for protein uptake. in 5th Internat. Congr. for Electron Microscopy, Phila., 1962, N.Y. Academic Press (Breese, S.S., Jr., ed.). vol. 2, LL-4.
Rouget, C.: Note sur la terminaison des nerfs moteurs dans les muscles chez les reptiles, les oiseaux et les mammifères. C.R. Acad. Sci. (Paris) 55:548-552, 1862.

Rouget, C.: Not sur la terminaison des nerfs moteurs chez les crustacés et les insectes. C.R. Acad. Sci. (Paris) 59:851-853, 1864.

Rowinski, P.: Sul significanto funzionale delle localizzazioni dell' acetilcolinesterasi nella differenziazione del musculo striato di embrione de pollo. Boll. Soc. Ital. Biol. Sper. 35:2228-2229, 1959.

Rule, A.H. Bartlett, P. and Osserman, K.E.: Studies in myasthenia gravis: Active antigenic sites related to humoral antibody induction. J. Immunol. 110:401-407, 1973.

Ruska, H.: Elektronenmikroskopischer Beitrag zur Histologie des Skelettmuskels kleiner Säugetiere. Z. Naturforsch. 9(B):358-371, 1954.

Russell, D.S.: Histologic changes in striped muscles in myasthenia gravis. J. Path. Bact. 65:279-289, 1953.

Sabatini, D.D., Bensch, K. and Barrnett, R.J.: Cytochemistry and electron microscopy. The preservation of cellular ultrastructure and enzymatic activity by aldehyde fixation. J. Cell Biol. 17:19-58, 1963.

Saito, A.: Experimental histological study of denervation and reinnervation in intercostal muscle of the dog. J. Jap. Orthoped. Assn. 41:181-198, 1967.

Saito, A. and Zacks, S.I.: Fine structure of neuromuscular junctions after nerve section and implantation of nerve in denervated muscle. Exp. & Mol. Path. 10:256-273, 1969a.

Saito, A. and Zacks, S.I.: Fine structure observations of denervation and reinnervation of neuromuscular junctions in mouse fast muscle. J. Bone and Jt. Surgery 51:1163-1178, 1969b.

Saito, A. and Zacks, S.I.: Ultrastructure of Schwann and perineural sheaths at the mouse neuromuscular junction. Anat. Rec. 164:379-390, 1969c.

Sakimoto, T. and Cheng-Minoda, K.: Fine structure of neuromuscular junctions in myasthenic extraocular muscles. Invest. Opthal. 9:316-324, 1970.

Salpeter, M.M.: Electron microscope radioautography as a quantitative tool in enzyme cytochemistry. The distribution of acetylcholinesterase at motor endplates of a vertebrate twitch muscle. J. Cell Biol. 32:379-389, 1967.

Salpeter, M.M.: Electron microscope radioautography as a quantitative tool in enzyme cytochemistry. II. The distribution of DFP-reactive sites at motor endplates of a vertebrate twitch muscle. J. Cell Biol. 42:122-134, 1969.

Salpeter, M.M., Plattner, H. and Rogers, A.W.: Quantitative assay of esterases in end plates of mouse diaphragm by electron microscope autoradiography. J. Histochem. Cytochem. 20:1059-1068, 1972.

Samojloff, A.: Zur Frage des Uberganges der Erregung vom motorischen Nerven auf den quergestreiften Muskel. Pflügers Arch. Ges. Physiol. 208:508-519, 1967.

Samuel, E.P.: The mechanism of silver staining. J. Anat. (Lond.) 87:278-287, 1953.

Samuels, A.J.: Differences in the incorporation of radioactive phosphate into gross fractions of muscle during denervation and tenotomy. Am. J. Phys. Med. 36:78-89, 1957.

Samuels, A.J., Boyarsky, L.L., Gerard, R.W., Libet, B. and Brust, M.: Distribution exchange and migration of phosphate compounds in nervous system. Am. J. Physiol. 164:1-15, 1951.

Samuels, A.J. and Gorevic, P.: Evidence suggesting a retardation of denervation atrophy upon injection of trophic brain proteolipids. Life Sciences 7:1169-1179, 1968.

Santa, T., Engel, A.G. and Lambert, E.H.: Histometric study of neuromuscular junction ultrastructure I. Myasthenia gravis. Neurology 22:71-82, 1972a.
Santa, T., Engel, A.G. and Lambert, E.H.: Histometric study of neuromuscular junction ultrastructure. II. Myasthenic syndrome. Neurology 22:370-376, 1972b.
Sanz Ibánez, J.: Estudios sobre el comportamiento de las cepas A y B del virus Coxsakie. Trab. Inst. Cajal Invest. Biol. (Madrid) 43:165-188, 1951.
Sávay, G. and Csillik, B.: The effect of denervation on the cholinesterase activity of motor endplates. Acta Morph. Acad. Sci. Hung. 6:289-297, 1956.
Sávay, G. and Csillik, B.: Lead reactive substances in myoneural synapses. Nature 181: 1137-1138, 1958.
Sawyer, C.H., Davenport, C. and Alexander, L.M.: Sites of cholinesterase activity in neuromuscular and ganglionic transmission. Anat. Rec. 106:287-288, 1950.
Sayen, A.: Comparative histologic changes at myoneural junctions, terminal axons, spindles and tendon organs of muscle after local cold injury. J. Neuropath. & Exp. Neurol. 21:348-363, 1962.
Sayen, A., Meloche, B.R., Tedeschi, G.C. and Montgomery, H.: Experimental immersion foot: Observations in the chilled leg of the rabbit. Clin. Sci. 19:243-256, 1960.
Schaefer, H.: Wietere Untersuchungen zum Mechanismus und zur Therapie des Wundstarrkrampfs. Arch. Exp. Path. u. Pharmakol. 203:59-84, 1944.
Schantz, E.J.: Paralytic shellfish poisoning and saxitoxin in Neuropoisons Their Pathophysiological Actions 1:159-167, 1971 (Simpson, L.L., ed.). Plenum Press, New York and London.
Schlaepfer, W.W. and Hager, H.: Ultrastructural studies of INH-induced neuropathy in rats. I. Early axonal changes. Am. J. Path. 45:209-219, 1964.
Schmidt, C.G.: Das Verhalten der Cytochromoxydase im denervienten atrophischen Muskel. Biochem. Z. 323:266-274, 1952.
Schmidt, J. and Raftery, M.A.: Purification of acetylcholine receptors from Torpedo Californica electroplax by affinity chromatography. Biochem. 12:852-855, 1973.
Schmidt, W.J.: Polarisationsoptiche Analyse des submikroskopischen Baues von Zellen und Geweben, in Handbuch des Biologischen Arbeitsmethoden (Abderhalden, E., ed.). Abt. V 10:435-665, 1938.
Schneider, W.C. and Hogeboom, G.H.: Intracellular distribution of enzymes. V. Further studies on the distribution of cytochrome C in rat liver homogenates. J. Biol. Chem. 183:123-128, 1950.
Schotté, O.E.: Nouvelles preuves physiologiques de l'action du systeme nerveux sympathique dans la regeneration. C.R. Soc. Phys. Hist. Nat. (Geneve) 43:140, 1926.
Schotté, O.E. and Butler, E.G.: Phases in regeneration of the urodele limb and their dependence upon the nervous system. J. Exp. Zool. 97:95-121, 1944.
Schröder, J.M.: Zur pathogenese der Isoniazid-Neuropathie II Phasen contrast und elektronen mikroskopische Untersuchungen am Rückenmark, an Spinalganglien und muskelspindeln. Acta Neuropath. 16:324-341, 1970.
Schröder, J.M.: Sarcolemmal indentations resembling junctional folds in myotonic dystrophy. in Muscle Diseases Proceedings of an International Congress, Milan, 1969 (Walton, J.M., Canal, N. and Scarlato, G., eds.). Excerpta Medica, Amsterdam, pp. 109-111, 1970.
Schübel, K.: Über das Botulinus Toxin. Arch. Exp. Path. u. Pharmakol. 96:195-226, 1922.

Schueler, F.W.: A new group of respiratory paralyzants. I. The "hemicholiniums." J. Pharmacol. & Exp. Therap. *115*:127-143, 1955.

Schulka, P.L. and Aitken, J.T.: Formation of motor endplates in denervated voluntary muscles of the rat. J. Anat. (Lond.) *97*:152P, 1963.

Schwarzacher, H.G.: Zur Lage der motorischen Endplatten in den Skelettmuskeln. Acta Anat. *30*:759-774, 1957.

Schwarzacher, H.G.: Untersuchungen über die skeletmuskel-Schnenverbindung. II. Histochemische Lokalisation der Acetylcholinesterase und Untersuchungen über ihre mögliche Funktion an der Muskelfasen-Schnenverbindung. Acta Anat. *42*:318-332, 1960.

Seecof, R.L., Teplitz, R.L., Gerson, I., Ikeda, K. and Donady, J.J.: Differentiation of neuromuscular junctions in cultures of embryonic *Drosophila* cells. Proc. U.S. Nat. Acad. Sci. *69*:566-570, 1972.

Senay, L.C., Imig, C.J. and Hines, H.M.: Neuromuscular damage resulting from exposure of the hind limbs of rats and hamsters to cold. Am. J. Phys. Med. *35*:170-176, 1956.

Shafiq, S.A., Gorycki, M.A., Asiedu, S.A. and Milhorat, A.T.: Tenotomy effect on the fine structure of the soleus of the rat. Arch. Neurol. *20*:625-633, 1969.

Shanthaveerappa, T.R. and Bourne, G.H.: The perineural epithelium: A metabolically active, continuous protoplasmic cell barrier surrounding peripheral nerve fasciculi. J. Anat. (Lond.) *96*:527-537, 1962.

Shanthaveerappa, T.R. and Bourne, G.H.: The effects of transection of the nerve trunk on the perineural epithelium with special reference to its role in nerve degeneration and regeneration. Anat. Rec. *150*:35-50, 1964.

Shanthaveerappa, T.R. and Bourne, G.H.: Histological and histochemical studies of the choroid of the eye and its relations to the pia arachnoid mater of the central nervous system and perineural epithelium of the peripheral nervous system. Acta Anat. *61*:379-398, 1965.

Shanthaveerappa, T.R., Hope, J. and Bourne, G.H.: Electron microscopic demonstration of the perineural epithelium of sciatic nerve. Acta Anat. *52*:193-201, 1963.

Sheff, M.F., Perry, M. and Zacks, S.I.: Unpublished observations, 1963.

Shen, S.C.: Changes in enzymatic patterns during development. *in* The Chemical Basis of Development (McElroy, W.D. and Glass, B., eds.). Johns Hopkins Press, Baltimore, pp. 416-432, 1958.

Sheridan, M.N., Whittaker, V.P. and Israël, M.: The subcellular fractionation of the electric organ of *Torpedo*. Z. Zellforsch. *74*:291-307, 1966.

Sherman, R.G. and Fourtner, C.R.: Ultrastructural features of synaptic regions in walking leg muscles of the horseshoe crab, *Limulus polyphemus*. J. Ultrastr. Res. *40*:44-54, 1972.

Sherrington, C.S.: The central nervous system and its instruments, *in*: Sir Michael Foster's A Text Book of Physiology, 7th ed., Macmillan & Co., Ltd., London, 1897.

Sherrington, C.S.: The Integrative Action of the Nervous System. Charles Scribner's Sons, New York, 1906.

Shimada, Y.: Suppression of myogenesis by heterotypic and heterospecific cells in monolayer cultures. Exp. Cell Res. *51*:564-578, 1968.

Shimada, Y.: Early stages in the reorganization of dissociated embryonic chick skeletal muscle cells. Z. Entwickl-Gesch. *138*:255-264, 1972.

Shimada, Y., Fischman, D.A. and Moscona, A.A.: Formation of neuromuscular junctions in embryonic cell cultures. Proc. U.S. Nat. Acad. Sci. 62:715-721, 1969a.

Shimada, Y., Fischman, D.A. and Moscona, A.A.: The development of nerve-muscle junctions in monolayer cultures of embryonic spinal cord and skeletal muscle cells. J. Cell Biol. 43:382-387, 1969b.

Shimada, Y. and Fischman, D.A.: The morphological and physiological evidence for the development of functional neuromuscular junctions in vitro. Developmental Biology 1973 (in press).

Shimada, Y. and Kano, M.: Formation of neuromuscular junctions in embryonic cultures. Archiv. histol. japon. 33:95-114, 1971.

Shulman, S., Lang, R., Beutner, E. and Witebsky, E.: Precipitation of autoantibody from patients with myasthenia gravis. Immunology 10:289-303, 1966.

Shy, G.M., Engel, W.K., Somers, J.E. and Wanko, T.: Nemaline myopathy. Brain 86:793-810, 1963.

Shy, G.M. and Silverstein, I.: A study of the effects upon the motor unit by remote malignancy. Brain 88:515-528, 1965.

Sica, R.E.P. and McComas, A.J.: An electrophysiological study of limb-girdle and facio-scapulo-humeral dystrophy. J. Neurol. Neurosurg. Psychiat. 34:469-474, 1971.

Silver, S.: A histochemical investigation of cholinesterases at neuromuscular junctions in mammalian and avian muscles. J. Physiol. (Lond.) 169:386-393, 1963.

Simpson, J.A.: Myasthenia gravis: a new hypothesis. Scot. Med. J. 5:419-436, 1960.

Simpson, L.L.: Effects of intraperitoneally injected botulinum toxin on rat cerebral cortex levels of acetylcholine. J. Neurochem. 15:359-360, 1968.

Simpson, L.L.: Ionic requirements for the neuromuscular blocking action of botulinum toxin: implications with regard to synaptic transmission. Neuropharmacol. 10:673-684, 1971.

Simpson, L.L. and Rapport, M.M.: Ganglioside inactivation of botulinum toxin. J. Neurochem. 18:1341-1343, 1971.

Singer, M.: The nervous system and regeneration of forelimb of the adult *Triturus*. II. The role of the sensory supply. J. Exp. Zool. 92:297-315, 1943.

Singer, M.: The invasion of the epidermis of the regenerating forelimb of the urodele, *Triturus*, by nerve fibers. J. Exp. Zool. 111:189-210, 1949.

Singer, M.: Induction of regeneration in the forelimb of the postmetamorphic frog by augmentation of the nerve supply. J. Exp. Zool. 126:419-472, 1954.

Singer, M.: The influence of nerves on regeneration, in Regeneration in Vertebrates (Thornton, C.S., ed.). University of Chicago Press, Chicago, 1959, pp. 59-80.

Singer, M.: The acetylcholine content of the normal forelimb regenerate in the adult newt, *Triturus*. Devel. Biol. 1:603-620, 1959.

Singer, M. and Caston, J.D.: Neurotrophic dependence of macromolecular synthesis in the early limb regenerate of the newt, *Triturus*. J. Embryol. & Exp. Morph. 28:1-11, 1972.

Singer, M. and Craven, L.: The growth and morphology of the regenerating forelimb of adult *Triturus* following denervation at various stages of development. J. Exp. Zool. 108:279-308, 1948.

Singer, M., Davids, M.H. and Arkowitz, E.S.: Acetylcholinesterase activity in the regenerating forelimb of the adult newt, *Triturus*. J. Embryol. & Exp. Morph. 8:98-111, 1960.

Singer, M., Davis, M.H. and Scheuing, M.R.: The influence of atropine and other neuropharmacological substances on regeneration of the forelimb in the adult urodele, Triturus. J. Exp. Zool. *143:*33-45, 1960.

Singer, M., Flinker, D. and Sidman, R.L.: Nerve destruction by colchicine resulting in suppression of limb regeneration in adult Triturus. J. Exp. Zool. *131:*267-300, 1956.

Sjöstrand, F.S. and Hanzon, V.: Membrane structures of cytoplasm and mitochondria in exocrine cells of mouse pancreas as revealed by high resolution electron microscopy. Exp. Cell Res. *7:*393-414, 1954.

Sjöstrand, F.S. and Rhodin, J.: The ultrastructure of the proximal convoluted tubules of the mouse kidney as revealed by high resolution electron microscopy. Exp. Cell Res. *4:*426-456, 1953.

Slotwiner, P., Song, S.K. and Anderson, P.J.: Spheromembranous degeneration of muscle induced by vincristine. Arch. Neurol. *15:*172-176, 1966.

Smith, C.W., Metzger, J.M., Zacks, S.I. and Kase, A.: Immune electron microscopy. Proc. Soc. Exp. Biol. & Med. *104:*336-338, 1960.

Smith, D.S.: On the significance of crossbridges between microtubules and synaptic vesicles. Phil. Trans. Roy. Soc. B. (Lond.) *261:*395-405, 1971.

Snell, R.S. and McIntyre, N.: Changes in the histochemical appearance of cholinesterase at the motor endplate following denervation. Brit. J. Exp. Path. *37:*44-48, 1956.

Sokoll, M.D. and Thesleff, S.: Effects of pH and uranyl ions on action potential generation and acetylcholine sensitivity of skeletal muscle. Europ. J. Pharm. *4:*71-76, 1968.

Solandt, D.Y., Partridge, R.C. and Hunter, J.: The effect of skeletal fixation on skeletal muscle. J. Neurophysiol. *6:*17-22, 1943.

Sonesson, B. and Thesleff, S.: Cholinesterase activity after DFP application in botulinum poisoned, surgically denervated or normally innervated rat skeletal muscles. Life Sciences *7:*411-417, 1968.

Song, S.K.: Electron microscopic study of terminal nerves, motor endplates and sarcoplasmic reticulum in denervated skeletal muscle. J. Neuropath. and Exper. Neurol. *27:*108 abs., 1968.

Sperry, R.W.: The effect of crossing nerves of antagonistic muscles in the hind limb of the rat. J. Comp. Neurol. *75:*1-19, 1941.

Sperry, R.W.: Chemoaffinity in the orderly growth of nerve fiber patterns and connections. Proc. U.S. Nat. Acad. Sci. *50:*703-710, 1963.

Spicer, S.S.: Histochemical differentiation of sulfated rodent mucins. in Proc. First Internat. Cong. Histochem. and Cytochem. (Paris), Pergamon Press, Oxford, London, N.Y. and Paris, *92:*1960.

Spicer, S.S. and Jarrels, M.H.: Histochemical reaction of an aromatic diamine with acid groups and periodate engendered aldehydes in mucopolysaccharides. J. Histochem. Cytochem. *9:*368-379, 1961.

Spicer, S.S. and Meyer, D.B.: Histochemical differentiation of acid mucopolysaccharide by means of combined aldehyde fuchsin-alcian blue staining. Am. J. Clin. Path. *33:*453-460, 1960.

Sprague, R.G., Power, M.H., Mason, H.L., Albert, A., Mathieson, D.R., Hench, P.S., Kendall, E.C., Slocumb, C.H. and Polley, H.F.: Observations on the physiologic effects of cortisone and ACTH in man. Arch. Int. Med. *85:*199-258, 1950.

Stedman, E., Stedman, E. and Easson, L.H.: Choline-esterase. Biochem. J. *26:*2056-2066, 1932.

Steidl, R.M., Oswald, A.J. and Kottke, F.J.: Myasthenic syndrome with associated neuropathy. Arch. Neurol. 6:451-461, 1962.
Stein, J.M. and Padykula, H.A.: Histochemical classification of individual skeletal muscle fibers of the rat. Am. J. Anat. 110:103-125, 1962.
Steindler, A.: Direct neurotization of paralyzed muscles, further study of the question of direct nerve implantation. Am. J. Orthoped. Surg. 14:707-719, 1916.
Steinert, H.: Myopathologische Beiträge: I. Über das klinische und anatomische Bild des Muskelschwunds der Myotoniker. Deutsche Z. Nervenh. 37:58-104, 1909.
Stelzner, D.J.: The relationship between synaptic vesicles, Golgi apparatus, and smooth endoplasmic reticulum: A developmental study using the zinc-iodide-osmium technique. Z. Zellforsch. 120:332-345, 1971.
Stevenson, J.W.: Bacterial neurotoxins. Am. J. Med. Sci. 235:317-336, 1958.
Stewart, D.M.: Changes in protein composition of muscles of the rat in hypertrophy and atrophy. Biochem. J. 59:553-558, 1955.
Stewart, D.M. and Martin, A.W.: Hypertrophy of the denervated hemidiaphragm. Am. J. Physiol. 186:497-500, 1956.
Stirnemann, H. and Brönnimann, R.: Erfahrungen in der Tetanusbehandlung Bericht über die im letzten Jahr behandelten 12 Fälle. Langenbeck's Arch. klin Chir. 286: 335-350, 1957.
Straus, W.L., Jr. and Weddell, G.: Nature of the first visible contractions of the forelimb musculature in rat fetuses. J. Neurophysiol. 3:358-369, 1940.
Strauss, A.J.L., Seegal, B.C., Hsu, K.C., Burkholder, P.M., Nastuk, W.L. and Osserman, K.E.: Immunofluorescence demonstration of a muscle binding, complement fixing serum globulin fraction in myasthenia gravis. Proc. Soc. Exp. Biol. & Med. 105:184-191, 1960.
Streter, F.A.: Effect of denervation on fragmented sarcoplasmic reticulum of white and red muscle. Exper. Neurol. 29:52-64, 1970.
Stromblad, B.C.R.: Cholinesterase activity in skeletal muscles after botulinum toxin. Experientia 16:458-460, 1960.
Szobor, A. and Petrányi, Gy.: Immunosuppressive therapy of myasthenia gravis. Acta Med. Acad. Sci. Hung. 27:397-411, 1970.

Takamori, M. and Gutmann, L.: Intermittent defect of acetylcholine release in myasthenia gravis. Neurology 21:47-54, 1971.
Takeno, K., Nishio, A. and Yanagiya, I.: Bound acetylcholine in the nerve ending particles. J. Neurochem. 16:47-52, 1969.
Takeuchi, A.: Neuromuscular transmission of fish skeletal muscles investigated with intracellular microelectrode. J. Cell Comp. Physiol. 54:211-220, 1959.
Takeuchi, A. and Takeuchi, N.: On the permeability of endplate membrane during the action of transmitter. J. Physiol. (Lond.) 154:52-67, 1960.
Takeuchi, N.: Some properties of conductance changes at the endplate membrane during the action of acetylcholine. J. Physiol. (Lond.) 167:128-140, 1963.
Tannenbaum, A.S. and Rosenbluth, J.: Myoneural junctions in larval ascidian tail. Experientia 28:1210-1212, 1972.
Tasaki, I. and Mizutani, K.: Comparative studies on the activities of the muscle evoked by two kinds of motor nerve fibers. Jap. J. Med. Sci. 10:237-244, 1944.

Taxi, J.: Action du formol sur l'activité de diverses préparations de cholinestérases. J. Physiol. (Paris) *44:*595-599, 1952.

Taylor, D.B., Steinborn, J. and Lu, C.: Ion exchange processes at the neuromuscular junction of voluntary muscle. J. Pharm. Exp. Therap. *175:*213-227, 1970.

Tello, J.F.: Terminaciones en los músculos estriados. Trab. Inst. Cajal Invest. Biol. (Madrid) *4:*105-114, 1905.

Tello, J.F.: Dégénération et régéneration des plaques motrices apres la section des. nerfs. Trab. Inst. Cajal Invest. Biol. (Madrid) *5:*117-149, 1907.

Tello, J.F.: Génesis de las terminaciones nerviosas motrices y sensitivas. I. En el sistema locomotor de los vertebrados superiores. Histogenesis muscular. Trab. Inst. Cajal Invest. Biol. (Madrid) *15:*101-199, 1917.

Tello, J.F.: Die Entstehung der Motorischen und sensiblen Nervendigungen. I. In dem lokomotorischen System der Höheren Wirbeltiere. Anat. Entwickl.-Gesch. *64:*348-440, 1922.

Tello, J.F.: Gegenwärtige Anschauugen über den Neurotropismus. Vortr. u. Auf. über Entwicklungsmech. *33:*1-73, 1923.

Tello, J.F.: Sobre una vaina que envuelve toda la ramificación del axon en las terminaciones motrices de los músculos estriados. Trab. Inst. Cajal Invest. Biol. (Madrid) *36:*2-59, 1944.

Tennyson, V.M. and Brzin, M.: The appearance of acetylcholinesterase in the dorsal root neuroblast of the rabbit embryo. J. Cell Biol. *46:*64-80, 1970.

Teräväinen, H.: Carboxylic esterases in developing myoneural junctions of rat striated muscle. Histochemie *12:*307-315, 1968a.

Teräväinen, H.: Electron microscopic and histochemical observations on different types of nerve endings in the extraocular muscles of the rat. Z. Zellforsch. *90:*372-388, 1968b.

Teräväinen, H.: Development of the myoneural junction in the rat Z. Zellforsch. *87:* 249-265, 1968c.

Teräväinen, H.: Electron microscopic localization of acetylcholinesterase in small multiple endings in the extraocular muscles of the rat. Experientia *25:*389, 1969a.

Teräväinen, H.: Localization of acetylcholinesterase in the rat myoneural junction. Histochemie *17:*162-169, 1969b.

Teräväinen, H.: Axonal protrusions in the small multiple endings in the extraocular muscles of the rat. Z. Zellforsch. *96:*206-211, 1969c.

Teräväinen, H. and Huikuri, K.: Effect of oculomotor and trigeminal nerve section on the ultrastructure of different myoneural junctions in the rat extraocular muscles. Z. Zellforsch. *102:*466-482, 1969.

Thesleff, S.: Motor endplate "desensitization" by repetitive nerve stimuli. J. Physiol. (Lond.) *148:*659-664, 1959.

Thesleff, S.: Supersensitivity of skeletal muscle produced by botulinum toxin. J. Physiol. (Lond.) *151:*598-607, 1960.

Thesleff, S.: Nervous control of chemosensitivity in muscle. Ann. N.Y. Acad. Sci. *94:*535-546, 1961.

Thesleff, S.: Acetylcholine utilization in myasthenia gravis. Ann. N.Y. Acad. Sci. *135:* 195-206, 1966.

Thesleff, S., Zelená, J. and Hofmann, W.W.: Restoration of function in botulinum paralysis by experimental nerve regeneration. Proc. Soc. Exp. Biol. & Med. *116:*19-20, 1964.

Thies, R.E.: Neuromuscular depression and the apparent depletion of transmitter in mammalian muscles. J. Neurophysiol. 28:427-442, 1965.

Thomsen, J.: Tonische Krämpfe in willkürlichen beweglichen Muskeln in Folge von ererbterpsychischer Disposition (Ataxia muscularis?). Arch. Psychiat. u. Nervenkr. 6:706-718, 1875-1876.

Thron, C.D., Durant, R.C. and Friess, S.L.: Neuromuscular and cytotoxic effects of holothurin A and related saponins at low concentration levels. III. Toxicol. and Appl. Pharmacol. 6:182-196, 1964.

Tiegs, O.W.: A study be degeneration methods of the innervation of the muscles of a lizard (Egernia). J. Anat. (Lond.) 66:300-320, 1932.

Tiru-chelvam, R.: Demonstration of sites of snake venom localisation by immunoflorescence techniques. J. Path. 107:303-305, 1972.

Titeca, J.: Étude des modifications fonctionelles du nerf au cours de la degenerescence Wallerienne. Arch. int. Physiol. 41:2-56, 1935.

Todd, T.J.: On the process of reproduction of the members of the aquatic salamander. Q. J. S. Arts & Lit. 16:84-96, 1823.

Toivonen, T., Ohela, K. and Kaipainen, W.J.: Parathion poisoning; increasing frequency in Finland. Lancet 2:175-176, 1959.

Torda, C. and Wolff, H.G.: On the mechanism of paralysis resulting from toxin of Clostridium botulinum. The action of the toxin on acetylcholine synthesis and on striated muscle. J. Pharm. & Exp. Therap. 89:320-324, 1947.

Torrey, T.W.: The relation of taste buds to their nerve fibers. J. Comp. Neurol. 59:203-320, 1934.

Toussaint, D., Coërs, C. and Toppet, N.: Heredopathia atactica polyneuritiformis (syndrome de Refsum): constatations cliniques et biopsiques. Bull. Soc. Belg. Opthal. 122:383-402, 1959.

Tower, S.S.: Atrophy and degeneration in skeletal muscle. Am. J. Anat. 56:1-43, 1935.

Tower, S.S.: Trophic control of non-nervous tissues by the nervous system: a study of muscle and bone innervated from an isolated and quiescent region of spinal cord. J. Comp. Neurol. 67.241-268, 1937.

Tower, S.S.: The reaction of muscle to denervation. Physiol. Rev. 19:1-48, 1939.

Trams, E.G. and Lauter, C.J.: Properties of electroplax protein. Biochim. Biophys. Acta 83:296-304, 1964.

Treherne, J.E. and Smith, D.S.: The metabolism of acetylcholine in the intact central nervous system of an insect Periplaneta Americana. J. Exp. Biol. 43:441-454, 1965.

Tsunoda, T.: Morphologische Studien über die Innervation der willkürlichen Muskeln. Virchow's Arch. Path. Anat. 267:413-420, 1928.

Tuček, S.: Motor nerve and the activity of choline acetyltransferase in the skeletal muscle. Biochim. Biophys. Acta 170:457-458, 1968.

Tuček, S.: Choline acetyltransferase activity in rat skeletal muscles during postnatal development. Exper. Neurology 36:378-388, 1972.

Tuffery, A.R.: Growth and degeneration of motor endplates in normal cat hind limb muscles. J. Anat. 110:221-247, 1971.

Tuncbay, T.O.: Histochemistry of esterases of the motor endplates and the lumbar motorneurons of the cat after sciatic neurectomy followed by primary and secondary anastomosis. Neurology 14:657-667, 1964.

Tuncbay, T.O., Ketel, W.B. and Boshes, B.: Cortisone effects on myoneural junctions. Neurology 15:314-320, 1965.

Tyler, H.R.: Pathology of the neuromuscular apparatus in botulism. Arch. Path. 76:55-59, 1963.

Uchizono, K.: Characteristics of excitatory and inhibitory synapses in the central nervous system of the cat. Nature 207:642-643, 1965.
Uchizono, K.: Morphological background of excitation and inhibition at synapses. J. Elect. Microsc. (Jap.) 17:55-66, 1968.
Usherwood, P.N.R. and Grundfest, H.: Peripheral inhibition in skeletal muscles of insects. J. Neurophysiol. 28:497-518, 1965.
Usherwood, P.N.R. and Machili, P.: Pharmacological properties of excitatory neuromuscular synapses in the locust. J. Exp. Biol. 49:341-361, 1968.

Valentin, G.: Über den Verlauf und die letzten Enden der Nerven. Nova Acta Phys. Med. Acad. Leopoldino-Carolinae 18:51-240, 1836.
Vandenburgh, H.H., Sheff, M.F. and Zacks, S.I.: Muscle sarcolemma — solubilization and characterization. Fed. Proc. 32:555Abs, 1973.
Van Ermengem, E.: Contribution a l'étude des intoxications alimentaires. Recherches sur des accidents à caractères botuliniques provoqués par du jambon. Arch. Pharmocodyn. 3:213-276, 1897.
Van Harreveld, A.: Reinnervation of denervated muscle fibers by adjacent functioning motor units. Am. J. Physiol. 144:477-493, 1945.
Van Harreveld, A.: Reinnervation of paretic muscle by collateral branching of the residual motor innervation. J. Comp. Neurol. 97:385-403, 1952.
Van Harreveld, A. and Tachibana, S.: Innervation and reinnervation of cricothyroid muscle in the rabbit. Am. J. Physiol. 201:1199-1202, 1961.
Varga, E., Szigethy, J. and Kiss, E.: The hydrolysis of acetylcholine in the presence of pure myosin. Acta Physiol. Acad. Sci. Hung. 5:383-392, 1954.
Veneroni, G.: Formation de novo and development of neuromuscular junctions in vitro. Anat. Rec. 160:503, 1968.
Veneroni, G. and Murray, M.R.: Formation de novo and development of neuromuscular junctions in vitro. J. Embryol. exp. Morph. 21:369-382, 1969.
Vetters, J.M., Simpson, J.A. and Folkarde, A.: Experimental myasthenia gravis. Lancet 1:28-31, 1969.
Viets, H.R. (ed.): Myasthenia Gravis. The Second International Symposium Proceedings. Charles C. Thomas, Springfield, Ill., 1961.
Visintini, F. and Levi-Montalcini, R.: Relazione tra differenziazione Strutturale e funzionale dei centri e delle vie nervose vell' embrione di pollo. Schweiz. Arch. Neurol. Psychiat. 43:381-393, 1939.
Vos, J.K., Kuriyama, K. and Roberts, E.: Electrophoretic mobilities of brain subcellular particles and binding of γ-aminobutyric acid, acetylcholine, norepinephrine and 5-hydroxytryptamine. Brain Res. 9:224-230, 1968.
Vrbová, G.: The effect of motorneurone activity on the speed of contraction of striated muscle. J. Physiol. (Lond.) 169:513-526, 1963.

Waggener, J.D. and Beggs, J.: The membrane coverings of neural tissues: An electron microscopic study. J. Neuropath. & Exper. Neurol. 26:412-426, 1967.

Wagner, R.: Neue Untersuchungen über den Bau and die Endigungen der Nerven. Leipzig. Cited in Ranvier, L.: Lecons sur l'Histologie du Système nerveux. Savy, Paris, 1878.

Wake, K.: Motor endplates in developing chick embryo skeletal muscle: Histological structure and histochemical localization of cholinesterase activity. Arch. histol. jap. 25:23-41, 1964.

Walker, M.B.: Treatment of myasthenia gravis with physostigmine. Lancet 1:1200-1201, 1934.

Walker, S.M.: Electron microscopic study of sarcoplasmic reticulum and myofilaments of tenotomized rat muscle. Am. J. Phys. Med. 44:176-192, 1965.

Walton, J.N.: Amyotonia Congenita. Lancet 1:1023-1028, 1956.

Walton, J.N. and Adams, R.D.: Polymyositis. E. and S. Livingstone, Edinburgh and London, 1958.

Walton, J.N., Geschwind, N. and Simpson, J.A.: Benign congenital myopathy with myasthenic features. J. Neurol. Neurosurg. & Psychiat. 19:224-231, 1956.

Warnick, J.E., Albuquerque, E.X., and Sansone, F.M.: The pharmacology of batrachotoxin. I. Effects on the contractile mechanism and on neuromuscular transmission of mammalian skeletal muscle. J. Pharm. Exp. Therap. 176:497-510, 1971.

Waser, P.G. and Hadorn, I.: Relations of cholinergic receptors to acetylcholinesterase of endplates in denervated muscle. Bibl. Anat. 2:155-160, 1960.

Waser, P.G. and Lüthi, U.: Über die Fixierung von ^{14}C-Curarin in der Endplatte. Helv. Physiol. Acta 20:237-251, 1962.

Watkins, J.C.: Pharmacological receptors and general permeability phenomena of cell membranes. J. Theoret. Biol. 9:37-50, 1965.

Watson, W.E.: Centripetal passage of labelled molecules along mammalian motor axons. J. Physiol. (Lond.) 196:122-123P, 1968.

Watson, W.E.: The response of motor neurones to intramuscular injection of botulinum toxin. J. Physiol. (Lond.) 202:611-630, 1969.

Webster, H.D., Spiro, D., Waksman, B. and Adams, R.D.: Phase and electron microscope studies of experimental demyelination: Schwann cell changes in guinea pig sciatic nerves during experimental diphtheritic neuritis. J. Neuropath. & Exper. Neurol. 20. 5-34, 1961.

Wechsler, W. and Hager, H.: Elektronenmicroskopische Befunde bei muskelatrophie nach nervendurchtrennung bei der weissen Ratte. Beitr. Path. Anat. 125:31-53, 1961a.

Wechsler, W. and Hager, H.: Elektronenmikroskopishe Untersuchungen bei myotonischer Muskeldystrophie. Arch. f. Psychiat. u. Zeits. f. Neurol. 201:668-690, 1961b.

Wei, L.Y.: Electric dipole theory of chemical synaptic transmission. Biophys. J. 8:396-414, 1968.

Wei, L.Y.: Role of surface dipoles on axon membrane. Science 163:280-282, 1969.

Weiss, P.: Eine neue theorie der Nervenfunktion. Nicht durch gesonderte Bahnen, sondern durch spezifische Formen der Erregung schaltet das Nervensystem mit den Muskeln. Naturwissenshaft. 16:626-636, 1928.

Weiss, P.: In vitro experiments on the factors determining the course of the outgrowing nerve fiber. J. Exp. Zool. 68:393-448, 1934.

Weiss, P.: Experimental innervation of muscles by the central ends of afferent nerves (establishment of a one-neuron connection between receptor and effector organ), with functional tests. J. Comp. Neurol. 61:135-174, 1935.
Weiss, P.: Nerve patterns: the mechanics of nerve growth. Growth 5:163-203, 1941.
Weiss, P.: An introduction to genetic neurology, in Genetic Neurology (P. Weiss, ed.). University of Chicago Press, Chicago, 1950, pp. 1-39.
Weiss, P. and Edds, M.V., Jr.: Spontaneous recovery of muscle following partial denervation. Am. J. Physiol. 145:587-607, 1946.
Weiss, P. and Hoag, A.: Competitive reinnervation of rat muscles by their own and foreign nerves. J. Neurophysiol. 9:413-418, 1946.
Weiss, P. and Taylor, A.C.: Further experimental evidence against "neurotropism" in nerve regeneration. J. Exp. Zool. 95:233-257, 1944.
Weiss, P., Taylor, A.C. and Pillai, P.A.: The nerve fiber as a system in continuous flow: microcinematographic and electron microscopic demonstrations. Science 136:330, 1962.
Weller, R.O. and McArdle, B.: Calcification within muscle fibres in the periodic paralyses. Brain 94:263-272, 1971.
Welsh, J.H.: Evidence of a trophic action of acetylcholine in a planarian. Anat. Rec. 94:421, 1946.
Welsh, J.H.: Concerning the mode of action of acetylcholine. Bull. Johns Hopkins Hosp. 83:568-579, 1948.
Welsh, J.H.: Composition and mode of action of some invertebrate venoms. Ann. Rev. Pharm. 4:293-304, 1964.
Welsh, J.H. and Taub, R.: The action of choline and related compounds on the heart of Venus mercenaria. Biol. Bull. 95:346-353, 1948.
Welsh, J.H. and Taub, R.: Molecular configuration and biological activity of substances resembling acetylcholine. Science 112:467-469, 1950.
Werdnig, G.: Zwei fruhinfantile hereditäre Fälle von progressiver Muskelatrophie unter dem Bilde der Dystrophie ober auf neurotischer Grundlage. Arch. Psychiat. & Nervenh. 22:437-480, 1891.
Werman, R., Carlen, P.L., Kushnir, M. and Kosower, E.M.: Effect of the thiol-oxidizing agent, diamide, on acetylcholine release at the frog endplate. Nature New Biology 233:120-121, 1971.
Westmorland, B.F., Ward, D. and Johns, T.R.: The effect of methohexital at the neuromuscular junction. Brain Res. 26:465-468, 1971.
Whittaker, V.P.: The isolation and characterization of acetylcholine-containing particles from brain. Biochem. J. 72:694-706, 1959.
Whittaker, V.P.: Origin and function of synaptic vesicles. Ann. N.Y. Acad. Sci. 183:21-32, 1971.
Whittaker, V.P. and Gray, E.G.: The synapse: Biology and Morphology. Br. Med. Bull. 18:223-228, 1962.
Wiesendanger, M. and D'Alessandri, A.: Myasthenia gravis mit fokaler infiltration der Endplattenzone. Acta Neuropath. 2:246-252, 1963.
Willis, T.: De Anima Brutorum. 404, 1672.
Wilson, A. and Wilson, H.: The thymus and myasthenia gravis. Am. J. Med. 19:697-700, 1955.

Wilson, I.B.: Acetylcholinesterase. XI. Reversibility of the tetraethyl pyrophosphate inhibition. J. Biol. Chem. 190:111-117, 1951.

Wilson, I.B.: Acetylcholinesterase. XIII. Reactivation of alkyl-phosphate-inhibited enzyme. J. Biol. Chem. 199:113-120, 1952.

Wilson, I.B. and Ginsburg, S.: A powerful reactivator of alkyl-phosphate-inhibited acetylcholinesterase. Biochem. et Biophys. Acta 18:168-170, 1955.

Windle, W.F. and Baxter, R.E.: Development of reflex mechanisms in the spinal cord of albino rat embryos. Correlations between structure and function, and comparisons with the cat and the chick. J. Comp. Neurol. 63:189-209, 1935.

Wirsen, C. and Larsson, K.S.: Histochemical differentiation of skeletal muscle in foetal and newborn mice. J. Embryol. Exp. Morph. 12:759-767, 1964.

Wohlfart, G.: Regenerative phenomena in the muscle nerves in connection with poliomyelitis and amyotrophic lateral sclerosis. Nord. Med. 54:1075-1078, 1955.

Wohlfart, G.: Collateral regeneration from residual motor nerve fibers in amyotrophic lateral sclerosis. Neurology 7:124-134, 1957.

Wohlfart, G.: Collateral regeneration in partially denervated muscle. Neurology 8:175-180, 1958.

Wolman, M.: Studies on the impregnation of nervous tissue elements. III. Mechanism of impregnation of astroglia and the nature of the compound responsible for the impregnation. Lab. Invest. 6:551-557, 1957.

Wolter, J.R.: Thin nerves with simple endings containing cholinesterase in striated human eye muscles. Neurology 14:283-286, 1964.

Woltman, H.W. and Wilder, R.M.: Diabetes mellitus: Pathological changes in the spinal cord and peripheral nerves. Arch. Int. Med. 44:576-603, 1929.

Woolard, H.H.: The nature of the structural changes in nerve endings in starvation and beri beri. J. Anat. (Lond.) 61:283-297, 1926-27.

Woolley, D.W.: Extraction and assay in vitro of an "acetylcholine receptor (?)". Fed. Proc. 18:461, 1959.

Woolf, A.L.: Chronic degeneration of the lower motor neurons studied with vital staining and histochemical techniques. Excerpta. Med. (Neurol. and Psychiat.) 8:877-878, 1955.

Woolf, A.L.: Changes in the nervous systems in vitamin B deficiency. J. Clin. Path. 9:388, 1956.

Woolf, A.L.: Carcinomatous neuropathy. J. Clin. Path. 10:216, 1957.

Woolf, A.L.: Biopsy study of the pathology of the lower motor neurone. Am. J. Phys. Med. 38:26-35, 1959.

Woolf, A.L., Dagnall, H.S., Bauwens, P. and Bickerstaff, E.R.: A case of myasthenia gravis with changes in the intramuscular nerve endings. J. Path. Bact. 71:173-178, 1956.

Woolf, A.L. and Malins, J.M.: Changes in intramuscular nerve endings in diabetic neuropathy; a biopsy study. J. Path. Bact. 73:316-317, 1957.

Woolf, A.L. and Till, K.: The pathology of the lower motor neurone in the light of new muscle biopsy techniques. Proc. Roy. Soc. Med. 48:189-194, 1955.

Wright, G.P.: The neurotoxins of *Clostridium botulinum* and *Clostridium tetani* Phar-Rev. 7:413-456, 1955.

Yamada, K.: Effects of oxidation upon alcian blue staining of acid mucopolysaccharides. Nagoya J. Med. Sci. 26:217-220, 1964.
Yarom, R. and Meiri, U.: Effect of scorpion venom on ultrastructure of frog sartorius muscle. Toxicon 10:291-294, 1972.
Yasargil, G.M.: Systematische Untersuchung der motorischen innervation des Zwerchfells beim Kaninchen. Helv. Physiol. et Pharm. Acta, suppl. XVIII:5-60, 1967.
Yellin, H. and Guth, L.: The histochemical classification of muscle fibers. Exper. Neurol. 26:424-432, 1970.
Yntema, C.L.: Relations between innervation and regeneration of the forelimb in urodele larvae. Anat. Rec. 103:524, 1949.
Young, J.Z.: The functional repair of nervous tissue. Physiol. Rev. 22:318-374, 1942.

Zacks, S.I., Bauer, W.C. and Blumberg, J.M.: Abnormalities in the fine structure of the neuromuscular junction in patients with myasthenia gravis. Nature 190:280, 1961.
Zacks, S.I., Bauer, W.C. and Blumberg, J.M.: The fine structure of the myasthenic neuromuscular junction. J. Neuropath. & Exper. Neurol. 21:335-347, 1962.
Zacks, S.I. and Blumberg, J.M.: Observations on the fine structure of mouse and human neuromuscular junctions. J. Biophys. & Biochem. Cytol. 10:517-528, 1961a.
Zacks, S.I. and Blumberg, J.M.: The histochemical localization of acetylcholinesterase in the fine structure of neuromuscular junctions of mouse and human intercostal muscle. J. Histochem. & Cytochem. 9:317-324, 1961b.
Zacks, S.I. and Blumberg, J.M.: Accidental and suicidal parathion poisoning in man. A report of four cases with histochemical and toxicological observations. Unpublished data, 1961c.
Zacks, S.I., Lipshutz, H. and Elliott, F.: Histochemical and electron microscopic observations on "onion bulb" formations in a case of hypertrophic neuritis of 25 years duration with onset in childhood. Acta Neuropath. 11:157-173, 1968.
Zacks, S.I., Metzger, J.F., Smith, C.W. and Blumberg, J.M.: Localization of ferritin-labelled botulinus toxin in the neuromuscular junction of the mouse. J. Neuropath. & Exper. Neurol. 21:610-633, 1962.
Zacks, S.I., Pegues, J.J. and Elliott, F.A.: Interstitial muscle capillaries in patients with diabetes mellitus: a light and electron microscope study. Metabolism 11:381-393, 1962.
Zacks, S.I., Rhoades, M.J. and Sheff, M.F.: The localization of botulinum A toxin in the mouse. Exper. Mol. Path. 9:77-83, 1968.
Zacks, S.I. and Saito, A.: Uptake of exogenous horseradish peroxidase by coated vesicles in mouse neuromuscular junctions. J. Histochem. Cytochem. 17:161-170, 1969.
Zacks, S.I. and Saito, A.: Direct connections between the T system and the subneural apparatus in mouse neuromuscular junctions demonstrated by lanthanum. J. Histochem. Cytochem. 18:302-304, 1970.
Zacks, S.I., Saito, A. and Sheff, M.F.: Cytochemical properties of the basement lamina of myofibers and neuromuscular junctions. Internat. Acad. Path. Monograph. Muscle (Pearson, C., ed.). (in press) 1973.
Zacks, S.I. and Sheff, M.F.: Tetanus toxin: fine structure localization of binding sites in striated muscle. Science 159:643-644, 1968.

Zacks, S.I. and Sheff, M.F.: Tetanism: Pathobiological aspects of the action of tetanal toxin in the nervous system and skeletal muscle. *in* Neurosciences Research *3:*210-306, 1970 (Ehrenpreis, S. and Solnitzky, O.C., eds.). Academic Press, New York.

Zacks, S.I. and Sheff, M.F.: unpublished data, 1970.

Zacks, S.I. and Sheff, M.F.: Biochemical and physiological aspects of tetanus intoxication *in* Neuropoisons their pathophysiological actions *1:*225-262, 1971 (Simpson, L.L., ed.). Plenum Press, New York.

Zacks, S.I. and Sheff, M.F.: unpublished data, 1972.

Zacks, S.I., Sheff, M.F., Rhodes, M.A. and Saito, A.: MED myopathy. A new hereditary myopathy. Lab. Invest. *21:*143-153, 1969.

Zacks, S.I., Sheff, M.F. and Saito, A.: Structure and staining characteristics of myofiber external lamina. J. Histochem. Cytochem. *21:*703-714, 1973.

Zacks, S.I., Shields, D.R. and Steinberg, S.A.: A myasthenic syndrome in the dog: A case report with electron microscopic observations on motor endplates and comparisons with the fine structure of endplates in myasthenia gravis. Ann. N.Y. Acad. Sci. *135:* 79-97, 1966.

Zacks, S.I., Vandenburgh, H. and Sheff, M.F.: Cytochemical and physical properties of myofiber external lamina. J. Histochem. Cytochem. (in press) 1973.

Zacks, S.I. and Welsh, J.H.: Cholinesterases in rat liver mitochondria. Am. J. Physiol. *165:*620-623, 1951.

Zaimis, E.J.: Motor endplate differences as a determining factor in the mode of action of neuromuscular blocking agents. J. Physiol. (Lond.) *122:*238-251, 1952.

Zalewski, A.A.: Effects of reinnervation on denervated skeletal muscle by axons of motor, sensory and sympathetic neurons. Am. J. Physiol. *219:*1675-1679, 1970.

Zelená, J.: Development of acetylcholinesterase activity at muscle-tendon junction. Nature *205:*295-296, 1965.

Zelená, J. and Lubinská, L.: Early changes of acetylcholinesterase activity near the lesion in crushed nerves. Physiol. bohemoslov. *11:*261-268, 1962.

Zelená, J. and Szentagothai, J.: Verlagerung der lokalisation spezifischer cholinesterase während der entwicklung der muskelinnervation. Acta Histochem. *3:*284-296, 1956.

Zenker, W. and Anzenbacher, H.: On the different forms of myoneural junctions in two types of muscle fiber from the external ocular muscles of the rhesus monkey. J. Cell Comp. Physiol. *63:*273-285, 1964.

Zenker, W. and Gruber, H.: Über Form, Anordnung, Zahl and Grosse der myoneuralen Synapsen multipel innervierter Skelettmuskelfasern. Z. mikrosk-anat. Forsch. *76:* 361-377, 1967.

Zenker, W. and Krammer, E. Untersuchungen über Feinstruktur und innervatien der inneren Augen-Muskulatur des Huhnes. Z. Zellforsch. *03:*147-168, 1967.

Zlotkin, E. and Shulov, A.S.: Recent studies on the mode of action of scorpion neurotoxins. A review. Toxicon *7:*217, 1969.

Zupančič, A.O.: The mode of action of acetylcholine: A theory extended to a hypothesis on the mode of action of other biologically active substances. Acta Physiol. Scand. *29:*63-71, 1953.

Župančič, A.O.: On the chemical distinctions between cholinesterase and cholinoreceptor. Life Sciences *8:*989-992, 1969.

Index

Absolute "terminal innervation ratio," 366
Acetyl CoA, 157, 160
Acetyldisulfide, 132
Acetylcholine (see Ach)
Acetylcholine receptor (see AchR)
Acetylcholinesterase (see AchE)
Acetylselenocholine, 135
Ach,
   exocytotic release of, 164-166
   hydrolysis of, 196
   interactions with AchR, 189-193
   localization of, 153
   packaging of, 158-159
   packets, 167
   release, effect of ions on, 170-174
   sensitivity, extrajunctional, 274
      of myofiber membrane, 263-264
   synthesis, in electroplax, 156-157
      in myasthenia gravis, 346-347
      in synaptic vesicles, 159
   synthesis of, 153, 158-160
AchE, 134
   development of, 35-36
   in denervated muscle, 260-261
   in musculotendinous junctions, 137
   in sarcolemmal tubes, 94
   induction of, 270
   membrane localization of, 133
   NMJ location of, 123
   release by collagenase, 87

AchE sites, number in NMJ, 139
AchR, 107, 152, 181, 316
   changes in denervated muscle, 183-185
   chemistry of, 185-187
   conformational changes in, 193-194
   cooperative binding in, 194-195
   development of, 182-183
   effect of pH changes on, 191
   in denervated muscle, 265
   interactions with Ach, 189-193
   localization of, 181-182
   phospholipoproteins in, 192
   protein nature of, 186
   similarities to AchE, 187-189
   surface density of, 191
Acrolein, fixation with, 72
Acrylamide polyneuropathy, 330
Actinomycin, 184, 348
Affinity labelling, 188, 191
Age changes in NMJ, 320-321
A-1 junction, 69
Alizarin, 174
Alcoholic neuropathy, 240
Amitosis, 34
Amphibian toxins, 312-314
Amyotonia congenita, 329, 334, 340-341
Amyotrophic lateral sclerosis, 328-329
Animal model, of myasthenia gravis, 361-364
Aniline fuchsin, 53

Anodonta, 113
Anolis carolinensis, 53
Anticholinesterases, 105, 135-288, 151
  DFP, 135, 288
  E600, 135, 288
  eserine, 105, 151
  HETP, 285
  Iso OMPA, 135
  parathion, 285
  soman, 288
  tabun, 288
Antimuscle globulins, 347-348
Antivenin, fluorescein-labelled, 317
Aposynaptic granules, 110
Arborization nuclei, 12
ATBD, 129
Atrophy, peroneal muscular, 332
Atropine, 174, 189
ATTD, 129
Axialbaum, 6, 18
Axon, flow in, 281-282
  mitochondria in, 154
  ultraterminal sprouting of, 238
Axon sprouting, 237
  in tetanus intoxication, 305-306
  stimulus for, 238
Axonal protrusion, 63
  retraction, 49
Azathioprine, 348

Bacterial toxins, 291-307
Basement lamina (see external lamina)
Batonnets, 58
Batrachotoxin A, 312-314
Bernstein model, 176
Bioelectric currents, generation of, 175-178
Birefringence, of lead reactive substance, 103-108
Black widow spider venom, 163-164, 309-310
Blocking agent 342
Borstensaum, 7
Botulinum intoxication,
  morphological changes in, 296-300
  Q10 of, 296
  recovery from, 297-298

Botulinum toxin, 263, 269, 292-300
  ferritin labelled, 294-295
  fluorescein labelled, 295, 298
  lethal dose of, 296
  localization of, 294-296
  mode of action of, 293-294
  site of action of, 292
Bungarotoxin, 185-186, 192, 265, 316
Butyrylcholine, 141

Calcium, binding sites of, 102
  release of by NMJ, 174
Calcium gluconate, in myasthenia gravis, 346
Calvacin, 383
Carbamylcholine, 190, 192-193
Carcinomatous neuromyopathy, 337-338
Catecholamines, 173
  in dense core vesicles, 80
Cephalotoxin, 309
Cell coat, 85
Cell theory, 1
ChE, in extraocular muscle NMJ, 27
Checkerboard pattern, 43, 256-258, 271
  formation of, 43-44
Choline, 160, 165
  as blocking agent, 343
  radioactive, 159
Choline acetyltransferase, 153-154, 156
  histochemical localization of, 157
  in nerve fibers, 157
Cholinesterase,
  development in organ culture, 145
  in morphogenesis, 142-145
  in regenerating newt muscle, 50, 144
  myosin, 137
  radioautographic localization of, 142
  site of origin, 145-146
Ciliary ganglion, 69
Citrate synthetase, 160
Cleft, secondary synaptic, 57
Cleft, synaptic, 57
  (see also subneural apparatus)
  size of, 57
Close junction, 113
Coated vesicle, 63, 74
  fine structure of, 77-78

location of, 78
  uptake of horseradish peroxidase by, 79
Cobrotoxin, 316
Coelenterate toxin, 308
Coenzyme A, 347
Cold injury of NMJ, 319
Collagenase, 90
Collateral, branching, 147
  regeneration, 320
  reinnervation, 237-242, 269
  sprouting, 354
    in disease, 325-327
Colloidal, iron, 85
  thorium, 85
Combined staining, of NMJ, 147
Congenital myasthenia gravis, 353
Cords of Bungner, 18
Cortisone acetate, 291
Coxsackie virus, 333
Cross innervation, 271-273
Crotoxin, 316-317
Curare, 181, 283-284
  poisoning, 293
  radioactive, 265
Cyclic AMP, 174
Cyclohexamide, 184, 281

Dale theory, 81, 133
Decamethonium, 345, 356
Dedifferentiation, of urodele limbs, 49
Demyelination, segmental, 336
Denervation,
  classical studies of, 198-206
  esterase activity after, 137
  fine structure changes, 206-213
  membrane changes during, 228
Denervated muscle,
  changes in AchE activity, 260-261
  enzymes in, 254
  histochemistry of, 255
  myofiber types in, 255-258
Denervated NMJ, esterase activity in, 217-225
Denervation atrophy, 324
  histopathology of, 249-250
  species differences, 250-251
Dense core vesicle, 49, 74, 80

catecholamines in, 80
  in en grappe NMJ, 63
Density gradient centrifugation, 154
DFP (see diisopropyl fluorophosphate)
Diabetes mellitus, 240
Diabetic, myopathy, 337
  neuropathy, 325
Diamide, 173
Diisopropyl fluorophosphate, 135, 288
Dimethylene phenylene diamine stain, 84
Diphtheria polyneuritis, 292
Dissociated cell culture, 45-46
Distal neuronitis, 330, 339
Dithiothreitol (see DTT)
DMBTA, 126
DTT, 188
Dual fixation, 75
Duchenne muscular dystrophy, 368
Dying back neuropathy, 330
Dysplastic NMJs, in myasthenia gravis, 352-353
Dystrophic NMJs, in myasthenia gravis, 350
Dystrophy, myotonic, 365-366
  progressive muscular, 367-371

E600, 135, 288
Eaton-Lambert syndrome, 338
Electric eel, 153
Electroplax, 156-157, 188
Elolidina paradoxa, 2
Embryonic NMJ, fine structure of, 36-43
Eminence of Doyere, 12
En grappe NMJ, 12, 65, 100, 272
  denervation of, 214-217
  esterases in, 143
  fine structure of, 63
En plaque NMJ, 12, 24, 48, 272
Endocytosis, 73, 164
Endomysium, 99
Endoneural sheath, 12
Endoplasmic reticulum, 75, 281
Endplate potential (see EPP)
Epilemmal theory, 9
EPP, 152, 166, 180
EPSP (see excitatory postsynaptic potential)

Erabutoxins, 316
Escaped fibers, 205
Eserine, 106, 151
Esterase, early studies of, 117
  histochemical demonstration of, 117-141
  in fast and slow muscles, 141-142
  kinds of, 134-136
Esterase activity, in en grappe NMJ, 141
  species differences in NMJ, 142
Esterase histochemistry, 117-133
  acetylthiocholine, 122-125
  azodye methods, 119-121
  criteria for, 118
  DMBTA, 126
  Gomori methods, 118-119
  indoxyl acetate, 121-122
  osmiophilic polymer methods, 126-127
  specificity of, 134-136
  thiolacetic acid methods, 130-133
Excitatory postsynaptic potential, 178
Exocytosis, 79
Exploring fibers, embryonic, 33
External lamina, 4, 37, 43, 61, 63, 81
  chemistry of, 83, 94
  enzymes in, 86
  formation of, 81
  glycoproteins in, 85
  histochemistry of, 82-87
  hydrolysis by enzymes, 89-90
  in denervated NMJs, 107
  in musculotendinous junctions, 30
  in snail NMJs, 114
  LIS extract of, 95-96
  metal binding by, 87-89
  staining by alcian blue, 83
    with aldehyde fuchsin-alcian blue, 84
    by ruthenium red, 83
  water in, 95
Extraocular muscle, 69, 141

False transmitter, 347
Familial periodic paralysis, 324
Fascioscapulohumeral dystrophy, 369
Felderstruktur, 28
Fibrillenstruktur, 28
Fish toxins, 312

Fixation, with acrolein, 72
  with formalin, 121
  with glutaraldehyde, 72
  with permanganate, 80
Fluorescence, of catecholamines, 80
Functional innervation ratio, 23, 327, 354
Fundamental nuclei, 12
  embryonic, 35
Fuzzy vesicle (see coated vesicle)

Gap substance, 81
  (see also external lamina)
Gas chromatography, 94
Glutaraldehyde, fixation with, 72
Glutathione, 173
Glycogen, 280
  content of denervated muscle, 254
  in soleplate, 110
Gold, thiocholine method, 125
  thiolacetic acid method, 132
Golgi apparatus, 75, 110
Granules, aposynaptic, 110
Guillain-Barre syndrome, 327

Hemicholinium, 160, 344
  radioactive, 157
Henle's sheath, 54
  role in reinnervation, 232
HEPES reagent, 157
HETP, 285
Hexazonium pararosanilin, 121
Histochemical methods, P-acetylthiolbenzene diazonium, 411-412
  acetylthiocholine, Couteaux, 402-403
  azodye, 408
  combined with silver, 415-417
  for esterases, 399-417
  gold acetylthiocholine, 406-407
  gold thiocholine, 404-406
  gold thiolacetic acid, Koelle and Gromadzki, 414-415
  indoxyl acetate, 409
  thiocholine ferricyanide, 403-404
  thiocholine, Koelle, 399-402
  thiolacetic acid, Barrnett and Palade, 412-413
  2-thiolacetoxybenzanilide, 410-411

2-thiolpropionoxylbenzanilide, 410-411
Histrionicotoxin, 187
Hodgkin-Huxley model, 176
Holothurin, A, 308
Horseradish peroxidase, uptake
  by frog axons, 165
  by lobster axons, 165
  by vesicles, 79
HRP (see horseradish peroxidase)
Hyperglycemia, 336
Hyperneurotization, 240, 169, 336
Hypolemmal theory, 9

Idiopathic myoglobinuria, 324
Imbibition curve, 104
Innervation, band, 22
  cross, 271-273
  ratio, defined, 21
  terminal, 23, 238
  trophic influences of, 248
Intermediate junction, 37
Ionophore, 186
Isoniazid neuropathy, 289
Isoprenaline, 173
IsoOMPA, 135

Janus green B, 16

Key-Retzius sheath, 12, 323

Lamprey larva, 75
Landouzy-Dejerine dystrophy, 369
Lanthanum, tracing with, 101-103
LDH, in denervated muscle, 258
Lead poisoning, 288
  reactive substance, 103-108
Limb regeneration, effect of nerves on, 275-279
Lipoprotein, in subneural apparatus, 106
LIS (see lithium diiodo salicylate)
Lithium diiodo salicylate, 95
Lymphocytes, 348
Lymphorrhage, 353-354

Maculotoxin, 309
MED myopathy, 376-382
  EMG in, 380
  protein synthesis in, 381
  ultrastructure pathology of, 379
Membrane complex, layers of, 59
Membrane potential, 176-178
MEPP, 76, 152, 163, 166-170, 265, 293, 302
  characteristics of, 166
  effect of drugs on, 168-169
  effect of ions on, 169
  effect of lanthanum on, 163
  effect of solvents on, 173
  in denervated NMJs, 207-209
  in myasthenia gravis, 344
  restoration of after denervation, 210-211
Mesoerythrite, 348
Methotrexate, 348
Methylene blue, staining with, 10
Methyl xanthines, 174
Micelles, membrane, 107
Microsomes, 153
Milnesium tardigardum, 1
Mitochondria, in axon, 154
  in pigeon brain, 154
  in soleplate, 109
  in terminal axons, 52, 71
Mitochondrial granules, in tetanus intoxication, 303-307
Monolayer culture, 48
Motor endplate, defined, 4
  disease, 376-382
Motor unit, 20-21
  diseases of, 340
  formation of, 20
Mouse muscular dystrophy, 371-372
MTJ (see musculotendinous junctions)
Mucocytic degeneration, 350
Multiple innervation, 243
  evolution of, 29
  in vocalis muscle, 27
Muscarinic receptor, 151, 187
Muscle atrophy,
  biochemical changes in, 253-254
  checkerboard pattern of, 20
  contraction speed, neural regulation of, 271-275
  spindles, in vocalis muscle, 27
Muscular dystrophy, 324
  in mouse, 371-372

NMJ pathology in, 369-370
progressive, 367-371
pseudohypertrophic, 368
Musculotendinous junctions, 30-31, 262, 274
esterases in, 30-31
Myasthenia gravis, 238, 311, 342-361
Ach synthesis in, 346-347
animal model, 361-364
antimuscle globulins in, 347-348
blocking agents in, 349
calcium gluconate in, 346
denervation in, 358
dysplastic NMJ in, 352-353, 355
EMG in, 349
false transmitter in, 347
immunopathology, 347-349
myofiber atrophy in, 360-361
nature of defect, 342-346
NMJ, esterases in, 354-355
fine structure of, 356-361
pathology of, 350-356
postsynaptic defect, 343-345
presynaptic defect, 342, 345
role of Mg++ and Ca++ in, 346
treatment with immunosuppressive drugs, 348-349
Myasthenic defect, 342
Myasthenic dog, EMG from, 362-363
NMJ fine structure of, 364
Myasthenic syndrome, 337
Myelin, 155
Myeloma, 369
Myoblast, Ach sensitivity of, 48
Myofiber atrophy, in myasthenia gravis, 360-361
cell membrane, 99
fast, 65
red, 65
slow, 65
specialization of, 100
types, 43
unit membrane of, 100
white, 65
Myopathy, diabetic, 335-336
MED, 376-382
nemaline, 372-373

thyrotoxic, 369
vacuolar, 372-376
Myosin cholinesterase, 137
Myositis, 369, 382
NMJ in, 382-383
Myotonia congenita, 365
Myotonic dystrophy, 238, 324, 365-366, 372
NMJ in, 366
Myotube, 37, 246

Naja haje, 317
β-Naphthyl acetate, 119
Necturus, 26
Nemaline myopathy, 372-373
Neurilemma, 14
Neurocladism, 238, 326, 366
Neurofilaments, 9, 71, 331
Neuromuscular junction, defined, 4
(see also NMJ)
Neuromyopathy, carcinomatous, 337-338
steroid, 290-291
Neuron, diseases of, 323
doctrine, 10, 149
Neuropathy, 354
alcoholic, 240
diabetic, 335-336
dying back, 330
isoniazid, 289
vincristine, 290
Neurosecretion, 318
Neurotubule, 37, 74-75
Newt, NMJ regeneration in, 246
Nicotinic receptor, 151, 174
NMJ, AchE, in myotonic dystrophy, 366
age changes in, 320-321
blood supply of, 19
cholinesterases, solubility of, 136
cold injury of, 319
combined staining of, 147
comparative anatomy of, 24-27
de novo formation of, 46, 242-245
ultrastructure of, 245-247
desensitization of, 264
dysplastic, in myasthenia gravis, 352-353
dystrophic, in myasthenia gravis, 350
embryogenesis, postsynaptic membrane changes in, 37

en grappe, 12, 100, 272
en plaque, 12
esterases, localization in, 136-139
evolution of, 29-30
fine structure of myasthenic, 356-361
formation, in cell culture, 45-48
in regenerating muscle, 49-51
in *Amphioxus*, 116
in arthropods, 115-116
in *Ascaris*, 112
in chick embryo, 143-144
in crustacea, 114-115
in Eaton-Lambert syndrome, 338
in extraocular muscles, 26
in fast and slow muscles, 28
in fish, 26
in *Helix*, 114
in human, 26
  fine structure of, 61-62
in *Hydra*, 112
in insects, 116
in intrinsic ear muscles, 69
in lizard, 25
in MED myopathy, 379
in molluscs, 113
in muscular dystrophy, 369-370
in myasthenic dog, 364
in nemaline myopathy, 373
in *Nereis*, 112
in snake, 25-26
in vacuolar myopathy, 375-376
in vocal muscles, 27
induction of, 269
mammalian, 25
myasthenic, pathology of, 350-356
myoseptal localization of, 29
myositic, 354
nonspecific esterase in, 136
pathology in myositis, 382-383
polar innervation, 29
replacement of, 240-242
rodent, 26
size of, 23
  relation to myofiber, 23
soleplate of, 109-111
staining methods for, 4
  with gold, 5

with silver, 8
structure and function, correlations of, 65-69
supersensitivity of, 264
transmission, chemical, 150
  electrical, 150
NsE, 134
Nuclear magnetic resonance, 189
Nuclei, arborization, 12
  soleplate, 62
  vaginal, 12

Octopus toxin, 309
Osmium black, 127
Ostrea, 113

2-PAM, 139
Papain, 91
Paraphenylene diamine, 383
Parathion poisoning, 285
  case report, 285-286
  histochemical demonstration of, 287
  symptoms of, 285
PCMB, 188
Perineural epithelium, 14, 54
  in nerve regeneration, 232
Peripheral neuropathy, 327, 333
  (see also neuropathy)
Periterminal network, 62, 110
Permanganate, fixation with, 80
Peroneal muscular atrophy, 332
Phosphotungstic acid, 85
Photochromic activation, 191
Physostigmine (see eserine)
Plaque terminale, 3
  (see also terminal plaque)
Plasmocid, 383
Poliomyelitis, 238, 323, 325, 328
Polymyositis, 238, 382
Polyneuropathy, acrylamide, 330
  diphtheritic, 292
  due to B^{12} deficiency, 334
Postsynaptic defect,
  in myasthenia gravis, 343, 345
  membrane, 42, 152
Presynaptic defect,
  in myasthenia gravis, 343, 345

stimulatory potential, 152
Primary synaptic cleft, 41
Primitive eminence, 34
Progressive muscular atrophy, 328
Pseudohypertrophic muscular dystrophy, 368

Ranvier, node of, 54
Reactive sprouting (see collateral sprouting)
Red tide, 307
Regeneration, of urodele limbs, 49
Reinnervation,
  chemotactic factors in, 230
  collateral, 237-242
  consequences of delayed, 202-206
  fine structure of, 213
  guidance problem in, 229-232
  mechanical factors in, 231
  selective, 232-234
  time required for, 228-229
Replacement of NMJ, 240-242
Resonance theory, 236
Retraction space, 206
Ribosomes, in neuron, 160
  in soleplate, 110

Sarcolemma, 15
  definition of, 97-100
  width of, 98-99
Sarcolemmal tubes, 90-96
  AchE in, 95
  chemistry of, 92-94
Sarcoplasmic reticulum, 313
Saxitoxin, 307-308
Schiff reagent, 83
Schwann cell, 37, 43, 138, 227
  AchE in, 223
  as source of Ach, 209-211
  at NMJ, 54
  fibrogenesis by, 205
  in denervated NMJ, 208-209
  in isoniazid neuropathy, 290
  phagocytosis by, 211
Schwann tube, 235, 238
Scorpion venom, 311
Secondary synaptic cleft, 180

Selective reinnervation, 232-234, 236
Sensory nerve, effect on limb regeneration, 278
Sheath, Henle, 13
  Key-Retzius, 12
  Schwann, 14
Shell fish intoxication, 307-308
Silver staining, mechanism of, 8
Snake bite, symptoms of, 314
  venoms, actions of, 314-317
Soleplate, 7, 12, 35, 203, 205, 348
  fine structure of, 62-63
  pathologic changes in, 324
  size of, 12
Soman, 288
Spinal nerve compression, 339
Staining method,
  aldehyde fuchsin-alcian blue, 393-394
  combined, for axons and AchE, 147
  gold, Carey, 386
    Cole, 385
    Ranvier, 384
  Janus green B, 392
  lanthanum, 397-398
  lead, Savay and Csillik, 394-395
  methylene blue, Coers, 390
    Denz, 389
    Evans, 391
  paraphenylene diamine, 393
  ruthenium red, 396-397
  silver, Addison, 388-389
    Gray, 386
    Gros-Bielschowsky, 387
  zinc-iodide-osmium, 398-399
Steroid neuromyopathy, 290-291
Subneural apparatus, 17, 53, 57, 62, 67, 247
  connections with T system, 101-103
  in myasthenia gravis, 358
  in seahorse, 100-101
  in urodele limbs, 49
  lead reactive substance in, 103-108
Succinylcholine, 345
Suicide, with anticholinesterases, 284-285
Superinnervation, rejection of, 267-268
Synaptic cleft, 59
  (see also subneural apparatus)

Synaptic vesicles, 40, 69, 72, 74, 75-77, 215
  changes after denervation, 207-208
  effect of electric current, 163-164
    of ions on, 162-163
  experimental alteration of, 160-164
  fate of membrane, 164-165
  fusion of, 164
  in guinea pig ganglia, 161
  in rabbit retina, 161
  in slug NMJ, 113
  location of, 75-76
  membrane of, 75
  origin of, 75
  sedimentation of, 155
  shapes of, 76
  storage of Ach, 167
  uptake of Ach by, 159
  zinc iodide staining of, 77
Synaptoplasm, 158
Synaptosome, 159
  defined, 155

T system, 43, 176, 306
  connections with subneural apparatus, 101-103
  in ear muscles, 69
Tabun, 288
Taste bud, 280
Tdf, 188, 190-191
Telodendria, in myasthenia gravis, 350
Teloglia, 13, 54
Telolemma, 14, 54
Tensilon test, 356
TEPP, 285
Terminaisons en ligne, 24
Terminal, innervation ratio, 23, 238
  plaque, 4
Tetanus antitoxin, 303
Tetanus intoxication,
  action on muscle, 303
  effect on NMJ, 301-303
  localization of, 306
  morphologic changes in, 303-307
  spinal inhibition in, 302
Tetramine, 308
Tetrodotoxin, 184, 312
Thiamine, 282

deficiency, 331
Thin layer chromatography, 94
Thiocholine methods, modifications of, 125-126
Thorium dioxide, 73
Thyrotoxic myopathy, 326, 369
Thymin, 348
Thymoma, 347
Thymus, 348
Tick paralysis, 311
Tonic myofiber, 100
Torpedo, 153, 156, 164, 186
Toxin, amphibian, 312-314
  bacterial, 291-307
  botulinum, 165, 292-300
  coelenterate, 308
  fish, 312
  from *Physalia*, 308
  insect, 309-311
  invertebrate, 308-309
  snake, 314-317
  tetanus, 300-307
Triorthocresylphosphate, 290, 330
Trypsin, 90
Tubocurarine, 107, 174, 185
  (see also curare)
Twitch myofiber, 100

Ultraterminal branching, stimulus for, 235
Unit membrane, of myofiber, 100

Vacuolar myopathy, 373-376
Vaginal nuclei, 12
Vaginula soleiformis, 113
Vagusstoff, 151
Venom, of black widow spider, 163-164
  of snake, 314-317
Vesicle, dense core, 40
  of soleplate, 111
  pinocytotic, 43, 73
  synaptic, 40
    (see also synaptic vesicle)
Vincristine, 288
  neuropathy, 290
Vitamin B, deficiency of, 334
  deficiency of, 340

Wallerian degeneration, 323
Werdnig-Hoffman disease, 323, 329, 350
Wobbler mouse, 330
Zinc iodine stain, 75
    method for, 77